Alcoholism Treatment Marketing: Beyond T.V. Ads and Speeches

The *Health Marketing Quarterly* series, William J. Winston, Editor:

- *Marketing the Group Practice: Practical Methods for the Health Care Practitioner*
- *Marketing for Mental Health Services*
- *Marketing Long-Term and Senior Care Services*
- *Innovations in Hospital Marketing*
- *Marketing Ambulatory Care Services*
- *Marketing Strategies for Human and Social Service Agencies*
- *Health Marketing and Consumer Behavior: A Guide to Basic Linkages*
- *Professional Practice in Health Care Marketing: Proceedings of the American College of Healthcare Marketing Symposium*
- *Alcoholism Treatment Marketing: Beyond T.V. Ads and Speeches*

Alcoholism Treatment Marketing: Beyond T.V. Ads and Speeches

Donald R. Self
Editor

Routledge
Taylor & Francis Group
LONDON AND NEW YORK

Alcoholism Treatment Marketing: Beyond T.V. Ads and Speeches has also been published as *Health Marketing Quarterly*, Volume 6, Numbers 1/2/3 1988.

First published 1989 by
The Haworth Press

Published 2013 by Routledge
2 Park Square, Milton Park, Abingdon, Oxon OX14 4RN
711 Third Avenue, New York, NY 10017, USA

Routledge is an imprint of the Taylor & Francis Group, an informa business

Library of Congress Cataloging-in-Publication Data

Alcoholism treatment marketing : beyond t.v. ads and speeches / Donald R. Self, editor.
p. cm.
"Has also been published as Health Marketing Quarterly, Volume 6, Numbers 1/2/3 1988."
Bibliography: p.
ISBN 0-86656-889-1

ISBN 978-0-866-56889-0 (hbk)

1. Alcoholism – Treatment – Marketing. I. Self, Donald R.
RC565.N454 1989
362.2'928'0688 – dc19 89-1745
CIP

Dedication

This volume is dedicated to
Barbara Craun,
Administrative Secretary, Department of Marketing,
without whose help this project could not have been completed.

Alcoholism Treatment Marketing: Beyond T.V. Ads and Speeches

CONTENTS

II. PROGRAM DEVELOPMENT, IMPLEMENTATION, AND EVALUATION

ABOUT THE CONTRIBUTORS

(All are employees of Auburn University at Montgomery, except as noted.)

Donald R. Self, DBA (Marketing, Louisiana Tech), is Professor and Head of the Department of Marketing.

Cathleen A. Owens is a Graduate Research Assistant in the Department of Marketing and completing an MBA.

Daniel M. Blucker, MSM (Boston University-Vrije Universitie, Brussels, Belgium), **MLS** (North Texas State University), is acting Dean of the library.

Ingram Gomillion, MBA (Auburn University at Montgomery), was Director of Planning and Research for the Alabama Department of Mental Health and Mental Retardation at the time of this writing. He is currently Executive Director of the Chilton/Shelby County Mental Health Center.

Jerry J. Ingram, PhD (Marketing, University of Arkansas), is Professor of Marketing.

Vaughan C. Judd, MBA (University of Rochester), is Assistant Professor of Marketing and is writing his dissertation at North Texas State University.

Teri Kline, MBA (Auburn University at Montgomery), is Instructor of Marketing.

Robin S. McCullin, MA (Communications, University of Georgia), is a doctoral candidate and Graduate Research Assistant in the Department of Management at Georgia State University.

William I. Sauser, Jr., PhD (Psychology, Georgia Tech), was Head of the Department of Management. He is currently Associate Vice-President for Extension, Auburn University.

Michael Jones, PhD (University of Missouri), is Associate Professor of Marketing at Auburn University at Montgomery.

ABOUT THE EDITOR

Donald R. Self is Professor and Head of the Department of Marketing at Auburn University, Montgomery, Alabama. An active health care and wellness consultant, Dr. Self has worked with various health care facilities, trade associations, and the U.S. Army. He has published widely in professional journals, including *Health Marketing Quarterly*, *Journal of Marketing for Mental Health*, *Journal of Hospital Marketing*, and *Journal of Professional Services Marketing*. Dr. Self received the Doctorate of Business Administration degree in Marketing at Louisiana Tech University.

Preface

This special text was prepared by Donald Self at Auburn University in association with many fine faculty in Montgomery, Alabama. It has been a pleasure to witness such an excellent and worthwhile niche being filled by this text.

It consists of fifteen excellent articles on various aspects of marketing alcoholism programs to the general public and to professionals. Considerable amounts of research and analysis went into the various studies presented.

The area of alcoholism marketing is relatively new and is gradually developing into a specialty. The specialty has emerged as substance abuse became a significant problem in our society and around the world. It is important to remember that the tools and techniques used for marketing alcoholism programs are also applicable for other forms of substance abuse services.

It is the hope that this special text will be a springboard for additional research, writings and publications which will enhance the use of marketing techniques in substance abuse programs throughout the country.

It has been my pleasure to work with Dr. Self and his associates with this publication and we sincerely hope it will contribute to the development of the field.

William J Winston
Senior Editor for Marketing & Health Services Administration
The Haworth Press

Acknowledgements

Thanks are extended to:

Cathleen A. Owens
Editorial Assistant

Teri A. Kline
Section Editor

Vaughan C. Judd
Section Editor

Introduction

This volume contains some fifteen separate articles focused on Alcoholism Treatment Marketing (ATM), and is the first attempt to produce such a focused set of research. Literally thousands of articles and proceedings papers were reviewed to determine the extent of current theory development, along with several hundred in-depth interviews with ATM representatives and a wide variety of referral sources.

The articles are eclectic in nature, drawing from a wide variety of databases and sources. Several articles are dominated by an attempt to provide a synopsis of a cross section of current research, and several are descriptive of the authors' primary research. Finally, other articles focus on the adaptation of marketing tools by ATM facilities.

MARKET BEHAVIOR AND MARKET SEGMENTATION

The first section, "Market Behavior and Market Segmentation," includes five articles, the first of which is a flow process model of the alcoholization/dealcoholization process (Self), which integrates several of the later articles. The second article (Sauser and Self) defines the theoretical models currently in use to describe the alcoholization process.

The following three articles in the section outline three types of markets (groups of clients): the direct consumer market (Judd, Owens, and Self), the direct organization markets (Judd, Self, and Owens), and the indirect referral markets (Kline and Self). From this section the reader should benefit from an enhanced understanding of the theory of alcoholization and the specific markets for ATM. This section provides the basis for understanding and developing a set of ATM consumer behavior and promotion channels literature.

PROGRAM DEVELOPMENT, IMPLEMENTATION, AND EVALUATION

Section II discusses the treatment process from both a theoretical and empirical basis. The first article (Sauser and Self) discusses the various generic services available for ATM including enforced temperance. spontaneous remission, and various types of therapy. In the second article in the section, Kline and Self describe ATMs, providing a distribution system classification model and descriptions of typical specific services offered by particular centers.

Self, McCullin and Kline then discuss the various measures of success in treatment, the characteristics of successful treatment and failure in treatment.

Gomillion and Self complete the section with a case study of a successful PPO utilizing the Alabama Mental Health System to provide services for Alabama teachers and state employees.

TOOLS AND TECHNIQUES

Although not designed to be a total "marketing management" tutorial, this section applies several elements of the marketing process to ATM, with articles on marketing research, promotion, and pricing.

In the first two articles, Ingram et al. present articles on estimating demand and measuring needs and progress of clients. Blucker, Judd, and Self provide an array of sources for secondary research. The final two articles discuss promotion (Jones et al.) and pricing considerations (McCullin, Self, and Kline). The final Epilogue (Self et al.) discusses the transition toward a client-centered (marketing-oriented) facility.

SUMMARY

Without the assistance of several individuals, this volume could not have been completed. Barbara Craun, our department secretary kept the process moving forward along with Cathleen Owens, our graduate research assistant. Suzanne Clemens, Gail Green and Michelle Hendrix provided additional manuscript preparation, library research, and proofreading.

Manuscript revisions and editorial comments were provided by the editors and reviewers. The School of Business at Auburn University at Montgomery provided resources in the form of manuscript preparation and graduate assistants. The AUM Library provided research support from both the reference department and the government documents section. The National Clearinghouse for Alcohol Information provided literally thousands of abstracts, from which we started this entire project.

This volume is not intended to be a handbook of ATM. However, these articles serve as a starting point in that direction. Unfortunately, the deep splits in treatment theory, public vs. private controversies, and inpatient vs. outpatient proponents would make this a hard task.

I take the blame for all errors and omissions, and proudly give the credit to my colleagues and co-authors.

Donald R. Self

I. MARKET BEHAVIOR AND MARKET SEGMENTATION

A Model of the Alcoholization/ Dealcoholization/Maintenance Process

Donald R. Self

PURPOSE

The intent of this article is to present the ideas developed in a recent (Self et al., 1988) flow process model which will be further developed by various authors in this volume. Rather than "reinvent the wheel," this article relies heavily on previous research, which is presented in tabular form throughout the text.

Some Existing Models

Several input-output models exist to describe the process of alcoholization and dealcoholization (see, for example, Armor et al., 1978, pp. 165-168; Denzin, 1987, pp. 135-202).

The Denzin model (1987), as well as several others, specifies Alcoholics Anonymous as the primary agent for the establishment and maintenance of sobriety. These models are not all-inclusive in at least two respects. First, competing treatment philosophies are not considered. Armor et al. (1978, pp. 12-26), and others, however, have identified a wide variety of competing alcoholism theories based on psychological and socio-cultural variables, as well as the physiological/biological underpinnings of the AA philosophy. Further, the "abstinence" requirement of the AA philosophy has been found to be non-required in at least some cases. These two characteristics were observed as early as the 1960s, when Pattison (1966) observed from empirical evidence that (1) to be effective, alcoholism treatment must address multiple aspects other than drinking alone, and (2) abstinence, per se, has a low correlation with successful rehabilitation. Other models focus on other causative factors, such as "life problems" based dependencies (see for example, Simmermacher, 1981, p. 13). While these models provide partial views, contradictory conclusions may be drawn from a cross-philosophy comparison.

The Armor model (1978) presents a three-part flow process model of the alcoholization/dealcoholization process including client inputs, treatment inputs, and outcomes for recovery. This model does an excellent job of describing the salient characteristics for initial treatment evaluation, for which the model was designed, and provides some of the components for the model presented below. However, several characteristics are not included, such as the process of recidivism during treatment, elements of the socio-cultural model, and the problem recognition/search process.

TOWARD A COMPREHENSIVE MODEL

A five-step decision process has been frequently referenced in the marketing literature (Assael, 1987, p. 28; Harrell, 1986, pp. 19-20; Hawkins, Best, and Coney, 1986, pp. 33-36; Mellott, 1983, p. 509; Mowen, 1987, pp. 31-32; Wilkie, 1986, pp. 496-498). John Dewey (1910) is credited as the original source of the multi-step decision process concept (Assael, 1987, p. 28; Engel, Blackwell, and Miniard, 1986, p. 23). A review of Dewey's work (1910, Chapters 1 and 8) documents the framework for a five-step decision process with sub-steps of internal and external search as well as the suggestion of evaluative criteria as a basis for alternative selection.

The process attributed to Dewey has been described as (1) problem recognition; (2) search (both internal and external); (3) evaluation; (4) purchase; and (5) post-purchase evaluation. The flow process model in Figure 1 incorporates these steps as applied to the alcoholization/dealcoholization process, and is the basis for this volume.

Prior to discussing the sequential development of the model, it is important to differentiate between two competing philosophies of

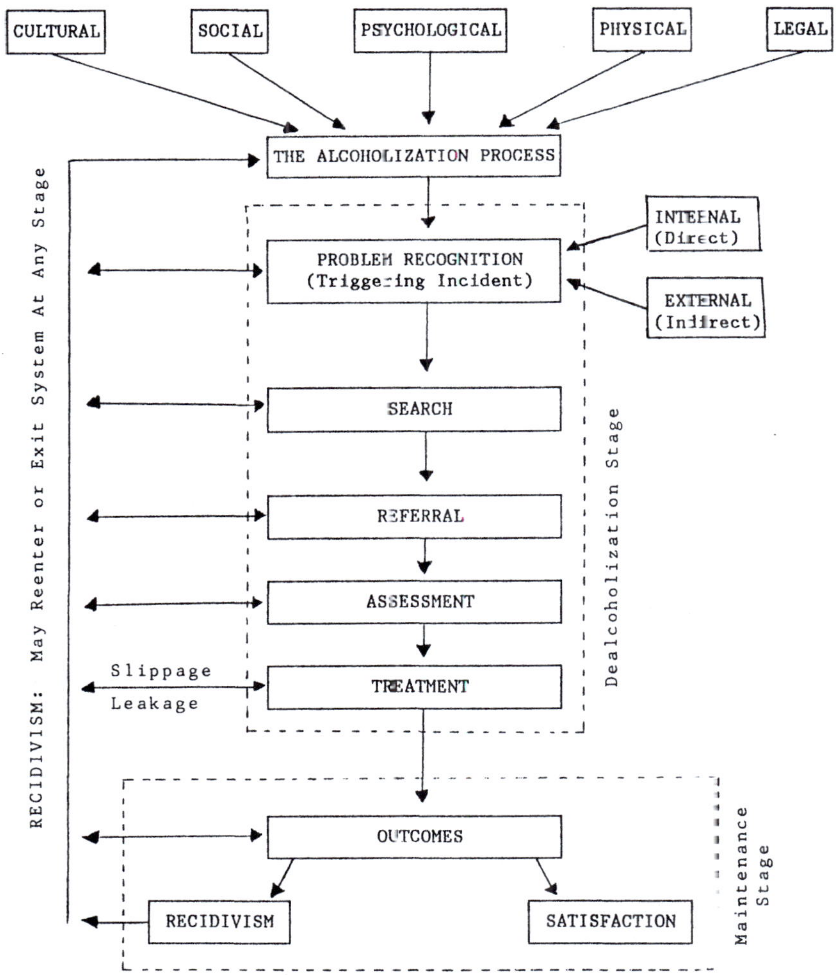

FIGURE 1. A Model of the Alcoholization/Dealcoholization Variables Affecting Alcoholization

anti-alcoholism and the historical development of alcoholism treatment.

EVOLUTION OF TREATMENT AND PREVENTION

The development of the alcoholism treatment discipline closely parallels our earlier description (Self, Ingram, McKinney, and Buchanan, 1987) of the evolution of change-oriented disciplines of (1) change-agent, (2) professional client, (3) marketing-oriented or "chain-link fence," and (4) societal marketing. This evolutionary model, presented in Table 1, is developed from various disciplines, and proposes that human change organizations start as change-agent or "idealism-oriented" organizations. From the development of the temperance movement through prohibition repeal, the goal of the "movement" was the limitation of alcohol use, focusing on change of the system. With the advent of Repeal of Prohibition and the formation of Alcoholics Anonymous, the focus changed to treatment, with AA or treatment centers adopting the role of "professionals" and the alcoholic as client. The goal of the treatment was abstinence.

With the publication of several major provocative studies in the 1960s (see especially Davies, 1962, and Pattison, 1966), several revolutionary changes have occurred in the discipline, including the questioning of the "disease" model of alcoholism and the related previous "requirement" of complete abstinence on the part of all former patients.

Both the increase in population growth and the rising number of alcoholics in America contribute to the rising number of individuals seeking treatment for alcoholism and alcohol related problems. Data from a number of sources indicate that alcoholism treatment services and number of people in treatment continue to increase; more than half a million people were reported to be in treatment in September, 1984 (Harwood et al., 1985; Noble, 1985). The State Alcohol and Drug Abuse Profile (SADAP) reports that alcohol client admissions increased by 6 percent from 1984 to 1985 (Butynski, Record, and Yates, 1986).

Prompted, perhaps, by the growing number of well-known individuals who have chosen to speak out about their alcohol problems and the role of treatment in their recovery, the stigma of alcoholism appears to be slowly diminishing (NIAAA, 1987). Korcok (1985) attributes the rise in treatment demand partially to the changing perceptions of alcoholism treatment from a marketing standpoint. In the rapidly changing health care marketplace, alcoholism treatment has become a dynamic and popular "product line." It is a good seller for hospitals, and a good buy for third-party payers and corporate purchasers of health services.

In virtually all parts of the nation, print and broadcast messages now promote varying types of alcoholism services such as hospital inpatient programs, outpatient services, residential facilities, programs that involve the entire family, and programs designed specifically for teenagers.

Treatment vs. Prevention

Prevention is viewed by many authorities as an alternative, or even conflicting orientation toward alcohol and health. Gusfield (1982, p. 403) defines three subsets of prevention:

1. Primary prevention: actions to prevent agents from causing disease or injury.
2. Secondary prevention: early detection and treatment of alcoholics or problem drinkers.
3. Tertiary prevention: preventing further deterioration and reducing disability.

The focus of this volume is on treatment. For definitional purposes, the definitions of the response sought, target market and characteristics contained in Table 2 are used in this volume. For the interested reader, an excellent history, overview and resource list on prevention is contained in the *Prevention Action Manual* listed in the bibliography (see Saulter and Leaque, 1986).

ELEMENTS OF THE MODEL

Cultural Inputs

We have proposed elsewhere (Self, Buchanan, and Ingram, 1987) that customer orientation and satisfaction are often not dominant considerations for not-for-profit service organizations and pro-

TABLE 1. Evolution of Alcoholism Treatment Philosophy

Era	Change/Agent	Client/ Professional	"Social Marketing"
Time Period	1800s-Prohibition Repeal	1930s-Present	1970s to Present
Marketing Evolution Stage	Product	Sales	Marketing
Goal	Eliminate Alcohol Use	Treatment of Alcoholism	-Treatment of Alcoholism and other problems -Intervention -Prevention
Major Philosophies	Alcohol is deviate substance responsible for accidents, crimes, moral relapse	Abstinence is required	-Preventative medicine -Multivariate approach -Chain link fence
Major	Temperence Movement	A.A.	

Alcohol Consumption	Increased until 1900s. Remained high until 1920 (Prohibition)	1933 (Repeal) to 1945: increased to pre-prohibition level. 1940-1960: level consumption. 1961-1971: 30% increase.	1971 to Present: relatively stable
Focus of Attention	Sobriety	Abstinence on part of alcoholics	Spectrum of alcohol problems (DWI, productivity, marital strife, medical ailments)
Characteristics of Era	Political Conflict	Medicalization of Alcoholics	Integrated drinking by some former alcoholics
Relationship with Alcohol Industry	Antagonistic	Defusing of political conflict	Increasing cooperation
Limitations	Lack of treatment orientation	Minimizes consequences of drinking /drunkeness in general population	Lack of research data

TABLE 2. Treatment vs. Prevention

	Treatment	Prevention
Response Sought	Curing of unhealthy	Erodication/minimization of occurence
Target Market	Those who deviate from normal conditions	Those who might become alcoholic
Characteristics	Individualistic Remedial	Collective, Environmental

pose that the rationale used also fits profit-oriented intervention organizations such as alcohol treatment centers. Multiple publics often dictate operation strategies which may not be in the best interest of customers (Lovelock and Weinberg, 1978; Rados, 1981). The very fact that many non-profit or change-oriented organizations are created to deliver unwanted services negates, in large measure, the customer orientation normally associated with the marketing concept—customer needs which are considered desirable from the customer's perspective. Levitt (1973) emphasized that non-profit social-action groups act as change-agents in advancing their causes. Lovelock and Weinberg (1984, p. 567) define "manipulation" of customer behavior as the basis for social behavior (change-agent) marketing.

Alcoholism may produce greater costs to society than any other public health problem since its effects are not only medical and physical, but also psychological, spiritual, social, vocational and legal (Costello, 1982). The economic burden alone of alcohol abuse and alcoholism in 1980 in the United States was an estimated 89.5 billion dollars. Lost employment and reduced productivity (54.7 billion) accounted for more than half of this amount (NIAAA, 1987). The United States Department of Health and Human Services calculated that the cost to society of alcohol abuse in 1983 was 116.7 billion dollars. This figure includes estimates from lost wages, productivity, property damage from car crashes and other accidents, and for health and welfare programs tied to alcoholism.

A basic assumption of the economic theory underlying the concepts used here is that resources are finite or scarce. Therefore, when resources are allocated to the production of certain goods and services they are consumed and cannot be used in the production of other goods and services. The loss of the opportunity to use resources for another purpose is the opportunity cost.

Economic or opportunity costs may be measured from various perspectives. Employers incur costs when treatment is provided at company expense for employees with alcoholism or other health problems, or when production is lost due to factors such as lowered productivity or absenteeism. Costs are borne by an entire society as current resources are used for prevention, treatment, and rehabilitation, and as potential resources are lost due to lowered productivity, absenteeism, or withdrawal from the work force due to death or disability.

Although health care costs have risen significantly, the aggregate measures of the economy have improved over the last several years (Ricardo-Campbell, 1986). Inflation has fallen from double digit levels and unemployment is hovering around 6 percent. The velocity of money has slowed and the money supply has not shown dramatic changes. Corporate profits continue to rise. The big area of growth in U.S. business is in the service sector, including financial services. The health industry, classified as a service, has been growing rapidly, spurred by third party reimbursement by government and business. The health delivery industry with about 7 million employees is the second largest service industry in the United States, exceeded only by the education industry.

The Alcoholism-Chemical Dependency Market

A rapidly growing segment of this industry is in the area of alcohol and chemical dependency treatment and services. Although alcohol consumption in the United States is declining, alcohol remains the most widely used and abused drug in the United States. The number of alcoholics has risen as have the number and types of treatment available to the alcohol abuser or dependent person, and the number of individuals seeking treatment.

Purchasers of health care in the United States are generally paying from 7-10 percent of claim dollars on mental and substance abuse claims, with the vast majority (80%) of the dollars expended on inpatient treatment rather than the less costly outpatient care (Lee, 1987). Gunby (1987) reports that the total 1986 alcohol and drug abuse market was 1.6 billion, of which 73.4% was spent on treatment.

Legal Inputs

During recent years various legal mechanisms have been invoked to reduce alcoholism in the U.S. and in other countries such as Russia (Kirn 1987A, 1987B). Examples include drinking driver referral, others whose public assistance is conditional on entering treatment, and others whose mandate involves probations and parole (Panepinto and Simmons, 1986). This increase in public attention has increased the number of persons entering treatment and has caused a broadening of and restructuring of the definition of alcoholism. The recent Kentucky school bus accident in which over two dozen occupants of the bus were killed by a drunk driver and other similar incidents are predicted to cause increased legal inputs.

What is Alcoholism? – Physiological/Biological, Psychological, and Socio-Cultural Inputs

Three major streams of theory have evolved in attempts to define alcoholism (see Table 3). These include the physiological or biological approach, from which the dominant "disease" concept has developed; the psychological approach, including the psychoclynomic trait, and learning models; and those approaches which stress the demographic factors of a cultural or sociological basis. The next article in this volume (Sauser and Self) develops each of these theoretical constructs, and the third article in this volume (Judd, Owens, and Self) uses each of these approaches in a demographically based segmentation classification.

THE ALCOHOLIZATION STAGE

As previously mentioned, various models have been developed to describe part or all of the alcoholization/dealcoholization process, with variations based on the theoretical constructs used by the different authors. The most widely accepted model of the alcoholization part of the process is the Jellenik Phase Model, which is presented in Table 4.

TABLE 3. Major Etiological Alcoholism Theories

Theory	Physiological/ Biological	Psychological	Socio-Cultural
Thesis	Intoxication is necessary and sufficient condition for ever increasing drinking craving and pathology. (Internal focus)	Alcoholics share certain traits or personality structures which are of causal significance in development of alcoholism. (Internal focus)	Recognizes internal determinants (physiological and psychological) but stress demographic predictors of alcoholism. (External focus)
Types of Theories	1. Genotrophic Theory - inherited metabolic defect. 2. Endocrine dys-function. 3. Normalizing Effect 4. Genetic Models	1. Psychodynamic Theories a. Freudian b. Immaturity/ Regression c. Dependency/ Autonomy Conflict 2. Personality Traits 3. Learning Models	1. Culture/ Socialization Theories 2. Cultural Stress 3. Familial Patterns 4. Instability & Crisis

Developed from: Armor, D. J., J. M. Polich, and H. B. Stambul, *Alcoholism and Treatment*, New York: John Wiley and Sons, pp. 12-26, 1987.

TABLE 4. The Jellenik Phase Model of Alcoholism

STAGE	PRE-ALCOHOLIC	PRODOMAL	CRUCIAL	CHRONIC
Change Occuring	Progression from occasional to almost daily relief drinking	Preoccupation with alcohol.	Loss of drinking control (physical demand - chain reaction).	Periods of prolonged intoxication (Benders).
Important Charateristics	1. Tolerance Development	1. Surreptitous Drinking	1. Aggressive behavior	1. Impaired thinking
	2. Increased Consumption	2. Gulping of Drinks	2. Drinking rationalization	2. Indefinable fears
	3. A stage of (evening) relief from emotional stress.	3. Blackouts*	3. Remorse	3. Tremors
		4. Guilt feelings	4. Periods of obstinence.	4. Psychomotor inhibition
		5. Heavy but not conspicuous drinking.	5. Morning drinking	5. Loss of tolerance.
			6. Usually intoxicated by evening.	

* This characteristic has been disputed by several researchers who propose that blackouts occur (1) in nonalcoholic drinkers and/or (2) later in the developmental sequence.

Developed from: Rudy, David R., *Becoming Alcoholic*, Carbondale and Edwardsville, Il: Southern Illinois University Press, pp. 81-88, 1986.

Jellenik grouped the alcoholization process into four stages. The *Pre-Alcoholic Stage* involves the progression to almost daily drinking, leading to a preoccupation with alcohol (*Prodomal Stage*). Eventually the person loses control of the drinking (*Crucial Stage*), leading to periods of prolonged intoxication (*Chronic Stage*). Some alcoholics develop periods of sobriety between benders, while some continue to drink on a daily basis. Knott (Chapters 3 and 4, 1986) presents excellent chapters on these last two stages. Brown (1985) presents a similar progression involving (1) increasing isolation, constriction and narrowing of the individual's environment; (2) struggle for control; (3) acceptance of failure; (4) loss of control; and (5) hitting bottom.

Armor et al. (1978) presents a similar model, focusing on the external environment. Table 5 demonstrates this model, which utilizes the socio-cultural contexts of culture and values predicating the decision to drink or abstain (Stage I); the social environment and lifestyle at least partially determine the amount of drinking (Stage II); and substantial factors such as a crisis or heavy drinking friends influences onset of alcoholism (Stage III).

THE DEALCOHOLIZATION STAGE

This part of the process (see Figure 1) involves (a) problem recognition, (b) search for alternatives, (c) referral, (d) initial assessment, and (e) treatment.

Problem Recognition

Some authorities (see Brown, 1985 for example) maintain that an alcoholic must "hit bottom" or admit a total loss of control before becoming not-dependent on alcohol. The problem recognition may be done by the individual or a wide variety of potential referral sources (internal or external). Various physical cues, as demonstrated in Table 6 are available for identifying the problem.

The Search

Little research has been done concerning the search process for appropriate treatment. Location, cost, types of programs offered, and privacy appear to be important characteristics used by external referral sources (Alabama Voice, 1986). (For an in-depth discussion of salient characteristics of treatment centers as perceived by various referral sources, see Kline, Self, and Ingram, 1987.)

TABLE 5. A Multi-Stage Model of Alcoholism and Recovery

STAGE I The Decision to Drink or Abstain

Determining Factors: Culture, Values

Salient Findings: Abstention is positively correlated with region (South), religion (Protestant), lower socio-economic class, female, older.

STAGE II The Amount of Drinking

Determining Factors: Social Environment, Life-Style

Salient Findings: Heavier drinking associated with drinking context (drinking in bars), marital status (unmarried), rare (black), socio-economic class, older (if in drinking population).

STAGE III Onset of Alcoholism and Problem Drinking

Determining Factors: Situational Factors, e.g. Crisis

Salient Findings:

Cluster A: Marital break-up and unemployment

Cluster B: Drinking context - Bars, heavy drinking spouses and friends.

STAGE IV The Recovery Process

Determining Factors: Individual Factors (Decisions)

Salient Findings: Successful decision-making process requires (1) experience of "costs" of alcoholism that outweigh short-run reasons for drinking, (2) breakdown of psychological barriers (e.g. denial) enabling a recognition of the problem, (3) commitment to change.

Source: Armor, D. J., J. M. Polich, and H. B. Stambul, *Alcoholism and Treatment*, New York: John Wiley and Sons, pp. 165-168, 1978.

TABLE 6. Alcohol-Related Disorders or Symptoms

Disorder	Symptoms	Possible Cause(s)
Alcoholic Fatty Liver	Smooth, non-tender enlargement of liver with or without abnormal liver functions.	In connection with drinking episode means higher intake of ethanol than liver can metabolize.
Pancreatis	Severe, constant abdominal pain and tenderness sometimes radiating to the back.	Pancreatic inflammation due to too many years of excessive drinking
Gastritis	Anorexia, nausea, and vomiting (sometimes bloody)	Toxic effect of alcohol on stomach lining with associated erosions and ulcerations
Nutritional Deficiencies	Impaired absorption of nutrients, changes in intestinal motility to diarrhea	Drinking bouts, inattention to proper nutrition
Poor Immune Response	Pulmonary infections	Failure of immune defense systems - inattention to proper hygiene while drunk
Neurological Changes	Diminished touch, temperature, pain, and position sensations: Atrophy and pain of calf muscles early in course of excessive drinking	Peripheral neuropathy-increased patellar reflex Hematologic Abnormalities

TABLE 6 (continued)

Disorder	Symptoms	Possible Cause(s)
Hematologic Abnormalities	-Folate deficiency producing megaloblastosis or macrocytosis -Sicleroblastic anemia -Thrombocytopenia and bleeding	Alcohol overuse
Myopathy	Lower extremity muscle aches, weakness, cramping, and tenderness.	-Alcoholic myopathy early in evolution of drinking career; -Cardiomyopathy (late evidence of alcoholism)
Skin Changes	1) Face may be puffy, the cheeks and nose flushed; conjunctival vessels injected; the tongue smooth and red.	Excessive drinking (early stages)
	2)Rhinophyma, acne rosacea and spider nevi.	Vitamin B deficiency
	Cigarette burns, contusions, and bruises.	Alcoholic stupor
	Insect bites & frostbite.	Spending nights outdoors in an alcoholic coma
Blackouts	Loss of recall for a period of time: Amnesia during a drinking bout may occur shortly after drinking has commenced & recur during subsequent sprees.	Heavy drinking: sometimes, but not always, an indicator of alcoholism

Impotence & Loss of Libido	Male impotence	Acute & chronic consequence of considerable drinking. Alcohol blocks synthesis of testorone in the gonads.
	Libido decrease	Later symptom resulting from low levels of testerone availibility, or its conversion to estrogen-like substances.
Cancer	Increased risk of cancer of the tongue, mouth, pharynx, larynx, esophagus and liver	Heavy drinking (alcohol may either act as a carcinogen or as a solvent for cancer-producing polyaromatic hydrocarbons)
	Increased rate of head and neck cancers	Heavy alcohol and tobacco use.

Source: Cohen, S., *The Substance Abuse Problems*, New York: The Haworth Press, Inc., 1981.

The Referral System

The referral process used in a particular case is particularly dependent on the willingness of the potential client to enter treatment. As is shown in Figure 2, the "exchange process" involved between the alcoholic and potential referral sources, may involve begging, persuading, negotiating or commanding the alcoholic to seek treatment. The fourth article in this volume (Judd, Self, and Owens) describes the employer and judicial referral markets (the coercive or calculative compliance system), and the fifth article (Kline and Self) describes the less coercive or more voluntary referral systems.

Once referred, getting the potential client to go to the treatment is not automatic. Dubinsky (1986) reports that approximately one-fifth will not report for the appointment in an outpatient setting.

Assessment

Although assessment of the client's needs is an ongoing process (see Ingram in this volume) the initial assessment of the client's needs will determine the treatment format. Conventional wisdom

FIGURE 2. The Exchange Process Continuum

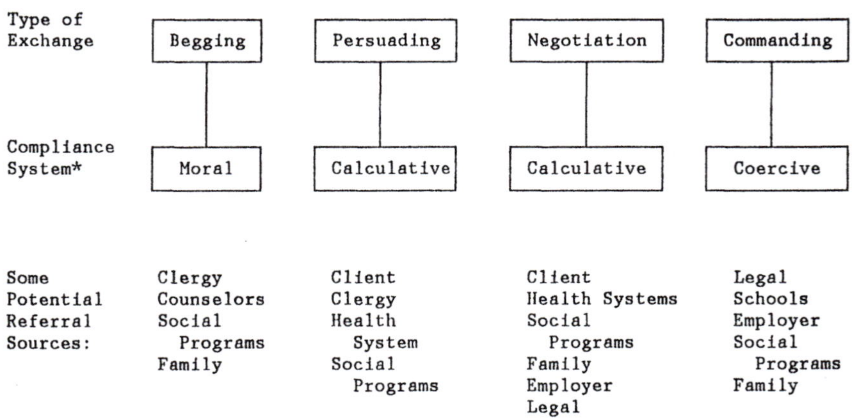

As developed by: Etzioni, A., *A Comparative Analysis of Complex Organizations*, Glencoe, IL: Free Press, 1969.

indicates an alcoholism dependence continuum in which alcoholism exists in varying degrees of severity (Shelley-McIntyre, 1987).

Treatment

Although some alcoholic individuals may recover without formal treatment (Prugh, 1986), formal treatment does produce increases in the probability of improvement. The first two articles in Section II of this volume detail the theoretical basis for the various treatment programs (Sauser and Self), and provide a classification system for the facilities based on such variables as location and length of stay, basis for funding, programs offered, and characteristics of clients (Kline and Self).

While inpatient care may be required for the initial detoxification stage, most recent studies mirror the findings of Longabaugh et al. (1983) that more costly inpatient programs do not produce significantly higher results. Exceptions include clients with concurrent psychological or health problems.

The first stage in the improvement process has been labelled as "transition," (Brown, 1985) in which there is a shift to not-drinking and acceptance of loss of control. During the first 12-96 hours after the last drink, the client will probably undergo a wide variety of withdrawal symptoms as indicated in Table 7.

Most clients will undergo the Stage I withdrawal symptoms and a few will also undergo the Stage II symptoms of hallucinations and/or amnesia. Very few will undergo the very serious Stage III symptoms.

Most authorities divide the post-transition period into two stages. Brown (Table 8) refers to these as *early recovery*, where the focus is on increasing isolation from alcohol, and the ongoing process.

THE MAINTENANCE STAGE

Abstinence is the goal of most programs, although there is limited research to validate the efficacy of a return to normal drinking on the part of some individuals. The third article in Section II of this volume (Self, McCullin, and Kline) summarizes research on these two outcomes and discusses the relative effectiveness of various

TABLE 7. Withdrawal Symptoms

STAGE I -	psychomotor agilation; autonomic hyperactivity consisting of hypertension, tachycardia, diaphoris, anorexia, insomnia, and illusions.
Time -	usually within 12-36 hours of last drink, up to 72-96 hours after last drink. Lasts from a few hours to one to two days.
STAGE II -	
Symptoms -	Stage I symptoms, plus hallucinations leading to paranoid ideations and behavior. Possible partial or total amnesia of hallucinatory experiences.
STAGE III -	
Symptoms -	Stage I and II's symptoms plus disorientation, delusions, and delirium. May be seizure activity. Infections especially respiratory; hypoglycemia; multiple drug tendencies, pancreatitis.
Other Observations:	Relatively rare unless there are concommitent conditions. Usually associated with medical-surgical disorder.

Source: Knott, D. H., R. D. Fink, and J. C. Morgan, Intoxication and the alcohol abstinence syndrome, in Schwartz, G. R., Sofar, P., Stone, J. H. et al. (eds.): *Principles and Practice of Emergency Medicine*, Philadelphia: Saunders, pp. 1345-1350, 1978.

types of programs. Labelled "The (Un)Finished Product," this article focuses on the very real phenomenon of attrition during treatment and the potential for one or more relapses.

Relapse

A major function of the later stages of a formal treatment program and of aftercare is the teaching of the skills and self-discipline to prevent relapse. Relapse begins with internal fears about one's ability to remain sober which may cause one or more external signs, leading to post acute withdrawal (Carlson, 1986) and invariably leading to a relapse. Dramatic mood changes characterize this pre-relapse stage, also labelled as the "dry-drunk." Hunter and Salomone (1987) classified these symbols (based on the AA model) as is shown in Table 9.

TABLE 8. Brown's AA-Based Model of Alcoholism Recovery

Basic Constructs: Four stages (Drinking, transition, Early recovery, Ongoing Recovery) in which three components (alcohol emphasis, environmental interactions, interpretations of self and other interact).

Stage I Drinking

1. Salient Characteristics: Increasing isolation, constriction and narrowing of individual's worlds; struggle for control; acceptance of failure; loss of control, hitting bottom.

Stage II Transition

1. Salient Characteristics: Shift to not-drinking, acceptance of alcoholic status, acceptance of loss of control leads to conversion.

Stage III Early Recovery

1. Salient Characteristics: interactions with others and the environment without alcohol presence; improved work and home relations; expanded world view; active dependency; need for support.

2. Alcohol Focus: Increasing personal isolation.

Stage IV Ongoing Process

1. Salient Characteristics: support from interdependent, sharing relationships and self-reliance; strong internalization of AA principles.

2. Alcohol Focus: Identification as an alcoholic with loss of control extreme dependence on external prevention, substitution of AA for alcohol.

Source: Brown, S., "Models of Alcoholism," *Treating the Alcoholic*, New York: John Wiley and Sons, 1985.

The importance of adjustment to external cues is extremely important. Binkhoff (1986) based on a control-group study involving alcohol cues reported increasing levels of self-anxiety and physical reaction were present. Even for individuals with psychiatric problems, external cues are very important.

Studies of the probability of relapse give widely varying predictions. In one recent study of 658 clients discharged from a residential treatment center (Pickens et al., 1985), 44% reported relapse, with the peak at about 6 months following treatment. Of those who

TABLE 9. Dry-Drunk Symptoms

1. Failure to appreciate the disease concept of alocholism
2. Guilt
3. Denial
4. Dishonesty
5. Isolation
6. People, places, and things
7. Cross-Addiciton
8. H.A.L.T. (Hungry, Angry, Lonely, Tired)
9. Resentments
10. Self-pity
11. Intolerance
12. Anxiety
13. Stress
14. Failure to feel good about one's self
15. Expecting too much too soon from others
16. Problems related to family needs
17. A lack of spirituality (not religiosity)
18. Omnipotence
19. Complacency
20. Slackening of self-discipline

Source: Hunter, T. A., and P. R. Salomone, "Dry Drunk Symptoms and Alcoholic Relapse," *Journal of Applied Rehabilitation Counseling*, Vol. 18(1), pp. 22-25, 1987.

relapsed, almost half (42%) reported a subsequent return to abstinence.

Various models of relapse have been proposed, most of them mirroring one of the biological/psychological/social models of addiction. The biological model has been well advanced by such authors as Donovan (1986), Donovan and Chancey (1985), and Gorski and Miller (1986).

In Table 10, Gorski (1986) presents a well developed model of the recovery period which gives indicators for appropriate prevention methods.

TABLE 10

I. THE PRETREATMENT PERIOD
During the pretreatment period, the alcoholic will typically attempt both periods of controlled use and periods of abstinence. The major cause of relapse during this period is the testing of personal control.

II. THE STABILIZATION PERIOD
Patients often find themselves unable to cope with the stress and pressure of these symptoms. They often use alcohol and drugs to relieve such distress. The major cause of relapse during the stabilization period is the lack of withdrawal management skills.

III. THE EARLY RECOVERY PERIOD
Early recovery is marked by the need to establish a recovery program that provides a social structure support of long-term sobriety.

IV. THE MIDDLE RECOVERY PERIOD
Middle recovery is marked by the development of a balanced lifestyle. This is a time of stress as the person begins applying basic recovery skills to real-life problems. The major cause of relapse during this period is the stress of life change.

V. THE LATE RECOVERY PERIOD
Late recovery is the time when a lifestyle that is balanced between recovery activities and normal, stable life activities is established. The major cause of relapse during this phase of recovery is either the inability to cope with the stress of unresolved childhood issues or evasion of the need to develop a functional, low-stress personality style.

VI. THE MAINTENANCE PERIOD
The physiology of addiction persists for the rest of a person's life. Any use of alcohol or drugs will reactivate previously damaged physiological processes. They must guard against relapse warning signs, continue to live productively, and strive to actualize sobriety-centered values within their lifestyles.

VII. "STUCK POINTS" IN RECOVERY
Although some patients progress through the stages of recovery without complications, the majority of recovering alcoholics do not. Most alcoholics get stuck somewhere in midstream. A "stuck point" can occur during any period of recovery and generally is caused either by the refusal or inability to complete recovery tasks or by the development of special problems that interfere with progress in recovery.

When patients encounter "stuck points," either they will recognize that they have a problem and take action, or they will deny that a problem exists. If patients deny that problems exist, stress will begin to build. Eventually, the stress will reach an intensity sufficient to trigger a state of internal dysfunction.

Source: Gorski, Terrence T., "Relapse Prevention Planning," Alcohol, Health, & Research World, pp. 6-11, Fall 1986.

General Theories of Alcoholic Behavior

William I. Sauser, Jr.
Donald R. Self

INTRODUCTION

Why people behave the way they do is a subject that has fascinated scientists and laymen alike for centuries, with many theories having been proposed to explain human behavior. For example, the belief that abnormal-appearing behavior is caused by demonic possession or magical forces has been espoused through the ages. Other explanations include chemical imbalances within the body, inherited behavioral tendencies, childhood experiences, cultural influences, patterns of reward and punishment, and environmental conditions.

Psychology is the field of science devoted to the study of behavior, and as such psychological theories which claim to explain a variety of human behaviors are called personality theories. While literally hundreds of personality theories have been developed over the years—each claiming to explain variations and nuances in human behavior—these theories can be grouped into relatively few categories for the purpose of discussion. Common categories include physiological/biological theories, psychodynamic theories, trait and type theories, learning (conditioning) theories, and sociocultural theories. Some broad theories cut across these categories, while others combine characteristics from several categories.

Since the consumption of alcohol is a human behavior, it has been a topic of interest to personality theorists from all five of the major schools of thought listed above. Thus, each of the theories of alcoholism discussed in this chapter has its roots in the more general theories of behavior mentioned above.

The purpose of this article is to familiarize general readers with five major theoretical approaches to understanding human behavior, and to show how each of these approaches deals with the specific behavior of interest in this volume—the consumption of alcohol. Professionals who treat alcoholics are generally well versed in these schools of thought, and their approaches to treatment are typically heavily influenced by the tenets of one or more of these theories.

Consumer Behavior Models and Product Line Models

Professional marketers are expected to be very familiar with their own product lines, as well as those of their competitors. They should know the strengths and weaknesses of all the products or services in their area of specialty, and should be able to identify and explain competitive advantages of their own line. The sixth article in this volume, "Alcoholism Treatment Philosophies and Theories," will present the specific characteristics of each of the major approaches to the treatment of alcoholics. These treatment philosophies are closely aligned with the more general theories of the alcoholism process described in the present article. Thus, the theories described here may be thought of as the theories of consumer behavior which underlie the more specific treatment approaches (products or services) discussed in the later article.

PHYSIOLOGICAL/BIOLOGICAL THEORIES

From one perspective, a human being may be viewed as an extremely complex system of individual, specialized cells. This viewpoint, called *reductionism* (Pronko, 1984, p. 45) suggests that to understand a human being's behavior, one must examine the metabolic processes, chemical and electrical changes, and other physiological phenomena which occur within the physical body of that human being.

A key concept of the physiological/biological theories of behavior is *homeostasis*—the tendency of the body to maintain many of its internal physiological processes at certain optimal levels (Morgan, King, & Robinson, 1979, p. 644). The tendency for the body to maintain this homeostatic balance has long been recognized as the basis for such primary human behaviors as drinking, eating, and breathing (Grossman, 1984, p. 43). Special receptors in that portion of the brain known as the *hypothalamus* are believed to monitor the body's needs for water and other nutrients, and to signal the body to seek and consume foods and liquids containing those nutrients when the body's internal supply falls below an acceptable homeostatic level (Grossman, 1984).

The phenomenon of *specific hungers* (Richter, 1943, 1947) has been documented in experiments with laboratory animals. Kalat (1984) defines a specific hunger as "an increased preference for foods that contain a specific nutrient, such as a mineral or a vitamin, under conditions of increased need for that nutrient" (p. 354). Clearly, if the body develops a specific hunger for ethanol, then the consumption of alcoholic beverages could be viewed as a behavior influenced heavily by internal, physiological processes. This is the basis of the popular concept of alcoholism as a physiologically addictive disease (Jellinek, 1960).

Possible Causes of Need

If one accepts the theory that the consumption of alcohol is driven by internal, physiological mechanisms, then the question becomes "What determines the physiological need for alcohol?" Several answers to this question have been suggested, including inherited metabolic defects and various endocrinal dysfunctions (Armor, Polich, and Stambul, 1978, pp. 13-17). These and other explanations will be explored following a description of the earliest and most popularly accepted physiological/biological theory of alcoholism—Jellinek's (1952, 1960) disease model.

Jellinek's Disease Model

Rudy (1986) states that Jellinek's (1945, 1952, 1962) phase model and his other writings on alcoholism "have heavily influenced most conceptualizations of alcoholism and its treatment within the past several decades" (p. 81). In fact, Rudy claims that despite recent criticisms of the model, many writers "view Jellinek's phase model and disease definitions of alcoholism as the most profound influence on the alcoholism field to date" (p. 83). Smith, Milkman, and Sunderwirth (1985) note that Jellinek's (1960) concept of alcoholism as a progressive and potentially fatal physiological disorder "has been embraced and promoted by Alcoholics Anonymous, the National Council of Alcoholism, the National Institute on Alcohol Abuse and Alcoholism, and the American Medical Association" (p. 146).

Table 1, adapted from Rudy (1986, pp. 81-82) provides descriptions of each phase of Jellinek's model.

Clearly, Jellinek's medical model is based in the physiological/biological tradition of explaining human behavior, since it conceives of alcohol consumption as a process designed to satisfy a physiological craving over which the addicted individual has little or no control. Armor, Polich, and Stambul (1978) offer praise for the model for removing the stigma of moral turpitude (p. 10) and thus making it possible "to provide medical and psychological

TABLE 1. The Phases of Jellinek's Model

I.	Prealcoholic Symptomatic Phase: characterized by a progression from occasional to almost daily relief drinking; that is, drinking to relieve tension. During this phase, individuals develop a tolerance to alcohol and generally drink "fairly heavily"....
II.	Prodromal Phase: marked by "blackouts." These losses of memory occur after a moderate amount of alcohol has been consumed; although persons affected may be able to carry on complex activities, they fail to recall them the following day....
III.	Crucial Phase: initiated by loss of control over drinking.... Although drinkers can control whether they will drink or not, they cannot control the quantity once they have initiated drinking....
IV.	Chronic Phase: begins when drinkers begin to engage in benders or periods of prolonged intoxication. Other features of this phase include impairment of thinking, indefinable fears, tremors, psychomotor inhibition, and loss of tolerance. During this phase, individuals control these symptoms by drinking.

treatment in place of punitive measures" (p. 10). However, these same authors also present several major criticisms of the model (pp. 10-11). Basically, the Jellinek disease model can be criticized for:

a. Placing alcoholism within the medical tradition of either-or differential diagnosis;
b. Placing causation "inside-the-man," thereby taking inadequate account of sociocultural factors that may play a causal role;
c. Directing responsibility for treatment to medical practitioners who perpetuate the doctor-patient relationship, encouraging the latter to assume a passive role;
d. Promoting a "sick role" which in some cases makes alcoholics worse, not better; and
e. Creating a self-fulfilling prophecy which frightens problem drinkers away from early treatment.

Jellinek's disease model has been the focus of strong support and heavy attack, and its implications for theories of treatment will be considered further in the following article. Jellinek's model, as described above, does not fully explain the physiological mechanisms which influence the consumption of alcohol. Other physiological/biological theories, however, have focused primarily on identifying these mechanisms. Four such approaches, as classified by Armor, Polich, and Stambul (1978), are discussed below.

Genetotrophic Theory—Inherited Metabolic Defects

Armor, Polich, and Stambul (1978) state that the genetotrophic theory, as advanced by Williams (1947, 1959):

> . . . postulates that alcoholism results from an inherited metabolic defect that causes the need for certain dietary substances in excess amounts to those provided in the ordinary diet. Since alcohol has caloric value, ingestion is thought to temporarily alleviate the symptoms of the dietary deficiency but not to provide necessary nutriments. (p. 14)

In terms of the homeostatic balance concept discussed earlier, this theoretical approach holds that some persons have an *inherited* metabolic defect which produces needs for far more of certain nutrients than they can satisfy by eating normal meals. Thus, they consume alcohol, which provides more calories and temporarily relieves the homeostatic pressure; yet, since the alcohol does not actually possess the craved nutrients, homeostasis is not really achieved, and more alcohol is consumed.

While Armor, Polich, and Stambul (1978) cited several theorists who supported the genetotrophic theory, they personally tended to dismiss it, claiming that "it remains unproven and has been met with criticism on theoretical and empirical grounds" (p. 14).

Interestingly, in a more recent review, Smith, Milkman, and Sunderwirth (1985) present a very convincing argument for the genetotrophic approach to understanding alcoholism, and claim that "the inheritance of addictive disease can best be understood using alcoholism as an example" (p. 148). While a full explanation of their technical findings is beyond the scope of this article, they claim that genetic abnormalities in the enzymes which help metabolize alcohol account for the alcoholic's inappropriate response to alcohol.

Whereas Armor, Polich, and Stambul (1978) claimed that "no unique metabolic pathways for alcohol as a nutrient distinct from other food substances have been discovered" (p. 14), more recent research on the genetotrophic theory has been more fruitful. For example, Talbott (1984) claims that alcoholism is a chronic, multidisciplinary, genetically linked disease. "The basic defect is a biochemical defect in the hypothalamic instinctual control center in the endorphic and encephalon systems" (p. 155). Clearly, this physiological/biological theory has progressed over the past decade.

Endocrine Theory

Armor, Polich, and Stambul (1978) review some evidence to indicate that alcoholism may be related to endocrine dysfunction, particularly hypoglycemia and hypothyroidism. However, their conclusion is that this approach has not been particularly fruitful: "No strong evidence for the causality of endocrine dysfunction has been obtained'' (p. 14).

Normalizing Effect Theory

A far more productive line of research from the physiological/biological viewpoint, according to Armor, Polich, and Stambul (1978), has been the examination of the ''normalizing effect'' of alcohol on physiological measures:

> [A] host of empirical studies exist that document physiological, biochemical, and neurophysiological parameters that differentiate alcoholics from nonalcoholic control samples. . . . [I]n most instances alcohol ingestion by alcoholics has a normalizing effect. Thus, in a ''dry'' state, alcoholics indices differ significantly from those of nonalcoholic controls; following their ingestion of alcohol, the alcoholics' indices change in the direction of greater normality. (p. 15)

The research reviewed by Armor et al. suggests that alcoholics tend to experience intense sensory stimuli more acutely than nonalcoholics, and also show differences from nonalcoholics in such measures as resting electroencephalograph (EEG) alpha wave activity, sleep patterns, salivary flow, glucose tolerance, and water balance. In all of these instances, by ingesting alcohol, alcoholics were able to move toward greater normality.

While this approach strongly suggests a physiological/biological basis for alcoholism, the primary question, as noted by Armor et al., is whether these physiological phenomena are the cause or the result of alcohol abuse. ''Until there is conclusive evidence to demonstrate the proper causal sequence, the physiological normalizing model of addiction remains a speculative proposal'' (p. 15).

Research conducted during the decade since Armor, Polich, and Stambul (1978) presented their review suggests that many of the physiological symptoms described above result from the process of classical conditioning (Marlatt, Baer, Donovan, and Kivlahan, 1988). Initial ingestion of alcohol produces changes in the chemical signals transmitted within the central nervous systems; these changes produce initial pleasurable feelings, but also have physical side effects. Tolerance for alcohol is increased, and withdrawal effects appear when alcohol is withheld. According to Marlatt et al.:

> [C]lassical conditioning processes play an important role in the development and elicitation of withdrawal and the experience of craving. . . . Increased drinking is predicted to achieve a previously obtained drug-related effect or to avoid the aversiveness of withdrawal distress. (p. 235)

Thus this theoretical approach holds that after repeated ingestion of alcohol the body acquires a new homeostatic balance point through the learning process known as classical conditioning. Alcohol is then sought and consumed to maintain this new point of balance. Since the absence of alcohol will result in craving and withdrawal symptoms, the body has become dependent upon the drug for continuation of a feeling of "normalcy."

Genetic Models

Evidence abounds that alcoholism is a familial disorder. Goodwin and Guze (1974) found that the relatives of alcoholics are far more likely than the general population to be alcoholics themselves. Tarter and Edwards (1986) reviewed research which indicated that 25 percent of the sons of alcoholics, even if reared away from their biological parents, will become alcoholic. Bower's (1986) review of research conducted in Denmark, Sweden, and the United States shows that sons of alcoholics are three to four times more likely to be alcoholic than are sons of nonalcoholics. Marlatt et al. (1988) note that "the current literature frequently states that children of alcoholics are four times as likely to develop alcoholism as children of nonalcoholics, based on data derived from adoption and twin studies" (p. 227). Furthermore, Smith, Milkman, and Sunderwirth (1985, p. 149) report evidence of racial differences in sensitivity to alcohol.

All of this evidence seems to point to the operation of genetic mechanisms in the transmission of a predisposition toward alcoholism. The genetotrophic theory, previously discussed, suggests that the inherited factor may have to do with metabolic processes. Other explanations have also been forwarded. For example, Edwards (1982) suggests that "the mode of operation may be through inheritance of a depressive tendency or high anxiety levels, rather than a direct transmission of a taste for alcohol or a metabolic predisposition" (p. 19).

The Physiological/Biological Model – A Partial but not Complete Assumption

The physiological/biological approach to investigating the causes of behavior has clearly been helpful in understanding alcoholism. It is apparent that alcohol has definite physical effects, and that such concepts as tolerance, withdrawal, and addiction are useful in explaining alcohol consumption. The disease model has both detractors and supporters, but has certainly had a major impact on the understanding and treatment of alcoholism. Several physiological conditions have been explored as explanations of alcoholism, including inherited metabolic defects, endocrine dysfunctions, normalizing effects, and genetic predispositions.

While the physiological/biological explanations of alcoholism are very compelling, there are other useful theoretical approaches which take into consideration psychological and sociocultural factors. It has already been shown above how classical conditioning – one form of learning – relates to the physiological explanation of alcoholism; other forms of learning have also proven to be powerful explanations of alcohol consumption. Our attention is now turned to these other theoretical approaches.

PSYCHODYNAMIC THEORIES

Whereas the physiological/biological theories discussed above are based in the philosophy of *reductionism* – the identification of actual physiological mechanisms which underlie behavior, psychodynamic theories make heavy use of *hypothetical constructs* – imaginary phenomena which can be used to explain the dynamics of behavior. Such hypothetical constructs as fixations, feelings of inferiority, and defense mechanisms (discussed below) have been found particularly helpful in understanding alcoholic behavior. Indeed, Light (1986) has argued that it is essential to have a working knowledge of abnormal psychology and psychodynamic theory in order to fully understand alcoholic behavior.

The Freudian Model

Sigmund Freud, whose pioneering work spanned the last decade of the nineteenth century and the first four of the twentieth century, postulated the existence of three hypothetical constructs—the *id*, the *ego*, and the superego, which constitute the individual's personality. (See Table 2, which is adapted from Hall and Lindzey, 1970, pp. 32-35.) According to Hall and Lindzey (1970), ". . . the id may be thought of as the biological component of personality, the ego as the psychological component, and the superego as the social component" (p. 35).

The id was conceptualized by Freud as being completely *unconscious*—beneath the level of awareness. The ego and the superego, both of which developed from the id, were partially unconscious and partially conscious. An individual's behavior, according to Freud, is determined by the complex interplay among these three hypothetical entities.

Freud postulated that the id, the ego, and the superego developed over time in response to the biological functioning of the individual (Zeigler, 1984). Furthermore, social experiences at each stage appear to leave a permanent mark on the personality in the form of attitudes, traits, and values (Hjelle and Ziegler, 1981). Table 3, adapted from Ziegler (1984, pp. 91-92), describes Freud's hypothesized oral, anal, phallic, and genital stages of personality development. Ziegler (1984) notes, "A period of *latency* intervenes between the latter two psychosexual stages but, strictly speaking, it is not to be understood as a stage" (p. 91).

As noted in Table 3, the ego is often strained while trying to integrate conflicting demands from the id, the superego, and the external world. The ego sometimes finds it useful to invest some of its psychic energy into defending itself from the strain created by these demands. In collaboration with his daughter, Anna Freud, Sigmund Freud identified a number of ego defense mechanisms. Table 4, derived from Holmes (1984, pp. 347-350), describes some of these defense mechanisms. According to Holmes (1984, p. 348), defense mechanisms are used to avoid or reduce negative emotional states, typically involve a distortion of reality, and are used unconsciously.

TABLE 2. Freud's Three Personality Systems

(Adapted from Hall & Lindzey, 1970, pp. 32-35)

The Id. The id is the original system of the personality; it is the matrix within which the ego and the superego become differentiated. The id consists of everything psychological that is inherited and that is present at birth, including the instincts It is the reservoir of psychic energy and furnishes all of the power for the operation of the other two systems. It is in close touch with the bodily processes from which it derives its energy.... [It] represents the inner world of subjective experience and has no knowledge of objective reality.

The id cannot tolerate increases of energy which are experienced as uncomfortable states of tension. Consequently, when the tension level of the organism is raised, ... the id functions in such a manner as to discharge the tension immediately and return the organism to a comfortably constant and low energy level.

The Ego. The ego comes into existence because the needs of the organism require appropriate transactions within the objective world of reality....The basic distinction between the id and the ego is that the former knows only subjective reality of the mind whereas the latter distinguished between things in the mind and things in the external world....

The ego is...the executive of the personality because it controls the gateways to action, selects the features of the environment to which it will respond, and decides what instincts will be satisfied and in what manner. In performing these highly important functions, the ego has to try to integrate the often conflicting demands of the id, the superego, and the external world. This is not an easy task and often places great strain upon the ego.

The Superego. [The superego] is the internal representative of the traditional values and ideals of society as interpreted to the child by his parents, and enforced by means of a system of rewards and punishments imposed upon the child. The superego is the moral arm of personality; it represents the ideal rather than the real and it strives for perfection rather than pleasure. Its main concern is to decide whether something is right or wrong so that it can act in accordance with the moral standards authorized by the agents of society.

TABLE 3. Freud's Stages of Personality Development

(Adapted from Ziegler, 1984, pp. 91-92)

The Oral Stage. During the oral stage of psychosexual development, which lasts approximately throughout the first year of life, the primary erogenous zone is the mouth. Through activities associated with the mouth -- sucking, swallowing, biting -- infants experienced their first continuous source of pleasure, and thus the mouth region becomes a focal point of rudimentary psychosexual satisfaction. As is true of the subsequent pregenital stages, either overgratification or deprivation during the oral stage may result in fixation at that stage; either too much or too little oral satisfaction results in some instinctual energy remaining devoted to the concerns of this stage, thus leaving indelible imprints upon subsequent personality formation and adult behavior.

The Anal Stage. During the second and third years of life, the anal stage, the primary erogenous zone is the anus. Children at this stage are thought to derive considerable pleasure from temporary retention...or expulsion of feces.... With the onset of parentally controlled toilet training, however, the child's pleasures in this regard encounter the stiff opposition of social restraints, and various fixations may thus occur.

The Phallic Stage. The genitals become the primary erogenous zone during the phallic stage of psychosocial development, which extends from the fourth through the fifth years of life.... [This] period of life serves as the stage [for]...the Oedipus complex.... Boys unconsciously want to seduce their mothers and remove their fathers; girls unconsciously desire their fathers and want to dispose of their mothers.... In the Freudian scheme of things,... the Oedipus complex and its degree of resolution leave permanent imprints upon subsequent personality formation and adjustment.

The Genital Stage. With the onset of puberty,...genital sexuality is reawakened and the genital stage of psychosexual development, extending from puberty until death, begins.... [The] adult genital personality type, the successful end product of psychosexual development in psychoanalytic theory, is characterized by capacity for mature heterosexual love, responsible concerns beyond the self, and productive living in society.

TABLE 4. Some Defense Mechanisms

(Derived from Holmes, 1984, pp. 347-350)

Regression --	the selective forgetting of material associated with conflict and stress.
Suppression --	avoiding stressful thoughts by not thinking about them.
Denial --	changing the interpretation of the situation so as to perceive it as less threatening.
Projection --	attributing personality characteristics or motivations to other persons as a function of one's own personality characteristics and motivations.
Displacement --	expressing a feeling toward one person or object that in fact should be expressed toward another person or object.
Regression --	returning to an earlier stage of life in which the person was secure, and in so doing avoid the present conflict or stress.
Identification --	taking on the personal characteristics of another person.
Compensation --	attempting to overcome the feelings of inferiority and related anxiety by devoting additional effort to the area of the inferiority.
Reaction Formation --	reinforcing repression by using behaviors diametrically opposed to the kinds of behaviors that would result from the repressed material.

Implications of the Freudian Model

Clearly, the Freudian model is rich with potential explanations of alcoholic behavior. The alcoholic may have fixated in the oral stage, and is thus seeking gratification through drinking. Conversely, the alcoholic may have fixated in the anal stage and is drinking to rebel against authority; or may have never resolved the Oedipus complex and is drinking to escape feelings of guilt. The alcoholic may be drinking to aid the processes of repression or regression, or to compensate for feelings of inferiority.

Unfortunately, the Freudian model proposes so many possible explanations of alcoholic behavior that research seeking to confirm or disconfirm Freudian explanations becomes very difficult to perform. Indeed, this is one of the weaknesses of Freudian theory from a scientific perspective: since it is based upon a set of unobservable hypothetical constructs, it is very difficult to study from an empirical perspective.

Other Psychodynamic Models

While Freud was the pioneer of the psychodynamic approach to the study of personality and behavior, he was by no means the only theorist to work out a complex system of hypothetical constructs. For example, Jung proposed a "collective unconscious" containing a set of "archetypes"; Adler discussed "feelings of inferiority"; Erickson extended Freud's idea of stages through adulthood and into old age. A full description of these and other psychodynamic models is beyond the scope of this article; the interested reader is referred to Hall and Lindzey (1970), Cartwright (1979), and Brenman-Gibson (1984).

Application to Alcoholic Behavior

Armor, Polich, and Stambul (1978, pp. 17-21) point out the difficulty of carrying out sound research from the psychodynamic perspective, but do cite several studies which suggest some evidence consistent with the psychodynamic model. They note three particularly interesting explanations of alcoholic behavior derived from the psychodynamic viewpoint which seem to be supported by empirical research:

> A relatively new formulation of the motivation for excessive drinking is derived from the psychoanalytic approach. According to this new hypothesis, the functional significance of alcohol lies in its ability to maintain and enhance regression and denial in individuals whose personalities function at an immature level. . . . This formulation focuses on the tendency of alcoholics (while intoxicated) to express impulsively their dominant mood or emotion while simultaneously suppressing incompatible motives, a behavioral mode presumed to be regressive. (p. 18)
>
> A second psychodynamic formulation holds that alcoholism results from enhanced feelings of self-esteem and prowess that the ingestion of . . . alcohol provides. In this view, alcoholics are individuals who suffer from pervasive feelings of inferiority and powerlessness coupled with unusually strong inhibitions against expression of hostile or aggressive impulses. For such individuals, the exaggerated aura of competence and the disinhibition of impulses provided by alcohol have special value. (p. 19)
>
> A final psychodynamic approach . . . focuses on the intrapsychic conflict between intense dependency needs and parallel strivings for autonomy and independence. . . . Drinking presumably provides reinforcement for the opposite motives simultaneously. . . . [and] the sedative property of ethanol is thought to diminish the effect of logical inconsistencies and enables denial of the dynamic conflict. (p. 20)

Gomberg (1982, p. 188) believes that the psychodynamic approach has made a valuable distinction between what Knight (1937) describes as "the essential alcoholic"—egocentric, hedonistic, and incapable of maintaining intimate relationships with others—and "the reactive alcoholic" who is more mature and better adjusted, but compulsive. Gomberg also identifies Menninger's (1938) description of the self-destructiveness of alcoholics as a major contribution of the psychodynamic approach.

Frosch (1985) prompts us to consider the next major approach to understanding alcoholic behavior—trait and type theories—by providing a description by psychoanalysts of individuals with addictive behavior as characterized by impulsivity, difficulty tolerating feelings and delaying gratification, and an antisocial personality style. A disposition to sensation seeking is also commonly reported.

TRAIT AND TYPE THEORIES

While they are different in many respects, both physiological/biological theories and psychodynamic theories share one thing in common—they focus on identifying the underlying causes of behavior and as such, are basic to developing a process-model of consumer behavior. The third approach to understanding behavior—trait and type theories—has a somewhat different focus. This approach is oriented more toward the *measurement* and *prediction* of behavior than the *explanation* of behavior. These theories may be helpful in identifying market segments for varying promotional messages.

Morgan, King, and Robinson (1979) define a *trait* as "an aspect of personality that is reasonably characteristic of a person, is relatively consistent over time, and distinguishes that person in some way from other people" (p. 661). Courage, laziness, ambition, stubbornness, intelligence, and physical strength are but a few examples of traits; Morgan et al. estimate that there are at least 170 *unique* traits which have been identified (p. 513).

Trait theorists typically perform their research by choosing one or more traits to examine; carefully constructing tests, questionnaires, or other instruments to measure these traits; applying these instruments to measure a group of people; and finally using these measures to study relationships among traits and even to predict behaviors in given situations.

Some theorists also use their measurement devices to sort people into *types*—classes of individuals grouped together because they share certain personality *traits*. The "Type A, Type B" characterization of individuals in terms of likelihood of heart disease (Friedman and Rosenman, 1974) is an example of a type theory.

This approach to the study of behavior has been very popular and very fruitful; thousands of instruments have been devised to measure traits and sort people into types. Furthermore, many of these instruments have been demonstrated to predict, with a fair amount of accuracy, what people will do in given situations. It is beyond the scope of this article to describe in detail any of the major trait or type theories; the interested reader is referred to Hall and Lindzey (1970) and Cartwright (1979) for discussions of the theories of Murray, Allport, Sheldon, and Cattell.

Application to Alcoholism

The major contribution of trait and type theories to the study of alcoholic behavior has been the construction of instruments to measure proneness to alcoholism, identify potentially effective treatments for alcoholics, and assess progress in therapy.

Major Findings—The Antisocial Personality

Armor, Polich, and Stambul (1978) report that research focused on determining a consistent set of traits that correlate with the onset of alcoholism has not been successful: "A large number of studies have generally failed . . . to identify any specific personality traits that clearly differentiate alcoholics from other deviant groups or from persons judged to be normal" (p. 21).

However, the longitudinal research which does exist seems to be fairly consistent. Gomberg (1982) reviews three follow-up studies which indicate that children who later became alcoholic displayed serious antisocial behavior as youngsters. For example, McCord and McCord (1982) studied 200 boys who later became alcoholics, and described them as "apparently self-contained, outwardly self-confident, undisturbed by abnormal fears, indifferent toward their siblings, and disapproving of their mothers. Also, they more often evidenced unrestrained aggression, sadism, sexual anxiety, and activity rather than passivity" (p. 427).

A recent study by Stabenau, Dolinsky, and Fischer (1986) found that regardless of gender, alcoholics with antisocial personality diagnosis drank significantly more alcohol than non-antisocial personality alcoholics. Based on their review of recent research, Marlatt et al. (1988) concluded the following:

> The most consistent finding is that many substance abusers have a history of antisocial behavior (e.g., nonconformity, acting out, and impulsivity) and a high level of depression and/or low self-esteem. (p. 231)

Armor, Polich, and Stambul (1978) noted that "while most writers agree that no unique, premorbid alcoholic personality has been discovered . . . , there exists some empirical evidence to suggest that alcoholics show a cluster of personality traits once their drinking patterns have been established" (p. 21). Traits included in this cluster are low stress tolerance, dependency, perceptual dependence, negative self-image, and feelings of isolation, insecurity, and depression. These characteristics provide implications for a wide variety of marketing functions, from treatment design, information for staff training programs, and promotional message design.

LEARNING (CONDITIONING) THEORIES

The next general theory of human behavior to be applied to the understanding of alcoholism is learning theory, sometimes called conditioning theory. This approach recognizes that some human behavior is *reflexive*, and that a few human behaviors may even be *instinctive*, but that the vast majority of the things people do have been *learned*. Three forms of learning—classical (Pavlovian) conditioning, operant (instrumental) conditioning, and social learning—are described below, and their implications for understanding alcoholism are explored. As with the other approaches to understanding human behavior discussed in this article, it will be impossible to describe each of the many forms of learning theory that have been mentioned in the psychological literature. Such sources as Hilgard and Bower (1975) and Estes et al. (1954) provide excellent descriptions of the many versions of learning theory.

Classical (Pavlovian) Conditioning

During his famous experiments with dogs during the late 1890s, Ivan Pavlov found that when a previously neutral signal, such as a bell, was paired with the provision of food, dogs would learn to salivate when they heard the bell. From this pioneering research he developed the principles of classical (sometimes called Pavlovian or "respondent") conditioning theory.

It is now known that almost any human reflexive behavior can be classically conditioned to occur in the presence of signalling cues. For example, if a whistle is paired over time with a puff of air to a boy's eye, he will become classically conditioned to blink every time he hears the whistle. If a woman eats lunch every day at noon, her stomach will become classically conditioned to begin contracting and "rumbling" shortly before noon. If she smokes a cigarette after every meal, her body will become classically conditioned to crave nicotine toward the end of each meal.

The importance of classical conditioning theory to the understanding of alcoholism has been noted earlier in this article during the discussion of the "normalizing effect" version of the physiological/biological theory of alcoholism. Marlatt et al. (1988, p. 235) claim that the withdrawal symptoms faced by the alcoholic who is trying to abstain have been acquired through the classical conditioning process.

Armor, Polich, and Stambul (1978) describe succinctly the classical conditioning theory of alcoholism, and also point out how the theory can be used to treat alcoholics:

> [According to the Pavlovian model,] alcoholic behavior is seen as caused and maintained by the simple association of alcoholic ingestion with positive, rewarding experience. Accordingly, modification of alcoholism should occur through changing the stimulus value of alcohol from positive to negative by pairing drinking with aversive consequences. (p. 22)

Aversion therapy (see Sauser and Self "Alcoholism Treatment Philosophies and Theories" in this volume), based on the classical conditioning principle described by Armor et al., is a very effective means of treatment for some alcoholics.

Operant (Instrumental) Conditioning

Classical conditioning is a very useful concept for understanding how an individual can learn to respond reflexively to previously neutral stimuli. However, not all human behavior is reflexive; indeed, most of the things people do are under their conscious control and are performed "of their own free will." These behaviors are called "operant behaviors."

The law of effect, originally formulated by Thorndike (1911), holds that the likelihood of performing operant behaviors is influenced by the effects these behaviors produce. For example, behaviors which produce positive effects (i.e., are rewarded) are more likely to be repeated, while those which produce no effects (i.e., are ignored) or negative effects (i.e., are punished) are less likely to be repeated. For the past 50 years, B. F. Skinner and his followers have been demonstrating the enormous power of rewards for reinforcing and shaping behavior.

Armor, Polich, and Stambul (1978) claim that "the major causal assumption of most behavioral models is that alcoholics begin and continue drinking because alcohol ingestion is followed by a reduction in anxiety, psychological stress, or tension" (p. 22). In operant conditioning terms, the ingestion of alcohol is rewarding because it reduces tension, thus the individual learns to drink alcohol when in a stressful situation. Armor et al. cite several studies which support the tension-reduction reinforcement model, but note that "the theoretical reliance on tension and its reduction as the sole causal factor controlling alcoholic behavior does not seem warranted by the empirical evidence" (p. 23).

Bandura's (1969) two-stage learning model suggests that alcoholism develops in stages. Anxious individuals find that drinking helps them relieve tension, thus they learn to drink when anxious. The relief alcohol provides reinforces the habit of drinking. However, this habit produces aversive consequences—such as feelings of guilt or even loss of a job—which create more anxiety, and thus lead to more drinking. The effects of alcohol on the metabolic processes then create a physiological addiction, and drinking is continually reinforced because it staves off aversive withdrawal symptoms.

Social Learning Theory

The two previous versions of learning theory require persons to experience directly the consequences of an experience in order to learn from it. However, we know that people can also learn *vicariously*—by observing, reading about, or hearing about the experiences of others. Social learning theory extends operant theory to take into consideration such concepts as observation, imitation, modeling, and cues.

If you are watching television or a movie and you see people drinking and having a good time, you may begin to associate alcohol with fun. If you observe someone you admire taking a drink, you may desire to imitate that person by also drinking. If your friends are drinking and pressure you to join them, you may yield to peer influences and begin drinking also. Situational cues, such as cocktail parties, bars, and some sporting events, can influence the onset of alcohol consumption. Advertisers are well aware of the power of social learning theory, and make effective use of it to influence people to purchase alcoholic beverages.

People have been told repeatedly—through advertising, films, books, television, and other media—that alcohol is a "magic elixir" (Marlatt, 1987). "Alcohol is expected to enhance social and physical pleasure, enhance sexual performance and responsiveness, increase power and aggression, increase social assertiveness, and reduce tension" (Marlatt et al., 1988, p. 234). Numerous recent studies cited by Marlatt et al. (1988) have found strong evidence to support the social learning theory.

People do indeed have strong expectations regarding the consequences of alcohol, and choose to drink or not to drink based on the evaluations of these expectations. For example, Berglas (1986) suggests that alcohol has a performance-inhibiting reputation that can be exploited by individuals seeking to avoid the negative implications of failure—the "self-handicappers." Laberg (1986) concluded that expectations of the effects of alcohol exert an even greater influence on craving than do the pharmacological effects of alcohol.

Perhaps the best formulation of the social learning theory of alcoholism is the model presented by Hodgson and Stockwell (1985). This model is built around the following six assumptions, which are supported by evidence cited within Hodgson and Stockwell's paper: (1) Drinking alcohol is mainly functional; (2) Drinking is learned; (3) Learning to drink heavily will be influenced by compensatory adaptive processes; (4) A learned habit can become a learned compulsion; (5) Cognitive control will tend to be impaired; and (6) The nature of the relapse process will change as drinking progresses. Hodgson and Stockwell (1985) suggest that there *is* such a thing as an "alcohol dependence syndrome," and that it can best be understood from the social learning perspective.

SOCIOCULTURAL THEORIES

While the social learning theory described above certainly acknowledges the importance of role models and environmental cues, it shares in common with the other psychological models a primary focus on the *individual* as the key to understanding the onset of alcoholism. Gomberg (1982) views this "person centeredness" as "a major limitation to psychological theories" (p. 193). She believes a clearer picture of alcoholic behavior is revealed when the social environment—the culture—in which people behave is considered. She notes:

> People have families, kin networks and friends. They go to a workplace along with other people, they affiliate with educational, religious and political institutions, and they come into contact with health-concerned and leisure-concerned institutions as well. They belong to groups which influence not only value systems and social attitudes and voting behavior and child-rearing patterns, but attitudes toward alcohol and drinking behavior as well. (pp. 196-197)

Sociocultural theories thus focus not on the individual's personality or biological processes as the major cause of alcoholic behavior, but rather upon sociological, anthropological, and cultural variables, such as "the traditional demographic variables of age, socioeconomic status (SES), urbanization, ethnic origin, and religion" (Armor et al., 1978, p. 24) which have been found to predict quite well problem drinking among males (Cahalan and Room, 1974).

Armor et al. (1978) conclude from their review of the literature that psychological and physiological variables are significant causal factors in the process of alcohol addiction; yet, due to their predictive power, "the contribution of sociocultural variables to the etiology of alcoholism merits consideration" (p. 24). Their four classes of sociocultural models—(a) Culture and Socialization, (b) Cultural Stress Factors, (c) Familial Patterns, and (d) Instability and Crisis—are considered below.

Culture and Socialization

Citing the exceedingly low rates of alcoholism among Jews, Mormons, and Moslems—and the high rate of chronic alcoholism among the Irish—Armor et al. (1978) claim that "the 'appropriate' use of intoxicants, attitudes toward alcohol, mores regulating drinking practices, and environmental support for drinking are largely determined by cultural setting. Children are socialized into culturally prescribed beliefs, attitudes, and practices regarding the use and consumption level of alcohol" (p. 25).

Edwards (1982) concurs with this viewpoint, and provides the following recommendation:

> To understand any adult's use of alcohol it is certainly necessary to take note of his attitudes to drinking which his particular culture inculcated. His culture may for instance have taught that "a real man" is "a good drinker," while a man who drinks moderately or is an abstainer is suspect. When that person moves from his original culture to another part of the country or goes abroad, he takes these attitudes with him, while at the same time in the new environment he may be

> freed from previously controlling social and cultural influences. (p. 16)

Edwards also points out the important role such influences as occupations and leisure habits have on the predisposition to drink. Consider the following two passages from his work:

> People who work in the entertainment world are often at risk, and in many occupations the bar may be the place to make useful contacts. The salesman may see entertaining as essential to his obtaining business and he may drink along with his clients. The executive may enjoy an expense account and part of the prestige of his job may be a cocktail cabinet in his own room, while the directors' dining-room can encourage lunch-time drinking. (p. 17)
>
> Clubs of every variety may be influences towards heavy drinking. . . . Drinking may be written into the social life of the student, with the Fraternity House or the bar in the Students' Union the hub of social activities. A family may change its drinking habits because of a new circle of friends, new patterns of entertaining, a different group of people with whom to play cards. (p. 18)

Edwards' examples, combined with the evidence cited by Armor et al. regarding the power of sociocultural variables to predict the onset of alcoholism, certainly create a strong case for the consideration of the culture and socialization model. Marketers of alcohol rehabilitation programs should pay particular attention to this finding, since it is these same factors which might influence the individual's choices regarding whether to seek treatment, or which type of treatment to seek.

Cultural Stress Factors

Armor et al. (1978, p. 25) note that cultural factors – such as the insecurity or anxiety level of a culture – may contribute to the degree of stress felt by members of that culture, and thus to their drive to drink. They cite Bales' (1946) three major contributing factors to the incidence of alcoholism in a given society: (a) the degree of stress and inner tension produced by the culture, (b) the attitudes toward drinking fostered by the culture, and (c) the degree to which the culture provides substitute means of satisfaction and coping with anxiety.

Familial Patterns

The familial patterns of alcoholism cited earlier to support genetic influences may also be used as evidence for the sociocultural approach. Armor et al. (1978) suggest, "Sociocultural factors also operate by structuring familial patterns that in turn provide role-modeling and social learning experiences for children" (p. 25). A recent study by Monteiro (1986) produced results which gave further support to the hypothesis that children model the drinking behavior and attitudes of their parents.

Instability and Crisis

The final sociocultural theory presented by Armor et al. (1978) is labeled "Instability and Crisis":

> Social factors may also contribute to conditions of environmental stress that precipitate the onset of heavy consumption. Alcoholism has been reported to develop during "crisis periods," when significant changes in an individual's life situation or social role lead to instability, confusion, and stress. (p. 26)

Situational changes which might lead to the onset of heavy drinking include menopause, loss of employment, death of a spouse, marital instability, divorce or separation, and retirement. Commenting on the impact of situational change on the onset of drinking behavior, Gomberg (1982) notes:

> Evidence is accruing which indicates a strong relationship between certain types and periods of stress and heavy drinking. Women under 35 who are experiencing or have recently experienced marital disruption appear to be under some risk for heavy or problem drinking. The relationship between eco-

> nomic strains and economic hardship and drinking for stress relief has been explored. And there is some evidence of high risk status among elderly men experiencing the double loss of widowerhood and retirement. (p. 197)

Marlatt et al. (1988), in their summary of recent research on alcoholism and other addictive behaviors, state, "A host of other studies have begun to specify the roles of stressful life issues, self-derogation, and role status and social environments within broad multivariate frameworks" (p. 229). Clearly, marketers and others interested in the factors which contribute to alcoholism must look beyond the individual; the environmental context must also be considered.

Armor et al. (1978) provide this final comment regarding the power of the social context:

> A cyclical relationship exists between social instability and alcoholism. Heavy consumption of alcohol may occur in response to changes in one's social environment that create aversive stress; this excessive drinking in turn results in further deterioration of social adjustment, creating even greater stress and perpetuating the alcoholic process. (p. 26)

EXCESSIVE DRINKING HAS MULTIPLE CAUSES

Each of the general theories of alcoholic behavior presented above seem to make sense and are supported by research findings and clinical experience. There is strong evidence for a biological/physiological component in the onset of alcoholism. Similarly, the psychodynamic, trait and type, and learning theories seem to have validity for understanding alcoholism. And how can the power of the sociocultural theories for explaining the onset of heavy drinking be denied?

Which theory is right? What is the *real* cause of alcoholism? Perhaps the following passage from Edwards' (1982) work provides the best answer to these questions:

> That a single, isolated cause should ever exist for a person's excessive drinking is unthinkable. There is always a multiplicity of causes. Not only do several causal factors operate at any one time, but present causes influence drinking behavior which was shaped by factors in the past. It would be wrong therefore to interpret the reasons for excessive drinking . . . as mutually exclusive influences. It is necessary to see these factors as interactive both in cross-section of time and longitudinally. (p. 13)

Convincing arguments for multivariate or interactionist models to explain alcoholism have been presented by Jellinek (1952), Trice (1956), and Plaut (1967). Armor et al. (1978) conclude:

> It has now become apparent to most theorists and researchers in the field that a great range of sociological, cultural, and psychological variables can be invoked to account for variance in problem drinking and alcoholism. The full range of such factors and their possible interactive effects with one another and with various clinical interventions must be considered in any comprehensive model of causation, treatment, and cure. (p. 27)

Marlatt et al.'s (1988) recent phase model is an example of the modern comprehensive theoretical approach to understanding alcoholism referred to in the passage above. Their model considers physiological, psychological, and sociocultural factors which influence each of the following stages in the onset and treatment of alcoholism: (a) Initiation, (b) Transition and maintenance of addictive behavior, (c) Initiation of the change process, (d) Active change process, and (e) Maintenance of successful change.

IMPLICATIONS FOR MARKETERS

Since alcoholism is now known to have multiple causes, it is important for marketers of alcohol treatment facilities and services to have a working knowledge of the physiological/biological, psychological, and sociocultural theories of the onset of alcoholism.

Each theoretical approach has significant merit, but none stands alone as the key to the understanding and treatment of alcoholic behavior. Treatment facilities and services which are based upon only one of these approaches may not be complete—they may not be treating the entire problem, and thus may not provide a satisfactory outcome.

The article in this volume entitled "Alcoholism Treatment Philosophies and Theories" (Sauser and Self) describes a variety of treatment methods. Each one is described in terms of its relationship to the general theories of alcoholism presented in this article. The marketer should appreciate the strengths and weaknesses of each general theory and treatment theory, since these represent the aspects of consumer behavior of interest and the product and service lines which have been created to impact upon that behavior.

Market Segmentation of Alcoholics: A Demographic/Psychographic Approach

Vaughan C. Judd
Cathleen A. Owens
Donald R. Self

INTRODUCTION: MARKETING STRATEGY AND PLANNING

Recent literature on the characteristics and treatment of alcoholism reflects a growing recognition that alcoholics are not a homogeneous population, and that treatment is more effective when tailored to fit the needs of the individual sub-groups found among alcohol-dependent persons. This trend suggests the basis for a marketing strategy orientation in providing treatment for alcoholics.

A marketing strategy entails a unique marketing program developed for a specific market, or a particular group of potential customers. Marketing strategy starts with an organization's statement of its reason for existing (mission statement) and its organizational goals. The marketing strategy is shaped by an assessment of the organization's resources and the organization's evaluation of opportunities in the market. The tactical components of a marketing strategy involve a marketing mix—a marketing program which includes a product (good or service), pricing strategies, place or distribution strategies, promotional strategies, and a target market (McCarthy, 1960).

The development of a marketing plan is both an extension and documentation of the process of creating a marketing strategy. The marketing plan is a written statement of a marketing strategy together with a specified time frame, statement of expected results and provision for control procedure. (For a recent practical guide to marketing planning see: William Winston, *How to Write a Market-*

ing Plan for Health Care Organizations, New York: The Haworth Press, 1985.)

The key elements of a marketing plan are the marketing mix and target market. The marketing mix elements, widely known as the "four P's of marketing," are viewed as controllable by the marketing organization. If an organization is targeting more than one market segment, a different marketing mix is developed for each segment. It is the marketing mix which forms the basis for the customer's perception of the organization, while it is market segmentation which determines which potential customers constitute the target markets.

Target Marketing

Three interrelated concepts form the basis for successful implementation of target marketing. These ideas relate to customer needs, organization objectives, and competitive advantage. Bagozzi (1986) suggests that all organizations have two broad marketing goals: satisfaction of customer needs, and achievement of competitive advantage. Achievement of a competitive advantage results from successful differentiating of one's organization (or marketing mix) along any dimension which is important to the buyer. The significance of differentiation has been pointed out by Levitt (1983, p. 128) who stated:

> If marketing is seminally about anything, it is about achieving customer-getting distinction by differentiating what you do and how you operate. All else is derivative of that and only that.

The goal of satisfying customers' needs is at the heart of the client-centered organization. An organization with a marketing or client orientation will strive to implement the "marketing concept"; a concept which embraces the notion of serving the customer while achieving the goals of the organization (Pride and Ferrell, 1985; Stanton and Futrell, 1987).

The decision concerning which customers will be served is determined by three questions the customer-oriented organization should ask itself as it begins to develop its marketing strategy:

1. to whom are we planning to market?
2. where are they and what are they like?
3. what are their current perceptions and needs? (Kotler and Andreason, 1987)

In order to answer these questions the marketer must recognize that within the total market for the product lies groups that have similar product needs or other important similarities (e.g., media habits) for the purpose of designing a marketing mix (strategies concerning pricing, promoting, and distributing the treatment or services) to more precisely match the needs of individuals in a selected segment. Thus we have the concept of *market segmentation*.

MARKET SEGMENTATION

The total market for any service or product is established by the individuals and/or organizations which have the need, ability, willingness, or authority to purchase the service. Inside the total market several conditions must be present for effective segmentation.

1. Consumers' needs for the service must be heterogeneous.
2. The segments must be identifiable and divisible.
3. The total market should be segmented in such a way that the segments can be compared with estimated sales potential, costs, and profits. For non-profit ATMs costs will be the topic of concern since they are "mission"-oriented rather than profit-oriented.
4. At least one segment must be big enough (in a profit-seeking sense) or dictated by the organization's "mission" statement to justify developing and maintaining a special marketing mix.
5. The segment must be reachable by the marketing mix (e.g., media, insurance, etc.). (Adapted from Pride and Ferrell, 1987)

It must be recognized that there is always the alternative of not segmenting the market, i.e., treating members of the market as though they were all alike in terms of important dimensions. To do so is "mass marketing," (McCarthy and Perreault, 1987) which may ignore significant differences among members of the potential market. If a marketer uses a segmentation approach, a decision must be made as to whether a single segment or multiple segments will be targeted. These options are outlined in Table 1.

Within the total market for Alcoholism Treatment Services exist two broad categories for markets. First, the Consumer/Client market which consists of those individuals who directly benefit from alcoholism treatment. In general marketing literature, this segment is typically represented as having the need, ability, willingness, and authority to purchase; however, for ATM the willingness for direct purchase is not always present, which leads to the importance of the second major category—the Referral Markets. These include individuals and organizations with influence over the decisions of the consumers, and are considered in the next two articles.

Segmentation Strategies

When segmenting the consumer client market, several categories of variables are available for dividing the total market: these include demographic, geographic, social unit, psychographic and behavioral-based characteristics. The basis for segmentation may be a single variable, or more commonly, a multi-variable approach, involving several segmentation bases. For example, a marketer may target households in the northern regions of the United States with an annual income of $50,000 or more. In the example, two demographic variables—households and income—and one geographic variable have been used.

Table 2 summarizes the method of segment classification used in this article. As indicated by the table some of the characteristics can be objectively observed while others may be inferred.

Demographic Variables

Some of the characteristics which may be included in this category are age, sex, marital status, employment status (working/retired), spouse's employment status, number of children, national origin, religion, occupation, and education. Demographic characteristics are commonly used to divide markets, especially since they are readily measured through observation. These variables may also be closely related to consumers' product needs and purchasing be-

TABLE 1. Strategies to Select Target Markets

Total Market or Mass Marketing Approach	Single Segment Approach	Multi-Segment Approach
	DEFINITION	
Target Market is Total Market	Market is divided into relatively homogeneous segments for targeted marketing mix. Organization markets to one segment.	Similary to concentrated approach. Organizations markets to more than one segment.
	CHARACTERISTICS	
A large proportion of customers have similar product needs	hetergeneous markets	hetergeneous markets
The organization can develop and maintain a single marketing mix to meet those needs	specialization allows more efficient and effective marketing	specialization allows more efficient and effective marketing
Product differentiation often used simultaneously to establish perceived superiority and preferability	small organization can compete with larger organizations	sales may be increased by focusing on more than one approach
	If segment declines, the organization's strength declines.	may allow excess capacity utilization
		may require separate processes/skills. May have higher operating costs.
		distinct promotion plans and distribution system may increase marketing costs.
	EXAMPLES	
Many AA-based programs	outpatient program VA hospitals Adolescents	multi-drug facilities integrated systems

TABLE 2

		CUSTOMER CHARACTERISTICS	
		General	Situation Specific
MEASURES	Objective	Demographic Factors Geographic Factors Social Unit	Consumption Patterns Brand Loyalty Patterns Buying Situations
	Inferred	Personality Traits Motives Lifestyle	Attitudes Perceptions & Preferences

havior. In alcoholism treatment literature, segments have typically been divided in this manner, with special emphasis on age, sex, and national origin (for example see Knott, 1986, and Gomberg et al., 1982).

Geographic Variables

This category covers such characteristics as place of residence (rural vs. urban), region of country, population density, and subcultural values.

Social Unit Variables

Family life cycle and social class are two common characteristics in this category.

The types of variables discussed so far are common methods of segmenting. Table 3 is a study based on a regression analysis which shows these three categories of variables used in establishing the typical characteristics of different drinking patterns in males.

Psychographic Variables

The three most common factors included by researchers using this category are personality characteristics, motives, and lifestyle.

Personality characteristics include such "labels" as compulsive, gregarious, competitive, extrovert, introvert, ambitious, and ag-

TABLE 3. Regression Analysis of Males

Abstainer tend to be:	Drinkers tend to be:
Protestant	Catholic
Southern	Northern
Older	Younger
Low Socioeconomic Status	Higher Socioeconomic Status
Light Drinker tend to be:	**Heavy Drinkers tend to be:**
Married	Unmarried
Younger	Older
In a nondrinking context (spouse drinks, bars)	In a drinking context
Problem Drinkers tend to be:	**Alcoholics tend to be:**
Unemployed	Unemployed
Unmarried	Unmarried
In a drinking context	Southern
	Lower Socioeconomic Status
	Protestant

STABILITY FACTORS: Marital status and employment are important indicators of problem drinking

Source: Armor, Polich, and Stambul, 1978.

gressive. Segmentation based on these characteristics is useful in cases where the product is similar to competing products (as is the case with alcoholism treatment).

In traditional marketing literature, the effectiveness of segmentation based on personality is considered to be limited due to the difficulty in measuring personality types, in reaching individuals of a specific type, and in recognizing their effect (if any) on consumer purchases. However, due to the more controlled nature of alcoholism treatment, this type of variable may have more significant impact on segmenting, using commonly accepted tests.

An abundance of literature recounting clinical testing of personality types exists for alcoholism treatment. One type of study argues that pure types of alcoholics do not exist but that alcoholics represent mixtures of "types" characterized by rebelliousness, thought disturbance, neuroticism, defensiveness, and a combination of these factors. Partington and Johnson (1969) identified five such classes. Possibly the most important label for psychological-type segmentation is the Anti-Social Personality (ASP) which has been found to make up 25% of the alcoholic population, yet only 3% of the total population (Gomberg, 1982).

Another important factor which has been included in this area is lifestyle, which may be defined as how consumers spend their time and money, based on their surroundings, beliefs, and socioeconomic factors. Lifestyle as a variable is of interest to marketers when there is a relationship between lifestyle characteristics and the consumption patterns of individuals.

The third psychological factor is motive, described as the internal energizing force that drives the consumer toward a goal (Pride and Ferrell, 1987). This type of segmenting can be seen in Jellinek's model of 4 types of alcoholics, presented in the previous article, "General Theories of Alcoholic Behavior" (Sauser and Self).

Behavioral Based Variables

These are the situation specific factors shown in Table 2. Typical characteristics included on an objective, or observable, level are consumption patterns, brand loyalty patterns, and buying situations: the other factors are those which must be inferred including attitudes, perceptions and preferences.

How the consumers use or apply the product may be used as a basis for segmentation. (Recall in Table 3 that the categories being studied were based on consumption levels of alcohol for the population, ranging from abstainer to alcoholic.) These population segments assist in establishing characteristics of persons with a need for treatment: those persons who have the tendencies of heavy alcohol consumption and/or alcohol dependence.

Another focal point of alcoholism treatment research is the binge drinker vs. the continuous drinker as two segments of the drinking population. Connors et al. (1986) have described continuous drinkers as those who drink five or more days per week, with little variability from week to week. Binge drinkers are those who typically drink for several consecutive days, weeks, or months, separated by periods of abstinence. Binge drinkers were found to be significantly more likely to have reported parental alcoholism, and also tend to have a greater number of alcohol-related arrests and hospitalizations.

On the inferred level, the concept of attitude has been widely researched as a variable influencing human behavior. An attitude (Fishbein and Ajzen, 1975, p. 6) is "a learned predisposition to respond in a consistently favorable or unfavorable manner with respect to a given object." It is this relationship between attitude and response which is of interest to marketers, and marketers have looked to the behavioral sciences in an endeavor to find models that capture the relationship between attitudes and behavior. Two popular models are the tri-component model and the multi-attribute model.

The tri-component attitude model consists of cognition, affect and conation (Sherif and Cantril, 1945; Ostrum, 1969). In this model, cognition (knowledge and perceptions) is presumed to lead to beliefs as to whether the attitude-object possesses various attributes and whether specific behavior will lead to specific outcomes. The affect component captures feelings or emotions with respect to a particular object and is expressed as either favorable or unfavorable feelings. Whether an individual will take a specific action or behavior with regard to the attitude-object is proposed to be a function of the conative (likelihood or tendency) component of the model.

A number of other researchers support multi-attribute models. These models treat the affective component of the tri-component models as the attitude itself, and downgrade cognition and conation to supporting roles as shown in Figure 1.

While there are several variations of this type of attitude model, much of the work in marketing has focused on models developed by Martin Fishbein—the most recent of which is a behavioral intentions model which incorporates an element of normative or social influence on behavior in addition to attitude (Fishbein and Ajzen,

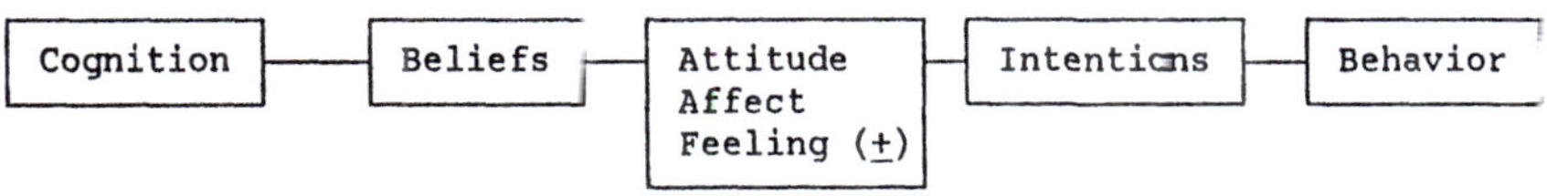

FIGURE 1. Generalized Multi-Attribute Model

1975). An analysis of this and other multi-attribute models is beyond the scope of this article. It is important to recognize, however, that there are linkages between and among knowledge, beliefs, attitudes, intentions, social influence, and behavior.

The multi-attribute models suggest strategies for changing an individual's behavior by changing his/her knowledge base and by social influence. Also, it is important to note that there is a body of literature which suggests the possibility for behavioral change to precede attitudinal and cognitive changes. From a market segmentation viewpoint, a marketer might attempt to measure according to favorable, unfavorable or neutral feelings toward the product or the marketer.

At the American Marketing Association's 18th Attitude Research Conference, two key points were made regarding behavioral-driven segmentation: (1) whatever dimensions are used to segment a market, the resulting segments are most significant if they respond in different ways to marketing inputs, and (2) needs-benefit segmentation and attitude segmentation (if there is a demonstrated useful relationship between attitudes and behavior) are practical variables predicting what consumers will do in the future (*Marketing News*, 1987, p. 40).

As mentioned previously, demographic variables are the strongest measures for segmentation due to their ready observation and measurability. The other categories of the proposed segmentation matrix (Table 2) are best used in understanding the individual demographic groups' makeup on a more intimate level. Of course, many of these segments will overlap in terms of shared characteristics, e.g., among elderly persons many other groups are found including men, women, black, Hispanic, etc. All of these variables can be taken into account to further the marketer's understanding of his target markets.

RECOGNIZED CONSUMER/CLIENT MARKETS

The following tables are composed of research findings in the area of alcoholism treatment. These groups have been recognized as segments among the alcoholic population with different dependency characteristics and treatment needs. These are not the only segments found among alcohol-dependent persons, but are a sampling of the substantial research material available which can be useful to the marketer as he/she profiles his/her chosen target markets.

The information included in the tables is drawn from research based largely on psychological and physiological aspects of alcoholism. The statements have been entered in the most appropriate categories of the segmentation matrix (Table 2) for purpose of identifying the marketing aspects of the findings. These tables can serve as a starting point and a guideline for further such research by the marketer.

The customer characteristics from Table 2 are listed as follows for the purpose of these tables: Category I—demographic, geographic, and social unit factors; Category II—consumption patterns, brand loyalty patterns, and buying situations; Category III—personality traits, motive, and lifestyle; and Category IV—attitudes, perceptions, and preferences.

ADOLESCENTS
CUSTOMER CATEGORY I

- 1. Average age of initial alcohol ingestion appears to be 11 years.
  2. Since 1965 there is a trend toward alcohol consumption at an earlier age.
  3. There is no evidence that more adolescents are using alcohol now than in previous generations.
  4. Since 1975, it appears that more adolescent females are using alcohol, and male-female ratio in terms of numbers of users is approximately 1.
- Problem drinking is more highly correlated with an urban setting and a higher Socioeconomic Status (SES) of the family.
- The major factors that influence teenage drinking are peers, family and parents, sociocultural background, contexts of drinking, and the personality of the drinker.
- One estimate of the economic costs of alcohol-related traffic accidents runs over $55 billion, and a disproportionate number of these accidents occur among young men.
- Studies have demonstrated that adolescents being treated for ad-

dictions are more likely to live in a 1-parent home, usually headed by the mother.

- Alcohol addiction affects 20% of adult Americans and most of these individuals developed the pattern of problem drinking in adolescence.

ADOLESCENTS
CUSTOMER CATEGORY II

- Four Differential Groups (based on survey by Adolescent Alcohol Involvement Scale by Mazer and Filstead):
  1. Adolescents who completely abstain or use alcohol at a minimum level – 5%.
  2. Adolescents who use alcohol but do not experience or display any associated behavior problems – 71%.
  3. Adolescents who use alcohol and experience associated problems (social, legal, family, academic) – 19%.
  4. Adolescents who use alcohol and experience problems to the degree found in patients being treated for alcohol dependence – 5%.
- There appears to be a trend toward increased amount of alcohol consumed by adolescents, partly due to an earlier initial drinking age.
- The drinking cohort is composed of friends and peers more than parents and relatives.
- In regard to social setting and influences, the *home* is the most frequent location for drinking.
- Heavier drinking among adolescents is apparently related to drinking outside the home, with age peers, and – more rarely – drinking alone.

ADOLESCENTS
CUSTOMER CATEGORY III

- The psychological characteristics reported in adolescent problem drinkers include: unhappiness, boredom, aggressiveness, frustration, and dissatisfaction. (Since so many of these characteristics are shared with unhappy adolescents in general, early intervention programs should look to [1] the drinking behavior itself, and [2] associated problem behaviors, particularly antisocial behavior.)

- In contrast to nonproblem drinkers, problem drinkers (a) place less value on academic achievements; (b) place greater value on independence and personal autonomy; (c) place greater value on independence relative to achievement; (d) have lower expectations of achievement; (e) are more tolerant of deviance; (f) are less religious; (g) place more importance on the positive than the negative functions of drinking.
- In contrast to nonproblem drinkers, problem drinkers (a) are more involved in deviant behavior; (b) smoke more marijuana; (c) are less involved in religious activities; and (d) have a lower academic achievement.
- It is important to remember that primary alcohol dependence can be manifest during adolescence when there is a positive family history of primary alcohol dependence and especially when alcohol use begins at an earlier age.
- Secondary alcohol abuse/dependence can be manifest in the adolescent, particularly in those with primary diagnosis of identity disorder, schizoid disorder, affective disorder, borderline syndrome, attention deficit disorder, or anxiety disorder.
- When the causative conditions involved with adolescent alcohol use and abuse are explored, the following are considered important factors: (1) peer group pressure and/or family breakdown; (2) need for symbolic expression of rites of passage into adulthood; (3) solving of moral dilemmas; (4) search for identity (including a sexual identification); (5) rejection of social norms and values; (6) coping with aggressive impulses (boredom or apathy); (7) overcoming personal inhibition, anxiety, and depression generated in a competitive society; (8) increased sociability—entertainment; (9) an alternative to drugs; (10) a search for the meaning and purpose of life.
- When drinking is introduced to the adolescent (or child) by parents, there may be fewer problems than if drinking were introduced by peers.
- Diagnostically, one must remember that alcohol use and problem drinking in the adolescent is a part of a general development adaptation to self, others, and situations rather than an isolated and necessarily distinct pathological entity. Developmental issues must be addressed in formulating an individualized treat-

ment approach. Although it may appear self-destructive—imperative to identify the *secondary* gains of such behaviors as they relate to developmental issues.

- The number of adolescents seen in alcoholism treatment facilities remains small but it may very well be that youngsters who have problems associated with their drinking, e.g., objections from significant others, are more likely than others to develop alcoholism in their twenties, thirties and forties.
- Adolescent problem drinking is associated with child-parent relationships characterized by rebelliousness, less parental disapproval of drinking and more parental heavy drinking, and with a lack of interest, affection from parents.
- Adolescent problem drinkers are more responsive to peers than to parents and frequently have friends who drink heavily and show other problem behavior. Such friends are supportive of heavy drinking.
- Heavy drinking among adolescents has been linked to precocious sexual behavior, poor school performance, acting out behavior in the classroom, family problems, truancy, and high drop-out rates from school.

ADOLESCENTS
CUSTOMER CATEGORY IV

- Attitudes toward alcohol use appear to be formed at an early age, i.e., 8-10 years.
- In contrast to nonproblem drinkers, problem drinkers: (a) perceive less compatibility between their peer group and their parents; (b) are more easily influenced by their peers than parents; and (c) perceive more pressure for drinking and drug use.
- It is important to realize that attitudes and early drinking behaviors are usually shaped by the parents and relatives rather than the peers; subsequently, the adolescent seeks that peer group whose attitudes, behaviors, and values are compatible with those already formed through parental influence. Adolescents who tend to seek peer groups that are involved with problem drinking generally come from homes in which there is less parental disapproval of drinking and in which the parents are less involved with and less affectionate toward the adolescent.

- Family and social factors at an early adolescent age appear to be highly significant in the development or non-development of problem drinking, such significance having important treatment and prevention implications.
- Adolescent and young adult AA groups have been very helpful in shifting social support systems and peer influence. Generally, adolescents do not relate well to AA groups with older adults.
- Treatment of problem-drinking adolescents is usually best accomplished in a milieu with other adolescents rather than in a mixture of adults and adolescents.
- Because early attitudes and drinking behaviors are significantly influenced by parents (or caretaking relatives), involvement of these persons in the treatment process is important.

Sources: Braught, (in press); Gharderian, 1979; Gomberg, 1982; Knott, 1986.

WOMEN
CUSTOMER CATEGORY I

- There is a broader knowledge base in regard to alcohol-dependent women from lower socioeconomic backgrounds, particularly those in state hospitals and prisons, since it is their drinking that attracts more public attention.
- Among employed women, the heaviest drinkers in general are those with jobs in the service fields.
- The association between drinking practices and socioeconomic status is more pronounced for women than for men.
- Alcohol-dependent women in the middle and lower socioeconomic status groups are usually younger, experience more childhood and marital disruption, have more unstable employment histories, more familial alcoholism, more medical complications, and are more prone to binge drinking.
- Alcohol-dependent women in a higher socioeconomic status are generally older, experience a later age of onset of alcohol dependence, are more likely to be continuous drinkers than binge drinkers, are less likely to lose friends or a job, are less likely to be arrested, and are hidden by their families to a greater degree.
- Current estimates place male-female ratio for alcohol depen-

dency at 4:1, although this number may approach 2:1 or even 1:1 in private practice.

- Rate of divorce is higher among alcohol-dependent women, than non-alcohol dependent women.
- Morbidity and mortality among women appears to be higher in the alcohol-dependent.
- Women usually start drinking and begin drinking heavily at a later age. Although this trend may be reversed by the emerging class of young working women.
- In 1982, approximately 60% of women admitted to British hospitals for treatment were aged 40 and under; a marked increase of alcoholic women of child-bearing age over the past decade.
- Recent studies suggest risk indicators for women may include the following: recent marital disintegration experienced by women under age 35; "dual role stress" for women of all age groups who deal with double responsibilities, working outside and working at home; non-white young women who are the head of the family and raising young children with little financial and social support; and recently widowed.
- Women begin drinking later, experience their first intoxication later, develop alcoholism later, and come to treatment with briefer histories than do men. There are some recent data which suggest that these sex differences are minimal when younger alcoholics are compared.

WOMEN
CUSTOMER CATEGORY II

- Women are more often solitary drinkers and experience fewer drinking binges.
- Abuse of psychoactive drugs in combination with alcohol is more common in women.
- Women in general are more often prescribed drugs than men and more often take psychoactive drugs, and significantly more women alcoholics appear to be polydrug misusers. Drug histories may be more similar among young men and women alcoholics than middle-aged alcoholics.
- Women drink alone much more than do men, partly because of social role and guilt, partly because of stigmatization. When

women alcoholics do not drink alone, they are most likely to be drinking with a significant other. Far fewer women alcoholics drink in public places than do men alcoholics.

WOMEN
CUSTOMER CATEGORY III

- Clinical observations suggest that alcohol-dependent women have lower self-concepts and more sexual identity problems than do alcoholic men.
- Genetic factors in addition to arly deprivation may help explain the higher incidence of affective disorders (particularly depression) in women. Secondary alcohol dependence superimposed on an underlying affective disorder occurs more frequently in women, which can explain why alcohol-dependent women are more likely to be admitted to hospitals as psychiatric patients.
- The impact of family factors on the developmental phase of women who became alcohol-dependent may be more influential than for men. During childhood women who become alcoholics sense a greater loss associated with deprivation and disruption, such as loss of parent by desertion, divorce or death. In addition, the parental background of alcohol-dependent women is often characterized by a cold dominating, rejecting, mother and a rather passive, indulgent (frequently alcoholic) father. Such women lack preparation to assume the responsibility of an adult.
- There is a general assumption that alcohol-dependent women are "psychologically sicker and more deviant" than alcohol-dependent men, supported by the argument that if excessive drinking by women is viewed culturally as a social taboo and an obvious deviation from accepted behavior, only women with significant psychopathology would exhibit such behavior.
- There has been a consensus that the incidence and extent of medical complications is more serious in women than in men.
- Women drinkers suffer a relatively higher incidence of severe liver disease (cirrhosis and alcoholic hepatitis), anemia, and peripheral neuropathy.
- There appears to be a significantly higher mortality rate among female than male alcohol-dependent persons. The apparent increase in both morbidity and mortality in alcohol-dependent

women places greater importance on early diagnosis and aggressive intervention for the population.

- Certain physiological mechanisms (levels of hormones during pre- and post-menstrual phases) may partially explain the clinical observation that the response to alcohol in women varies more from drinking episode to drinking episode and is less predictable with an established dose of alcohol than noted in men.
- Women achieve a higher blood alcohol concentration with a given gram per kilogram dose of alcohol than men.
- Four theories of etiology of alcohol-dependent women:
  1. One theory suggests that women who are alcohol-dependent are overwhelmed by intense and unresolved dependency needs and conflicts, with a repressed, but unresolved need for maternal care. One explanation for the larger number of men vs. women alcoholics is that women are better able to be dependent in our society.
  2. The theory of need for power prevails with regard to male alcohol-dependence; however, with the changing posture of women in our society to that of a more competitive role, the disinhibiting effects of alcohol in regard to enhancing aggressive behaviors and fantasies of omnipotence may become increasingly important.
  3. A third theory suggests that the alcohol-dependent woman has a strong ambivalence toward her femininity and doubts about her adequacy as a woman. Theoretically, alcohol ameliorates this ambivalence and doubt, and enhances her sense of femininity, making the woman drinker feel more "womanly."
  4. Another theory holds that alcohol is used by women in coping with life crises—particularly those that may be defeminizing. Life crises that have been associated with the onset of heavy drinking in women are: (a) separation and divorce; (b) death of the mate; (c) extramarital affair of the mate; (d) obstetrical and gynecological problems (spontaneous abortion, infertility, mastectomy, hysterectomy); (e) the "empty nest syndrome," a time when the role of the woman as a wife and mother is undergoing radical change; and (f) death of a parent, particularly the mother, who characteristically has been cold and dominating.

- Women experience fewer "blackouts" but more suicide attempts.
- The course of alcohol-dependence appears to be more telescoped in women, i.e., a more rapid psychological-physiological-social deterioration.
- Women are less aggressive, exhibit less drunken-driving behavior, and are arrested less frequently for alcohol-related offenses. (This may represent a selective bias on the part of law enforcement officers.)
- Comparison of men and women alcoholics shows that an alcoholic spouse or lover occurs much more frequently in female alcoholism. Women alcoholics are often married to alcoholics but the histories suggest the transmission is most usually male to female.
- Medical complications of alcoholism are a significant issue and it would appear that women alcoholics are more vulnerable to severe medical complications. Health concerns are important motivations for women to seek treatment.
- Little evidence has been found of the association of female alcoholism and sexual promiscuity. Women who drink in public places may be more vulnerable to sexual assaults.
- Women cite stressful events as precipitating their alcoholism more frequently than do men, which may be due to defensiveness, sex differences in reporting, or greater vulnerability to environmental stress and to loss.
- Women in alcoholic marriages perceive a conflicted childhood relationship with their fathers, unlike women in non-alcoholic marriages.
- Women are more inclined than men to describe their current drinking in ways which minimized its harmfulness.

WOMEN
CUSTOMER CATEGORY IV

- A factor contributing to women's perception of their drinking as unproblematic or as not serious enough to warrant help-seeking was supported by the reactions of their spouses. Several women reported past attempts by partners to prevent help-seeking and to encourage the woman to continue drinking even when she herself had begun to worry about it.

- Interviews have revealed that many men and women have experienced difficulty in identifying their own behavior with the stereotypes of "the alcoholic" or of a "drink problem" which they had. For both sexes the assumed indicators of a drink problem were similar:
  1. Certain kinds of alcoholic drinks were regarded as not really harmful.
  2. Alcoholics were people with a constant craving for drink.
  3. To have a problem meant you had to consume large quantities and it was only when alcohol was clearly seen to impair the performance of family or work roles that it became a problem.
- Women are especially concerned to emphasize, that their drinking has not diminished their ability to fulfill their roles as wives and mothers. In particular, the provision of food for the family was given as "evidence" that all was well.
- Although a modest increase in the incidence of female dependence may be occurring, other factors such as a new awareness of women, increased visibility of women, the ability of women to drink more openly without being stigmatized, and an increased willingness of these women to seek treatment play important roles in the recognition of alcohol-dependency in women.
- There is no such things as the "typical woman alcoholic."
- Studies indicate that women view alcohol as an aphrodisiac despite their physiological and behavioral responses indicating otherwise.

Sources: Connors et al., 1986; Gomberg, 1982; Hill, 1982; Knott, 1986; Mishara and Kastenbaum, 1980; Thom, 1985.

ELDERLY
CUSTOMER CATEGORY I

- Senior citizens (age 65 and older) are the second fastest growing population group in the U.S. today. They comprise 10% of the total population and exceed 22 million persons. It is estimated they will comprise 16% of U.S. population within the next 20 years.

- It is estimated that 10-15% of the elderly who contact the health care delivery system for assistance have an alcohol-related problem.
- In recent studies, at least 5% of those persons observed over the age of 65 clearly suffer from alcohol dependence.
- As one grows older, the lean body mass decreases, adipose tissue increases, and total body water decreases, therefore, there is a smaller space for the distribution of alcohol—resulting in higher blood alcohol levels. Not only does tolerance to alcohol decrease, but higher blood alcohol levels are achieved with standard gram per kilogram dose than would have existed at a younger age.
- Erroneous assumption that "most of the elderly live in nursing homes"—Only 4-5% of persons over 65 reside in institutions, primarily nursing homes. Of those in nursing homes, 50% have no living relatives.
- 17% of elderly men live alone or with non-relatives; 45% of women live alone or with non-relatives; 77% of men and only 48% of women over 65 are married—loneliness is an extremely severe stress for elderly women.
- Average years of education in 9.5 years—there is a trend toward higher education levels which will have an impact on health care education and planning for this group.
- Survey reported that older men, recently retired and recently widowed, are at a higher risk for alcohol problems and for suicide as well.

ELDERLY
CUSTOMER CATEGORY II

- Surveys indicate that the absolute number of abstainers increases and that the consumption of alcohol decreases with age.
- In the later years, the number of abstainers increases, the proportion of heavy drinkers decreases among both sexes at about age 50 and there is a second decrease among men around age 65.
- Not only do persons become abstinent as aging progresses, but alcohol users consume less alcohol due in part to physiological changes.
- Controversy still rages concerning the alleged benefits of the

"moderate use of wine" in the elderly: heart disease and diabetes mellitus (2 very common maladies among elderly) mandate against use of any alcohol. In addition, there appears to be an association between the incidence of cancer and alcohol use in the geriatric population. The physician must view with great caution the statement that the "moderate use of alcoholic beverages has advantages in the the elderly." This assumption in based on short-term studies, which have been unable to distinguish between the advantages of the social setting and the advantage of alcohol per se. It is perfectly legitimate for the physician to advise abstinence from alcohol for the elderly rather than prescribe "moderate" alcohol use.

- Potential for Alcohol/Drug Interactions – Older people receive about a quarter of all prescriptions. Alcohol frequently diminishes the effectiveness of medical management of these patients.
- Heavy, problematic drinking, when of recent origin, is likely to be associated with depression, loss, and isolation.

ELDERLY
CUSTOMER CATEGORY III

- There appear to be two distinct alcohol-dependent groups in the geriatric population.
  1. Group composed of persons whose alcohol dependence had its onset at an early age and who have "survived," to an old age – mainly the *Primary Alcohol Dependent* person. Approximately 2/3 of elderly alcoholics fall into this category.
  2. Group exhibits late onset of the disease, i.e., after age of 55 (1/3 of elderly alcoholics) – mainly the *Reactive Type* of alcoholic.
- In clinical diagnosis, one should suspect alcohol dependence in the geriatric patient who is diagnosed as "senile dementia." If indeed the signs and symptoms of dementia are secondary to alcohol-dependence, treatment of alcoholism will frequently lead to dramatic improvements: the prognosis is much worse in persons with true senile (irreversible) dementia.
- Many researchers have observed that neuropsychological deficits that occur in the central nervous system (CNS) as a function of the aging process are seen in alcohol-dependent patients at a

younger age. This has led to the hypothesis that heavy alcohol use actually accelerates the aging process: Alcohol dependence may lead to both premature aging and to organic mental disorders (brain damage) superimposed on the intrinsic aging process.

- Due to effect of aging on the CNS, elderly alcohol-dependent patients are more prone to develop both classical and atypical alcoholic psychoses:
  1. Schizophrenic symptoms such as auditory/visual hallucinations and delusions, if caused by alcohol, will generally clear when alcohol problem is treated.
  2. Many of these patients have an acute delirium characterized by disorientation for time and place, impaired consciousness, retardation, and exhaustion—in all cases, alcohol must be considered as a possible cause, since this is a form of reversible delirium with proper diagnosis and treatment.
- Depression is frequent among elderly—can stem from pharmacological effects of alcohol abuse; consequence of retirement (boredom, loss of income); change from productive to non-productive status; health problems, etc. All too frequently, medication is prescribed for the depression although these important factors have not been adequately addressed.
- Social isolation and alienation certainly plague the elderly.
- Generally, older alcoholics are probably most visible to spouse, family, friends, and neighbors, and those networks appear to be a primary source of casefinding. Health problems associated with excessive drinking loom large so that physicians' offices, emergency rooms, hospital wards, and services may also be significant casefinding settings.
- Older men with alcohol problems are less likely to be visible than younger men because fewer are in the workplace. Older people who drink excessively at home tend to be overlooked, particularly if they have withdrawn from family and friends. There is less belligerence among older alcoholics than among younger ones but older men alcoholics do tend to be picked up by the police, primarily for public intoxication rather than for being drunk and disorderly. Older men alcoholics are most visible in hospital wards and emergency rooms, or as public intoxication offenders. Elderly women alcoholics appear to be invisible—ex-

cept for family, friends, neighbors, or visiting welfare workers who may spot them.

ELDERLY
CUSTOMER CATEGORY IV

- The most important obstacle to overcome in the treatment of the elderly alcohol-dependent patient is the attitude that advanced age is incompatible with active treatment and a favorable prognosis. Because of this, identification and diagnosis of the elderly alcoholic have been approaches with limited enthusiasm.
- Those persons suffering the onset of alcohol dependence later in life (after age of 55) appear to respond better to treatment than do those "survivors" who have a long history of alcohol dependence.
- Although the elderly may not require the intensive detoxification often necessary for younger persons, the amount of time required for detoxification may be longer, and although no "special" treatment methods have been identified as universally applicable to the elderly alcohol-dependent population, there are certain guidelines that have proven helpful.
  1. Behavior psychotherapy may be more helpful than in-depth, dynamically oriented psychotherapy.
  2. It is essential to offer the full range of medical services for the treatment not only of alcohol-related complications, but of other chronic disease as well.
  3. The use of sedative-hypnotics should be minimized.
  4. Addressing the need for decreasing the loneliness and social isolation is essential. Redefining a social support system, which can include volunteer activities, recreational programs, and in some cases, vocational rehabilitation improves the prognosis.
  5. Intensive follow up and after care, even with home visitation, are important.
- Education should not only emphasize the medical-psychiatric risks of alcohol use, but also should deal with the anticipated loneliness, isolation, loss of income, increase in free time, inevitability of death, health problems associated with aging, and cul-

tural issue of "being old" as critical issues that demand the acquisition of new coping skills.

- Although educational effects in the name of Prevention have met with only limited success in younger age groups it is feasible that education thru media might be more effective with the elderly, since their exposure to newspapers, radio and TV is more intense than it is in younger age groups.
- Many agencies and therapists are not particularly responsive to the needs of older alcoholics although there is evidence that older alcoholics are very responsive to help, particularly to the social therapies. It is believed that shame and denial play a significant role in keeping older problem drinkers away from sources of help; this is consistent with their underrepresentation at community mental health centers.
- It appears that the later years are a time of decision and indecision about drinking (as in the adolescent years).

Sources: Bailey et al., 1965; Brody, 1982; Gomberg, 1982; Knott, 1986; Maletta, 1982; Mishara and Kastenbaum, 1980; Vestal, 1977.

PHYSICIANS
CUSTOMER CATEGORY I

- Medical specialties in which alcohol/drug-related dependence is proportionally greater include family practice, obstetrics and gynecology, psychiatry, and anesthesiology. (However it is found in all specialties.)
- Average age of onset of depression (linked to alcohol/drug) is 40 years which is also the average age when alcohol/drug-dependence appears to become clinically manifest.
- If onset before 40—personality more serious psychopathology (usually borderline type)
- If onset after 40—organic mental disorders and depression predominant.
- 75% of alcohol/drug-dependent physicians report sexual difficulties in marriage.
- A significant number of physicians' wives suffer psychological

and alcohol/drug-dependencies problems—onset at 40 years of age like physicians.
- Many physicians who become impaired are from lower income families and have difficulty handling their economic success.
- Range of 60-85% recovery, defined as "serene sobriety" and effective re-entry into community, family and practice of medicine.
- 10-12% of physicians suffer a degree of impairment sufficient to compromise their work.
- The major problems have been identified as alcohol-dependency, drug-dependency and suicide, with alcohol- and drug-dependency as the primary problems. (Alcohol often precedent to drugs.)
- Alcoholic physician also suffers the medical complications associated with alcoholism.

PHYSICIAN CUSTOMER CATEGORY II

- Consumption patterns (of treatment)—Most physicians who enter treatment are coerced with the threat of licensure suspension or revocation. (Can assist the treatment team in dissolving the consummate denial so characteristic of the physician patient.)

PHYSICIAN CUSTOMER CATEGORY III

- Physicians are perhaps more vulnerable to alcohol- and/or drug-dependence and psychological problems (especially depression) than the non-physician population.
- Physician is difficult patient:
  1. generally there are more medical-psychiatric complications in the physician-patient because he or she resisted intervention until the impairment has become overtly obvious to everyone.
  2. even with impairment, physician has not relinquished the self-imposed and society imposed omniscience and omnipotence; thus accepting patient role is difficult.
  3. hostility, denial and manipulation of the therapist and treatment staff often results in minimizing the severity of the condition and/or underdiagnosing the problem.

- Sequential deterioration in physician as measured by performance in (1) community, (2) family, (3) employment, (4) physical function, (5) office function, and (6) hospital function.
- Psychological traits of impaired physician:
  1. obsessive-compulsive behaviors often of neurotic dimensions.
  2. secondary anhedonia for the sake of "doing all for everyone."
  3. self-perceived feelings of omniscience, omnipotence, and indispensability.
  4. inability to tolerate failure.
  5. lack of creativity and flexibility (these traits are usually apparent during the medical school and post graduate training periods).
- Nearly 75% of alcohol/drug-dependent physicians experience emotional impoverishment during childhood and adolescence. They often describe a distant relationship with the father and a compromised relationship with the mother, who typically is characterized as being rigid, domineering, perfectionist, puritanical and impersonal.
- Depression has been observed in over 60% of physician presenting alcohol/drug-dependency.
- Psychodiagnostic Categories
  (separating alcohol/drug-dependent physician)
  Study involving 50 addicted physicians
  36% High-level personality organization groups (personality disorders if obsessive-compulsive, histrionic or mixed varieties.
  32% Intermediate-level personal organization groups (narcissistic, avoidant or schizoid varieties).
  28% Borderline personality organization.
  4% Psychotic state (schizophrenia, manic psychosis).
- Other social behaviors of impaired physician extramarital affairs, excessive spending on material things, overinvolvement in high-risk investments, inappropriate business ventures and gambling.
- The suicide potential of the impaired physician is high, particularly after confrontation and early phases of treatment: indicates a need for in-patient treatment.

PHYSICIAN
CUSTOMER CATEGORY IV

- Early efforts by impaired physician programs were to address tertiary prevention. As knowledge increased about the profile of the impaired physician, attention was directed at secondary prevention (early case finding) and primary prevention.
- Physicians are notorious for treating themselves for alcohol-related diseases – this often permits the alcohol-dependence to be more progressive since intervention is not afforded until the later stages of their diseases.
- Medical schools may cultivate alcohol abuse through their tolerant attitudes (e.g., practice of lunchtime drinking in medical settings).

Sources: Knott, 1986; Talbott and Beson, 1986.

AMERICAN INDIANS/NATIVE ALASKANS
CUSTOMER CATEGORY I

- Native people in Alaska (including Eskimaux, Indians and Aleuts) comprise 17% of the population of Alaska but account for 60% of the deaths due to alcoholism.
- Alcohol figures prominently in arrest records: Los Angeles Police Department data from a 15-year period show that of all adult Indian arrests, 90% were for intoxication.
- 58% of the boys and 30% of the girls at a reservation school reported "regular drinking" before age 12 (boys reported drinking at an earlier age than girls, both boys and girls reported regular drinking by the age of 13).
- Life expectancy is shorter than for other groups and death rate from alcohol is high. Among American Indians 35% of mortality is alcohol-related.
- Alcoholism among Indians is 2-4 times the national level and is higher than for any other minority group.
- Male Indians drink more and have more problems related to drinking, but the female Indian drinking rate is also at a high level, equal to white Anglo males.
- Indian drinking patterns vary markedly from tribe to tribe.

- 60% of Navahos are complete abstainers from alcohol.
- Urban Indians consume less alcohol than rural Indians and styles tend to conform to their social class as much as to their tribal origin.
- Among rural Indian alcoholics, boredom, hopelessness, and the periodic need to release suppressed feeling must contribute to the binge-type drinking observed there.
- 76% of all adult American Indians' arrests are alcohol-related.

AMERICAN INDIANS/NATIVE ALASKANS CUSTOMER CATEGORY II

- It is believed Indians adopted their drinking practices from the frontiersman and later the cowboy who tended to drink rapidly till drunk and then exhibit unrestrained or violent behavior. It is possible these role models still influence current consumption styles.
- Indians never had the opportunity to learn how to drink moderately or to develop social taboos against drunken comportment.
- Group drinking is a norm, solitary drinking is infrequent.

AMERICAN INDIANS/NATIVE ALASKANS CUSTOMER CATEGORY III

- Alcohol-related suicide rates among American Indians are considerably higher than they are for the general U.S. population.
- A recent discussion argues for a "Community-based phenomenon" in which alcohol problems are not psychological but based on the impact of urban, industrial living on Indians who lack "the necessary sacred social controls." BREAKDOWN OF TRADITIONAL CUSTOMS

AMERICAN INDIANS/NATIVE ALASKANS CUSTOMER CATEGORY IV

- Although there was a possibility of getting in trouble, 7th and 8th graders studied expressed *positive* attitudes toward drinking.
- Recent trends in alcoholism treatment with native peoples have moved toward emphasis on native cultures and customs.
- The image of the "drunken Indian" is a widely held stereotype

and American Indians themselves see excessive drinking as one of their major social problems.
- A traditional AA group conflicts with the Indian tradition of not discussing personal problems and confessing in public.

Source: Gomberg, 1982; Hedin, 1986.

BLACK AMERICANS CUSTOMER CATEGORY I

- Black alcoholics tend to be younger than white alcoholics.
- Urban blacks tend to drink more than rural blacks.
- In 15-30 age range, the black male is most likely to be a victim of alcohol-related homicide.
- Black and white adolescents in the South have similar drinking rates.
- There is a high rate of liver disorders among black women alcoholics and recent research indicates serious biomedical consequences of excessive drinking among blacks of both sexes.
- High rates of hypertension among blacks compound the medical problems associated with heavy drinking.
- The black family is often intimately involved with the drinking problems and treatment of the alcoholic family member.
- Black females show even stronger motivation for sobriety than black males.
- Blacks admitted for treatment have been found to be younger than whites admitted, and tend to be morning drinkers.
- Median age of both black males and females admitted to psychiatric facilities for alcoholism in a midwestern state over three years was 38 years. (Median age for white males and females was 46 and 44, respectively.)
- Black alcoholism must be viewed in the context of the social status in a given black community. Depending on the direction of the black community change, alcoholism may increase or decrease.
- The high availability of alcohol in black residential communities compared to traditionally white residential communities has economic, political, and therapeutic implications.

BLACK AMERICANS
CUSTOMER CATEGORY II

- Black alcoholics utilize treatment facilities less than do white alcoholics (although it is a question whether that would be true for facilities designed for outreach in the black community).
- Black college men often drink heavily on weekends in group settings.
- Many blacks drink in public or in outdoor places, e.g., street corners, automobiles, in front of stores or residences.
- Blacks tend to drink more frequently and heavily during weekends.
- Black women 58% abstainers (white women—39%); Heavy drinkers black women—11% (whites—4%).
- Surveys in the 1960s and more recent surveys have shown little difference in the drinking pattern of black and white men: 38% blacks/31% white report abstinence and 19% blacks/22% white heavy drinking.
- Rural black families tended to treat or deal with their alcoholic family members at home.

BLACK AMERICANS
CUSTOMER CATEGORY III

- Demonstrate strong association of problem drinking with health and social problems, particularly in black ghettos.
- Clear relationship between alcohol and homicide among black men and women homicide offenders.
- Violent consequences of alcohol use are much more serious for blacks, especially black men.
- The lifestyles of black and white skid row alcoholics differ: blacks are younger, less likely to be homeless, less likely to get jobs or utilize welfare resources and they tend to identify with the black community.
- Blacks often use alcohol for social celebrations and sexual activity.
- Blacks tend to be group rather than solitary drinkers.

- Black women reported heavy drinking at home and drinking with family members (just as white women who are heavy drinkers).
- Black women alcoholics are less apt to be churchgoers than other black women.
- Studies indicate that black alcoholics who volunteer for alcohol treatment tend to be more highly motivated than their white counterparts.
- Some authorities say the race of the therapist does not affect treatment of black alcoholics, yet others maintain that blacks (and other racial or ethnic groups) respond better to therapy administered by blacks or someone thoroughly knowledgeable and understanding of their background and behavior.
- Blacks are more likely than whites to enter alcoholism treatment through the legal system (e.g., arrests and/or court referral).
- Researchers suggest close examination of the religious experience in the black community for those aspects which provide spiritual and material strength for personality development.

BLACK AMERICANS CUSTOMER CATEGORY IV

- Compared with whites, black alcoholics admitted to hospitals and clinics show stronger motivation for treatment, fewer complaints and more cooperation during the treatment process.
- Heavy drinking black women are less oriented toward respectability, more permissive about drinking by men, more apt to drink in public places, and drink more often for reasons of escape.
- Blacks are unlikely to view excessive drinking as a problem requiring professional help.
- A large proportion of rural blacks are much more concerned about social problems associated with problem drinking (possible arrests/prison and waste of needed family money on alcohol) than with health problems resulting from alcoholism.
- Some cultural concerns that may impede blacks' usage of treatment include language usage hampering communication with therapist of other background, negative reactions and discriminatory actions of treatment personnel and law enforcers, and suspicious reaction of black alcoholics to white counselors, middle-class black counselors, and traditional AA programs.

- Outreach counseling appears to be very important in the treatment of black alcoholism.

Source: Gomberg, 1982.

ASIAN AMERICANS
CUSTOMER CATEGORY I

- First generation Japanese Americans are considerably less permissive about drinking than second generation, etc.
- Chinese and Japanese Americans have low arrest rates in general, but if a member is arrested, it is very likely to be an alcohol-related offense.
- Asian Americans are generally concentrated in Hawaii and the West Coast.
- Relatively small in number and maintain a "low profile."
- Low rates of alcohol problems.
- May have an allergic sensitivity to alcohol.

ASIAN AMERICANS
CUSTOMER CATEGORY II

- Relatively low level of consumption in general.
- Among Oriental adolescents it appears that those who drink often drink heavily (these may be acculturated, multi-problem young people).
- Research indicates that, on the whole, Asians drink less than Europeans, and that more Asian Americans, both adolescents and adults are abstainers.

ASIAN AMERICANS
CUSTOMER CATEGORY III

- The idea of counseling services is alien to a traditional Oriental emphasis on the role of the *family* in dealing with its members' problems.
- Urbanization, changes in family structure, economic mobility, cultural conflict and acculturation are likely to push drinking and problem rates upward.
- They have cultural taboos against heavy drinking.

ASIAN AMERICANS
CUSTOMER CATEGORY IV

- There is a shame attached to a family member's deviant behavior.
- Asian Americans underutilize mental health services in general.

Source: Gomberg, 1982.

HISPANIC AMERICANS
CUSTOMER CATEGORY I

- Lower proportion of drinkers among young Hispanics than young Anglos.
- High proportion of abstainers among Spanish women.
- Higher rates of death from cirrhosis among Hispanics than in the general U.S. population.
- Alcohol-related automobile accidents are also higher among Hispanics.
- The high rates of alcohol problems among Hispanic Americans are indicated by statistics of arrests for DUI, public drunkenness and alcohol-related offenses of all kinds. The statistics may be qualified by the differential likelihood of arrest as lower status people are more likely to be arrested by the police and both Mexican Americans and Puerto Ricans are overrepresented in the low income brackets.
- Rates of alcohol consistent with high rates of alcohol in country of origin.
- Cuban immigrants have concentration of elderly.
- Puerto Ricans concentration in service organization in Northeast.
- Heaviest concentrate of Mexican Americans is South and Southwest
  - —younger than general population
  - —lower education and income than general population
  - —Mexican Americans have high birth rate

HISPANIC AMERICANS
CUSTOMER CATEGORY II

- Indicator of Alcoholism—Above average concentrations of alcohol outlets in Spanish-speaking communities.

HISPANIC AMERICANS
CUSTOMER CATEGORY III

- The few treatment outcome studies available suggest that Spanish-speaking patients do at least as well and generally better than Anglo patients.
- Few Hispanic women apparently develop alcohol problems but there is some suggestion that increasing acculturation is associated with the breakdown of tradition sanctions against women drinking.
- A high degree of stress is theorized among those who show a pattern of abandoning their root culture with little opportunity to achieve social status and identify with the dominant culture.
- High ratings of alcoholism as a community problem.
- Some evidence that acculturation stress and higher rates of alcoholism are linked.

HISPANIC AMERICANS
CUSTOMER CATEGORY IV

- Perceptions—Hispanics are more likely to view alcoholism as a moral weakness, not as a condition requiring treatment.
- The underrepresentation of Hispanics in treatment facilities is consistent with their underutilization of mental health facilities in general and probably indicates an unwillingness to use the institutionalized psychological approach of most treatment programs.
- Discrimination, prejudice and low social status have been linked to alcohol problems.

Source: Gomberg, 1982.

The Direct Organization Markets: Some Industrial Marketing Principles and Recommendations from Clients

Vaughan C. Judd
Donald R. Self
Cathleen A. Owens

INTRODUCTION

A key target market for Alcoholism Treatment Marketers are those organizations which have the right to "refer," either on a voluntary or involuntary basis. The organization market is the Alcoholism Treatment Marketing (ATM) version of the traditional industrial market, and can be classified into three distinct sub-markets: the Primary (Direct) market, the Reseller market, and the Voluntary system. Each category consists of those organizations with enough social power to "force" the unwilling addict to seek treatment.

The concept of social power is defined rather consistently throughout marketing literature. French and Raven (1959) originally suggested and defined five bases of power which have become generally adopted: reward, coercion, legitimate, expert and referent.

Power as a Basis for Market Identification

Reward power is based on the belief that the influencer has the ability to mediate rewards, usually manifested in financial gains—either perceived or actual. Coercive power stems from expectations of punishment for failure to conform to influencers' attempts. *Ex-*

pert power is based on the perception of an influencer's special knowledge or advice. *Referent* power has its basis in an identification or a feeling of oneness with the influencer. *Legitimate* power stems from internalized values giving a feeling that the influencer has the "right" to exert influence.

In the *Voluntary Referral System,* the referral source has little or no economic or coercive power. Some, therefore, must provide services based on expertise (expert power), an example being a professional counsellor, or through some other non-coercive power base like referent power, which might apply to clergy and significant others. These organizational markets are considered in the next article in this volume (see Kline and Self).

The *Reseller Market* consists of integrated systems such as Health Maintenance Organizations and Preferred Provider Organizations. (See Gomillion and Self elsewhere in the volume for a case study of implementing a mental health/substance abuse PPO for state employees.) It also includes Insurance Companies and Third Party Administrators (TPA). Self (1988) profiles TPAs as professional services wholesaler operations representing vertical integration of the financing and delivery of health care systems for the employer organizations (and sometimes for insurance firms). TPAs perform administrative, cost reduction and marketing tasks for self-insuring organizations. Market shares of TPAs have increased dramatically in recent years, at the expense of insurance companies.

This article deals with the *Primary (Direct) Markets*. The dominant organization of this type is the employer organization, which may be commercial, institutional, or governmental (including the military). Also included are educational organizations which mirror the functions of employee organization for the adolescent population, and can provide increased clientele for ATMs. Included are several basic concepts from the field of industrial/organizational marketing which are relevant to ATMs, including market segmentation and the process by which organizations procure the goods and services they need. Also included are recent studies about the characteristics of the employer organization markets using employee assistance programs (Hewitt Associates, 1986), and of EAP coordinators, military referral, educators, and courts and attorneys.

MARKET SEGMENTATION

Several broad market segmentation variables have significance for ATMs. These are demographic-type variables which relate to industry classification, organization size, and geographic location.

SIMILARITIES AND DIFFERENCES BETWEEN PRIMARY, RESELLER, AND CONSUMER MARKETS

Reeder and Reeder (1987) constructed a table (Table 1) illustrating the chief differentiation between traditional industrial (primary), reseller, and consumer markets on the basis of market characteristics, uses of products purchased, and nature of buying behavior involved. Most notable information for ATMs include the degree of geographic concentration, number of buyers, customization of brands, and status of the buying center (one person in industrial versus committee involvement in reseller). Another point of interest is the importance of personal selling for both industrial and reseller markets, as opposed to an advertising emphasis for promotion to the consumer market.

Industry Classification

An ATM may have data which indicates that some occupations or industries have higher rates of alcohol dependency than do others. For example, Mannello and Seaman (1979) estimated the prevalence of problem drinking among railroad workers overall to be 19% while among railroad engineers and conductors the rate was estimated at 23%. The railroad industry, consequently, would be considered a high-incidence industry which an ATM might want to select as a target market.

Information on any given industry is available to marketers from a number of government and private sources. Access to much of this information is provided through the federal government's Standard Industrial Classification (SIC) system described in the *Standard Industrial Classification Manual* (United States Executive Office of the President 1987). Every organization (establishment) in the United States is assigned a code which reflects the main type of product produced or activity undertaken at that location. At the

TABLE 1. Areas of Similarities and Differences Between Industrial, Reseller, and Consumer Markets

	Industrial Markets	**Reseller Markets**	**Consumer Markets**
Market Structure	Geographically Concentrated Relatively fewer buyers Oligopolistic competition Oligopsonistic Buying Power	Geographically dispersed Relatively fewer buyers Monopolistic competition Oligopsonistic Buying Power	Geographically dispersed Mass markets Monopolistic competition
Products	Technical complexity Customized Service, Delivery, and availability very important	Customized for private brands Service, delivery, and availability very important	Standardized Service, delivery, and availability somewhat important
Buyer Behavior	Functional involvement Rational/task motives predominate Technical expertise Stable, interpersonal relationships Supplier evaluation	Committee involvement Rational/task motives predominate Limited technical expertise Stable, interpersonal relationships Supplier evaluation	Family involvement Social/psychological motives predominate Less technical expertise Nonpersonal relationships

Decision Making	Distinct, observable stages	Distinct, observable stages	Unobservable, mental stages
Channels	Shorter, more direct, fewer linkages	Direct/indirect, linkages	Indirect, multiple linkages
Promotion	Emphasis on personal selling	Emphasis on personal selling	Emphasis on advertising
Price	Competitive bidding Negotiating on complex purchases List prices on standard items	Negotiating on discounts, promotional allowances, transportation, and handling terms	List prices

Source: Reeder and Reeder, 1987

broadest level the SIC system divides establishments into ten industry divisions which include:

- Agriculture, Forestry & Fishing
- Construction
- Manufacturing
- Transportation & Public Utilities
- Wholesale Trade
- Retail Trade
- Finance, Insurance & Real Estate
- Services
- Public Administration
- Nonclassifiable Establishments

The ten divisions are further broken down into major groups, groups and individual industries represented by a series of two-, three-, and four-digit numerical codes—the more digits used, the more detailed will be the industry description. For example, line-haul operating railroads which are represented by SIC 4011, are found in the Railroads group—SIC 401 within the major group. Railroad Transportation—SIC 40, which is part of the industry division denoted as Transportation and Public Utilities.

Alcoholism Treatment Marketers can use the SIC system to obtain statistical data on the industries of interest to them. Such information on individual industries is available from the United States Department of Commerce in the form of economic censuses and the census of agriculture. The series of economic censuses, taken every five years, covers manufacturers, retail and wholesale trade, transportation, mineral, construction and service industries and governments. In 1982, the economic censuses together with the census of agriculture covered over 800 of the approximately 1,000 individual industries within the SIC system.

Generally, the most detailed census data are published at the national level. Additionally, most statistics are available for states and many for counties, metropolitan areas, cities and other places (United States Department of Commerce, 1984). *County Business Patterns,* an annual publication of the United States Department of Commerce, has potential planning significance for ATMs. It presents state and county data for 2-, 3-, and 4-digit SIC levels on all areas of the economic censuses. It also provides information on numbers of establishments by size, number of employees, and payroll.

While neither the economic censuses nor *County Business Patterns* report information on individual companies or establishments, publishers of private directories such as *Dun & Bradstreet's Million Dollar Directory*, *Standard and Poor's Register, Directory of Corporate Affiliation*, and *Thomas Register* provide information on individual companies. In most directories, companies are listed according to their four-digit SIC number; and each company's address is given, together with the product produced, sales volumes and names of key executives. Usually a geographic listing of companies is also provided.

The previously mentioned directories are national in scope. At the state and local level, a variety of industrial directories provides marketers with useful information on individual companies. These directories generally use the SIC system and provide information similar to that contained in the national directories. Telephone directory "yellow pages" also provide limited information on local companies under topical categories, rather than SIC number. The SIC system then provides ATMs with a method for identifying individual organizations within a specific industry as well as means of obtaining statistical information regarding that industry. An example of this latter type of information relates to measures of concentration, based on the size of the organization.

Organization Size

Organization size is relevant to those attempting to market goods or services to organizations. Generally the larger the organization's size—as measured by employments, shipments, sales, value added, etc.—the greater will be the quantity demanded of the goods and services it requires.

Buying power, in terms of demand for goods and services, is concentrated in the hands of a relatively small number of large organizations. The "20/80" principle is a generalization based on the assumption that 20% of the entities represent 80% of the output. In practice, it is often found that approximately 20% of the establishments in a particular industry or industry division account for approximately 80% of the activity of that industry. Two examples based on data from the economic censuses substantiate the generalization.

Example 1A: There were 1,731,055 retail establishments (stores) operating in the United States during 1982, with a combined sales volume of over one trillion dollars ($1,010 billion). The number of retail establishments with 7 or more employees was 425,727 in 1982. These stores represented only 25% of all retail stores, however, they accounted for $735.4 billion in sales, or 73% of all retail sales—which is a close approximation of the 20/80 principle. (U.S. Department of Commerce 1985C, Table 2.)

Example 1B: Grocery stores (SIC 5411) are one of the individual industries within the retail trade industry division. During 1982, 121,039 grocery stores operated in the United States. Of these stores, 26,561 or 22%, operated with 20 or more employees. These same stores accounted for $167.4 billion in sales, or 78% of total grocery store sales. That is, grocery stores with 20 or more employees represent only 22% of all grocery stores, but they accounted for 78% of all grocery sales.

Example 2: In 1982, there were 248,285 manufacturing establishments (plants) in the United States employing a total of 17.8 million people. The number of manufacturing establishments with 50 or more employees was 61,753 in 1982. These plants represented only 18% of all manufacturing plants, however, they accounted for combined employment of 14.7 million people, or 82% of all people employed in manufacturing—another approximation of the 20/80 principle. (U.S. Department of Commerce 1985A, Table 1.)

Account Size Classes

These three examples suggest that an ATM interested in marketing to retail or manufacturing establishments might target only the larger firms—thereby dramatically reducing the number of organizations to be contacted, yet retaining most of the market potential. It is common for a marketing firm to classify their accounts by size, using designations such as "A," "B," or "C" accounts. Respective annual sales or billing potential ranges for an alcoholism treatment marketer, for example, might be $150,000 or more (A accounts), $50,000 to $149,999 (B accounts) and less than $50,000 (C accounts). Primary emphasis might be placed on A and B accounts, and the C accounts treated as secondary accounts, with less emphasis on personal selling and increased emphasis on mass marketing techniques. The ATM might want to market through Preferred Provider Organizations to reach the secondary account.

Buying Decision Location

It is useful to make a distinction between a company, an establishment, and single- and multi-unit companies. Some companies are single-unit companies. For example, a manufacturing company may have only one establishment (plant); therefore it is considered a single-unit company. Manufacturing companies with two or more plants are considered multi-unit companies. Our concern for single-unit vs. multi-unit companies is associated with buying decisions.

When an ATM is dealing with a multi-unit company, it is imperative to determine at which location the decision is made to provide treatment for alcohol-dependent employees. In some multi-unit companies, many decisions are made at the headquarters location; while other multi-unit companies provide more autonomy to their various units and a great deal of buying decision making occurs at the local level. In still other multi-unit companies, decision making with regard to a particular purchase is shared between the headquarter location and the local unit. Each company differs in the degree to which these decisions are centralized or decentralized. It is necessary for the ATM to ascertain where the decision makers—with regard to alcoholism treatment for employees—are located.

With companies, as with establishments, there is concentration of buying power among the larger companies; that is, there is an approximation of the 20/80 principle. The *Census of Manufacturers* reports the percentages of industry shipments represented by the four, eight, twenty and fifty largest companies in each industry. The following example is an illustration from the furniture industry.

> *Example 3*: In 1982, there were a total of 2,430 companies producing wood household furniture, not upholstered (SIC 2511) in the United States. The fifty largest of these companies (2% of all the companies) accounted for 54% of the total shipments of industry SIC 2511. . . . (U.S. Department of Commerce 1985B. Table 2.)

Again in Example 3, the significance of larger organizations is demonstrated as a segmentation variable to be considered by Alcoholism Treatment Marketers.

Geographic Location

Alcoholism Treatment Marketers will, by necessity, focus their marketing efforts on a geographic area in the proximity of their facilities. Such geographic restriction amounts to a segmentation strategy, to the extent that geographical boundaries circumscribe organizational targets while essentially excluding organizations outside. Alcoholism Treatment Marketers might designate their local market area as their primary target market, the remainder of the state as their secondary market, and any or all other states as their tertiary market. Those ATMs located in Standard Metropolitan Statistical Areas (SMSAs) might define their primary market as those organizations located within the SMSA. For example, an ATM located in Chicago, Illinois, might define their primary market as the Chicago SMSA (Cook, DuPage, Kane, Lake, McHenry and Will Counties, Illinois) with emphasis on Cook County. Their secondary market might be described as the rest of northern Illinois plus southern Wisconsin or northwest Indiana, and their tertiary market as other outlying areas.

Marketers attempting to reach the organizational market typically use a combination of demographic segmentation variables. Accordingly, an ATM based in Chicago might define one of their target market segments as retail grocery stores (SIC 5411) with 20 or more employees located in the Chicago, Illinois SMSA. According to *County Business Patterns* (United States Department of Commerce, 1987), there were 2,272 grocery stores operating in the Chicago SMSA in 1985, of which 637 stores, or 28% of the total stores, employed 20 or more people. Based on national data shown in Example IB of this article, it would be expected that these 627 stores with 20 or more employees would account for approximately 80% of all grocery store sales in the Chicago SMSA.

ORGANIZATION BUYING PROCESS

The Decision Process

The ATM in many instances is faced with a two-pronged challenge in dealing with the primary organizational market. That is, the ATM may be marketing both the concept of referral systems/Employee Assistance Programs (EAPs) as well as the ATM's own treatment programs/facilities. An Employee Assistance Program is a planned systematic program designed to provide professional assistance to employees experiencing alcohol, drug, emotional, or other personal crises—problems which interfere with their job performance. Individual primary organizations have different levels of awareness with respect to alcohol-dependent employees or members and possible solutions to the problem. Primary organizations which have not already established a referral system or EAP must be sold on the need for participating in the process before they can be persuaded to select a particular ATM as a place to refer their employees. A three-stage model of the process is proposed in Table 2. The model is based on an individual's decision process (Dewey, 1910), and the eight-phase organizational buying process model popularized by Robinson, Faris and Wind (1967).

In the first stage of the process shown in Table 2, Problem Recognition, Step 1 deals with the awareness of alcohol-dependency problems within the organization. Recognition of the problem may come from within the organization—from a superior, subordinate or a peer, or it may come from outside the organization in terms of referrals from courts, attorneys, social programs, counselors or physicians (Kline, Self, & Ingram, 1987). Typically there is a significant role for marketers in uncovering needs unrecognized by organizations. In the case of ATMs, it is not their role to bring individual alcohol-dependency problems to the attention of an organization (Step 1). It might be argued, however, that there may be opportunities for making some organizations aware that there is a

TABLE 2. Organizational Decision Process Relating to Alcohol-Dependent Employees/Members

Stage	Steps To Be Taken
Problem Recognition	1. Aware that alcohol-dependency problems exist within the organization 2. Aware that there is a need for treatment ofalcohol-dependent employees/members
Alternative	3. Aware of organizations role in treatment by way of employee referrals or establishment of an EAP 4. Aware of the availability of one or more alcohol treatment programs
Solution Implementation	5. Have established either a referral system or an EAP 6. Have referred employees/members to an ATM
Outcome/Feedback	7. Determine satisfaction with an ATM´s program by observing employees under treatment or having completed treatment, or by feedback directly from these employees.

need for treatment of alcohol-dependent persons (Step 2). This type of activity is known as primary demand stimulation; that is, the marketer's role is to create a demand for the good or service category. An ATM at this step would be trying to stimulate an organization to provide treatment for alcohol-dependent employees without regard for the ATM's own treatment program. It is in the next stage that an ATM would attempt to stimulate secondary demand: that is, demand for the ATM's own treatment program.

Some organizations will have fully recognized the problem (Steps 1 and 2) and have a need for information regarding alternatives, while others have already passed through the alternative awareness stage and have established a referral system or an EAP and are referring alcohol-dependent persons to alcoholism treatment programs.

Alcoholism Treatment Marketers have an opportunity to serve the needs of client organizations by making them aware of alternatives (Steps 3 and 4) and for an organization which has already reached Step 6, marketers have an opportunity to persuade the organization to switch to their program if the organization is presently referring alcohol-dependent persons to other programs. For those organizations with a referral system, but no EAP, an ATM—once it is receiving referrals—might work with the organization in helping them establish an EAP. In that case, the establishment of an EAP would follow, rather than precede the sixth step shown in Table 2. At the final stage, "Outcome/Feedback," the organization evaluates its satisfaction with the success of the treatment program(s) to which it has referred employees. Successful outcomes generally indicate continuing referrals to that program.

Buying Classes

The "Buy grid" model of the organizational buying process developed by Faris and Wind (1967) is a useful framework for summarizing the various types of situations above. Faris and Wind referred to three different types of "buy classes" or situations: new task, modified rebuy and straight rebuy. Applying the "buy class" concept to alcoholism treatment marketing provides one basis for developing buying-situation based marketing strategy. The results are shown in Table 3.

Influences on the Organizational Buying Process

Organization buying is generally considered to be more rational than consumer buying because it is driven by economic-based needs rather than by social or psychological needs. Organizations typically procure goods and services which enable them to achieve their objectives which, in the case of commercial organizations, includes the primary objective of earning profits. Although the economic motive is dominant in organizational buying, it is, as Bonoma (1982) points out, the people in the company who do the buying, not the company; and as individuals they do have some sensitivity to the emotional dimensions of the buying situation. With regard to the involvement of individuals in the buying process, there are three interrelated concepts relevant to Alcoholism Treatment Marketers. These concepts involve the buying center, buying influences, and differences in evaluative criteria used by those individuals in the buying center.

Typically several people in an organization are involved in the decision to purchase a good or service. These individuals or "buying influences" play a set of roles which essentially are the same regardless of the products or the individual people involved. Bonoma (1982) suggests that the set of roles be thought of as "pigeonholes" into which different buying influences can be placed so that marketers can better understand the process. The individuals who take on these roles in a given situation are collectively referred to as the "buying center." Haas (1986, pp. 114-115) notes that the motivations of the buying influences may differ, and Hutt and Speh (1985, p. 71) observe that members of the buying center frequently use different criteria to evaluate suppliers. Table 4 summarizes the various buying decision roles and possible motives relevant in the selection of an ATM for alcohol-dependent employees.

From Table 4, it can be seen that several different organizational functions are represented in the various decision-making roles in a new buy situation. It is possible that individuals from secretaries (as gatekeepers) to company presidents (as initiators and/or deciders)

TABLE 3. Buying-Decision Based Segments of the Organizational Market

<u>New Buy Segment</u>

Includes organizations that are progressing through the three stages and six steps of the decision process for the first time.

This segment can be further sub-segmented according to the steps in the process already reached by the organization.

<u>Modified Rebuy Segment</u>

Organizations in this segment are already referring employees/members to alcoholism treatment programs. Those ATMs who are receiving the referrals from a given organization are the "in-ATMs," the others are the "out-ATMs." An "out-ATM" can consider a strategy of persuading the organization to rethink the present solution and consider them as an alternative alcoholism treatment provider. Such efforts would focus on Steps 4 and 6 of the decision process.

<u>Straight Rebuy</u>

An "in-ATM's" marketing strategy will focus on Step 6 of the decision process. The ATM will strive to maintain its relationship with the referring organization by providing a level of treatment congruent with the expectations of the organization, and seek periodic feedback from major client sources.

will be involved in the process as members of the buying center. Through experience, an Alcoholism Treatment Marketer will learn what types of people (by their function in the organization) will typically be involved in the decision regarding the selection of an ATM. These are the individuals within the target organizations to whom the marketing efforts should be directed. For each targeted organization, an ATM will have to identify, by name, those people who hold the functional positions known typically to be involved in the selection decision. These individuals will then be the focus of the ATM's marketing efforts and during the marketing process the ATM will have an opportunity to test the assumption that these individuals constitute the buying center. Although, not shown in Table 4, the individual treatment client may have a role in the buying decision as a possible "influencer" in a rebuy or modified rebuy situation. Based on the client's assessment of treatment received from the ATM, the organization will either be reinforced in its decision to continue using the ATM, be impelled to search for another, more effective ATM (modified rebuy), or discontinue the service.

The motives which influence the individuals in the buying center tend to vary by their functional responsibility and role in the buying decision. Table 4 suggests possible motives associated with the various roles. It is important for the ATM to recognize that members of the buying center are looking at the ATM from different perspectives based on how they view the problem of alcoholism within the context of the organization. Their motivations might range from improving the personal lives of employees and their families to increasing the on-the-job productivity of their employees. Although not reflected in Table 4, the evaluative criteria used in the selection of an ATM varies among the individuals in the buying center—that is they do not all necessarily evaluate the ATM on the same basis. Possible evaluative criteria include:

—initial familiarity with or attitude toward ATM
—success rate of treatment
—average length of treatment
—cost of treatment

TABLE 4. Buying Center Example: Roles and Motives Involved in Selection of an ATM for Treatment of Alcohol-Dependent Employees

Role	Description of Role	Possible Buying Decision Motives for: Adopting An ATM's Underline
Initiator	Person who recognizes that an employee alcoholism problem can be addressed by treatment. Could be the president, personnel director, company physician or someone else in the organization.	-Improve productivity of employees -Reduce accidents -Improve welfare of employees and their families
Gatekeeper	Anyone who is able to control the flow of information about alcoholism treatment into and through the organization. Could be a receptionist, secretary, or personnel director.	-May be in favor ATM for any of the motives mentioned for the other roles -May be against the ATM

TABLE 4 (continued)

Role	Description of Role	Adopting An ATM's Underline
Influencer	Persons who have a say in whether a referral system or EAP will be established and and to which ATM referrals will be made. Could be <u>company</u> . <u>physician</u>, <u>financial officer</u>, <u>legal counsel</u>, etc.	-Improve health of employees -Decrease costs from lost-time, tardiness, absenteeism -Reduce exposure to lawsuits and claims
Decider	Person or persons who will say yes or no to the ATM's proposal. Could be the <u>president</u>, <u>personnel</u> <u>director</u>, or other person(s).	-Improve productivity of employees -Improve welfare of employees and their families

Purchaser	The person who has the authority to formally complete the arrangements with the ATM when general agreement is reached.	-May be subject to any of the motives mentioned for the other roles -May be being directed by another individual(s) in the buying center
User "Referrer"	Persons in supervisory position who are in a position to refer alcohol-dependent employees for treatment....that is the supervisor is a user of the referral system	-Improve productivity of employees -Reduce accidents -Improve welfare of employees and their families -Enhance image as a supervisor

Empirical support for the first two criteria was found in survey results reported by Kline, Self and Ingram (1987).

The significance of the buying center concept for ATMs is the recognition that the decision is a multi-individual decision – that is, it is very likely that two or more individuals within an organization will be involved in the decision process. They will play different roles, have different information needs and have different expectations regarding the services provided by the ATM. Accordingly, successful ATMs will tailor their marketing communications to address the differing motives and concerns of the individuals involved in the decision process. (See Kline, etc. in this volume.)

ORGANIZATION USAGE AND VIEWS OF ATMs

There is a paucity of information about the usage of or attitudes toward ATMs by organization clients. Two recent studies provide some meaningful information. A survey by Hewitt Associates (1986) of 293 companies dealt with the extent to which companies provide mental health benefits (including coverage for alcoholism treatment) and EAPs for their employees. Hewitt Associates found that all but one of the companies surveyed provided some form of mental health benefits – (292 companies) and specifically EAPs (136 companies) – for their employees. Table 5 provides a summary of several significant findings from the survey.

From Table 5 it can be seen that the two most frequently mentioned reasons for offering mental health coverage are because companies feel morally obligated to do so and because their competitors do. Most (91%) of the companies' programs provide reimbursement for treatment of alcohol/substance abuse, and 16% of these companies required rehabilitation in a rehabilitation group. With regard to companies with EAPs, 91% of the programs cover alcohol/chemical dependency. The prevalence of various other components of EAPs is shown in Table 5.

The results of an empirical study of 64 organizations' observations to alcohol and chemical dependency treatment facility management were reported by Kline, Self and Ingram (1987). Table 6 provides a summary of some of the results of the study which have marketing implications. Included are the views of various direct

TABLE 5. Profile of Companies Providing Mental Health Benefits or EAPs for Employees (Source: Hewitt Associates, 1986)

Mental Health Coverage (292 Companies)

- Reasons Cited For Providing: Moral Obligation (37%), Competitive Practice (35%), Cost Management for Overall Medical Plan (15%)
- 91% of the companies indicated that their employees were eligible for reimbursement for treatment of alcohol/substance abuse.
- Of those companies that cover alcohol/substance abuse, 16% require rehabilitation in a rehabilitation group, while the other 84% do not.

EAPs (136 Companies)

Components of EAPs:

Cover susbstance abuse--alcohol/chemical dependency (91%)
Company policy statement in EAPs (77%)
Formal training sessions for Supervisory/Management personnel on referral of employee to EAP (64%)
Off-site Counseling -- private provider organization (64%)
Short-Term (limited number of sessions) Outpatient Counseling (53%)
Employee Assessment & Referral only (43%)
On-Site Counseling -- Employer-based (34%)
Inpatient Hospitalization Services (26%)
EAP Advisory Committee (22%)
Long-Term Outpatient Counseling (18%)

Source: Hewitt Associates, 1986

market organizations of employer (EAPs, educators, military) and courts and attorneys.

Table 6 provides some direction to ATMs in terms of where referrals are made and the main reason for referral choice. Interestingly, organizations in all four categories – EAPs, educators, military, and courts and attorneys – choose treatment facilities primarily because of their familiarity with the treatment facility. The other significant

TABLE 6. Observations and Recommendations by Organizations to Alcohol- and Chemical-Dependent Treatment Facility Management (Source: Kline, Self, and Ingram, 1987)

	EAPs	EDUCATORS	MILITARY	COURTS/ATTORNEYS
Where Referrals Are Made To	-Social programs	-Social programs -other educators	-Social programs	-Social programs
Main Reason For Referral Choice	-Familiar with program	-familiar with program	-Familiar with program	-Familiar with program
Other Important Reason(s) For Referral Choice	-Only program available	-Better Success Rate	--------	-Better success rate
Best Promotional Tools for ATMs to Use	-Open house -Public Speeches -Direct Mail	-Personal selling -Public Speeches	-Public speeches -Open House	-Public speeches -Open house

Important Services Sought in Adult Centers	-Follow-up Program -Individual Counseling	-Follow-up program -Individual counseling	-Follow-up program -Individual counseling	-Follow up program -Family therapy
Recommendations to Management of Adult Centers	-Maintain Close relationship with patients	-------	-Lowcr costs	-Maintain close relationship with patients
Important Services Sought in Adolescent Center	-Group Therapy -Staff specially trained in treatment of adolescents	-Staff Specially trained in treatment of adolescents	-Group therapy -Individual counseling	-Staff specially trained in treatment of

reason given for the referral choice is a better rate of successful treatment. Organizations view public speeches, open houses, direct mail and personal selling as effective means of communication for treatment facility marketers. The most important services sought in adult treatment organizations appear to be follow-up programs and individual counseling. For the treatment of adolescents, organizations seek specially trained staff, group therapy, and individual counseling.

The Referral System: Influencing the Influencers

Teri A. Kline
Donald R. Self

INTRODUCTION

A growing number of alternatives exists for individuals seeking alcoholism treatment. Because of increased levels of complexity and variety in the treatment delivery system (Nakao et al., 1986), individuals seek advice or recommendations concerning treatment from those persons or organizations they consider to be knowledgeable concerning treatment alternatives. These referral sources can be categorized into two basic groups: individual reference groups and organizational reference groups. The latter group includes employers, military and educational institutions. These referral sources and their role in the referral process are discussed in detail in the preceding article in this volume.

Individual reference groups will be the focus of this article. Whether a professional referral source (physicians, counselors, social workers, clergy, etc.) or a personal referral source (family and friends), this group is characterized by their role as either a buyer, decider or influencer in the decision process to "purchase" alcoholism treatment. Which role the referent takes in the process can vary depending on the individual situation. We find some amount of coercion with all referral groups.

The referral sources can be placed on a continuum of personal to professional sources (see Figure 1), with family and friends being the more personally—and courts and attorneys as the more professionally oriented. Referral sources are generally a result of personal relationships, emotional support, health association or legal connections. Social programs also show up in the referral process,

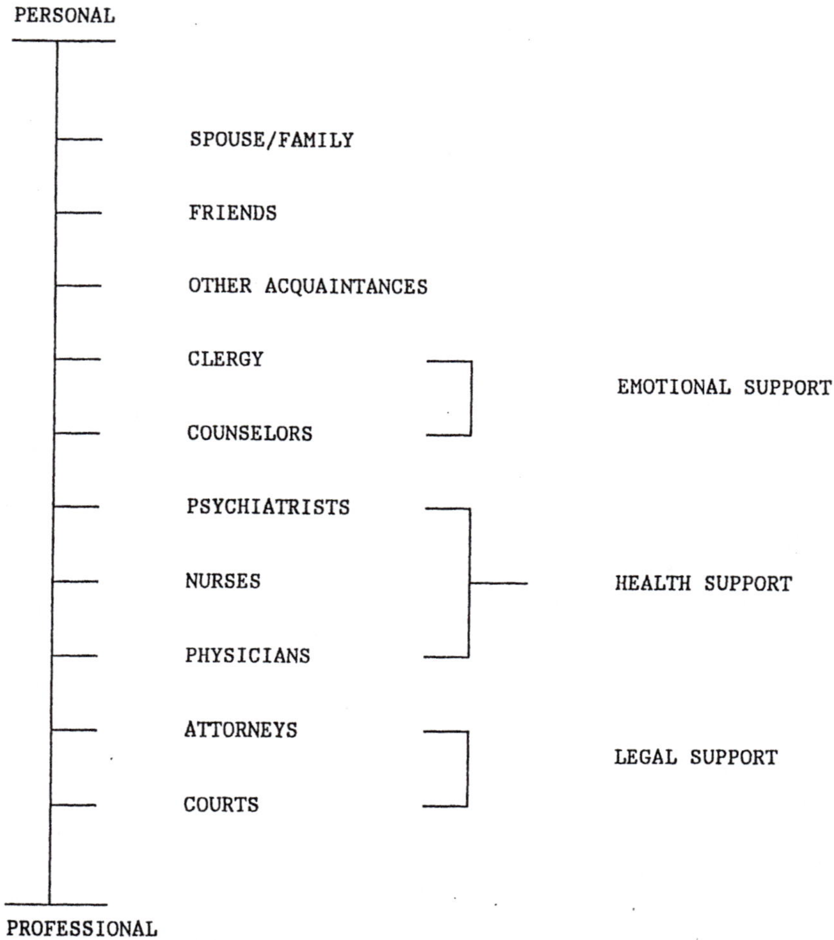

FIGURE 1. Individual Reference Group Continuum

however most often they are where the other referral sources refer potential clients for more information on alternatives (Alabama Voice, 1986). An in-depth look at each component of the continuum from personal to professional will provide a better understanding of referent groups. Much of the following primary data is from a 1986 survey of 150 referral sources. (For further analysis of these individual groups, see Self, Kline, and Ingram, 1987-88, or Kline, Self, and Jones, 1988.)

PERSONAL REFERENCE GROUPS

Family and/or spouse provide the greatest motivation to seek treatment. The intervention method (also known as confrontation or crisis precipitation) is an approach designed to work with alcoholics (or others with a chemical dependency) who deny the problem and their need for professional help. The program is designed to educate concerned others (family and friends) about alcoholism and get the alcoholic and personal referent actively involved in treatment. Intervention is conducted in an atmosphere of care and concern with factual information about the alcoholic's drinking patterns (Thorne & Baughan, 1986).

When the family has the role of convincing the alcoholic to get help, it forces them to bear the responsibility for the alcoholic getting help (Thorne & Baughan, 1986). Motivation for change must be present in the individuals *and* their families if a treatment program is to be successful (Kosnetz, 1986).

The family is an important referral source because the family often recognizes an alcoholism problem long before the patient. The spouse is usually the single most useful source in intervention (Getlon & Peyser, 1980). Peer support can also prove supportive of healthful behaviors and counteract the effects of unhealthful behavior, such as alcoholism (Gottlieb & Baker, 1986).

While family and close friends are shown to be most effective in referring the client to treatment, other personal contacts such as bartenders can serve as referral sources as well. Some hotel and eating chains train staff at manager and attendant levels to communicate effective referral procedures for patrons with excessive drinking which infringes on behavior limits of the establishment. Because a patron of a bar may establish an ongoing relationship with the bartender, the personal relationship can be used to refer the client.

PROFESSIONAL RELATIONSHIPS

Clergy, counselors, physicians and courts/attorneys are considered to be professional referral sources. The professional relationships can be further divided on the basis of those that provide *primarily* emotional support (clergy and counselors), health support (psychiatrists and physicians) and legal support (courts and attorneys).

The type of influence exercised and the success of referral may depend on the point of the continuum. At this point, the record of the helping professions in developing significant programs to confront alcoholism remains dismal (Googins, 1984).

Emotional Support

Clergy

Helping alcoholics and their families is an important facet of the ministry of counseling. The clergyman is in a strategic position to contribute significantly to the handling of alcoholism by:

a. helping bring hidden alcoholics out of hiding for help
b. creating openness to help
c. providing pastoral care and counseling with particular reference to the spiritual dimension of alcoholism
d. helping spouse and children during recovery
e. stimulating and supporting the development of community resources
f. heading the congregation in developing creative approaches to both prevention and treatment. (Clinebell in *Alcoholism* by Catnzaro, 1968)

In one study (Alabama Voice, 1986), 23% of clergy contacted reported making occasional referrals for alcoholism treatment. Most clergy refer fewer than six persons per year and most referrals are adults. The main reason clergy refer to a particular treatment program is familiarity with the program, indicating the need for informational visits to the clergy. Factors of importance to clergy are *type of facility*, *religious orientation* and *relative price*. *Individual counseling*, *family therapy* and the existence of a *follow-up pro-*

gram were also reported as important to clergy. Clergy are most likely to receive referrals from courts and attorneys and refer most often to social programs.

Because the clergy is in regular touch with many families and may be expected to call on homes without a special invitation, he or she is in a unique position to sense a potential problem. Clergy whose traditions encompass hearing confessions as a regular part of their function, have an excellent opportunity to identify hidden alcoholics.

Many people spontaneously turn to their minister when they encounter troubled times. One study found that 42% of all those who sought professional help with personal problems had gone to a minister (Gurin, 1960). The minister who is sensitive can help identify an alcoholism problem and motivate an individual to seek help.

Because alcoholism is often seen as a spiritual illness because of the spiritual factors often involved in both its cause and treatment, the clergy person can be an important work in the treatment and referral process, and should be actively contacted by the facility.

Counselors

Until the middle of the 1970s counseling was usually provided by physicians, nurses, and social workers, but in recent years increasing numbers of trained counselors have become available (Chafetz, 1983).

Of the counselors contacted in the Alabama survey (Alabama Voice, 1986), one-third make referrals for alcoholism treatment. Counselors contacted in the survey included persons listing themselves as counselors or psychologists in the Yellow Pages; most are Licensed Professional Counselors. On the average, counselors refer at least one adult to alcoholism treatment per month, with about half of the counselors contacted referring adolescents for treatment. *Familiarity with the program* and *success rates* are two of the main reasons reported by counselors for choosing a particular treatment alternative. *Group therapy*, *family therapy* and *follow-up programs* were rated as important facets to counselors, as well as *quality care* and *professional personnel*. Counselors primarily receive referrals from physicians and most often refer patients to a social program.

Health Support

Although physicians are viewed as the main referent in the health support system, psychiatrists, nurses and other health care professionals may also be important referral sources for ATMs. In one study (Potamianos et al., 1986) patients referred from psychiatric services had a greater reduction in their alcohol intake than did those from general medical services.

When compared with internists and surgeons, psychiatrists hold the most positive views on the treatability of alcoholism (Rander et al., 1987), and therefore may be more likely to make referrals. However, the most important overall referent is the general practitioner. More than half of all persons with chemical dependency and mental disorders obtain all their care from the general medical sector. In most cases the general practitioner is the first authority an alcoholic will consult (Kruse, 1985).

Because the family physician often has a pre-existing non-judgmental rapport with the patient, he or she can play a valuable role in intervention. By attending the initial intervention meeting with the client, the physician can dramatically underscore the gravity of the physical effects of continued drinking and demonstrate the depth of concern for the patient (Baughan, 1986). The family physician is in a unique position to recognize parental alcoholism, provide empathic concern for children and direct them to supportive programs (Harrigan, 1987).

While physicians are an important referral source they *may* at times actually enable a patient to remain dependent on alcohol and drugs by (1) not asking about the use of alcohol and other chemicals, (2) failing to diagnose alcoholism when its signs and symptoms are obvious, (3) failing to refer patients after the diagnosis is recorded or (4) prescribing narcotics, sedatives and stimulants. Physicians may become enablers simply through lack of knowledge or through difficulty in dealing with their own chemical dependency.

Nine out of ten physicians reported not being embarrassed in dealing with alcoholic patients, but one-third admitted that sometimes they do not take a drinking history (even when they thought they should) (Monbray & Kissel, 1986). Of the physicians contacted in the Alabama Study (Alabama Voice, 1986), 38% refer patients for treatment of alcoholism and chemical dependency. For the majority the number of patients referred is a low three to six persons per year.

Among those physicians who do refer, *success rate* of the program is the most important determinant of referral choice, although *familiarity with the program* and *method of treatment* are also important. The services physicians feel are most important are *group therapy*, *family therapy*, *individual counseling* and *follow-up programs*. Physicians stated the importance of a staff specially trained for the treatment of adolescents.

Legal Support

Courts and attorneys are the main referral sources in the legal support system. Most often persons come in contact with these referents as a result of DWI or some other legal infraction while under the influence of alcohol or drugs. While this area has the potential to be the most coercive of the referral sources cited, one study found that coerced alcoholics did no better or no worse than other alcoholics entering treatment without coercion (Flores, 1982).

In the Alabama Study, about one-fifth of the courts and attorneys contacted refer persons to treatment. However, of those who did refer, over half refer at least one person per month and one out of eight refer 50 patients or more per month. Half of the courts and attorneys listed *familiarity with the program* as their main reason for referral choice. *Family therapy* and a *follow-up program* were the most important services to the legal referents.

SOCIAL PROGRAMS

Although social programs may serve as the initial contact in the referral process, in most cases they are an intermediate referent. Other referent groups refer clients to social programs more often than any other referral source. In essence, the social program is the referral source's referral source.

In the Alabama Study (Alabama Voice, 1986), social programs tended to refer the highest number of patients referred per month for treatment compared to other referral sources. One out of five programs referred between 16-49 persons each month. As with other referral groups, *familiarity with a program* is an important determinant in referring a client. The services which social programs consider most important are *family therapy* and a *follow-up program*.

MARKETING IMPLICATIONS

An understanding of the different sources through which a person enters the alcoholism treatment process is essential for the alcoholism treatment facility. In many cases facilities have centered promotional and educational efforts on only personal referents while essentially ignoring the professional sources. The professional referents are often an important step in the treatment process. It is essential to identify those professional referral sources who are in contact with persons needing referral on a regular basis. For example, although as an overall group, courts and attorneys do not refer many clients (only 18%) a few are referring over 50 people each month.

By educating professional referents about treatment and specifically familiarizing them with the treatment facility, the client can more directly be referred to treatment (possibly bypassing referral through social programs). Time can be of the essence in translating the triggering incident into an appropriate treatment program for the chemically dependent client.

In each of the above groups, "familiarity with the program" is a key reason for referral. The reasons cited for referral and the program elements tested as important provide the basis for promotional programs aimed at the respective segments.

II. PROGRAM DEVELOPMENT, IMPLEMENTATION, AND EVALUATION

Alcoholism Treatment Philosophies and Theories: Basis for Service Strategies

William I. Sauser, Jr.
Donald R. Self

INTRODUCTION

An earlier article in this volume, "General Theories of Alcoholic Behavior," reviewed five major theoretical approaches to understanding the onset of alcoholism. As consumer behavior models, these theoretical approaches have heavily influenced the development of a number of techniques to "treat" alcoholics. These treatment techniques represent the full line of services available to the potential clients of alcoholism treatment centers.

Some treatment centers offer a variety of treatment techniques or a combination of techniques (broad product lines); some specialize in only one or a selected few techniques. However, marketers of alcoholism treatment centers should have a working knowledge of *all* available techniques, since they must be familiar with their strengths and weaknesses in order to identify and explain the competitive advantages of their own services.

The purpose of this article is to describe some of the techniques for treating alcoholics—in layman's terms—so that marketers can become more knowledgeable regarding the full line of services available from alcoholism treatment centers. There are so many individual techniques that describing them all in detail would fill volumes. Thus, the approach taken in this article is to group techniques into general categories and to discuss each category in turn. The categories of alcoholism treatment philosophies and theories reviewed in this article are (a) enforced temperance, (b) spontaneous remission, (c) crisis therapy, (d) charismatic therapy, (e) family therapy, (f) individual psychotherapy, (g) group psychotherapy, (h) aversive behavioral treatment, (i) contingency management, (j) medication, and (k) social work.

Before proceeding to descriptions of these treatment philosophies, however, it is useful to consider some of the relationships among them. The next section of this article presents a context for the descriptions of the specific philosophies. It contains a brief review of some of the classification models for alcoholism treatment techniques.

MODELS OF ALCOHOLISM TREATMENT

Four General Models of the Professional/Client Relationship

Brickman et al. (1982) classified approaches to understanding addictive behavior—such as alcoholism—based on the answers to two questions: (a) To what extent is the person held responsible for the initial development of the problem? (b) To what extent is the person held responsible for changing the behavior or solving the problem? Marlatt, Baer, Donovan, and Kivlahan (1988) describe the resulting four classifications as follows:

> Based on responses to these two attributional questions, four general models were derived: the *moral model* (person is held responsible for both acquiring and solving the problem), the *medical/disease model* (person is held responsible neither for the etiology nor for the solution), the *enlightenment model* (person is responsible for development of the addiction but is

> incapable of changing without the help of a "higher power"), and the *compensatory model* (although the person is not held responsible for etiology, change is considered to be a personal responsibility). (p. 225)

According to the *moral model*, the alcoholic is viewed as possessing a weak character, and excessive drinking is defined as a sin. Treatment approaches based on this model could be expected to be punitive; the "enforced temperance" treatment technique described below would fit into this category, as might the "spontaneous remission" approach. From the viewpoint of the *enlightenment model*, the alcoholic is also viewed as a sinner, but one who is seeking spiritual assistance in overcoming the addiction; the "charismatic" approach of Alcoholics Anonymous is based on this model. The *disease model*, heavily steeped in the tradition of the physiological/biological theories of alcoholism described in the earlier article, is the basis for the "medication" and "crisis therapy" approaches. Several of the other approaches, including "individual psychotherapy," "group psychotherapy," "aversive behavioral treatment," and "contingency management," would probably fit best into the *compensatory model*. Two approaches, "family counseling" and "social work," are based in the sociocultural theories described in the earlier article, and fit best under the biopsychosocial model described next.

The Biopsychosocial Model: Toward Multi-Determinism

In their recent review of the literature on research dealing with addictive behaviors, Marlatt et al. (1988) noted an emerging fifth model—a biopsychosocial model—which recognizes multiple determinants of alcoholism. They argue that the processes of becoming an alcoholic, then working to overcome the addiction, "appear to fall into discrete developmental stages" (p. 224). They describe their "stages of change" model as follows:

> Although terminology differs among investigators, the usual sequence includes the initiation of the addictive behavior (experimentation and the requisition of dependency), the transition to maintenance of ongoing use (sometimes called the

> "precontemplation stage"), and active change itself (attempts at reduction or cessation of addictive behavior). The behavior-change sequence (if it occurs) is further divided into three component stages: contemplation and motivation for change, active commitment to change (either self-initiated or treatment-aided), and finally postchange maintenance (successful change vs. relapse). (pp. 226-227)

Fleming's (1945) approach to treating alcoholics, described by Sugerman (1982), appears to be a pioneering treatment approach based on the biopsychosocial model. Fleming believed that alcoholics begin drinking excessively to obtain relief from symptoms of underlying physical, psychological, or social problems. Excessive drinking begets more such problems, which leads to more drinking, and eventually addiction to alcohol. Treatment consists of somehow breaking this cycle, then alleviating such medical and social problems as withdrawal symptoms, unemployment, homelessness, and poverty.

Clearly, the biopsychosocial model calls for a combination of treatments, such as crisis therapy, medication, psychotherapy, family therapy, and social work. According to this model, treatment will probably not be permanently effective until all of the problems underlying the patient's reliance on alcohol have been resolved.

The Multivariant and Multimodal Models

Sugerman's (1982) multivariant model is similar to the biopsychosocial model, but does differ in at least one regard:

> The multivariant model rejects the traditional concept of a unitary syndrome of alcoholism: that all persons afflicted are substantially the same, experience a similar progressive deterioration, and respond to a singular treatment which results in one specific outcome, abstinence. (p. 276)
>
> Since the population of individuals with alcohol problems is multivariant, treatment intervention must also be multivariant, addressing the severity of alcohol use, the particular problems and consequences of drinking, and the patient's ability to

> achieve specific treatment goals. The model recognizes that alcohol problems are usually related to other life problems, so that rehabilitation should aim at specific changes in drinking behavior suitable for each individual, and also at specific changes in problem areas of life function. (p. 227)

Sugerman's (1982) multivariant model has a major implication for marketers. In order to provide "full service," an alcoholism treatment center may need staff members or consultants or call in a variety of specialties, including medicine, psychotherapy, and social work. "Full service" alcoholism treatment centers may of necessity be similar to what Frye (1985) has described as the "multimodality" model for treating opiate addiction:

> Early multimodality programming consisted of an organized system of clinics with a central intake unit and special support units under one roof. Multimodality treatment approaches included services such as detoxification, mental health counseling, group therapy, confrontation therapy, therapeutic communities, methadone maintenance, narcotic antagonists, vocational counseling, social work, and religious counseling. (p. 175)

Indeed, Sugerman (1982) argues that current alcoholism treatment centers should be multimodal:

> Modern approaches to treatment are multimodal and multidisciplinary, so that different therapies are available to different kinds of patients, and different programs are available at different stages of the illness. (p. 263)

What treatments are available? Now that a context for understanding them has been established, below eleven major treatment philosophies and theories are reviewed.

ALCOHOLISM TREATMENT TECHNIQUES

Enforced Temperance – The Coercive Approach

The "moral model" of addiction views alcoholism as a character flaw, and its advocates generally urge alcoholics "to exercise greater will power to overcome their sins" (Marlatt et al., 1988, p. 225). Often advocates of this model will try to help alcoholics overcome their problem by pouring out or hiding alcoholic beverages, physically restraining or isolating the alcoholic, or using some other means to separate the alcoholic from ethanol. Unfortunately, since the alcoholic is rarely a willing participant in this activity, commitment to the program is weak, and the treatment rarely is effective unless combined with other approaches.

Strug, Priyadarsini, and Hyman (1986) indicate that the moral model was predominant during Prohibition: the United States' "grand national experiment" with enforced temperance. It is generally no more effective on the individual level than on the national level. The alcoholic whose liquor has been poured down the sink will seek, and generally find, another bottle somewhere. The drunk who is locked in jail will, upon release, probably get drunk again.

Spontaneous Remission

While enforced temperance generally fails due to a lack of commitment from the alcoholic, there is evidence that some alcoholics can recover on their own through self-imposed programs of abstinence (Keenan, 1984, pp. 23-25; Prugh, 1986) This has led to the concept of "spontaneous remission" – recovery without benefit of formal or institutional treatment.

Marlatt et al. (1988) comment that many individuals choose not to seek treatment for reasons of pride or fear of stigmatization. Some of them do recover, but this recovery is not necessarily "spontaneous," since many of them undergo extensive self-treatment. Marlatt et al. note:

> Self-change does not appear to be spontaneous, for a number of factors have been found to be related to the initiation of change efforts. These factors include a personal illness or accident, hitting a personal "bottom" (involving real or perceived humiliation, shame, despair, or loss), some meaningful religious experience, direct support from or intervention by family or friends, financial and/or legal problems related to substance use, or the alcohol-related death or illness of another person. (pp. 237-238)

Marlatt et al. point out that the internal motivation to change created by these external factors must be strong enough to overcome the power of the physical and psychological addiction. They comment:

> The individual must actively engage in a set of coping behaviors to maintain motivation, initially disengage from substance use, and persist in this change. Factors associated with successful self-change include public announcement, social support, alterations in one's social and leisure-time activities, general life-style changes to avoid cues that may elicit conditioned craving, strategies for coping with stress, and the generation of negative expectations of continued use and positive expectations concerning continued abstinence. (p. 238)

"Pulling oneself up by the bootstraps" is a difficult process for an alcoholic, but apparently it can be done without the aid of a formal treatment program. The treatment approaches described below are designed to help the alcoholic sustain the necessary motivation to improve, to overcome physical and psychological dependency on alcohol, and to alleviate the underlying problems which lead many alcoholics to seek comfort through excessive drinking.

Crisis Therapy

Since alcohol produces significant physiological effects, its overuse can create life-threatening situations. Sugerman (1982) comments, "The treatment of an acute episode is least controversial; it is generally agreed that this is a proper area for the application of the medical model and the use of the medications" (pp. 263-264). He notes:

> A patient in a coma after an overdose of alcohol must be treated as in serious danger of death from respiratory depression. Cardiopulmonary resuscitation may be required; the airway must be kept clear and ventilation supported if necessary. Intravenous fluids should be started and blood samples obtained to check levels of alcohol, electrolytes, blood gases and glucose, and hepatic and renal function tested. (p. 264)

In addition to coma, Sugerman (1982, p. 264) lists several other reasons for hospitalization relating to alcohol abuse. These include malnutrition, hepatic cirrhosis, polyneuropath, chronic obstructive pulmonary disease associated with excessive smoking, pulmonary tuberculosis, diabetes, heart disease, gastritis, and the most frequent reason: the alcohol withdrawal syndrome. This syndrome includes increased psychomotor activity, anxiety, tremors, sensory hyperacuity, hyperventilation, increased rapid eye movement and decreased delta sleep, hallucinations, delirium, and convulsions (Sugerman, 1982, p. 264).

Detoxification can be performed on an outpatient or inpatient basis, depending upon severity of symptoms and other factors. Treatment typically includes the use of anti-anxiety medication (such as Valium, Librium, Serax, and Ativan), careful medical supervision, daily vitamins, good nursing care, and strong psychological support (Sugerman, 1982, pp. 265-266).

Charismatic Therapy

Charismatic therapy is based upon the "enlightenment model"; alcoholics are viewed as helpless sinners who can overcome the disease of alcoholism only through spiritual assistance. Alcoholics Anonymous (AA), considered by Cohen and Callahan (1986) to be "the most potent of all sources of help for alcoholics" (p. 170), is the best-known source of charismatic therapy. Founded by a surgeon and a businessman in 1935, AA is based upon a basic set of beliefs, the "twelve steps":

1. We admitted we were powerless over alcohol—that our lives have become unmanageable.
2. Came to believe that a power greater than ourselves could restore us to sanity.
3. Made a decision to turn our will and our lives over to the care of God as we understood Him.
4. Made a searching and fearless moral inventory of ourselves.
5. Admitted to God, ourselves, and to another human being the exact nature of our wrongs.
6. We are entirely ready to have God remove all these defects of character.
7. Humbly, we ask Him to remove our shortcomings.
8. Made a list of all persons we had harmed, and became willing to make amends to them all.
9. Made direct amends to such people wherever possible, except when to do so would injure them or others.
10. Continued to take personal inventory, and when we were wrong, promptly admitted it.
11. Sought through prayer and meditation to improve our conscious contact with God as we understood Him, praying only for knowledge of His will for us and the power to carry that out.
12. Having had a spiritual awakening as the result of these steps, we tried to carry this message to alcoholics, and to practice these principles in all our affairs. (Cohen & Callahan, 1986, pp. 170-171)

Cohen and Callahan (1986) describe AA as "a unique organization: it has no organizational hierarchy: it has no officers; it owns no property; it espouses no political doctrine" (p. 170). Sugerman (1982) notes:

> The desire to stop drinking is the only qualification for AA membership. Would-be members may attend open AA meetings or contact AA in an emergency, when two members are sent as a crisis team to establish rapport, provide emotional support, help the problem drinker define his problem and clarify alternative courses of action. As in formal AA meetings the crisis team members may talk about their own personal experiences to illustrate their doubts at the beginning of their membership and how they were resolved. The potential member may identify with his rescuers and feel less unique and hopeless. He is given information on how to contact AA again. (p. 275)

Alcoholics Anonymous insists upon total abstinence as the treatment goal for all its members, yet emphasizes that an alcoholic is always recovering but never recovered. The AA member is viewed always as a potential drinker, no matter how long sobriety has been maintained. In addition to the "crisis team" approach described above, AA also holds open meetings at which members share their stories, develop new interpersonal relationships, establish role models, identify sponsors, and reinforce other members' efforts to maintain sobriety. "Help is always available, no matter how harshly the alcoholic judges himself or is judged by others" (Sugerman, 1982, p. 276).

Frye (1985) views AA as a charismatic group:

> The group members adhere to a consensual belief system, sustain a high level of social cohesiveness, are strongly influenced by behavioral norms, and impute charismatic power to the group or its leadership. The altered states of consciousness produced by charismatic therapy appear to be similar to those seen in the religious conversion experience, and relief from depression and anxiety may be experienced by the charismatic group member. (p. 177)

Maxwell (1982) claims that "continued growth is the most obvious fact" about AA (p. 295). His data "show that by the beginning of 1980 there were about 26,000 groups in the U.S. and Canada, including over 1200 groups in treatment facilities and over 1100 in correctional facilities. The total membership in the two countries was estimated to be about 800,000" (p. 295).

Armor, Polich, and Stambul (1978) comment, "Despite its very substantial membership and lengthy history, surprisingly little is known about the effectiveness of AA in a systematic way because the group has consistently avoided rigorous scientific study" (p. 35). After reviewing what research literature does exist regarding the effectiveness of AA, Glaser and Ogborne (1982) concluded that AA has not been demonstrated to be effective beyond what might be expected by chance. They found that AA was very effective for some persons, but not at all for others, and called for additional research to indicate when to use and when not to use the charismatic approach. Cohen and Callahan (1986) agreed that the AA approach might not work for everyone, but argued that it should be broadly applied:

> Attending AA regularly can be a part of every treatment regimen. Attendance appears to provide the emotional support necessary for some alcoholics to resist the strong internal and external pressures to drink. AA teaches that people should conceptualize the struggle as "one day at a time." (p. 171)

Family Counseling

Armor, Polich, and Stambul (1978) comment that, "A notable advance in the treatment of alcoholism has been the recognition that, in many cases, family interaction factors play a significant role in the chronic drinking problems of a family member" (p. 34). Family counseling is focused on reducing marital disharmony and stress; dealing with the emotional, social, and economic impact the alcoholic's behavior has on the family; and developing and integrating more adaptive coping behaviors by which the family can help the recovering alcoholic maintain sobriety.

Armor et al. claim that advances in family therapy "have led to the inclusion of family members in many alcoholism programs, either through direct family therapy or adjunctive treatment of family members (e.g., therapy for wives of alcoholics, etc.)" (pp. 34-35). For example, Al-Anon and Alateen—two groups affiliated with AA—"were created to assist family members of alcoholics to help themselves and their alcoholic parent, spouse, or relative in whatever way possible" (Cohen & Callahan, 1986, p. 171).

Walsh (1986) recently completed an outcome study of a nationally known family treatment center, and concluded:

> The results are interpreted as supporting the contention that family members are in need of psychological counseling and also support the hope that a family treatment approach can bring about a significant improvement in the emotional state of identified patient and codependent alike. (p. 393-B)

Individual Psychotherapy

Several of the general theories of alcoholic behavior discussed previously in this volume view alcoholism as the result of underlying psychological conflicts. The object of individual psychotherapy, as noted in the passage from Armor, Polich, and Stambul quoted below, is to alleviate these underlying causes.

> According to the psychodynamic and trait models, excessive alcohol consumption is a manifest symptom of underlying pathology. Treatment, therefore, is not aimed solely at the symptomatic behavior but rather seeks to uncover the intrapsychic conflicts and to achieve an ultimate care by altering the patient's basic personality structure. (pp. 28-29)

Specific Techniques

Frye (1985, pp. 176-178) has described several individual psychotherapeutic techniques which have been used to treat alcoholics, including stress management training, visual imagery, progressive relaxation, deep muscle relaxation, autogenic therapy, meditation, alpha brain wave conditioning and biofeedback, Ericksonian psychotherapy, neurolinguistic programming, cognitive-behavioral therapy, and rational emotive therapy. Armor et al. (1978, pp. 31-32) mention insight-oriented therapy, Freudian psychoanalysis, Rogerian client-centered therapy, and Transactional Analysis.

Sugerman (1982) describes the psychoanalytic approach as follows:

> The traditional psychoanalytic approach involves working backwards from the defenses—repression, denial and reactive grandiosity—to the underlying psychological conflicts. The process of therapy must uncover the unconscious conflict; it must be fully experienced in conscious awareness. The approach has not been very successful; the pharmacological effects of alcohol are too strong to be altered through insight alone, and the technique of uncovering produces anxiety which often leads to the craving to drink. (pp. 272-273)

For the reason stated above, Sugerman (1982) claims, "One of the most important principles in psychotherapy with alcoholics is that first the drinking must be terminated" (p. 273).

Group Psychotherapy

Group psychotherapy is an effective way to extend the therapeutic benefits of individual therapy. Frye (1985) suggests employing cognitive techniques such as "didactic lectures, seminars, workshops, and audiovisual presentations" (p. 178). Sugerman advocates the use of group therapeutic techniques during the post-withdrawal phase of the detoxification process:

> As the patient begins to feel well, perhaps for the first time in years, he will be ready to learn about his illness and what he must do to avoid further problems with alcohol. An inpatient unit can provide information lectures, films and discussions with a trained counselor, as well as the traditional individual and group psychotherapy, psychodrama, classes in relaxation techniques and auto hypnosis. (p. 267)

Environmental Management

Armor, Polich, and Stambul (1978) discuss the merits of "milieu" therapy, "in which the inpatient ward becomes a therapeutic community government itself, planning activities and supporting its members" (p. 30). They claim that this provision of an overall milieu of supportive communal living is also a major advantage of "halfway houses" for group therapy of recovering alcoholics:

> Recovering alcoholics in this setting are thought to experience the emotional warmth and support of a reconstituted family. Moreover, the setting provides its residents with adequate food, shelter, vocational guidance, and a structured environment. In turn, the halfway house requires continued abstinence by its residents. (p. 30)

Aversive Behavioral Treatment

Aversive behavioral treatment is based on the principles of classical conditioning as described in an earlier article in this volume, "General Theories of Alcoholic Behavior" (Sauser and Self). Aversive conditioning "involves pairing the sight, smell and taste of alcoholic beverages with an unpleasant stimulus such as electric shock or a chemical compound which induces nausea, vomiting or other distressing effects" (Sugerman, 1982, p. 269). This repeated pairing leads to a classically conditioned unpleasant response to alcohol, and the conditioned client will begin to abstain from use of alcohol in order to avoid these unpleasant conditioned effects.

Electroshock, injections of emetine hydrochloride, injections of succinylcholine (a chemical substance that induces temporary paralysis and respiratory arrest), and verbally induced aversions have all been employed within the context of aversive behavioral treatment (Armor, Polich, & Stambul, 1978, p. 33).

Frye (1985) claims that electrical and chemical aversion techniques may be difficult to apply to the typical addict. However, "covert conditioning or sensitization has gained some acceptance . . . and consists of the use of imagined scenes as aversive and rewarding events" (p. 179). Disulfiram therapy (described in more detail in the "Medication" section below) was originally designed as an aversive conditioning technique (Sugerman, 1982, p. 270).

Research on aversive behavioral treatment has been mixed. For example, Lemere and Voegtlin (1950) concluded that aversion therapy benefits mainly alcoholic patients in better socioeconomic circumstances; only occasionally does it help indigent, inadequate, psychopathic, or extremely neurotic patients. Nathan and Lipscomb (1979) found chemical aversion treatment to work well with highly motivated persons who wished to achieve and maintain abstinence;

they also concluded that electrical aversion appears to have little value of the treatment of alcoholism.

Contingency Management

Contingency management, also known as behavior modification, is based on another of the learning models described in the earlier article (Sauser and Self)—operant conditioning. The operant conditioning theory of alcoholism holds that drinking behavior is maintained because the consumption of alcohol is rewarding: It reduces tension and creates a state of well-being (Sugerman, 1982, p. 269).

Behavior modification therapy uses the principles of reinforcement to create alternatives to abusive drinking behavior. Whereas aversive conditioning employs the use of negative consequences (such as vomiting) to curb alcohol consumption, the contingency management approach employs rewards—such as a weekend pass or an enriched living environment—to reinforce sobriety or controlled drinking (Sugerman, 1982, pp. 270-271).

Specific Techniques

Frye (1985, p. 179) lists a number of techniques used by behavioral therapists, including anxiety-relief responses, assertive behavior facilitation, behavioral rehearsal, conditioned suppression, covert extinction, covert reinforcement, emotive imagery, implosive therapy, replication therapy, self-desensitization, shame aversive therapy, thought stopping, time out from reinforcement, and contingency contracting. Armor, Polich, and Stambul (1978, pp. 33-34) add to this list reinforcement through vocational activities and desensitization by reciprocal inhibition.

Sobell and Sobell's (1972, 1973; Pattison, Sobell, & Sobell, 1977) "individualized behavior therapy for alcoholics" is perhaps the best researched and best-known approach to the use of contingency management to treat alcoholism. Armor et al. (1978) describe this approach as follows:

> Essentially, this approach permits the patient to select his/her own treatment goal: either abstinence or moderate, controlled drinking. The choice is subject to review by the treatment staff. An individually tailored, stimulus-control program is then developed for each patient aimed, in the controlled-drinking case, at modifying behaviors that differ from those that are characteristic of social drinkers (e.g., gulping or ordering straight drinks are punished behaviors). In addition, the approach includes training the patient to identify the setting events for his excessive drinking and to devise and perform acceptable alternative behaviors. Patients also learn assertion techniques and behavioral repertoires that assist them in turning down proffered drinks and in ordering half-sized mixed cocktails. (p. 34)

Armor et al. (1978) describe Sobell and Sobell's approach as "highly controversial, since the specification of controlled drinking as a treatment goal is in direct contradiction to the traditional 'loss of control' model of alcoholism" (p. 34). There has been considerable research regarding the effectiveness of behavioral treatment of alcoholism. Sugerman (1982) summarizes this research as follows, "Although several elaborate studies have used behavioral therapy to teach controlled drinking to selected patients, we do not yet have enough information to enable us to select patients rationally for a program aimed at control rather than abstinence" (p. 271).

Medication

The use of medication to treat alcoholism is firmly based in the "disease model" and is typically employed by physicians. "It stresses the biological mechanisms of alcoholism with much less attention to the psychological and social. It emphasizes the use of medications such as antianxiety or antipsychotic agents and disulfiram" (Sugerman, 1982, p. 268). The use of medication to treat acute cases of alcohol abuse was described in the "Crisis Therapy" section. Medication may also be used in long-term sobriety maintenance treatment.

Armor, Polich, and Stambul (1978) describe three classes of medication which have been used to treat cases of alcoholism, typically in combination with other forms of therapy. They claim that "the most commonly used drugs in the treatment of alcoholism are the aversively protective agents, among which disulfiram (Antabuse) receives widest use in the United States" (p. 32). They describe the use of this medication as follows:

> Individuals who have ingested disulfiram and who subsequently consume even very small amounts of alcohol experience severe discomfort characterized by headache, flushing of the head and neck, rise in blood pressure, faintness, and nausea. Disulfiram is generally used as an adjunct to outpatient treatment to prevent the patient's resumption of drinking and to keep him/her available for therapeutic intervention. The efficacy of disulfiram treatment is obviously dependent on the patient's willingness to continue taking the medication. (p. 32)

The second class of drugs described by Armor et al. (1978) are tranquilizers, antidepressants, and antipsychotic compounds. "Among the most widely used are chlordiazepoxide, diazepam, meprobamate, imipramine, promazine, haloperidol, and lithium" (p. 32). These drugs are viewed as substitutes for the patient's chosen self-medication (alcohol) to treat such dysphoric symptoms as anxiety and depression.

Hallucinogenic agents, such as LSD, are the third group of drugs listed by Armor et al. (1978) as having been used in alcoholism treatment. "Such drugs are thought to disrupt the self-destructive alcoholic cycle by facilitating traumatic cathartic experiences and deep personal insight" (p. 33).

Research on the effectiveness of medication for the treatment of alcoholism has been mixed. For example, Sereny, Sharma, Holt, and Gordis (1986) found disulfiram (Antabuse) to be effective in maintaining sobriety for almost 60 percent of the 68 outpatient alcoholism clinic patients they studied. However, Fuller and Roth (1979), in their study of 128 alcoholic men, found that 21 percent of those receiving the regular dose of disulfiram and 25 percent of those receiving a pharmacologically inactive dose remained abstinent, while only 12 percent of those who did not receive the drug remained abstinent.

After reviewing the literature of research on the effectiveness of medication to treat alcoholism, Mottin (1973) reached the following conclusions:

> Consistent and extensive support does not exist in the research literature for any of the drug therapies used to reduce alcohol consumption. The research has focused on antidipsotropics (disulfiram, citrate calcium cyanamide, metronidazole), aversives (emetics, curariforms, sympathomimetics), ataractics, and hallucinogens. The deficiencies in research approaches hamper sound decision making about treatment and may also raise false hopes in patients and their families, make it more likely that potential toxicities are overlooked, and waste research and therapeutic time in duplicate studies. (pp. 444-472)

Social Work

The final alcoholism treatment technique discussed in this article is based on the sociocultural theory of alcoholism presented in the earlier article. This theoretical approach views alcohol abuse as being heavily influenced by culture and socialization, cultural stress, familial patterns, and instability and crisis in the alcoholic's social setting. Naturally, if one accepts the validity of the sociocultural theory of alcoholism, then one must advocate intervention in the cultural or social environment in order to remove the conditions which lead to alcohol abuse.

Armor, Polich, and Stambul (1978) list halfway house settings, milieu therapy, job counseling, and "alterations in fundamental social contexts" as "sociotherapies . . . derived from sociocultural models" (p. 29). Sugerman (1982) describes social work interventions which should be considered as part of a long-term treatment plan for an alcoholic:

> Marital or family problems may need to be addressed. Changes in family attitudes are very important if the alcoholic's change in lifestyle is to be maintained. If the patient is employed his job may be protected by informing his employer of his progress in treatment (this of course should only be done

with the patient's permission). If he is unemployed he may require educational and vocational training and assistance in finding work. If he is homeless or without income he should be helped to find shelter and welfare benefits. He may require legal or other kinds of professional assistance to help him return to adequate socioeconomic functioning. These are some of the many kinds of special problems which may require adjunctive help before long-term treatment can proceed. (pp. 267-268)

EFFECTIVENESS OF TREATMENT

Eleven types of alcoholism treatment philosophies, each represented by numerous specific techniques, were reviewed above. Do they work? How well do they work? Do some work better than others? Do some work with certain types of patients but not others? Are there combinations of techniques which work better than the application of a single technique? Hundreds of studies have been performed to answer these questions; some of the best reviews of this research literature include works by Baekeland (1977), Miller and Hester (1980), Skinner (1981), and Marlatt et al. (1988).

Skinner (1981) criticizes much of the outcome literature for failing to meet four basic design requirements for a technically feasible study: (a) Client types must be equally represented in alternative treatment conditions, (b) Treatment conditions must be distinct, well-defined, and controlled, (c) Multiple outcome measures must be used at several stages of follow-up (end of treatment, 6 months, 1 year, 2 years), and (d) Adequate statistical power is needed for the investigator to have a reasonable chance of detecting treatment effects.

Gottheil (1985) agrees that outcome studies prior to the 1960s "were few in number, were not well controlled, and lacked objectivity" (p. 1). However, he notes, "since that time, they have been increasing in both number and quality. The hypotheses and questions have become more precise and the research designs more sophisticated" (p. 1).

After reviewing much of this research, Baekeland (1977) found limited support of the effectiveness of outpatient treatment, Alcoholics Anonymous, behavioral psychotherapy, and drug treatment.

Miller and Hester (1980) reviewed the effectiveness literature for a number of alcoholism treatment techniques, including medication, aversion therapies, hypnosis, psychotherapy, Alcoholics Anonymous, group therapies, family therapies, controlled drinking therapies, and teaching alternative skills. Their conclusions were as follows:

> Treatment methods not supported by research to date include the use of tranquilizers, metronidazole, LSD, succinylcholine, insight-oriented psychotherapy, and routine multimodal treatment. Moreover, most treatment procedures for problem drinkers are unproved, largely due to inadequate research or inconsistent findings. Certain procedures are tentatively supported, however, even though there are questions as to whether the risks, costs, or discomfort involved outweigh the benefits. No treatment has been shown to be consistently superior to the absence of treatment or to alternative treatment in enough well-controlled studies.

Despite the lack of sufficient research to answer many of the questions posed at the beginning of this section, Gottheil (1985) has ventured to address the "bottom line" question:

> Does alcoholism treatment work? The question is put to us by patients, legislators, referring physicians, social planners, and many others. It is a simple question, and the simple answer is that it does. Experienced individuals working in the field of alcoholism indicate that treatment is helpful and that more clinicians, programs, facilities, and resources are needed to care for the large number of patients in this country with alcohol problems. After treatment many patients provide glowing testimonials about how their treatment helped them turn their lives around and saved them from skid row. A review of outcome studies reveals that the vast majority report beneficial results. (p. 1)

CONCLUSIONS AND IMPLICATIONS FOR MARKETERS

There are a variety of alcoholism treatment philosophies and theories. The first section of this article discussed some of the most commonly accepted models of alcoholism: the moral model, the medical/disease model, the enlightenment model, the compensatory model, the biopsychosocial model, and the multivariant and multimodal models. Furthermore, there is a vast array of specific treatment techniques based upon these models.

The marketer must be familiar with all of these models and techniques if he or she is to design a marketing plan based on competitive advantages of the technique or combination of techniques offered by the treatment center he or she represents. Unfortunately, the outcome research which has been performed to date does not point out many techniques with clearcut advantages over the others.

Fitting the Client to the Treatment?

In the absence of solid data upon which to base decisions regarding potential treatment effectiveness, how do treatment centers decide which technique or combination of techniques to employ? Armor, Polich, and Stambul (1978) provide an unsettling answer to this question:

> In principle, the preferred therapeutic technique used by a given facility or clinical practitioner reflects adherence to one of the general etiological models. In practice, treatment delivery for alcoholism tends to be based on one of two common policies. . . . In some treatment centers, a single modality is available (e.g., disulfiram, traditional insight therapy, etc.) and is uniformly implemented with each patient seeking help. When the patient "fits" the treatment, he is helped; if the fit between patient and therapy is not met, the effort is presumably in vain. Other treatment centers employ an opposite strategy: patients are exposed to a wide variety of treatments in . . . a "salad-like mixture." This latter approach to treatment seems to derive from the vague notion that "something" may work, in which case a certain subset of patients will be helped.

> In both treatment philosophies, there is considerable waste of resources, both human and money. (p. 29)

The Client-Centered Approach

Frye (1985) proposes an alternative to these two wasteful philosophies. His approach is based clearly in the multimodal and multivariant models:

> Treatment for addictive behavior may need to consist of a multimodality approach aimed at (1) using cognitive and behavioral modalities to achieve abstinence from the behavior or modification of that behavior, (2) using affective modalities to substitute other behaviors to help fill the void created by abstinence, and (3) using cognitive, behavioral, and affective modalities to provide skill training in altering consciousness to overcome perceived environmental impediments on a long-term basis. (p. 180)

Korcok (1985) documents a wide variety of multiple-services offerings provided by innovative ATM chains such as the Recovery Centers of America and the Republic Health Corporation. These chains offer a continuum of services, including intensive and subacute beds, structured outpatient and aftercare programs.

Marketers seeking to create a "full service" alcoholism treatment center should heed Frye's (1985) advice. Market researchers should also consider the potential of this approach for determining the best client treatment match. Since it captures the spirit of this article, Sugerman's (1982) conclusion to his overview of treatment models and methods is a fitting way to conclude this article as well:

> At the present time, the multivariant model appears to provide the most adequate conceptual approach to alcoholism treatment, and it is likely that research based on this model will provide the framework for selecting "the appropriate treatment for the appropriate patient." (p. 277)

Alcoholism Treatment Facilities: The Retailers

Teri A. Kline
Donald R. Self

INTRODUCTION

A major key to competitive action by any retailer is understanding the number of competitors, their relative size, and how they differentiate themselves from other competitors. The starting point in this analysis is the development of a classification system which will allow comparisons within a particular category. This classification system should be all-inclusive and mutually exclusive for providing comparisons among different types of retailers. From this system, appropriate strategies can be developed for location and distribution decisions, retail image and promotional strategy, service strategy, and retail pricing strategy.

The number of treatment centers in the U.S. has skyrocketed in the past few years. According to NIAAA figures, the number of treatment centers grew from 4,233 facilities in 1982 to 6,963 facilities in 1983 alone (Kim, 1986). Across the U.S., in addition to these facilities there are about 32,000 AA groups (Topolnicki, 1986). There is literally a cafeteria of choices, and picking the appropriate facility may involve a great deal of "shopping." Because of the myriad of choices available, a classification system is essential in organizing, comparing and contrasting the alternatives.

One of the primary considerations to the decider is cost, specifically whether one can afford privately funded treatment centers (which can cost as much as $20,000 for a 28-day treatment program) or whether it is necessary to use a publicly funded facility.

Common Classifications of Facilities

The location of the facility and the length of stay required are also important determinants in the purchase decision. These characteristics can be summed up in three broad categories:

1. *Outpatient*: "provision for non-residential, evaluative and alcoholism treatment services both on a scheduled and non-scheduled basis." (NIAAA, 1987)
2. *Long-term Residential (Intermediate)*: An institution that provides structured or supervised peer group living and/or limited health related services emphasizing social rehabilitation with support and guidance toward the goal of independent living and reintegration into the home, job and community for clients who have problems related to the use of alcohol.
3. *Inpatient*: "The provision of medical services and other supporting services for patients who require 24-hour supervision in a hospital or other suitably equipped medical setting for treatment of alcoholism or other problems related to alcohol use (NIAAA, 1987), generally for a period of less than one month. (NIAAA, 1987)

This classification system is developed from one described by Armor (1978), which groups treatment by the setting in which the treatment is offered. Armor describes various sub-sets of these three types of facilities.

Inpatient (Hospital Setting):

1. *Inpatient hospital*, traditional 24-hour/day service, based on a medical model but often including psychotherapy as well.
2. *Partial hospitalization*, day care in a hospital setting (not 24 hours/day), allowing the client to go home or to work at appropriate times.
3. *Detoxification*, a short "drying out" period for clients with serious toxic symptoms (e.g., delirium tremens), usually custodial in nature but occasionally including emergency medical measures.

Long-Term Residential (Intermediate):

1. *Halfway house*, a total-milieu facility providing living quarters and ancillary services (job counseling, psychotherapy, etc.) for clients in need of extended care but not requiring hospital treatment.
2. *Quarterway house*, a facility similar to a halfway house, but offering more intensive, often physical, care under more structured conditions.
3. *Residential care*, a facility providing living quarters but little or no other therapy.

Outpatient Setting:

1. *Individual counseling*, treatment sessions given by a paraprofessional (i.e., someone without a graduate degree in psychology, medicine, social work, or a similar relevant field).
2. *Individual therapy*, treatment sessions given by a professional (someone who holds a relevant graduate degree).
3. *Group counseling*, Group sessions led by a paraprofessional.
4. *Group therapy*, Group sessions led by a professional.

Although a classification system is essential for studying the facilities, most clients actually receive multiple treatments in a combination of settings (Armor et al., 1978). For example, a client may enter an inpatient facility for detoxification followed by outpatient treatment.

This grouping of facilities is simple and describes almost all treatment scenarios. The system used by the NIAAA broadens these categories but adds confusion to the system. The NIAAA Classification System also includes broad categories of Emergency and Intermediate Care. Emergency care may be handled by any type of facility although it is handled primarily through inpatient treatment programs. Since emergency care tends to be of a "temporary" nature and most often results in referral to a "total" treatment program, it is not included as a separate category. Intermediate care,

> the provision of care in a full residential or partial treatment setting or partial residential treatment setting for patients who have need of more intensive care and treatment than is available through outpatient settings or who, although not seriously debilitated, would benefit from supportive living arrangements (NIAAA, 1987)

may fall into either inpatient or residential treatment. Therefore this area also is not included as a separate category.

METHOD OF RESEARCH

Few definitive studies are available on which to draw broad conclusions concerning differences among the various types of facilities. The information in this article is based on both a literature review of treatment facilities and their services and a survey of the 65 treatment centers listed with the Alabama SHPDA as of 1985. The survey was conducted in 1986 by in-depth telephone interviews with the manager or director of each treatment facility. The information reported below is admittedly not all-inclusive, but adds various bases for comparison.

TYPE OF FACILITIES

General Information

While it has been noted that there is a growing number of alcohol and drug abuse treatment programs, it is not necessarily true that there is growth in every type of treatment. Various studies show different concentrations of programs at various times and among various samples. One study of hospitals responding to annual surveys in 1975-80, shows decreasing inpatient and increasing outpatient services for alcoholism and chemical dependence. Possible reasons cited are the changing economics of health care and patient preference (Knowles, 1983). According to Diesenhaus (1982), the number of freestanding detox and rehabilitation facilities has also increased. A lack of resources for treatment and inequalities in distribution of services to indigent populations exists, despite the growing availability and accessibility of treatment services and the increases and refinements of available options. Much of the inequality of distribution can be attributed to a lack of availability of first and third party reimbursement (Diesenhaus, 1982).

There are a wide variety of studies indicating little definitive evidence that any one treatment or treatment center is better than another. In comparing inpatient and outpatient care alone, there is little evidence for the superiority of either method, although continuing aftercare as an adjunct to short term intensive rehabilitation appears to be important (Korcok, 1985).

Many facilities have not opted for providing only one type of care, but instead have adopted a continuum of care similar to the diversification practiced by many retailers in other fields. This philosophy seems to be the emerging approach, especially among hospital based programs.

CLASSIFICATION BASED ON LOCATION AND LENGTH OF STAY

Outpatient

Outpatient facilities include: Alcoholism Day Programs; HMO Outpatient Alcoholism Centers; Industrial Alcoholism Clinics; Hospital Based Outpatient Clinics; Free Standing Outpatient Alcoholism Clinics; Community Mental Health Centers (NIAAA, 1987).

The "typical" outpatient facility in Alabama has a usage rate of 91-100% of the total capacity and has been in business for at least eight years. The staff at outpatient facilities typically includes one doctor, one nurse, three counselors and one or two administrative/support persons. However, it is not likely to have a public relations/marketing person or a teacher. The vast majority of outpatient facilities are publicly funded (Alabama Voice, 1986).

Not all patients can or will commit themselves to residential or inpatient treatment, and about 90% of alcoholics or drug addicts who receive professional treatment do so on an outpatient basis. Not all patients can or will commit themselves to residential or inpatient treatment. The flexibility of outpatient services allows the patient to maintain a job and other responsibilities in the home and community. For these reasons, outpatient treatment can be an attractive alternative (Knowles, 1983; Kirn, 1986; Battegay & Ladewig, 1986), and can become a major thrust in promoting the facility. There is evidence to suggest a favorable outcome under the "day hospital" or outpatient condition (Penk, Charles, & Van Hoose, 1978).

Limits to the Client Base

Several potential problems exist with treatment on an outpatient basis, particularly if detoxification and withdrawal are factors (Battegay & Ladewig, 1986). Success in such programs is dependent on the patient's active participation, continuous feedback and individualized treatment objective(s) (Ojehagan & Berglund, 1986).

Long-Term Residential Facilities (Intermediate)

This group includes the halfway house/recovery house although some quarterway houses may be included as well. Halfway houses provide extended care for people who would be especially likely to slip back into their old ways after a standard 30-day inpatient program. Normally, halfway house residents attend lectures and group therapy at separate outpatient clinics (Topoinicky, 1986). The basic concept of such a facility is the creation of a support environment for the addict, "a man particularly sensitive and vulnerable at the point of discharge from custody to the harsh imperatives of the outside world" (Geis, 1974). The need for such a facility is predicated on the observation that a high percentage of addicts revert to chemical dependency within the first six "post-institutionalization" months (Kaplan & Meyerowitz, 1969), and they may be required for individuals who are.

In one study where residents of a halfway house were required to be employed, to be responsible for their own meals, to pay room rent, and to continue to attend weekly group therapy meetings and to maintain social interaction, 58% of the residents were sober after 25 months (Stanhope, Gihlhaar, & Florio, 1986). In the same study 62% of the residents were employed after the two-year period. Although the halfway house experience may not totally eliminate subsequent drunkenness, it does tend to integrate residents into the healthcare network and encourage them to seek available services on their own (Annis & Liban, 1979).

The success of the halfway house as a model of treatment is contingent on factors such as location, types of residents, program leadership and various aspects of the therapeutic approach (Geis, 1974).

The typical long-term residential treatment center in Alabama has 20 adult beds, an occupancy rate of 90-100%, and has been in the business for over 12 years. The staff for treatment centers is made up primarily of administrative personnel along with one custodian. Very few long-term residential programs have a doctor, public relations person, or a teacher. Some programs employ counselors and nurses. Virtually all long-term residential facilities are publicly funded (Alabama Voice, 1986).

Inpatient Facilities

According to the NIAAA classification, all hospital based (general and specialized) and free standing programs with short-term residence are included in this category. This is the broadest classification with the most treatment options, but there is a common characteristic among the facilities of specialized emergency or intermediate medical care (NIAAA, 1987).

Although outpatient usage has increased dramatically, the use of inpatient care is still considered the traditional approach to mental health treatment (Pokorny, 1984). The majority of treatment centers are still offering 30-day Alcoholics Anonymous based inpatient treatment (Kirn, 1986).

Most inpatient clinics charge $100 to $300 a day for typical 21- to 28-day stays. Generally, insurance reimbursement for inpatient care is limited to 28 or 30 days per year long benefit period, with a lifetime cap of two benefit periods (Topolnicki, 1986).

There is considerable controversy surrounding length of stay. In a study comparing a two-week stay versus a seven-week stay, there was significant improvement on all drinking and non-drinking criteria (Walker, 1983). However, outcome following the two-week and the seven-week programs did not differ significantly, suggesting the value of briefer hospitalization when accompanied by aftercare. Annis et al. (1978) also found that inpatient programs lasting a few weeks to a few months show no higher success rates than do periods of brief hospitalization of a few days. Moreover, day treatment programs produce equal or superior results to inpatient hospitalization at one-half to one-third the cost.

Other studies which question the superiority of the inpatient treatment method include:

- 26 controlled comparisons consistently showing no advantages for longer over shorter inpatient programs. (Miller & Hester, 1986)
- Stressful conditions in the hospital are often worse than in the home. The hospital is an artificial environment and as such is no place to try to understand the patient's everyday difficulties. Furthermore, dissatisfaction with longer inpatient care is especially widespread with recognition of the effects of institutional isolation and loss of social role. (Porkorny, 1984)
- Controversy exists about the cash benefit value of continuing to invest in primary treatment of alcoholism in general and in psychiatric hospital inpatient units. (Diesenhaus, 1982)

This type of treatment program is the "new kid on the block" in Alabama. On the average, inpatient facilities have been in business less than five years. The average number of beds is 25 with an occupancy/usage rate much lower than outpatient or residential facilities (61-80%). Inpatient treatment facilities report having the largest number and variety of staff positions. On the average, personnel include at least one doctor, three or more nurses, one public relations/marketing person, three administrative positions, at least one custodian, three or more counselors and often at least one other employee. Inpatient facilities in this study were three times more likely to be privately funded than publicly funded (Alabama Voice, 1986).

CLASSIFICATION BASED ON FUNDING

The most dramatic increase in the alcohol and chemical dependency treatment units has been in the private sector. In the five-year period from 1978-83 the number of for-profit units with alcohol treatment centers increased by 290% and bed capacity by 368%, compared to a smaller increase in not-for-profit units with alcoholism treatment centers of 71% and an increased bed capacity of 99%. In 1978 only 5% of the nation's alcohol and chemical dependence treatment units were investor-owned for-profit units. By 1983 that number had increased to 16% (Korcok, 1985). Traditionally, much of the alcoholism treatment came from public, non-profit centers but there is a significant shift to treatment in private for-profit facilities.

Public Funding

One survey of patients treated at an outpatient facility of state supported alcoholism programs showed that only 20% of the patients attended the clinic for 10 or more visits, or continued to keep appointments as long as six months after the initial visit. One-third continued to be drinkers, one-third became abstinent or controlled drinkers, and the outcome was unknown on the remaining patients (Gerard & Saenger, 1966).

In Alabama there are slightly more public facilities than private facilities. The greatest number are outpatient, although nearly one-third of the public facilities are long-term residential (intermediate) units and another third are inpatient facilities. The typical public facility in Alabama has 14 beds and an occupancy rate of 86-100%. Public facilities have been in business between 6 to 20 years—on the average over 10 years. The personnel in public facilities consists of one nurse, two administrative persons, one custodian, two counselors and possibly one other employee. These facilities are not likely to have a public relations or marketing person or a teacher. Since the largest number of public facilities are long-term/residential care facilities, very few adolescents (who would need a teacher on premises) utilize the facility type (Alabama Voice, 1986).

Private Funding

The typical approach used by private facilities attempts to avoid the "One Flew Over the Cuckoo's Nest" image of mental hospitals. Patients' rooms do not look like hospital but rather hotel rooms (Gubernick, 1985). These private facilities tend to attract those persons with greater financial resources. Persons of high social status, even those with severe drinking problems, can contact private, less publicly visible and less stigmatizing services (Fitzgerald & Mulford, 1981).

The typical private facility in Alabama has 15 beds and an occupancy rate (50%) much lower than that of the public facility. Typically the private facility has been in business less than three years. The personnel at public facilities include two doctors, three or more nurses, one public relations or marketing person, at least two administrative persons, three counselors, and one other employee. These facilities are not likely to employ custodians since many are housed in hospitals and receive custodial services from the hospital facility. Only the adolescent units are likely to have a teacher (Alabama Voice, 1986).

PROGRAMS AND SERVICES OFFERED

By Facility

The services offered by facilities can best be distinguished by viewing the location and type of treatment program used. While there are some programs and services offered by practically all treatment centers (such as group therapy and individual testing) there are many other services that are typically offered only by a particular treatment center setting.

Inpatient Facilities

Overall, inpatient facilities tend to offer a wider array of services. Over half of the inpatient facilities surveyed in Alabama offer medical detox, social detox, short-term rehabilitation, lab facilities, radiology, lectures, group therapy, individual testing, psychological testing, family therapy, reading groups, physical recreation, meetings, speakers and family accommodations. In one study of an inpatient facility, telephone skills appropriate for contacting potential employers to obtain job interviews were effectively taught to unemployed alcoholics (Harris et al., 1986).

Long-Term Residential Facilities (Intermediate)

The treatment components prevalent in all residential facilities in Alabama include group therapy, individual testing, evening meetings, speakers and family accommodations. One study shows positive effects as a result of these components, but questions still arise about the correlation between length of stay and level of success. Longer stays have been associated with better posttreatment functioning within the halfway house program (Finney, Moos, & Chan, 1981).

Outpatient Facilities

Outpatient facilities focus primarily on individual testing, group therapy, family therapy and educational lectures. One model studied consisted of evening and weekend treatment of alcoholism in the workplace, and was based on six major concerns:

1. The individuality of alcohol cases
2. The inavailability of annual/sick leave
3. The question of re-entry into the work force after a 28-day absence
4. Insurance coverage
5. Children of single parents and the lack of treatment facilities provision of accommodation for children
6. The interdependence of EAPS and the treatment programs. (Masi, 1983)

Outpatient treatment is not only a growing segment in the U.S. market but internationally as well. A day care center for alcoholics was established in India in 1980 in the belief that alcoholism is a treatable disease. The program offers a three-phase program including detoxification, intensive 21-day outpatient program and aftercare (including attendance at Alcoholics Anonymous) (Cherian, 1986). In West Germany, local funding for outpatient facilities increased during the period from 1980 to 1985. Nearly all patients are counseled through either group therapy, individual therapy, marriage/family counseling, or counseling care of friends and relatives (Simon et al., 1986).

Specific Services

Group Therapy

Group therapy is probably the most advanced therapeutic method employed in the management of alcoholics (Burian, 1985). Practically all facilities surveyed in Alabama offer group therapy (Alabama Voice, 1986). Despite the diversity of techniques available for group therapy, there are commonalities including group size (five to ten members), a leader or therapist, and members seated in a circular pattern so that everyone can see and react to everyone else. Participants generally receive advice and guidance not only from the therapist but other group members as well. Typically, group members experience relief from knowing they share common adjustment difficulties (Milkman & Sunderwirth, 1987). Talking in the therapy sessions helps show patients that the experiences of which they are often ashamed of are, in fact, well known to both therapist and other patients. This experience assists in relieving the discomfort of patients disclosing experiences (Luderer et al., 1986).

Family Therapy

There is a growing interest in the inclusion of family therapy in treatment of alcoholics. In one 1964 study cited (Regan et al., 1983) only 2% of the treatment programs included family counseling. In the 1986 Alabama study, as many as 91% of the inpatient facilities, 89% of the outpatient facilities and 82% of the residential facilities included family counseling in the treatment program (Alabama Voice, 1986).

The stress caused by alcoholism can have devastating effects on the whole family so the emphasis on engaging the family in the recovery program is important (Kirn, 1986). Spouses tend to be the most likely recipient of such family treatment according to a study in Massachusetts. Children were much less likely to be involved in family treatment. Such treatment for children was most likely to occur in outpatient settings (Regan et al., 1983).

In one study (Honig & Spinner, 1986), treatment of spouses is viewed as essential whether or not the alcoholic is in treatment. Carlson (1986) states, "The treatment of the family is essential since a client cannot be expected to stay well in a sick family environment." Such treatment helps the spouse to lead an independent, productive and gratifying life. While spouse participation is effective in helping alcoholics decrease their drinking, those situations including alcoholics found spouse involvement plus behavioral marital therapy resulted in clients who were more compliant with homework assignments, decreased their drinking more quickly during treatment, relapsed more slowly after treatment and maintained better marital satisfaction (McCrady et al., 1986).

Outpatient programs which include family therapy have several advantages: re-entry into the real-world is easier; the family realizes their importance in the treatment process, there is the realization that leading a sober lifestyle is difficult and the patient can begin immediately to attend AA meetings in the community (Wegschneider, 1986).

A two pronged approach may be used to involve the family. First, there is an education process with the goal being to give families a sense of support to motivate them to use community resources. Second, there is the provision of family assessment and therapy services (Whitley & Zankowski, 1986).

Lectures/Education

Educational methods such as lectures and videotapes are used at various stages of the referral and treatment process. They may be used upon admission as reported by Stockman (1987), where male clients diagnosed as alcoholics admitted for trauma to a general hospital were shown a videotape depicting conversations among recovering alcoholics; 6% of the subjects sought professional treatment and an additional 27% reported abstinence or reduced consumption. There were self-reported rates of improvement higher than would be expected from natural remission, but rates of help-seeking did not exceed those of a national sample of alcoholics.

Educational programs are used as part of an inpatient program, sometimes with mixed results. Janke and Young (1986) reported that while participation in an eight-hour program did improve self-esteem, there was no reported increase in "alcohol knowledge scores."

Staff/Physical Environment

The physical environment and the staff at a facility may impact the client's perception of the treatment. Environmental features should be designed to incorporate spatial design concepts to match the treatment philosophy (Corey et al., 1986). One designer who specializes in health facility planning, programming and design seeks to develop conditions to:

1. attract users to the facility
2. make the user feel good at the facility
3. make the user want to return to the facility, and
4. encourage the user to talk up the facility within their own personal network. (Ruga, 1984)

Substance abusers are more likely to be attracted to a treatment program or facility which has their ethnic peers on its staff. While ethnic programs do not appear to have better treatment outcomes among its patients than do majority or non-ethnic programs, they do attract more minority people into treatment and thus help larger numbers of particular ethnic groups served (Westermeyer, 1984).

Characteristics suitable for other types of counseling activities are not necessarily optimal for alcoholic and addiction counselor (Thrower & Tyler, 1986).

CHARACTERISTICS OF CLIENTS

Age

The average age of clients tends to be higher at inpatient facilities than either outpatient or long-term residential facilities (Alabama Voice, 1986). Inpatient facilities are also the most likely to have specialized adolescent treatment available. Inpatient treatment is most effective in the short-term reduction of alcohol and other drug use among adolescents, but also has the potentially negative effect of increasing deviant identity. According to Moberg (1986), outpatient treatment results for adolescents are negligible. While short-term intervention may reduce levels of deviant identity, there are no significant effects of behavior.

Sex

Long-term residential and inpatient facilities in Alabama have more male clients than female clients while the typical outpatient programs on the average report an even number of male and female clients (Alabama Voice, 1986). Outpatient clinics allow women who are not able to take a month off from family duties in order to go through inpatient programs to still receive alcoholism treatment. The association of sex with incidence of admission to a hospital emergency department for self poisoning shows higher blood alcohol levels in female clients on weekdays and males on weekends. According to Varadaraj and Medonca (1986) blood alcohol levels of women arriving during high-risk times of 11:00 p.m.-7:00 a.m. were significantly higher than those of women arriving at other times.

Ethnic Background

Most treatment centers in Alabama report that the majority of their clients are white. Public facilities report more non-white clients than private facilities, and long-term residential facilities are the most likely to have black clients, although over half of the long-term residential facilities have more white clients than black clients (Alabama Voice, 1986).

There are programs in some geographic areas aimed at specialized ethnic groups. For example, in Los Angeles, California, one local hospital serves the Hispanic community through its Spanish language interdisciplinary team-inpatient program (Zepeda, 1986).

Socio-Economic Background

Private facilities in Alabama tend to attract more middle income clients while publicly funded facilities attract the lower income clients. Generally, inpatient facilities have more middle income clients while outpatient and long-term residential programs attract a client with a lower income (Alabama Voice, 1986).

Anonymous treatment was found to appeal to those clients with a high educational and professional level and with a high degree of familial and social adaption (Gulyamov, 1986). Such anonymity is more likely in a private facility.

Korcok (1986) reports that outpatient treatment is especially effective for alcoholics who are married, employed, socially stable, and have experienced only a few years of drinking.

Long-term residential facilities tend to receive a disproportionate share of clients of low socio-economic status. There is also a tendency for the hospital-only category (inpatient) to receive few of the disadvantaged clients. This could indicate a pattern in which relatively advantaged clients (who may tend to have a better initial prognosis) successfully complete inpatient treatment (Armor et al., 1978). Such a trend has implications in a comparison of success between types of facilities and persons of various socio-economic backgrounds. Fitzgerald and Mulford (1981) reported that persons identified as problem drinkers who did not contact one of Iowa's public alcoholism clinics had more education, higher incomes, and higher occupations than those who did, and were also less advanced in the alcoholism process.

GEOGRAPHIC DISTRIBUTION

Outpatient, long-term residential and inpatient facilities in Alabama are receiving the majority of their patients from an area local to the facility. However, outpatient facilities draw the largest percentage of patients from the local area. This situation is logical since the patients must travel to the center on a regular basis.

Long-term residential facilities are more likely to pull clients from outside the local vicinity of the center. Inpatient facilities obtain clients primarily from local immediate areas and areas within the state boundaries, although like long-term residential centers, these facilities may pull a small number of clients (10% or less) from outside the state.

TABLE 1. Distribution of Facilities in Alabama by Classification Characteristics

		Funding Method		
	n = 65	Public	Private	Total
Location and Length of Stay	Outpatient	22%	6%	28%
	Long-Term Residential	17%	-0-	17%
	Inpatient	15%	40%	55%
	Total	54%	46%	100%

TABLE 2. Characteristics of Facilities: Classified by Location/Length of Stay

n = 65	Outpatient n = 18			Residential n = 11			Inpatient n = 36		
	Mean	Median	Mode	Mean	Median	Mode	Mean	Median	Mode
Number of Adult Beds	3.7	0	0	23	11-20	11-20	25	11-20	11-20
Occupancy Rate	73%	91-100%	91-100%	90%	91-100%	91-100%	62%	61-80%	61-80%
Years in Business	8.4	6-10	11-20	12.4	11-20	11-20	4.6	3-5	0-2
Personnel:									
Number of Doctors	.89	1	0	.27	0	0	1.7	1	1
Number of Nurses	1.3	0	0	.82	0	0	3.3	5 or more	5 or more
Number of P. R. People	.61	0	0	.45	0	0	1.14	1	0
Number of Admin. Personnel (Including Secretaries)	1.64	1	1	3	3-4	3-4	2.8	3-4	3-4
Number of Custodial Employees	.5	0	0	.73	1	1	1.58	0	0
Number of Counselors	2.9	2-4	2-4	.91	0	0	3.36	2-4	2-4 and 5 or more
Number of Teachers	.055	0	0	.0	0	0	.21	0	0
Number of Other Employees	1.44	1	0	.82	0	0	.94	0	0

NOTE: Calculation of Mean by Grouped Data by Direct Method

TABLE 3. Characteristics of Facilities: Classified by Method of Funding

	Public n = 35			Private n = 30		
N = 65	Mean	Median	Mode	Mean	Median	Mode
Number of Adult Beds	13.9	11-20	0	15.33	11-20	21-50
Occupancy Rate	86%	91-100%	91-100%	52%	41-60	41-60
Years in Business	10.7	6-10	11-20	2.9	0-2	0-2
Personnel:						
Number of Doctors	.71	0-1	1	1.93	1	2-4
Number of Nurses	1.34	1	0	3.1	5 or more	5 or more
Number of P.R. People	.57	0	0	1.23	1	1
Number of Admin. Personnel (Including Secretaries)	2.61	2	1 and 3-4	2.38	2	1
Number of Custodial Employees	1.4	1	0	.53	0	0
Number of Counselors	2.29	2-4	0	3.1	2-4	2-4
Number of Teachers	.07	0	0	.2	0	0
Number of Other Employees	1.17	0	0	.93	0	0

TABLE 4. Programs and Services Offered by Facilities (% Offering Services)

	OUTPATIENT	RESIDENTIAL	INPATIENT
Medical Detox	28%	18%	83%
Social Detox	22%	18%	58%
Short term Rehabilitation	45%	46%	61%
Long term Rehabilitation	50%	67%	33%
Lab Facility	11%	9%	61%
Radiology	11%	9%	61%
Lectures	89%	73%	91%
Group Therapy	95%	100%	97%
Individual Testing	100%	100%	97%
Psychological Testing	66%	64%	86%
Family Therapy	89%	82%	91%
Family Accommodations	16%	100%	53%
Reading Group	27%	82%	81%
Physical Recreation	22%	64%	94%
Evening Meetings & Speakers	50%	100%	89%

TABLE 5. Characteristics of Patients

	OUTPATIENT	RESIDENTIAL	INPATIENT
Number of Adults (1985)	101-200	51-100	101-200
Number of Adolescents (1985)	0	0	0
Total Number of patients (1985)	101-200	51-100	101-200
Age (in years)	19-35	19-35	36-55
Sex of Most Patients	1/2 Male-1/2 Female	Male	Male
Ethnic Background of Most Patients	White	White	White
Income	Lower	Lower	Middle
Avg % of Local Patients	81-100%	41-60%	61-80%
Avg % In-State Patients/Not Local	0-10%	41-60%	21-40%
Avg % of Out of State Patients	0	1-10%	1-10%

The (Un)Finished Product: Measurements of Satisfaction and of Recidivism for Former Alcoholism Treatment Clients

Donald R. Self
Robin S. McCullin
Teri A. Kline

INTRODUCTION

The "end-product" of alcoholism treatment is the return of the client to a life-situation that is "satisfactory." In analyzing the success of a program, it is important to establish measurements of success or satisfaction. An examination of the satisfaction of alcoholism treatment clients actually reveals the existence of various definitions and measures of satisfaction. The three common models used to explain recovery and relapse for alcoholism are the abstinence model, the controlled drinking model, and the biopsychosocial dysfunction (ability to cope with life situations) model. Emrick (1974), in a review of 384 psychologically oriented studies spanning 1952-1973, found that self-reported drinking behavior was the major criterion in 80% of the studies, followed by work, family relations and outpatient treatment. Other outcomes include affective-cognitive symptoms, work, home relations, physical conditions, arrests, social situations and Alcoholics Anonymous (AA) attendance. Many of the measures currently used to gauge success overlap, and some are contradictory. In addition, measures of success also are affected by whose judgment determines success: the treatment center, the client, the client's family, the client's employer or third-party payer.

A second area to be examined concerns the effectiveness of treatment and those variables which impact upon treatment success. Treatment may be more successful in some treatment situations and less successful in others. Additionally, certain groups of people are more likely to experience recovery than others. Spontaneous recovery (an individual recovers from alcoholism without undergoing formal treatment) also happens in some cases. Finally, difficulties in measurement of treatment will be examined concerning the impact on research studies and results.

An area related to satisfaction is recidivism, which involves alcoholic clients returning to drinking and experiencing problems with alcohol after undergoing some type of treatment program.

MEASURES OF SATISFACTION – WHAT IS SUCCESS?

The most prevalent measures of satisfaction for former alcoholism treatment clients are abstinence and controlled drinking. Subsets of these measures of satisfaction include behavioral impairment and social functioning.

Abstinence

Abstinence has long been accepted as the standard measure of success or satisfaction for a client undergoing alcoholism treatment and is the traditional measure of successful outcomes in disease model programs. The abstinence approach, based on the philosophy of Alcoholics Anonymous, is the primary method of treatment for alcoholism in the United States today (Keenen, 1984). Historically, treatment centers have been evaluated primarily in the abstinence rates of their clients, and today, the majority of treatment centers are still offering 30-day abstinence, Alcoholics Anonymous based inpatient treatment (Kim, 1986). With this perspective, if patients use alcohol they are said to be in relapse. If not, they are said to be in recovery (Gorski, 1986).

Abstinence based programs involve removing the toxic product. An underlying assumption of this approach is that recovery is never totally achieved. Further, thinking about using alcohol and the return of the compulsion to use it are viewed as relapse warning signs (Gorski, 1986). Many patients will experience initial problems with sexual dysfunction, trust, and dysphoria when they become abstinent so many experts maintain (see Knott, 1986 for example) that abstinence should be achieved as soon as possible and maintained during treatment to minimize the length of time in which these negative by-products may impair the ability to function.

Emrick (1974) reports in his survey of the literature that typical results showed abstinence rates between 10% and 53% and total improvement between 48% and 84% of the sample treated. In general terms, two-thirds were improved or abstinent. These findings are fairly consistent with later research.

Limitations and Opposition

Although in widespread use, abstinence as a model has limitations in that it excludes a variety of factors other than alcohol use that significantly affect recovery and relapse (Gorski, 1986). Pattison (1966) initiated a great deal of controversy by concluding that abstinence as a necessary condition for successful treatment is an overstatement and abstinence as a criterion of successful treatment is misleading because it may be maintained at the expense of total life functioning. Further, abstinence may in itself present problems for the reformed alcoholic. Some evidence suggests that the abstinent alcoholic may be subject to periodic episodes of fatigue and depression and that enforced abstinence may have disastrous results for the personality organization of some people. In their review of the literature, Heather and Robertson (1981) conclude that "abstinence and improvement in life functioning exhibit a low correlation and abstinence may introduce psychological or sociophysiological problems that make relapse more likely."

Brandsma, Maultsby and Welsh (1980) summarize the problems or limitations associated with using abstinence as a criterion of success. These include (1) the fact that patient denial makes this a less reliable measure than occupational stability or legal troubles, (2) patients improve in some areas of functioning but not in others as a result of treatment, (3) abstinence is not necessarily related to other areas of life improvement, (4) despite mythology to the contrary (i.e., loss of control theory) some alcoholics become normal drinkers, and (5) drinking status has been shown to be highly variable in longitudinal studies. Brandsma et al. (1980) conclude that multifactorial outcome measures should be employed without an overreliance on any single one.

Controlled Drinking

Davies (1962) represents the first major departure from a total abstinence based program or treatment goal in his report of normal drinking in a small number of recovered alcohol addicts. Seven out of 93 alcohol addicts were found on follow-up to have been drinking socially for continuous periods of seven to eleven years after discharge from inpatient alcoholism treatment programs. All were socially better adjusted than they had been for a year before admissions. Further support for a controlled drinking treatment outcome comes from Sobell and Sobell's (1978) research which compared 20 alcoholics trained to drink moderately by behavioral methods with 20 who received conventional abstinence oriented treatment. They found that after two years the controlled drinking group was significantly improved on the number of days functioned well criteria, and were described as having successfully achieved and sustained social drinking.

Heather and Robertson (1981) add support to this view by reporting studies which show that normal drinking among recovered alcoholics is possible and that signs of loss of control and craving are no longer irreversible properties of the alcoholic's drinking behavior. They further assert that a controlled drinking treatment goal may be advantageous in the sense that adoption of total abstinence is a deviant role that might attract other social living problems.

The first Rand report (Armor, 1976), citing conclusions drawn from a study of 1,340 alcoholic males, indicated that certain alcoholics might be able to control their drinking. This report, however, drew widespread criticism because of the manner in which the data was obtained, i.e., the use of self-reports of drinking behavior with no validity check.

Controlled drinking as a feasible treatment goal for selected clients was reported by Rush and Ogborne (1986) to be used by 36.7% of all alcohol programs reviewed. Endorsement of nonabstinent goals was lowest for detoxification centers and residential treatment services and highest for nonresidential programs and assessment referral services. Endorsement of nonabstinence goals was higher among programs aimed at young people and those associated with the criminal justice system.

Limitations and Opposition

Criticism, however, has been leveled at the appropriateness of controlled drinking as a treatment outcome. Pendery, Maltzman and West (1982) assert that "a very considerable discrepancy exists between the Sobell's papers and that of Pendery et al." Of the 16 subjects who originally fulfilled criteria for gamma alcoholics, 13 had been rehospitalized within one year of completion of their social drinking training and the remaining three out of the 16 abused alcohol over the three years following treatment. Further, they contend the cases of apparent success of controlled drinking appear to be related to treatment of alcohol abusers who were not exhibiting physical dependence. In addition, Helzer (1985), in a follow-up of 1,289 alcoholics, reports that only 1.6% of them were able to maintain a moderate drinking level.

The second Rand report (Polich & Braiker, 1980) contained information obtained on 85% of the original 1,340 men in the original Rand survey and is regarded as the most extensive study made in terms of the number of alcoholics traced and the length of the follow-up. This study in essence contradicts the first Rand report (1976) by suggesting that abstinence is the most appropriate goal in the treatment of alcoholism and does not recommend that any alcoholic should resume drinking. However, the report does state that those individuals who were less dependent upon alcohol and were under 40 years old had a good prognosis if they engaged in nonproblem drinking.

Cohen (1985) asserts that in view of the disappointing results of the second Rand report and the Pendery et al. (1982) review of the Sobells' research, it is necessary to reevaluate the controlled drinking treatment program. According to Cohen (1985), controlled drinking is dangerous and rarely successful over the long term and contends that it may not be ethically justifiable to expose some alcoholics to a controlled drinking goal.

CHARACTERISTICS DETERMINING APPROPRIATE TREATMENT GOALS

Since such significant discrepancies exist concerning abstinence and controlled drinking as treatment goals or measures of success, it may be more beneficial to examine the characteristics of alcoholics which seem best suited to either abstinence or controlled drinking as a treatment goal.

The primary factor determining the appropriateness of controlled drinking as a treatment goal is the degree of alcohol dependence and the severity of the problem (Smart, 1978; Finney & Moos, 1981; Gallant, 1986; Gorski, 1986, Keenan, 1984; Taylor, Helzer & Robins, 1986, Edwards et al., 1983). Another important characteristic repeatedly found is that of social and other supports (Smart, 1978; Elal-Lawrence, Slade & Dewey, 1987). Other positive characteristics include the use of psychotropic medication (Elal-Lawrence et al., 1987), greater sense of well-being (Finney & Moos, 1981), less prior treatment for alcoholism (Finney & Moos, 1981), evidence of recent sustained normal drinking, no physical deterioration due to alcohol (Keenan, 1984), fewer lifetime alcohol-related problems (Taylor et al., 1986), and female sex (Gallant, 1986).

Abstinence appears to be the preferred treatment outcome when the individual experiences precarious health problems (Cohen, 1985), is a chronic alcoholic (Volger, Weissback & Compton, 1970), drinks excessively alone or socially, is referred by a specialist, has had previous contact with AA, has the goal of abstinence at discharge, and has sustained a medium period of previous abstinence (Elal-Lawrence et al., 1987).

Orford and Keddie (1986) claim that abstinence or controlled drinking outcomes of treatment depend more upon the personal persuasion of a client, the persuasions of treatment personnel, and the compatibility of these two, than other characteristics.

DOES TREATMENT WORK?

Views regarding the successfulness of treatment range from little to no success to great success depending on the standards by which treatment is judged. For example, Heather and Robertson (1981) conclude that treatment is "probably one of the least important determinants of recovery" and assert that major life circumstances such as marriage and employment are of much more importance. Saunders (1985) asserts that treatment must be viewed as not working because treatment has failed to contain or reduce the number of problem drinkers. The major studies casting doubt on the efficacy of treatment are those conducted by Emrick (1975), Edwards et al. (1977) and Armor, Polich and Stambul (1976). The basic criticisms raised against treatment are that studies do not attribute differences in drinking outcome to measured characteristics and that evidence points to minimal treatment being as effective as much longer periods of treatment.

A problem in assessing treatment effectiveness is the wide range of treatment approaches available to the alcoholic. Treatment approaches vary from systematic desensitization to group-insight oriented analysis while place of treatment includes inpatient, outpatient, halfway house, and industrial and prison settings (Emrick, 1974).

When establishing the effectiveness of treatment, the major variables considered have been (1) type of treatment, (2) amount of treatment, and (3) post-treatment measures of drinking problems. Armor et al. (1976) assert that when establishing the effectiveness of treatment, it must be shown that persons who received treatment fared better than similar persons who did not. In order to accomplish this, researchers must search out, after the fact, a group of alcoholics who received little or no treatment, and delineate them by a careful definition of nontreatment. Armor et al. (1976) further divide untreated clients into two groups: single contact (clients who made only one visit to a treatment center and who received no further treatment) and pre-intake (clients who made contact and received minimal services—usually detoxification—but who then left the center and never resumed contact). This classification is fairly representative of that used by other researchers.

Relative Effectiveness of Programs

One area in which treatment effectiveness can be assessed concerns the efficacy of the different types of programs. Armor et al. (1976) and Saunders (1985) found relatively uniform rates of remission for different treatment modes including AA, which tends to contradict theories maintaining that alcoholics must be treated by dealing with deeper psychological problems. Some researchers claim that differences in treatment modes have little effect on drinking behavior and propose that in some cases patients get better with no or minimal treatment (see for example, Emrick, 1974, 1975). Emrick (1974, 1975) reviewed 380 treatment studies published prior to 1974 and of the 72 studies deemed acceptable by Emrick, only five indicated that any one treatment approach was superior to its control method. Mandell (1975) found no significant differences in abstinence rates for alcoholics treated with group therapy, aversion therapy, realization therapy, various drug therapies or AA; there were no differences in abstinent rates for treatment and control groups. Clare (1977) concluded that different methods or treatment setting did not produce different recovery rates. In a more recent study, McLachlan and Stein (1982) compared outcomes at one year after treatment of patients in either inpatient treatment or a separate hospital program, and found that the two groups did not differ on any of the following outcome measures: mental, medical or legal status, or employment. However, the day clinic was 65% less costly to operate per patient treatment episode than the inpatient program. Longabaugh et al. (1983) in their research concluded that partial hospitalization was proven to be at least as therapeutic and more cost-effective than extended inpatient treatment. Polich et al. (1980) suggest that recovery from alcoholism may depend on mechanisms unrelated to the factors that led to the onset of excessive drinking.

Braunstein, Powell, McGowan and Thoreson (1983) report that their results show that within the context of conventional alcoholism outpatient treatment, patients improve regardless of treatment type if thought is given to matching patient and treatment variables. The findings of Pfrang and Schenk (1986) support this view by suggesting that treatment approaches should consider the patient's attitude to be able to determine appropriate treatment goals and provide adequate support during rehabilitation.

Amount of Treatment

While some controversy exists concerning the relationship between amount of treatment (intensity and duration) and treatment success, research has shown that different amounts of treatment lead to different outcomes (Armor et al., 1976; Robertson et al., 1986; Baekeland et al., 1975; Blane, 1977). The following relationships between treatment amount and subsequent outcomes have been reported: (1) staying in treatment longer is a significant predictor of success in a halfway house setting (Humbles, 1986), (2) minimal treatment is similar to no treatment (Emrick, 1975), (3) alcoholics receiving adequate amounts of treatment have success averages of 73%, 20% higher than clients receiving no treatment (Armor et al., 1978), (4) alcoholics receiving only small amounts of treatment have success rates (i.e., abstinence) only slightly higher than untreated alcoholics (Armor et al., 1978), (5) the longer the period of treatment, the more likely the patient is to be abstinent (Baekeland et al., 1975), and (6) alcoholics receiving intensive treatment demonstrate reduced consumption compared to alcoholics receiving minimal treatment (Robertson et al., 1986).

Research which fails to support the view that more treatment leads to greater success includes Orford and Edwards' (1977) finding of no significant effects between overall outcomes and amount of treatment in a study of 100 male outpatient attendees. Further, Clare (1977) reported that only a small proportion of "alcoholics" achieve abstinence after treatment, regardless of the intensity or prolonged nature of the intervention.

Relative Efficiency of Programs

Given the somewhat contradictory evidence that more intensive treatment is more effective, Longabaugh et al. (1983) recommend that costly treatment settings be systematically compared with less expensive ones. The uniformity of treatment findings, therefore, suggests that a policy of supporting or adopting the less expensive treatment would be the more cost-effective. Kirn (1986) reports that more and more people are enrolling in outpatient treatment because it is less costly, may be equally effective in some cases, allows a patient time with family and enables him or her to continue working. However, more research must be conducted on alternative treatments and on the role and importance of outcome criterion other than drinking behavior (Armor et al., 1976). The majority of individuals in treatment fail to achieve the goals set for them by that treatment and that those who achieve some measure of recovery consistently fail to cite treatment as being an important factor in the remission.

Characteristics of Clients Related to Treatment Success

Numerous studies have focused on those characteristics of the client which are associated with treatment effectiveness or success. Although there are contradictory findings, socioeconomic status, marital status, sex, employment status, and psychological variables are characteristics which have been found to impact upon success. Armor et al. (1978) stress the importance of client characteristics by noting "it is hard not to conclude that remission and eventual recovery depend to a major extent on the characteristics and behavior of the individual client than on treatment characteristics."

Socioeconomic Status

Baekeland et al. (1975) cite socioeconomic status as the single most important variable influencing treatment outcome. Higher socioeconomic class is a variable consistently found to be related positively to treatment success (Mandell, 1985; Blane, 1977; Bromet, Moos, Bliss & Wuthmann, 1977).

Marital Status

Marital status as a predictor of treatment completion was found to be significant by Marotta and Rale (1986). In a two part investigation to assess whether marital status was related to treatment completion they concluded that marriage and family variables play critical roles in the drop-out phenomenon and argue that the patient's family needs to be involved in treatment to help ensure treatment completion. Those married individuals who specifically mentioned marriage as a primary reason for seeking treatment were more inclined to complete treatment. Otherwise, however, single patients were most likely to complete treatment. Other studies citing marital status as a predictor of success include Humbles, 1986; Williams, 1985; Obinali, 1986; Pattison et al., 1968; Neubuerger et al., 1980; Bromet et al., 1977.

Sex

Although most findings suggest that males have a higher likelihood of completing treatment than females (see for example, Humbles, 1986; Williams, 1985), Obinali (1986) tentatively concluded that females may have a higher success rate than males. Sex, as a predictor of treatment success, may be less valuable because of the changing roles of men and women and the increasing number of women entering treatment for alcoholism.

Employment Status

Patients who are employed when seeking treatment have a higher treatment completion rate than do unemployed patients (Neubuerger, 1980; Obinali, 1986), and finding employment at discharge is positively related to treatment success (Humbles, 1986). In a related vein, Braunstein et al. (1983) found that periodic visits to a physician appeared to be as effective as drug treatment or multitherapy for the employed alcoholic.

Psychological Variables

Williams (1985) examined psychological variables such as self-esteem, depression, drinking attitude, resentment and anxiety but found none to be significant in differentiating or predicting success or nonsuccess in treatment. Roberts' (1986) study represents an extension of previous research on alcoholic personality subtypes and their response to treatment for alcoholism. He found that alcoholics with no history of psychiatric syndromes experienced fewer emotional and health care problems following treatment than other subtypes of alcoholics such as depressed or antisocial alcoholics. Findings suggest that alcoholics with no psychiatric history may respond more positively to treatment than alcoholics who exhibit significant psychopathology such as major depression or antisocial personality disorder. The presence or absence of coexisting psychopathology may be an important moderator variable that could have significant influence on response treatment among alcoholics and in determining types and lengths of treatment provided (Roberts, 1986).

Other Characteristics

Interestingly, Costello's (1975) search for treatment characteristics associated with favorable results found that a restrictive admission procedure produced more successful treatment results. This suggests that some treatments are successful because they are able to eliminate unpromising clients at the admissions stage. The possibility exists that better than average treatment results have more to do with the elimination of poor risk clients at selection than the treatment factors which follow.

Another factor related to treatment success is the initial motivation or lack thereof of the individual seeking treatment. Costello (1975) reports that in his research a high initial motivation to change is facilitated by very general features of treatment. This motivation would be the crucial client quality discerned at intake by treatment workers in Costello's most successful treatment group. Williams (1985) reports similar findings on the importance of developing positive motivation early.

Spontaneous Recovery

One problem in evaluating the successfulness of treatment is the possibility of spontaneous recovery, what Prugh (1986) describes as recovery "without benefit of formal or institutional treatment." Although several studies have examined spontaneous recovery and identified some of the reasons behind it, Prugh (1986) contends that spontaneous remission is the most narrowly studied and least well understood area in alcoholism research. According to Cooke (1980), critics still assert that it is a theoretical concept and that research supporting spontaneous recovery mistakes statistical artifacts for the real thing.

However, the existence of spontaneous recovery among both alcoholics and alcohol abusers is supported by research studies.

Smart (1975/76), in a literature review, concluded that spontaneous recovery does occur and that yearly recovery rates vary from 1% to 33%. Armor et al. (1976) found that their untreated sample had remission rates of about 50%, indicating a substantial spontaneous remission. Formal treatment, then, in some cases, may play only an incremental role in the recovery of alcoholism accounting for about 20-25% remission over and above what would be expected from no treatment.

Tuchfeld (1981) examined 51 spontaneous remitters and found the major reasons for changing drinking patterns to be personal illness or accident, religious experiences, drinking-related financial problems, intervention by family members, and "extraordinary" events. He also found that social conditions contributed vitally to the maintenance of the subjects' resolution of their drinking problems. Subjects appeared to restructure their lives so that social circumstances reinforced their new behavioral patterns. Stall (1983) reports that three general patterns of changing perceptions are seen among spontaneous remitters: (1) temporary period of problem denial associated with drinking, followed by decision to quit, (2) slowly but steadily increasing awareness of scope of drinking behavior and its consequences, and (3) sudden reorganization of perception sometimes following a significant incident.

Ludwig (1985), in a study of 29 spontaneous remitters consisting of teetotalers and relative abstainers, found that the subjective experience of "hitting bottom" regardless of the circumstances producing it was often crucial; 75% of the respondents were in dire straits emotionally or physically prior to the radical change in drinking patterns. Profound experiences of the opposite kind—i.e., religious or transcendental experiences—also set recovery in motion for a significant number of respondents. Most of the subjects "arrived at a common cognitive destination: mental associations to alcohol with very unpleasant, sickening, humiliating or distasteful experiences of a personal nature" (Ludwig, 1985).

Saunders and Kershaw (1979) also isolated a number of factors leading to spontaneous recovery including physical ill-health, marriage or re-marriage, job change and overall life circumstance change and attributed remission to the social milieu of the individual rather than the impact of treatment.

An additional factor related to spontaneous recovery appears to be the age of the individual. Fillmore and Midanic (1984) found that the likelihood of spontaneous recovery was significantly higher in younger individuals and argue that the key question raised by their research is how to identify those younger individuals who are likely to have unremitting alcohol problems later in life.

Smart (1975/76) asserts that additional study of spontaneous remitters might indicate "which social circumstances such as changes in marital status and jobs and life conditions may be most associated with the process of recovery."

ATTRITION

Recovery and rehabilitation are predicated on the ability to retain the alcoholic until treatment goals are realized. Yet, prematurely discontinuing treatment for a broad range of alcohol related problems is a phenomenon which alcoholism treatment facilities face. Currently there is a dropout rate of 52 to 75% before the fourth outpatient alcoholism treatment session and approximately a 14 to 39% attrition rate in inpatient settings (Baekeland & Lundwall, 1975). Attempts to understand the factors involved in early dropout have provided the impetus for many research studies.

Baekeland and Lundwall (1975), in a study of dropouts in outpatient treatment facilities, found the typical dropout to be a male who is dependent or counterdependent, highly symptomatic with psychopathic personality features, in the lower socioeconomic class, socially isolated, in an unstable marriage, and highly ambivalent about treatment and its worth.

In psychotherapy oriented programs, younger patients with an earlier amount of alcoholism and more unstable marriages were more likely to leave treatment (Baekeland, 1975). Psychological differences found included more hostility and aggression, less maturity, responsibility and emotional control. Dropouts had lower socioeconomic status and more self-doubt and were more socially dependent although isolated. Baekeland (1975) reports an overall view of the inpatient dropout as an advanced-stage alcoholic with more passive-aggressive and psychopathic features who relies on alcohol for relief of feeling and has difficulty in forming close relationships. Studies have produced a picture of the patient most likely to drop out: socially unstable and isolate, lower socioeconomic status, symptomatic dependent yet denying it, ambivalent about treatment and has psychopathic features (Brandson, Maultsby & Welsh). Younger persons are more likely to drop out of treatment.

Chafetz and Blane (1963) report that only 5% of lower socioeconomic patients referred to treatment from a hospital emergency room attended treatment. However, this was increased to 65% when a social worker was used to work out the arrangements. Research also shows that writing letters, telephoning, putting patients in groups and seeing families seem to mitigate against the patient dropping out (Brandsma et al., 1980). Interestingly, research points to the fact that although there are many factors associated with the problem of dropping out, the patient controls most of the variance (Brandsma et al., 1980; Baekeland et al., 1975; Kennedy et al., 1978; Zirich, 1981).

Shortcomings on the part of the provider of treatment services have also been examined in an effort to explain treatment attrition. Problems in interviewing skills, improper attention to countertransference or relationship issues, ineffectual handling of resistance, and lack of personal experience as a recovering alcoholic have all been cited as contributing to a facility's failure to retain the alcoholic patient (NIAAA, 1987).

Problems and Criteria Used in Evaluating Treatment Effectiveness

Although evaluation is a crucial component of determining treatment effectiveness, the methods and logistics of programs remain primitive (Costello, 1982). Further, although the most common evaluation strategy has followed the experimental model, problems of randomization and experimental control of extraneous variables made a quasi-experimental approach more appropriate (Costello, 1982).

Armor et al. (1980) identify two factors other than treatment which might cause differences among treated and untreated groups of clients. One potential problem is the possibility that the groups may have differed initially on some important characteristic. A second factor is that in the case of the Armor study, the clients voluntarily contacted an alcoholism treatment center, and hence there is good reason to suspect that they are different from the ordinary "untreated alcoholic." They may have recognized they have a drinking problem serious enough to require professional help and may be more motivated to control their drinking than alcoholics who do not volunteer. Therefore, self-selection is a factor which might be operating in some studies.

According to Gibbs and Flanagan (1977), sampling error, variance in definitions, differing treatments and inconsistency in outcome criteria may cause inconsistencies and contradictory results in alcoholism treatment studies. An additional problem is that the personal characteristics of alcoholics receiving treatment may interact with the type of treatment, thus making group results mask important treatment effects (Gibbs & Flanagan, 1977).

Miller (1986) identified the following guidelines that should be considered when evaluating a treatment outcome study for alcoholism:

1. Clearly document the treatment being evaluated and describe the treatment regimen in detail.
2. Be clear about who was studied and how the diagnosis was made.
3. Include patient's history, interviewing techniques, training of interviewers and demographic information.
4. Consider methods of analysis and data collection because there is no valid biological test to measure alcoholism treatment.
5. Obtain follow-up data and corroboration data to see how well the patient is doing for example, 2 years after treatment.

Saunders (1985) has criticisms of the quality of much of the evaluative research and summarizes the limitations for current approaches to treatment evaluation. One major problem is that the methodology appropriate to clinical medicine, particularly the controlled trial, is an inappropriate design for evaluating alcoholism treatment. A second problem is that the use of research designs and sampling methodology which obscure the individuality of the patient has also masked possible subtle patient treatment interactions.

RELAPSE

Studies within the United States and elsewhere have found that the majority of people treated for alcoholism relapse within one year of their treatment (Wells & Wainwright, 1985). According to Hunt et al. (1971), between 50 and 60% of treated alcoholics tend to experience relapse within the first three months after treatment. Vaillant (1983) reports that when examining lifelong alcoholism recovery patterns, 10-20% of alcoholics never relapse after their first serious request for help and an additional 2-3% will achieve stable sobriety with each additional year of attempted abstinence.

Gorski (1986) classified recovering alcoholics into three groups based upon their recover/relapse histories: recovery-prone (49% of all patients), transitionally relapse-prone (20%) and relapse-prone (40%). The relapse-prone patients are described as those patients that will develop a progressive pattern of periodic alcoholism with the relapse episodes becoming more frequent, longer and marked by more severe consequences. These individuals experience progressively lower levels of functioning during periods of abstinence.

Gorski (1986) further projects that as a result of these patterns of recovery, alcoholism treatment programs will continue to encounter more relapse-prone and transitionally relapse-prone patients. In his informal survey of treatment centers, Gorski found that 20% of the private sector treatment beds were occupied by patients previously treated in 21- or 28-day alcoholism rehabilitation programs; when the survey was conducted again in 1985, the proportion had risen to over 40%.

Elal-Lawrence, Slade and Dewey (1986) identify those patients most likely to relapse as being more likely to be unemployed, to have a history of AA attendance, to experience a short period of previous abstinence, and are most likely to have liver damage and therefore advised to abstain.

Post-Alcoholism Treatment

An additional question concerning alcoholism treatment is what happens to the alcoholic after treatment? Pettinati, Sugerman, Di Donato and Maurer (1982) assessed drinking status and life adjustment for four years after treatment in a 100% follow-up to provide a comprehensive profile of the natural course of events after alcoholism treatment. They found that a substantial percentage of patients were able to maintain abstinence and show an overall good life adjustment through the four years. Further, if this status was maintained for two consecutive years after discharge, it was likely to be maintained for the next two years. Consistent drinking over the four-year period occurred in only a small percentage of the alcoholics. More typically, a periodic drinking pattern emerged with very few individuals able to drink without any problems. Regular AA attendance for four years after treatment was significantly related to maintaining abstinence over the four-year period but other post-treatment interventions were not.

In their research, Edwards, Duckitt, Oppenheimer, Sheehan and Taylor (1983) found that 40% of 99 male alcoholics were doing well at a 10-year follow-up, while 47% continued to drink in alcoholic fashion with adverse consequences. Edwards et al. (1983) contend that the small proportion of alcoholics who were able to return to a pattern of stable social drinking appeared to be those who had never become severely dependent. Those drinking in an uncontrolled way were continuing to have serious problems stemming from drinking such as peptic ulcers, major brain damage, signs of depression, suicide attempts, drug misuse, marriage breakdowns, problems with the law, and hospital admissions for alcoholism treatment.

A Preferred Provider Organization (PPO) Case Study for Mental Health and Substance Abuse

Ingram Gomillion
Donald R. Self

INTRODUCTION

In the midst of efforts to control the rising costs of health care in the United States, insurance companies have employed a variety of "cost containment" techniques, many of which have proven relatively ineffective. In fact, the trend toward limiting or even eliminating certain health care insurance coverage is being considered by more and more employers at an alarming rate. New programs such as HMOs and other managed care approaches to controlling these rising costs have resulted many times in conflicting and confusing insurance benefits for employees and their dependents.

This trend extends to the mental health and substance abuse treatment field. Consequently, with reduced and/or eliminated mental health care insurance coverage, there is an increased reliance on the publicly funded mental health system which was developed to serve the *economically* indigent. As a result, these systems are inundated with the *medically* indigent – those without the insurance coverage to pay for adequate treatment but who do not qualify for publicly assisted treatment.

The Alabama Mental Health System, composed of the state hospitals, community mental health centers and freestanding substance abuse providers, provides mental health services and substance abuse services available to all citizens of the state of Alabama. At the same time, it aims to reduce the reliance on publicly funded programs resulting from the elimination and/or reduction of mental health/substance abuse insurance coverage by employers of the state. How then can these two conflicting goals be merged into a comprehensive strategy to achieve the desired results of each?

BACKGROUND

The Alabama Mental Health System has approached the goal of improved mental health services in the state through prevention programs, employee assistance programs (EAPs) and through legislative means. In 1985, a bill was introduced in the Alabama Legislature which would have specified that certain "minimum" mental health benefits be required in all group insurance policies of 25 or more employees. Even though this bill was narrowly defeated in the Legislature, the Department embarked on a different approach or strategy towards improving mental health coverage offered by employers in the state. Currently, Alabama law specifies that such coverage must be *available* to all group insurance policies but stops short of requiring coverage. This strategy would be based on the relative cost containment benefits of providing mental health coverage through means of a preferred provider mechanism in lieu of the traditional approach of limiting mental health insurance coverage. The strategy then would be a "pull" strategy of convincing employers of the benefits of adequate mental health coverage in contrast to the historical "push" approach of imposing legal requirements through mandated minimum mental health coverage.

PROGRAM DESIGN

In the summer of 1986, a Mental Health PPO proposal was presented to the largest self-insured program in Alabama, the combined State Employees Insurance Plan (SEIP) and the Public Education Employees Health Insurance Plan (PEEHIP). Both of the plans for state employees and teachers/support personnel, are administered by the Retirement Systems of Alabama, and provide coverage for over 88,000 employees and over 138,000 total covered individuals scattered throughout all of Alabama's sixty-seven counties. Any organization wishing to participate as a provider in these two plans must be able to provide services on a statewide basis. The network of mental health centers throughout the state is able to meet the requirement since there is a mental health center or satellite program located in each county.

The SEIP and PEEHIP Plans approved the implementation of this pilot preferred provider organization for mental health and substance abuse coverage as an alternative to the existing coverage. The basic assumptions of the PPO proposal included:

A. Costs associated with outpatient mental health services can be controlled through a *case-management* approach to treatment whereby the level of therapy can be individualized to provide a cost-efficient method of serving customer needs. Insurance benefits are often structured so that outpatient utilization for mental health and substance abuse problems are penalized through limits and copayments. For example, one major employer offers a benefit plan that pays 80% of physician outpatient charges, but 100% for the more costly inpatient care.

B. Costs associated with the *inpatient* psychiatric and residential substance abuse services can be reduced through a preadmission certification process aimed at avoiding unnecessary inpatient/residential treatment and providing instead outpatient and day treatment alternatives. Often a patient is hospitalized for treatment when less expensive treatment may be the more appropriate treatment setting. Advertising and marketing efforts may also result in excessive use of psychiatric and substance abuse inpatient care at the expense of the insurance plan.

C. When inpatient/residential care is appropriate and necessary, the length of stay is many times unchecked especially with respect to the twenty-eight-day substance abuse programs. The case management aspects of the PPO can eliminate the unnecessary lengthy stays through a continuing care evaluation process. As an example of the occurrence of unnecessary stays, one Alabama employer with approximately 16,000 employees and dependents experienced an increase of 456% in psychiatric admissions/stays for child and adolescent coverage between 1980 and 1984. In some instances, employers have experienced stays as long as one year for adolescent treatment.

D. When inpatient/residential care is essential, the overall costs of treatment can also be reduced through negotiated per diem rates. Per diems have in the past been calculated based upon the overall cost of the hospital including the more expensive costs of the surgical and intensive care units. However, negotiated rates for psychiatric and substance abuse care for the PPO will not include such inflationary factors and will be, on the average, 30% lower than traditional rates charged.

E. Costs of employee absenteeism and performance can be reduced through early intervention and treatment efforts. A study by Harwood, Kristiansen and Rachal (1985) showed that American businesses lost $36.3 billion through decreased productivity and increased absenteeism, medical expenses, disability claims and theft due to alcohol and drug abuse alone. The implications of such data should encourage utilization of mental health services when needed, as a hedge against even larger financial losses on the job.

Therefore, the proposal is a cost containment program, while at the same time, is aimed at improving the level of mental health services available to the employee and dependents. Table 1 is a summary comparison of the benefits available under the PPO option as compared with the traditional major medical benefits. In summary, the PPO Program called for cost containment efforts through early intervention, outpatient service priority and managed care.

IMPLEMENTATION

The community mental health centers (CMHCs) throughout the state serve as the "gatekeeper" to mental health and substance abuse services of those employees/dependents electing to utilize the PPO alternative. Additionally, the CMHCs provide outpatient care and residential substance abuse care. Services that the CMHCs do not provide (i.e., psychiatric inpatient and, in some instances, substance abuse residential treatment) are subcontracted to other facilities meeting program requirements and the discounted per diem requirements. These facilities are very carefully screened and selected

TABLE 1

SERVICE TYPE	PPO COVERAGE	TRADITIONAL MAJOR MEDICAL
Outpatient Care	80% Coverage 20% Employee Copay Maximum: 30 Visits	50% Coverage $100 Deductible $500 Limit
Inpatient Psychiatric Care	Preadmission Certification Required 100% Coverage Maximum: 30 Days	$100 Deductible 80% of First $2000 100% After $2000 Acute Care Only
Inpatient Substance Abuse Care	Preadmission Certification Required 100% Coverage Maximum: 30 Days	$100 Deductible 80% of First $2000 100% after $2000 Detox Only

through means of a PPO Oversight Committee composed of appointed CMHC Directors.

The use of the mental health centers has resulted in a major policy change over traditional reimbursement to eligible providers. It promotes cost containment without reducing the quality of care. In Alabama, most third-party reimbursement requires a physician or licensed PhD psychologist to provide all care for persons receiving treatment for mental and nervous disorders. In the case of mental health centers, the center is certified to provide the service, rather than individual clinicians. Minimum qualifications for the centers are to provide clinicians with master's degrees in psychology and counseling, plus two years of post master's degree clinical experience. All clinicians are under medical supervision in the mental health centers as required by Alabama Certification Law. However, there is a serious shortage of licensed psychologists and physicians with none practicing in 40 of Alabama's 67 counties other than those in the mental health centers. Therefore, this change promotes early intervention which may reduce more costly inpatient care.

Purchasing services through community mental health centers

has provided the Insurance Boards with the mechanism for purchasing a system that provides whatever level of care is needed, ranging from the physician to the master's level therapist. The state employees/public education insurance boards are self-insured which allows flexibility in developing the PPO for mental health/substance abuse services. Blue Cross/Blue Shield serves as third-party administrator for health insurance, and pays the claims for the PPO which is administered by the Insurance Boards. The centers have a policy committee that has established policies for operating the program including pre-certification and utilization review which were initially handled by the centers. This function was recently transferred to a utilization review firm with a successful track record.

Starting on October 1, 1986, these new PPO benefits were available to all state employees, teachers and covered dependents (except those electing HMO coverage) for the plan year, October 1, 1986, through September 30, 1987. However, the program did not become fully operational until January 1, 1987. All employees were notified of the available PPO in their insurance handbook and were provided additional information through their employing agency. Some of the CMHCs followed up with informational and other training programs in an effort to market this new service. Finally, a telephone number was also provided for additional specific information on the comparison of mental health and substance abuse coverage available through the insurance boards. While Blue Cross and Blue Shield of Alabama administered the payment system for both programs, virtually all calls received by Blue Cross relating to mental health and substance abuse were referred to the Research and Planning Office within the Mental Health Department for specific details.

INITIAL OUTCOMES

For the period October 1, 1986, through September 30, 1987, a total of 1,295 clients were served in the PPO program. Of that total, 1,080 clients were served in the outpatient setting and 215 clients received inpatient or residential substance abuse services. In contrast to the belief that open-ended mental health services will result in runaway mental health costs, the average number of visits for the first plan year was only 5.39 visits per client, despite the fact that a total of 30 visits was allowable under the PPO program. For those 1,080 clients receiving outpatient services, a total of 5,234 visits were in individual therapy, 372 visits in group therapy, and there were 246 preadmission certifications. The CMHC with the highest rate of visits per client averaged only 9.18 and the lowest rate was 2.71 visits per client.

The 215 inpatient/residential clients served accounted for 4,957 days for an average length of stay of 23.06 days and an average cost per day of $272.99.

In terms of penetration rate of the subscriber/covered dependent population, the PPO achieved an estimated .93% penetration of the 138,000 eligible persons. This rate is somewhat low, and was probably due to the slow start-up of a new optional service. Overall, the PPO program expenditures totalled $1,654,141 for the first year of operation, and closed out under expected budget during a time period which saw a 28.4% increase in general medical care costs of the two insurance programs.

SUMMARY

The Preferred Provider Organization concept is quickly becoming more popular because of its relative cost-effectiveness and recent successes. Managed care through means of this mental health and substance abuse PPO may well serve as the prototype for the general health care cost containment efforts of the future for the self-insured insurance plans for Alabama state employees and teachers.

The first year also revealed several problems in the original proposal especially with respect to the unintended attractiveness of inpatient/residential care. Consequently, copayment plans were added to dissuade unnecessary lengthy stays (see Table 2).

Second, a new quality assurance mechanism has been added to further evaluate the need for admissions to facilities, as well as for the need for continued inpatient treatment. The Alabama Quality Assurance Foundation (AQAF) began on January 1, 1988, conducting the preadmission certification on all admissions based upon criteria established jointly by AQAF and the PPO providers. In addi-

TABLE 2

LENGTH OF TREATMENT	EMPLOYEE COPAY
Days 10-14	$15/Day
Days 15-19	$20/Day
Days 20-24	$25/Day
Days 25-30	$30/Day

tion, AQAF will conduct continuing stay reviews at predetermined time periods to ensure that continued treatment in an inpatient setting is indeed necessary.

IMPLEMENTATION AND RECOMMENDATIONS

This case study presents an innovative link in an administered channel of distribution for alcoholism treatment. A major innovation includes the establishment of a third-party pay service line for the system of non-profit CMHCs, creating a positive cash flow which can be used to defray indigent care and other costs. A second major element is the consortium of both public and private providers participating as providers. The cost containment measures such as independent pre-certification assessment and long-term negotiated per client rates in the PPO allow for substantial economics of scale in the system.

This case study is prepared as a prototype for diffusion among other states or major employers, and is not limited to the public sector benefitting from the CMHC system.

III. TOOLS AND TECHNIQUES

Alcoholism Treatment Demand Estimation

Jerry J. Ingram

INTRODUCTION

Determining the alcohol treatment needs of a particular service area, such as a county or a state health planning region, is a difficult and complex undertaking. Planners are hampered in assessing the severity of various local alcohol problems by both the lack of available data and differing opinions as to which data are significant (Ryan, 1984/85). The National Institute on Alcohol Abuse and Alcoholism (NIAAA) has become increasingly aware of the necessity of developing reliable quantitative based computational techniques when estimating alcohol abuse and alcoholism treatment needs (AEDS, 1982). Resources for the treatment of alcoholism have, in many cases, been allocated on the basis of *utilization levels* of existing treatment facilities. This situation has resulted in little effort being exerted to identify the *unmet* needs of an area. Many state agencies still employ simplified "utilization approaches" for alcoholism needs assessment. These utilization approaches base current and future needs upon past utilization rates of alcohol facilities and services. A major limitation of this demand approach is the omission of various population subgroups who have a need for treatment but are currently not using the facilities/services.

Considerable advancements have been made in need assessment techniques for alcoholism over the past five years. However, these improved techniques have not found widespread utilization by state health planning agencies. Significantly, it is these state agencies which ultimately determine need and, hence, resource allocation for the treatment of alcoholism. There appears to be a need for planners to better understand the various need assessment models so that area needs can be (1) identified more effectively and (2) targeted with the proper type and level of treatment. It is against this background that a model has been developed by this author to simplify our understanding of alternative methods for assessing alcohol treatment needs. The model is presented and discussed following a review of some basic need assessment terminology.

NEED VS. DEMAND

The position of the NIAAA, as noted above, suggests that resource allocation will increasingly be based upon true *need determination* in the future. Thus, alcohol treatment agencies have great reason to understand the various interpretations of this concept. Health planners were first faced with the necessity of need determination with the passage of The National Health Planning and Resources Development Act of 1974 (Public Law 93-641, 1974). This legislation formalized the concept of certificate of need (CON) and has had a significant impact upon planning for health related facilities and programs. MacStrovic (1978) stated that the basic notion of this legislation is that capital expenditures in health services development which are not made in response to demonstrated need should be prevented.

When defining *treatment needs*, one must first resolve the issue of needs vs. demand. Some economists suggest that health professionals define health needs while consumers/users define their health *wants* (demand). Boulding notes:

> The concept of need which emerges from the criticism of demand is that of professional choice. It is implied to some extent in the very idea of the patient or the client and it is expressed in the aphorism that doctor (or father, or lawyer, or

> preacher, or president) knows best. One's demand for medical care is what he wants. The need for medical care is what the doctor thinks he ought to have. (Boulding, 1966)

As far as alcoholism is concerned, it has been noted that an area's alcohol problem profile is equivalent to its need for treatment while both its treatment resources and utilization of services is the effective demand for treatment (Ryan, 1984/85). For purposes of this analysis, need is defined to include those in need of treatment from problems related to alcoholism while *demand* for treatment includes those persons who are *participating* in a treatment program. Jeffers et al. (1971) have suggested that need is always greater than demand.

Methods for Assessing the Need for Alcoholism Treatment

One of the major difficulties in developing a program to deliver services to alcoholics and problem drinkers is determining how many persons in need are in the area served by the program (Marden, 1974). It is even more difficult to determine the profiles of those in need of treatment and to prescribe the proper type of treatment.

A survey of the literature on alcoholism reveals that a large number of models have been developed to assess the need for treatment of alcoholism. The models vary greatly in their level of sophistication and in their ability to accurately assess needs. At one extreme, efforts to estimate the number of persons in need of alcoholism services involve simply applying some standard percentage to the population under study. Using this methodology, treatment needs in a particular service area are estimated by multiplying the adult population of the area by, for example, five percent to arrive at a figure upon which to base programs for alcoholism. Obviously, the application of a single percentage to all areas assumes that all population subgroups have the same incidence of problems related to the use of alcohol. It has been determined, however, that problems of alcoholism vary by such basic demographic characteristics as age, sex, socioeconomic status, ethnicity, marital status, etc. (NIAAA, 1987). Recently developed need assessment models have focused upon utilizing advanced statistical technologies to identify high-risk groups and to determine alcoholism treatment needs. In an effort to simplify the understanding of need assessment, a framework is proposed for grouping and classifying the various models.

CLASSIFICATION OF ALCOHOLISM TREATMENT ASSESSMENT MODELS

Figure 1 below shows that treatment assessment models can be logically grouped into two broad strata—*demand* based models and *need* based models. Demand based models have a relatively long history in the health care industry and are essentially based upon facility utilization or treatment analysis. Data on facility and service utilization are normally readily available from state and national planning agencies. However, the major criticism associated with demand based models is that they do not address the actual need for treatment. Demand based models do little more than reveal the number of people currently utilizing (demand) a particular facility/service. Need based models are typically based upon the relationship of selected independent variables (e.g., liver cirrhosis) to treatment needs. Some of the need based models developed within the last few years are focusing upon need determination for population subgroups by utilizing statistical techniques such as factor analysis and regression models.

Classification of Need Based Models

Need based models go beyond estimating the existing utilization rates for alcohol services and attempt to identify variables such as social indicators that are correlated with needs. Figure 2 presents a classification system for needs based models. Some of the ideas for this classification scheme were developed from materials published by the National Institute on Alcohol Abuse and Alcoholism.

The need based models are classified into four broad subgroups: (1) survey based models, (2) mortality based models, (3) treatment and mortality based models, and (4) multi-factor statistical based models. In the discussion to follow, examples of each type model are presented and discussed. However, space is not available to discuss the works and contributions of all authors and organiza-

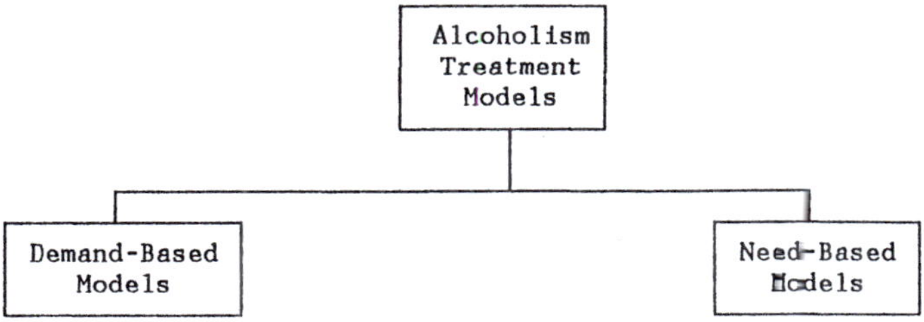

FIGURE 1. Models for Assessing the Need for Alcohol Treatment

tions. The examples presented are nonetheless representative of the field of alcoholism.

Survey Based Models

Utilization of survey based models are supported in the assumption that people in need must be directly approached in order to discover what their needs actually are (MacStravic, 1978). The Social Research Group (SAG) developed a general population survey based method for rating persons according to the severity of eleven problems associated with drinking (Cahalan and Room, 1972). From survey data, SAG has developed a Current Tangible Consequence Index (CTC). Using this index a person is considered to have a fairly high index of alcohol related problems when a current problem score of seven points or more is attained. Another example of a survey based model is the Frequent Heavy Drinking Index (FHD) used in the Federal Formula for State Grants. The FHD index is defined as the number of times that a persons takes five or more drinks on one occasion within one week (Marin et al., 1978).

Marden (1974) has proposed a method for estimating the potential clientele of alcoholism service programs using survey data combined with census data. The method uses national survey data on alcoholism developed by Cahalan and Room (1972) to estimate the prevalence of problem drinkers in selected demographic segments of the population. Once national prevalence data is obtained, the model user next determines the number of people in a selected demographic subgroup for a particular area. Thus, if a given service area has 10,000 males between the ages of 20-29 and national sur-

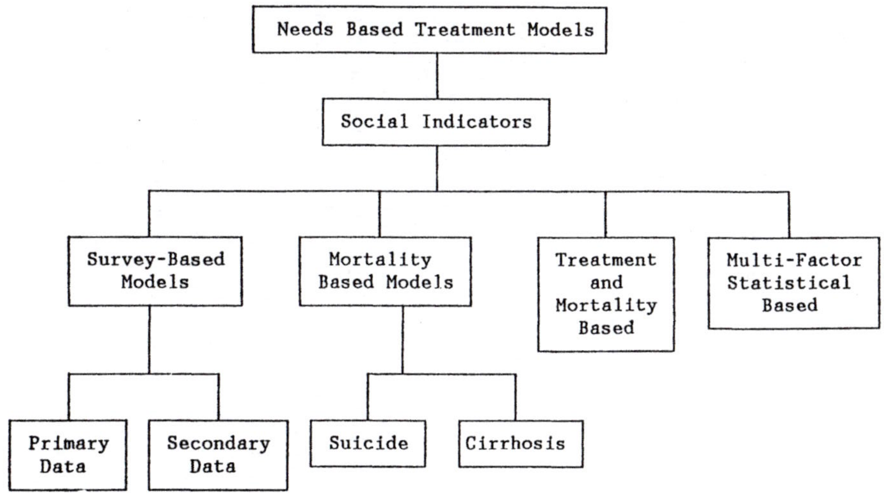

FIGURE 2. Needs Based Treatment Models

vey data indicates that .21 percent of this group are problem drinkers, the number of problem drinkers for that subgroup is equal to 2,100 (10,000 × .21).

The Marden procedure has been widely used for state planning purposes despite criticism that Marden's assumption (that the proportion of problem drinkers in any age, sex, or occupational group will be the same everywhere in the U.S.) is unwarranted (AEDS, 1982).

There are a number of problems associated with using surveys to estimate the need for alcoholism services. First, to be useful, surveys must be specific to a particular service area. The costs of such a large number of surveys is prohibitive. Secondly, it is questionable whether or not valid information on alcoholism can be collected through surveys. Third, some population subgroups (e.g., blacks) may be underrepresented in surveys due to such factors as low incidence of telephones.

Simple Mortality Based Models

Simple one factor based mortality models are distinguished from multi-factor models which incorporate several mortality indices in factor analysis and regression models (see discussion under multi-factor statistical based models). Mortality based models are divided into two subgroups, suicide and cirrhosis. Schmidt and deLint (1970) proposed a method for estimating alcoholism by observing that *suicide* is more frequent among alcoholics than among the general population. And, based on the number of suicides, the alcoholism level of an area could subsequently be determined. One possible problem with the suicide based procedure is that percentages of alcoholics among suicides may not always be known.

The *cirrhosis mortality* based procedure is based upon work originally conducted by Joliffe and Jellinek (1941). The so called Jellinek Calculation estimates alcoholism prevalence in a population based on liver cirrhosis mortality data. The use of a standard single figure to assess the need for alcoholism services is thought to be a major shortcoming of Jellinek's procedures. The original Jellinek model has been altered somewhat by various authors but the limitations still persist.

Treatment and Mortality

A treatment and mortality based model referred to as The Flow Model was developed by Creative Sociomedics Corporation under contract to the NIAAA (Creative Sociomedics, Inc., 1980). The procedure is based upon a mathematical model of the progression of a substance abuser through various events which occur to the abuse and end with death. The initial step in this model is the examination of individual treatment records and matching these with death data from vital statistics. From that analysis, an estimate of the life expectancy of the abuser is determined. Then, the rate at which deaths occur in a given year can be directly related to the incidence and prevalence of the abusing population. A major criticism of The Flow Model is that it includes alcoholics in remission in the estimation procedure which would lead to overstated estimates of prevalence.

Multi-Factor Statistical Based Models

One of the statistical based models which seems to hold a great deal of promise is the AEDS normative model. The model was developed in 1982 by The Alcohol Epidemiologic Data System (AEDS), under contract to NIAAA (Ryan, 1984/85). Even though this model is classified here as a needs based model, it actually combines demand analysis with needs analysis. In the actual model, need is determined using seven indicators of mortality, all of which involve alcohol as a cause of death in some percentage of cases. The seven indicators are: (1) liver cirrhosis, (2) alcoholic psychosis, (3) alcoholism, (4) alcohol poisoning, (5) automobile accidents, (6) suicide, and (7) homicide. Through statistical analysis of these seven indicators, AEDS had determined two indexes, The Chronic Health Index and The Alcohol Health Index. These two indexes summarize the data from these raw numbers and represent the relative prevalence of problems associated with chronic alcohol use and acute intoxication, respectively.

The Chronic Health Index summarized the mortality rates from liver cirrhosis, alcoholic psychosis, alcoholism, alcohol poisoning and homicide. The Alcohol Casualty Index includes highway fatalities, suicides and death from alcoholism. The values for the indexes for any county in the United States can be found in *County Alcohol Problem Indicators*, 1975-1977 (AEDS, 1981).

The complimentary component of the AEDS normative model is utilization levels and capacity (number of patients and number of beds or treatment slots, respectively). The utilization levels and capacity data represent the demand component of the AEDS model. The data for this part of the model is furnished by the National Drug and Alcohol Treatment Survey (NAATUS) conducted by NIAAA and NIDA.

The Chronic Health Index and The Alcohol Casualty Index are utilized in determining an area's *need* or estimates of *expected* treatment levels. An area's demand or actual treatment is determined by examining the number of patients/clients and the number of beds/treatment slots. The *need* figures are compared with the *demand* figures and efforts are made to explain any discrepancy. For example, when expected patients exceeds actual, this indicates the possibility of unmet treatment needs. One of the principal advantages of the AEDS normative model is that of providing estimates of utilization and capacity for seven different treatment modalities: Medical Detoxification, Social Detoxification, Rehabilitation, Custodial, Ambulatory, Limited Care and Outpatient. In addition, the advanced version of the AEDS normative model provides a breakdown of expected patient populations by age and sex, and estimated staffing patterns and a forecast of needed treatment capacity by modality (further delineated by age and sex) through the year 1990 (Ryan, 1984).

Schmittdiel and Ford (1983), using population based variables (e.g., total population, white and minority populations) and easily obtainable alcohol indicator variables (consumption, revenue, alcohol related deaths and arrest), developed regression models to predict state bed capacity data. The authors then produced prediction models for detoxification, quarterway and halfway houses, residential, hospital and outpatient services. Several variables, particularly total population, deaths and arrests, were found to be predictive of alcoholism service level by state. Based upon these findings, estimates of specific service needs within a geographical area can be made by varying the values of the independent variables in the models to reflect the characteristics of that area.

The real significance of the AEDS models and the Ford-Schmittdiel model is that professionals now have the ability to estimate the need for a range of alcoholism services with acceptable levels of statistical precision.

Demand Based Models

As shown in Figure 3, demand based models are based solely upon facilities/services utilization. A demand based model typically measures actual utilization, divides by service population to calculate a use rate, then projects that use rate against future population to predict future utilization (MacStravic, 1978). From a positive view, data are usually available and relatively inexpensive to obtain and analyze. However, the methodology can easily understate or overstate actual need. For example, some cases involving serious alcohol problems are not likely to come to the attention of any agency or hospital.

In their simplest form, demand based models apply utilization rates to the entire population under study. By treating the population as homogenous, professionals will not be able to effectively target resources to subgroups affected by alcoholism. Some utilization based models compute separate rates for subgroups in the population based upon relevant demographic groupings. However, the inability of this methodology to address the needs of those not already touched by treatment systems underscores the necessity of using need based models.

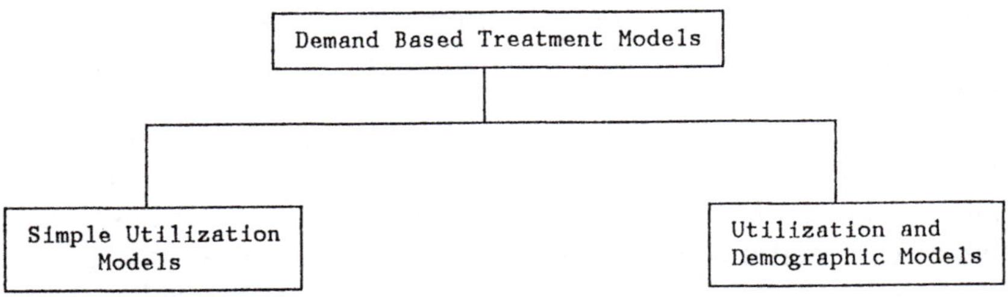

FIGURE 3. Demand Based Treatment Models

SUMMARY

There is a critical need to accurately determine the alcoholism treatment needs in a particular area so that treatment resources can be effectively allocated. Currently, many state planning agencies determine resource allocation based solely upon the population's utilization of existing treatment facilities. This demand approach for determining treatment needs omits the population subgroups who have need for treatment but may not be utilizing existing facilities. The preferred method of alcohol treatment assessment is to focus on need determination vs. demand measurement. For purposes of this paper, need is defined as those in need of treatment form problems reacted to alcoholism, while demand for treatment includes those currently participating in a treatment program.

In an effort to simplify the understanding of need assessment, a framework has been proposed for grouping and classifying the various alcoholism treatment assessment models. The initial phase of the model differentiates between demand vs. need assessment models. Next, need assessment models are grouped into four broad subgroups: (1) survey based models, (2) mortality based models, (3) treatment and mortality based models, and (4) multi-factor statistical based models. The final phase of the model presents a classification of demand based models. The demand based models include two types: (1) simple utilization models and (2) utilization combined with demographic models.

Assessment: Determination of Client Needs and Progress

Jerry J. Ingram
William I. Sauser, Jr.
Cathleen A. Owens

INTRODUCTION

It is the thesis of this article that the alcoholism assessment process can be made more clinically efficient by understanding the process from the perspective of a marketer. This contention is based principally on the realization that all organizations have marketing problems that can be aided by the application of marketing skills (Kotler, 1988). A discussion of some basic marketing concepts will demonstrate how alcoholism agencies can derive benefits from marketing technology.

Exchange Relationships

A principal mission of marketing activity is to understand and develop effective exchange relationships between an organization and its relevant publics. In short, successful exchanges mean that each party gives and receives something of value. Hence, alcoholism treatment agencies must establish viable exchange relationships with their client publics if organizational and client goals are to be realized.

Client Behavior and Motivations

To develop strategies and programs which result in mutually satisfying goal achievement, organizations must seek to understand the behavior and motives of their client publics. Marketers have developed and codified a large body of knowledge of consumer behavior. Futhermore, marketers have traditionally relied upon customer/user behavior analysis as the basis for strategy development.

Multiplicity of Influences on Client

In addition to the influence of customer/user motivations, many environmental variables impact upon "demand." These variables are cultural, social, economic, governmental, and political/legal in nature. Extensive treatment of the significance of environmental variables upon demand is found in marketing literature. The intricate understanding of these environmental variables by marketers can help alcoholism treatment agencies better assess treatment.

Market Delineation

Marketers have found that more effective and efficient strategies of market cultivation can be developed if smaller, more homogenous groups are targeted. This has led to the development of an extensive amount of market segmentation theory. It is the contention of these authors that effective applications of segmentation analysis can be made by alcoholism agencies.

These factors along with others are the basis for contemporary market cultivation and they have applications to all organizations desiring an effective and efficient exchange relationship with their relevant publics. The next section of this article will present an alcoholism assessment model from the perspective of a marketer. The basic components of the model have been derived from an intensive as well as extensive review of alcoholism assessment literature. The "abridged" terminology as well as the extensive attention to the impact of personal and environmental influences upon assessment and treatment represent the significant marketing influences upon the model. Following a presentation of the assessment model, a more detailed description of the marketing implications of the model will be presented. Finally, concluding comments will be made regarding the model's usefulness; and recommendations for future refinement will also be addressed.

ALCOHOLISM ASSESSMENT MODEL

The model depicted in Figure 1 represents a marketer's view of the alcoholism assessment process and is comprised of three basic components:

1. the assessment process,
2. personal and environmental influences, and
3. post exit activities.

The Assessment Process

The assessment process begins in the alcoholism market—a population of alcoholics and/or problem drinkers. This pool represents a heterogenous group with varying degrees of symptoms and problems. To be more useful in terms of effective assessment and treatment programs, this market must be subdivided into clinically meaningful subgroups. The marketing terminology for dividing markets into smaller more homogenous submarkets is market segmentation.

Efforts to segment the alcoholism market into more meaningful subgroups began in the mid 1800s. The earlier efforts to develop potential alcoholism typologies tended to focus on differences between alcoholics and nonalcoholics. But as noted by Alterman and Tarter (1986) the last two decades of typology research have produced an increased recognition of the heterogeneity of the alcoholic population. These authors point out that one implication of this awareness is that alcoholic individuals with different problems may respond differentially and be more susceptible to different treatments. Babor and Meyer (1986) have noted that to the extent that alcoholic types are readily identifiable, scientifically valid and clinically meaningful, they can be extremely useful for the purpose of diagnosis and treatment. Hesselbrook (1986) has stated that a growing number of clinical and research efforts have attempted to provide more accurate descriptions of the varied and complex factors involved in alcoholism. Hesselbrook further notes that many studies have employed multivariate statistical approaches (e.g., cluster analysis and factor analysis) to identify homogenous groupings of alcoholics based on various observations and measures. Other re-

Figure 1
ALCOHOLISM ASSESSMENT MODEL

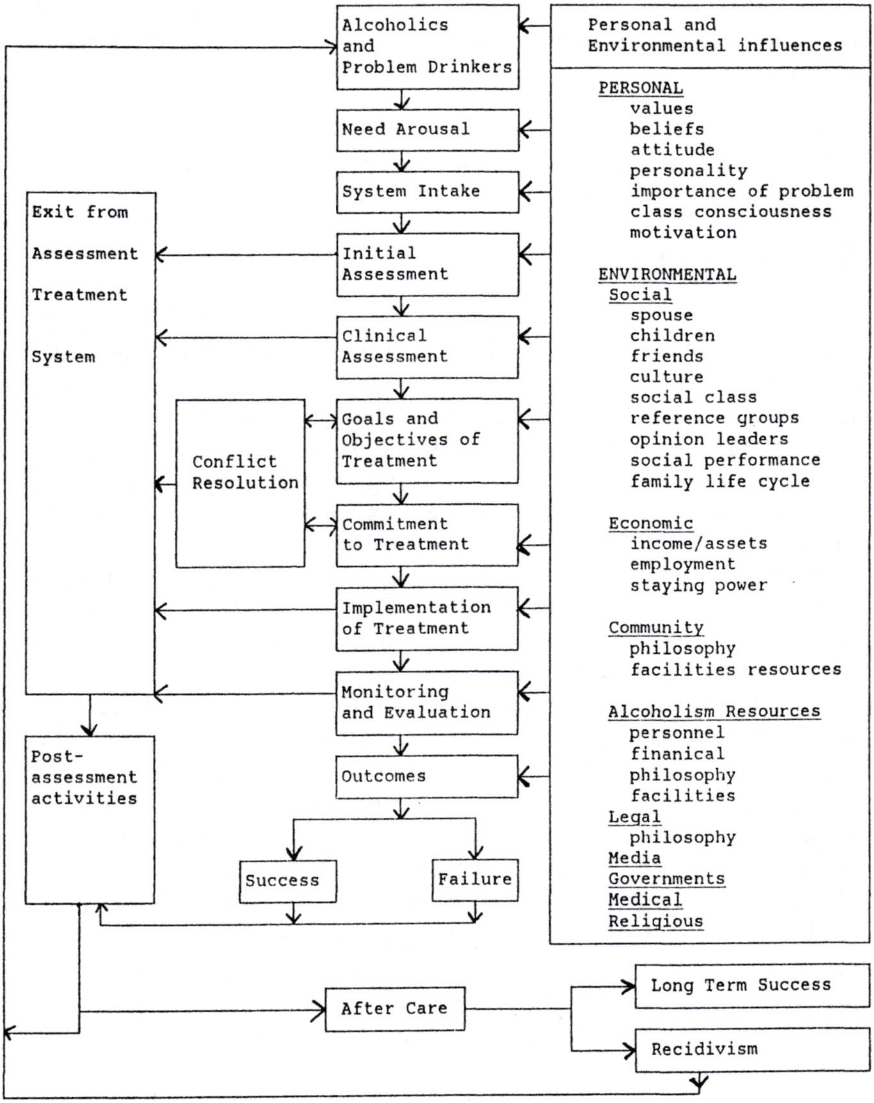

searchers advocating multiple assessment approaches to alcoholism have noted that such approaches allow the explanation of complex interactions among sociocultural, psychological and physiological processes thought to be important in the development and maintenance of alcoholism (Donovan, Kivlahan, & Walker, 1986).

Even though the adoption of advanced statistical analysis has assisted in the development of useful alcoholic typologies, some feel that more work needs to be done. As two authors have stated:

> Despite this encouraging development, it would be false to conclude that typology research has come of age. The current resurgence of interest in alcoholic typologies has not resulted in any compelling systematic theories. To a large extent the field is still characterized by disciplinary parochialism and methodological faddism. Typologies historically have been dictated more by the ideological biases of the typologists than by the rich clinical data available to the scientific observer. (Babor & Meyer, 1986)

It is interesting to compare the viewpoints of marketers vs. alcoholism researchers regarding the status of typological/segmentation research in their respective fields. Marketers have developed a generally accepted group of bases that are used in market division efforts, and research is conducted on a not too infrequent basis to determine the "typologies" for that particular market. No effort is made to segment all markets on the same bases. Hence, some markets may be segmented on the basis of income while others may be segmented on the basis of sex, geography, usage rate, etc. In other words, the marketer is not alarmed that the same segmentation basis does not suit all circumstances. On the other hand, those who are conducting typological research in alcoholism appear to be motivated to develop one grand segmentation scheme which is useful in classifying alcoholic subtypes in all circumstances. Given the heterogenous nature of the alcoholism market this may not be an achievable goal.

It may well be that alcoholism researchers will have to settle on a number of possible segmentation typologies with the most appropriate one in a given circumstance being determined after conducting research. However one views the alcoholism population, the first step toward assessment and treatment is need arousal or motivating the problem drinker to enter the assessment system.

Need Arousal

Marketers generally agree that all decision process behavior begins with need arousal or problem recognition. This is defined as the perception of a difference between the ideal state of affairs and the actual situation sufficient to arouse and activate the decision process (Engel, Blackwell, & Miniard, 1985) Need arousal may be internally or externally generated. It may be activated under desirable circumstances or from an unsatisfactory state of affairs. As shown in Figure 1, need arousal can be influenced by a large number of personal and/or environmental influences. The personal variables impacting upon need arousal include values, beliefs, attitudes, personality, importance of problem, class consciousness and motivation. In addition, environmental variables such as social forces, economic community attitudes, alcoholism resources, legal forces, governmental forces and the media can and do impact upon need arousal. Some of the environmental influences such as alcoholism agencies, religious organizations, legal institutions and family members may engage in *active* efforts to activate need arousal. Other environmental factors such as economic, community attitudes and governmental agencies may exercise a less direct impact upon need arousal. For example, those convicted of drunken driving violations may be required by a legal body to enter an alcoholism facility for assessment and treatment. On the other hand, a community which fosters a favorable environment for the treatment of problem drinkers will likely exercise a smaller level of influence upon need arousal.

It would appear that the alcoholism treatment industry should direct resources toward the identification of those personal and environmental variables which offer the greatest prospects for activating need arousal. For example, Mastrich (1988) conducted a study with Employee Assistance Program (EAP) personnel and found that motivational orientation, level of motivation, "triggering incident," and the number of motivators a client presented at intake were associated with significant differences in drinking behavior and job performance. Mastrich further noted that the differentiation quality of "triggering incident" suggests that EAP services and outreach efforts should be expanded with emphasis on encouragement of self-referrals.

Marketers Engel, Warshaw and Kinnear (1987) have noted that formalized promotional efforts have their greatest potential impact when problem recognition already exists. This would imply that organized efforts using the media and other resources to encourage alcoholics to admit themselves for assessment and treatment may not be particularly effective unless the person is already aware that he/she has a drinking problem. This may mean that such environmental factors as religion, family, legal, or targeted media could be more potent in the early stages of need arousal while mass media efforts may have their greatest impact following some realization that a problem exists.

Assessment

Once a client has been admitted into an alcoholism treatment system, the next step is to conduct an assessment so that appropriate treatment goals can be determined. For purposes of this article assessment has been divided into two phases, initial assessment and clinical assessment. Dean (1985) points out that an individual referred for assessment and possible treatment first enters the system through a brief intake procedure that includes demographic data collection for insurance and administrative purposes. Figure 1 reveals that both personal and environmental influences have some impact upon initial assessment. For example, lack of sufficient funds or insurance may indicate that the client cannot continue in the assessment system. An exit from the assessment process means that a client remains a part of the non-treatment population. From a marketing viewpoint initial assessment is synonymous to customers having their financial needs assessed by a financial planner for the first time. Before getting down to actual assessment there is a social phase of the meeting. Manning and Reece (1987) refer to the initial assessment as an approach which has three objectives: (1) make a good first impression, (2) capture the person's full attention, (3) generate interest in the product you are selling. Clifton Reichard (1985) suggests that sales representatives should develop an emotional relationship with buyers prior to moving on to other parts of the sales presentation. Stated differently the initial assessment phase in marketing generally emphasizes the development of social contact-building rapport. When making the transition from the initial social contact to the "business" relationship we need to focus on the client's dominant buying motive. The buyer must like what he or she sees and hears and must be made to feel that it will be worthwhile to hear more (Manning & Reece, 1987).

Dean (1985) notes that the second step in the assessment process is the clinical interview which has three objectives:

1. to establish positive client relationships;
2. to assess the case; and
3. to direct the individual to treatment.

According to Dean the chain of future therapeutic events is built on the clinical interview which employs testing instruments and the development of a case history. In some ways the clinical assessment is similar to the marketing researcher's responsibility of collecting and analyzing information about markets. The collected information is then used as a basis for developing strategy and plans of attack.

The clinical assessment process is a highly technical area with a large number of technical assessments instruments to select from. A sampling of alcoholism assessment instruments include:

- SADD Short Alcohol Dependence Data (see for example, Orford & Keddie, 1986; Davidson & Raistrick, 1986)
- SADQ Severity of Alcohol Dependency Questionnaire (see for example, Cosney et al., 1986; Davidson & Raistrick, 1986)
- MAST Michigan Alcoholism Screening Test (see for example, Dittrich, 1986; Babor & Mendelsohn, 1980; Selzer, 1971)
- EADS Edinburgh Alcohol Dependency Scale (see for example, Davidson & Raistrick, 1986)

–DIS	Diagnostic Interview Schedule (see for example, da Fonesca et al., 1986)
–AWRS	Alcohol Withdrawal Rating Scale (see for example, Brunning, Mumford, & Keaney, 1986)
–MMPI	Minnesota Multiphasic Personality Inventory (see for example, Dean, 1985; Hesselbrook, 1986)
–ISI	Intervention Stressor Inventory (see for example, Loneck, R. M., 1986)
–ATPS	Alcohol Treatment Profile System (see for example, Ryan, K., 1985)

This list of assessment instruments is not exhaustive but it does indicate the analytical tools available for those involved in clinical analysis.

The literature on alcoholism is abundant with research studies attesting to the validity and reliability of alternative assessment instruments. It is interesting to point out a major difference between assessment instruments in marketing research and alcoholism. Many of the alcoholism assessment instruments used to determine the nature and extent of clients' problems have been validated. Furthermore, when used by trained clinicians, these instruments have the ability to be effective in a number of circumstances. Marketers, on the other hand, do not enjoy the luxury of having several validated measurement instruments which can be effectively used under a variety of circumstances. Even the activities, interest, and opinion scales (AIO) developed to assist marketers with psychographic research are most effective when they are tailor-made for a particular product or service.

Even the casual observer would agree that several good assessment instruments in the alcoholism field have been developed, refined and validated. Some of the alcoholism assessment techniques rely upon self-reporting procedures as a basis for data gathering. Davidson and Raistrick (1986) have assessed the validity of the Short Alcohol Dependence Data (SADD) instrument and have concluded that there is sufficient evidence to justify its use on the basis of demonstrated construct, concurrent and content validity. These authors present SADD as a brief easy-to-administer, self-report assessment procedure that represents a comprehensive attempt to assess all the elements of the alcohol dependence syndrome within one questionnaire and that can be used in a research as well as a clinical setting. Other assessment "models" have been validated by researchers, and the emergence of computer-assisted testing provides the distinct advantages of individualized reporting, tailored testing, and statistically based diagnosis (Skinner et al., 1981). Even though clinicians have available validated "customer" needs assessment instruments, ultimately assessment must be executed to the satisfaction of both the client/customer and the professional. If this does not happen, the client may exit from the assessment/treatment system returning to the pool of untreated alcoholics.

From a marketer's perspective, if the client's needs have not been adequately assessed it makes the problem solution prescription a moot point. Hence, an inappropriate recommendation for problem resolution is accompanied by the liability of an increased probability that the customer will either go elsewhere seeking help or will simply exit from the search process. Assuming that the clinical assessment process has been carried out satisfactorily, however, the next phase of the assessment process is the determination of treatment goals and objectives.

Treatment Goals and Objectives

Not only are the treatment goals and objectives a function of the clinical assessment process but, as shown in Figure 1 they are influenced by both personal and environmental influencers as well. Hence, personal characteristics such as attitudes, class consciousness and motivation can easily influence the goals and objectives established for a particular client. In like manner, environmental factors such as income and "staying power" will influence the establishment of goals and objectives by the clinician. "Staying power" is defined as the financial strength to commit to treatment over the long run. Further, the alcoholism resources available in a particular setting may serve to limit objective and goal achievement.

Marketers typically differentiate between objectives and goals and it would appear that this distinction has some relevance for alcoholism assessment as well. An objective is expressed as a long-range purpose which is typically not quantified or limited to a time period (Jain, 1985). A goal is a measurable desired outcome for the organization, judged by an administrator to be attainable at some specific future date through planned actions (Jain, 1985). Thus, an objective of the assessment/treatment process is to achieve long-term recovery from alcoholism. On the other hand, a goal may be for clients to successfully complete a 28-day detoxification program as an inpatient. Since the objective of most treatment programs is long-term recovery, then clinical personnel have discretionary decisions to make principally in the area of goal setting. Pfrang and Schenk (1986) have concluded that treatment approaches should consider the patient's attitudes in order to determine appropriate treatment goals and to provide adequate support during the rehabilitation phase. This finding supports the theoretical constraints of the assessment model depicted in Figure 1, which indicates that attitudes do impact upon treatment goals. Orford and Keddie (1986) conducted a study in which they compared abstinence and controlled drinking-oriented treatment. After only an *initial* assessment clients were randomly assigned to one of three treatment groups. Following this experiment the authors concluded that it would be very difficult to make clear-cut recommendations about treatment goals at initial assessment except in a few cases. In another study Jordan et al. (1985) determined that including patients in the treatment planning process increases the likelihood of active participation. Specifically this study concluded that the treatment groups dealing with needs which were given higher priority by the patients were better attended. The prescription here is to involve the client in assessment and goal setting.

By involving clients in the prescription or goal setting phase of assessment, conflict resolution is likely to be expedited (see Figure 1). In addition, commitment to treatment as shown in the experiment conducted by Jordan et al. (1985) is also enhanced when the client has an input into the goal setting phase of assessment.

Commitment to Treatment

Loneck (1986) has noted that intervention is a highly specialized therapeutic technique used to bring about the alcoholic's acceptance of treatment. Hence, once a treatment plan (with objectives and goals) has been presented, the alcoholic must choose between acceptance or rejection of treatment. There is likely to be conflict generated at this phase of assessment due to a number of factors. Some of the conflict quite naturally may exist between the client alcoholic and the clinician concerning the prescribed treatment plan. Pattison (1979) has stated that the effectiveness of a specific treatment method is determined, in part, by the individual's desire to work with the treatment. Thus, it is important, notes Pattison, to have a choice of treatments available and to match the individual's indications and situational factors with an appropriate treatment.

Commitment to treatment can be influenced by personal and environmental variables. An individual's perception of the importance of the problem and his motivational level will likely impact upon commitment. Environmental factors such as social performance, spouse's attitude and financial ability of the client may likewise impact upon commitment to treatment.

Marketers have traditionally related the role of perceived risk to "go no-go" decisions. There is, for example, the possible existence of psychosocial risk. This implies that a purchase decision of significant consequences could prove embarrassing before family, friends, business associates, or neighbors. The risk that such discomforts will ensue is increased by the conspicuousness of the item under consideration (Berkman & Gilson, 1978). Taylor (1974) notes that because risk is anxiety producing and painful, consumers must deal with it in some way in order to make choices. In Taylor's view, any choice situation always involves two aspects of risks: uncertainty about the outcome and uncertainty about the consequences.

From a marketer's perspective it seems fruitful to study more completely the types and intensity of risks which a client alcoholic perceives in his decision to commitment to treatment. After the risk(s) have been identified and defined, alcoholism agencies can then proceed to develop a mix of "risk relievers." It may be, for example, that testimonials from famous personalities (e.g., Betty Ford) may be a potent risk reliever. In any event, commitment to treatment will be enhanced when alcoholics perceive fewer risks in terms of uncertainty about the outcome of treatment and uncertainty about the consequences of treatment. If perceived risks have been effectively handled, the likelihood of the client alcoholic exiting from the assessment/treatment system is reduced. Assuming that the alcoholic has committed to treatment, the implementations of treatment should proceed promptly.

Implementation of Treatment

After the alcoholic has made a commitment to the objectives and goals for the prescribed plan, actual treatment begins. From a clinical perspective, the process of implementing procedures to achieve treatment objectives and goals is put into motion. In this regard clinicians should have developed a detailed action plan for each phase of treatment. Not only should the action plan be specific in terms of facilities and treatment methods, but efforts should also be made to appropriately match the client and treatment situation with treatment personnel. The significance of the personnel aspect for treatment was noted by Pattison (1979) who stressed that treatment personnel should be matched in terms of their specific skills and values, with individual alcoholic clients who need those specific treatment skills and share similar values. Pattison found that matching therapist-client values is the most powerful predictor of successful outcome.

Marketers have stressed the necessity of expediting the terms and conditions of a sale in a timely manner (Balsley & Birsner, 1987). One of the principal reasons for expediting an agreement promptly and effectively is to minimize the possible complications of cognitive dissonance (assimilation). Festinger and Bramel (1962) have concluded:

> When a person chooses between two or more alternatives, discomfort or dissonance will almost inevitably arise because of the person's knowledge that while the decision he has made has certain advantages, it also has some disadvantages. That dissonance arises after almost every decision, and further, that the individual will invariably take steps to reduce this dissonance.

From a clinical perspective it is important to note that a dissonant customer (patient) will usually resort to one of two courses of action. The client may try to reduce the dissonance by abandoning or returning the product, or he may try to reduce the dissonance by seeking information that might confirm its high value (or avoiding information that might confirm its low value) (Kotler, 1988). Marketers have found that post-purchase communication with consumers in the form of follow-up calls, ads depicting satisfied purchasers, etc. to be effective in reducing cognitive dissonance.

As shown in Figure 1, client alcoholics can exit the treatment process during the implementation phase and return to the not-in-treatment pool. One way to minimize exiting from the treatment process is to be aware of and measure the level of post-commitment dissonance. Once dissonance has been detected programs should be implemented to reduce its severity. Not only should client dissonance be of concern immediately following commitment but efforts to detect dissonance should continue throughout the monitoring and evaluation phase as well.

Monitoring and Evaluation

Monitoring and evaluating a client's progress during treatment is essential if treatment objectives and goals are to be achieved. Moos and Finney (1983) have stated that researchers are addressing alcoholism evaluation issues within the context of a conceptually based, process-oriented evaluation framework which draws on current trends in evaluation research and behavioral medicine. Clinicians have employed a variety of evaluation techniques ranging from experimental research designs to urine simple analysis. Experimental designs as a tool by conducting alcoholism treatment evaluation studies have been criticized by Gottheil et al. (1981) and others. The criticisms of using experimental designs in the evaluation of alcoholism treatment programs is tied principally to the inability to draw representative random samples, as well as to measurement difficulties. On the other hand Peacey and Kapur (1986) concluded that urine sample analysis (the alcohol dipstick) proved to be a simple, inexpensive, and rapid alcohol measurement procedure.

Marketing researchers rely upon performance-monitoring research to track aspects of the marketing system (Kinnear & Taylor, 1987). For example, many business organizations utilize marketing research to track monetary measures such as sales, market share, and profit, as well as nonmonetary measures such as image, attitudes, and the like. Marketers typically accept the premise that a number of variables should be monitored and usually avoid the risk of relying upon single indicators.

Historically the abstinence criterion has been the most widely monitored variable in the treatment of alcoholics. However, as clinicians have seen the need to achieve other goals with alcoholics, variables which relate to the clients' social, marital, occupational and other areas of functioning are being monitored. As a consequence more clinicians are advocating multidimensional measures of treatment outcome. Gordis (1981) has pointed out the difficulties in setting up an evaluation study that shows a relationship between treatment and outcomes and notes that the basic measurement problem is the need for some type of biological or biochemical marker of alcohol consumption.

Outcomes

As noted previously, the outcomes of treatment programs are being based more on multidimensional measures rather than the single criterion of abstinence. This is due principally to the notion that patients who successfully recover control over their drinking also function well in non-drinking areas such as family life and the workplace (Billings & Moos, 1983). Hence the definition of a *successful* outcome is for a patient to control his use of alcohol so as to bring about long-term improvement in all aspects of life adversely impacted by alcoholism. The definition of a *failing* outcome for treatment would be a continuation of alcohol abuse which continues to impact adversely upon various aspects of the patient's life. If treatment outcome is classified as a failure (see Figure 1), this individual exits the assessment/treatment system and returns to the pool of alcoholics and problem drinkers. Due to a relatively high rate of recidivism among "cured" alcoholics, long-term success will not be experienced by all patients experiencing short-term success. The alcoholism assessment model proposed here indicates that after care is a type of post-treatment monitoring designed to increase the likelihood of a patient experiencing long-term success. In marketing terminology, this is synonymous to a salesperson staying in touch with a customer after the sale to promote long-term satisfaction.

Some of the patients returning to the pool of alcoholics and problem drinkers will be recycled at some later date. But as the number of alcoholics and problem drinkers continues to grow, there is a need to better understand the assessment process. It is the contention of this article that marketers can assist in rendering the system more effective. In order for this to happen marketers need to learn more about alcoholism and clinicians need to gain an appreciation of marketing processes.

SUMMARY AND RECOMMENDATIONS

This article has proposed an alcoholism assessment model developed with a marketing perspective. The marketing view emphasizes the importance of establishing viable exchange relationships between an organization and its relevant publics. The attainment of mutually gratifying exchanges hinges upon developing programs to deal with a large number of personal and environmental influences.

The actual assessment process begins with a detailed understanding of the heterogeneous pool of alcoholics and problem drinkers. The fact that the served market is heterogeneous is significant in terms of matching programs and treatments with specific needs. Need arousal is necessary if members of the pool of alcoholics and problem drinkers are to enter the assessment process. Strategies for initiating need arousal have been presented with emphasis placed upon the role of both personal and environmental variables.

Once the client has entered the assessment system two stages of assessment take place. Initial assessment is principally concerned with establishing rapport and trust and taking care of administrative matters. Clinical assessment is designed to test the nature of the alcoholic's problem(s) in a systematic and scientific manner. Following the technical assessment, the clinician is then in a position to develop objectives and goals tailored to the specific needs of the client.

Implementation of treatment then begins and a system is set up to monitor and evaluate the clients' progress toward recovery. Monitoring devices can range from sophisticated statistical designs to the simple alcoholism dipstick test. The treatment outcomes are conveniently classified as success or failure. A *failure* outcome means that the client remains in the alcoholism/problem drinkers pool, while a *success* outcome implies long-term control of alcohol consumption and improvement in areas of one's life adversely impacted by alcoholism. After care is a type of post-treatment monitoring designed to increase the likelihood of clients experiencing long-term success.

There remains the possibility that clients may exit the assessment/treatment system at any time following initial intake through monitoring and evaluation. By viewing the entire assessment process as an exchange relationship, agencies can better meet the client's treatment as well as nontreatment needs. This client-oriented approach has the possibility of reducing the assessment/treatment dropout rate.

The authors have presented the alcoholism assessment model as a starting point to assist both marketers and clinicians toward gaining a more conceptual understanding of the entire process. It is hoped that theoreticians in both disciplines will engage in research which not only evaluates the workability of this model but which improves upon this initial effort.

Secondary Information and Reference Sources for Alcoholism Treatment Marketers

Daniel M. Blucker
Vaughan C. Judd
Donald R. Self

INTRODUCTION–TYPES OF INFORMATION

Organizations—commercial, institutional, or governmental—need information to uncover market opportunities and to plan, implement, and evaluate programs and activities in pursuit of those opportunities. Alcoholism treatment marketers have needs for specialized information for these same reasons. Achievement of an alcoholism treatment marketer's objectives is contingent in part on how well the marketer researches for relevant information. Accordingly, this article deals with the general process of obtaining relevant information and with specific sources of information for alcoholism treatment marketers.

Information can be categorized as either primary or secondary information. Primary information is that which is "original" in the sense that it is not already available, and is generated to satisfy a specific need. Secondary information is that which is already published or available to the marketer from either internal or external sources. Information can also be categorized as being either statistical or non-statistical. Figure 1 represents the various types of information based on these two classification schemes.

External secondary data, as depicted in Figure 1, can be further subcategorized. In addition to being statistical or non-statistical, external secondary data can be either purchased from a vendor or obtained at no charge or a nominal charge from a library. It is the

Figure 1. Types and Examples of Marketing-Related Information from an Alcoholism Treatment Marketer's Perspective.

	Primary Data	Secondary Data	
		Internal	External
Statistical Data	Example: Conduct an original study using mail questionnaires to determine the percentage of employers who provide Employee Assistance Programs.	Example: Use existing client records to develop demographic profiles of past & current clients.	Example: Use U.S. government data (NIAAA) to develop a geographic profile of alcoholism treatment centers.
Non-Statistical Data	Example: Conduct research using focus groups to determine employers' attitudes toward ATMs in a particular market area.	Example: Obtain information from knowledgeable persons in the ATM's organization regarding the success of the organization's treatment programs.	Example: Use articles from publications such as Alcoholism Treatment Quarterly for information on alcoholism treatment issues.

external secondary data available through libraries which is the focus of this article.

THE AVAILABILITY OF LIBRARIES

Most readers will have a library close to their residence or place of work. The *American Library Directory* (1986) reports there are 31,475 libraries in the United States representing seven different types of libraries. For most readers, public libraries will be the type of library generally used since there should be at least one such facility in their locale. The *American Library Directory* (1986) shows that there are 8,865 public libraries in the U.S. and that 1,365 of these libraries operate a total of 6,350 branches—in total then, there are 15,215 public libraries in the United States. Public libraries vary widely in terms of their size and resources. As will be demonstrated later, however, the size of a library's collection is not necessarily a factor limiting the level of service it can provide its patrons.

Another type of library is the academic library found in public and private junior colleges, colleges, and universities. For some readers, an academic library might be more readily available than a public library. Academic libraries are typically open to the general public and their holdings are available for use on-premise. Others, for a fee, will provide a library card that allows members of the general public to borrow materials. In addition to public and academic libraries, there are other types of libraries including armed forces, government, law, medical, and special libraries. Although there may be a representation of several of the various types of libraries in the reader's local area, it is recommended that a public library be the first stop for secondary information.

While some readers may be skilled library users, others may be rather unfamiliar with library use or somewhat rusty in their library skills. For those who need guidance in the use of a library, the following sections on library organization and information sources and tools to access the information are provided.

LIBRARY ORGANIZATION AND INFORMATION SOURCES

The resources of a library are organized within several different departments or sections. A typical library will include reference and general books, serials, and possibly one or more other separate collections. Library staff in the reference section is available to provide patrons with general information and guidance on using the library. They are knowledgeable not only as to the holdings of their library and the services offered, but also as to relevant materials and services available elsewhere. A library's reference collection will include materials such as generalized and specialized encyclopedias and dictionaries, biographical sources, bibliographies, indexes, directories, almanacs, atlases, and statistical tools. Typically, the reference section also houses the card catalog, and interlibrary loan and on-line database search services.

The general book collection of a library is usually the largest section of the library and contains books arranged by categories such as literature, physical science, medicine, psychology, and business—according to either the Dewey Decimal or Library of Congress Classification System. In large libraries, the general collection may not only be departmentalized by category, but may also have specialized librarians in charge of individual subject areas such as fine arts, humanities, social science, and science and technology. In addition to the reference librarians, these specialists stand ready to provide assistance to patrons with regard to their respective subjects.

The serials section of the library contains publications such as newspapers, magazines, and journals. Most libraries have a serials librarian or a serials staff to help patrons locate specific publications in the collection. It should be noted that serials are available in several formats other than the traditional printed format. Larger libraries will have some of their serials holdings on microfilm or microfiche. Printed serials are usually housed in two different areas of the serials sections, current issues in one area and earlier bound volumes in another. Serials will be arranged either alphabetically according to the title or in accordance with the library's classification system. Serials of interest to alcoholism treatment marketers are noted in a later section of this article entitled "Journals."

Although there may be a number of separate collections in a particular library, one section which will be of special interest to the reader is the U.S. government documents section found in libraries designated as depository libraries. According to the U.S. Office of the Public Printer (1983), each state has at least one depository library. Forty states have at least one full or regional depository library which receives all publications designated as depository items. Other depository libraries are designated as "selective depositories" and receive only a portion of the available documents. Publications of the U.S. government range from topics of popular appeal to those more technical in nature. Information pertaining to subjects such as the environment, the economy, business, social problems, health, civil rights, education, energy, and crime is available. Government Documents Librarians are ready and willing to help patrons locate material which is usually classified according to the SuDocs system, a system different from that used to classify other materials in the library.

TOOLS AND SERVICES FOR ACCESSING INFORMATION

There are several tools and services available to library patrons that give them access to secondary information sources. Generally, these tools and services are found in the reference section of the library. The first tool is the card catalog which exists either in the form of a filing system of individual cards or an automated (computerized) catalog system. To find which books or serials a library owns, it is necessary to consult the library's card catalog. The catalog lists books by author, title, and subject, and serials by title and subject. On each card or record is the book or serial's call number. If a library has a government documents section, the documents may or may not be included in the main card catalog. Libraries use either the Library of Congress or the Dewey Decimal Classification System to develop call numbers. Call numbers indicate where in the library's collections the materials are physically located. Reference librarians are ready to assist patrons in using the card catalog system.

If you are looking for information in serials, which includes magazines, journals, or newspapers, you will want to use indexes. Most indexes examine several hundred serials. Serials dealing with business and marketing are indexed in the *Business Index* and the *Business Periodicals Index*. Serials dealing with alcoholism treatment are indexed in several indexes described in a later section of this article entitled "Indexes and Databases." Documents of the United States government are indexed in the *Monthly Catalog*, *CIS Index*, *American Statistics Index*, *Index to U.S. Government Periodicals*, and *Government Publications Index*. An index lists the articles in the serials it covers according to subject headings which reflect the subject content of the articles. The index supplies such information as an article's title and author as well as the title, publication date, and page number of the serial which contains the article. Indexes are published in several different formats including printed versions, optical and compact discs, film, and as on-line databases.

If a local library's collection does not contain the material needed by a patron, interlibrary loan service makes the collections of other libraries available to the patron. Most public libraries are linked with other libraries in various interlibrary loan systems which permit a patron to borrow books and obtain photocopies of articles in serials from other libraries. There is usually no fee charged for this service although in some instances a charge may be made by the lending library for photocopies of articles supplied. Interlibrary loan is one of two services which extends the local library's resources for the patron; the other service is on-line database searching which is available for a fee at most libraries. With the necessary computer equipment and minimal training, available from the vendors, an individual can perform their own on-line database searching at home or in the office. By way of a computerized hookup over long distance telephone lines between the searcher and the database vendor, information is accessed by the searcher. Databases of interest to alcoholism treatment marketers are included in this article under the heading of "Indexes and Databases." In addition to those databases listed, there are several databases covering business and marketing materials which might be of interest to Alcoholism Treatment Marketers. One such database is *ABI/INFORM* which provides general decision sciences information from approximately 550 primary publications in business and related fields. Whatever a patron's information needs, the world of database searching puts a wealth of information at the fingertips of the searcher. Trained librarian-searchers stand ready to make this wealth of information available to library patrons at a nominal fee.

There is a variety of sources of information related to the marketing of treatment programs for alcohol abuse: bibliographies, indexes, on-line databases, health care marketing and alcohol-related journals, organizations, associations, specialized self-help groups, and resource organizations. This chapter provides a list of references to those sources that the authors have found to be particularly useful due to their currency, reliability, and availability.

Bibliographies

A bibliography is a list of writings relating to a single subject or a specific author. There are some relatively comprehensive bibliographies available that list writings that address specific aspects of alcohol use and abuse. These bibliographies are available for use in most libraries as well as for purchase through local bookstores for quick reference use at home or the office. Selected for inclusion here are those bibliographies that are relatively current and comprehensive and that are arranged and indexed in ways that make finding relevant information easy.

Andrews, Theodora. *A Bibliography of Drug Abuse: Including Alcohol and Tobacco*. Littleton, CO, Libraries Unlimited, 1977.

This is an annotated bibliography of 725 titles. Part I lists "General Reference Sources," including bibliographies, journal indexes, directories, handbooks, guides, and journals. Part II lists "Source Material by Subject Area," including a section on "alcohol." The book concludes with "Author and Title" and "Subject" indexes.

Andrews, Theodora. *A Bibliography of Drug Abuse: Supplement, 1977-1980*. Littleton, CO, Libraries Unlimited, 1981.

This is a supplement to Andrews' 1977 work. It also is an annotated bibliography in two parts: "General Reference Sources" and "Source Material by Subject Area." This supplement lists 741 additional works, most published since 1976.

Barnes, Grace M., compiler. *Alcohol and Youth, A Comprehensive Bibliography*. Westport, CT, Greenwood Press, 1982.

This bibliography includes nearly 5,000 citations directly related to alcohol use among youth. The citations refer to books, journal articles, theses, government reports, and popular literature. The citations are listed alphabetically by the last name of the author. A subject index is provided.

Barnes, Grace M., Abel, Ernest L., and Ernst, Charles A. S., compilers. *Alcohol and the Elderly: A Comprehensive Bibliography*. Westport, CT, Greenwood Press, 1980.

This is a bibliography of more than 1,200 references related to alcohol consumption by the elderly, generally fifty-five years and above. Included are references to books, journal articles, and reports. The items in the bibliography are listed alphabetically by the last name of the author. A subject index is provided.

Barnes, Grace M., and Augustine, Diane K., compilers. *Alcohol and the Family: A Comprehensive Bibliography*. New York, Greenwood Press, 1987.

This bibliography attempts to be a comprehensive listing of the literature on alcohol and the family. There are over 6,000 references in all languages, including books, chapters, articles, reports, and government documents. The references are listed alphabetically by the last name of the first author. Where no author is given, references are listed alphabetically by the English title of the work. A subject index is provided at the end of the bibliography.

Chalfant, H. Paul, and Roper, Brent S., compilers. *Social and Behavioral Aspects of Female Alcoholism: An Annotated Bibliography*. Westport, CT, Greenwood Press, 1980.

This bibliography includes 488 annotated references to journal articles about the social and behavioral aspects of female alcoholism. The references are divided into nine subject categories. An author index is provided.

International Bibliography of Studies on Alcohol. New Brunswick, NJ, Publications Division, Rutgers Center of Alcohol Studies, 1966-1980.

"The general purpose of this work is to provide a broad multidisciplinary and interprofessional bibliography" (introduction) in three volumes. Volume I contains over 25,000 references from 1901-1950 arranged first by year and within year alphabetically by author's name. Volume II contains subject and author indexes to the references in the first volume. Volume III is a single listing of references for the period 1951-1960 arranged alphabetically by the first author's name. Subject and author indexes are included.

Kurtz, Norman R., Googins, Bradley, and Howard, William. *Occupational Alcoholism, an Annotated Bibliography* Toronto, Ont., Canada, Addiction Research Foundations, 1984.

This bibliography covers occupational alcoholism programs and related employee assistance programs and includes papers, reports, books, chapters, and journal articles. It is arranged in twenty subject categories. The authors have attempted to provide a comprehensive overview of the subject. Each citation is accompanied by an abstract. For citations reporting empirical research. the authors have attempted to include information on research design, sample size, instrument, and results. The alphabetical "Author Index" lists all authors' names. Using the same twenty subject categories, the "Category Index" lists each article under the primary and secondary topics covered.

Milgram, Gail Gleason. *Alcohol Education Materials: An Annotated Bibliography*. New Brunswick, NJ, Publications Division, Rutgers Center of Alcohol Studies, 1975-1981.

This title has been published five times covering different time periods; 1950-1973, 1973-1978, 1978-1979, 1979-1980, and 1980-1981. Included are references to books, curriculum guides, paperbacks, pamphlets, leaflets, periodicals, and miscellaneous items designed for alcohol education. The references are arranged alphabetically by author, or title if no author is given. There are four indexes; Title, Type of Publication,

Audience Level, and Major Contents of Texts. A list of publishers with addresses is also provided.

Watts, Thomas D., and Wright, Jr., Roosevelt. *Black Alcohol Abuse and Alcoholism: An Annotated Bibliography*. New York, Praeger, 1986.

The purpose of this volume is to bring together most of the written literature in the English language from the 1940s to the present on black alcoholism. Included are articles, books, and other published material. The citations with annotations are arranged first in chronological order by year and then alphabetical by author's name. The index lists authors, minority populations, agencies, tests or measurements employed, cities, and countries, but is not a true subject index. Following the bibliography are "Alcohol and Black Americans: Resource List" and "Directory of State and Territorial Alcoholism Program Directors."

Indexes and Databases

Because of the dated and static nature of a bound volume, the aforementioned bibliographies lack true currency. To access more current information than is available in the published bibliographies, printed and computerized databases have been made available. In printed form, these databases appear as indexes and abstracts and are available in many libraries. They are also available on a subscription basis to any individual or institution. Because of the time required in the printing and distribution process of these indexes, they lose some of their currency. To overcome this printing delay, the indexes are also available for on-line searching. These on-line databases are available from two of the major database vendors; *DIALOG Information Services* (3460 Hillview Avenue, Palo Alto, CA 94304, 800-3-DIALOG) and *BRS Information Technologies* (1200 Route 7, Latham, NY 12100, 800-2 ASK BRS). DIALOG provides access to more than 280 databases representing a broad scope of disciplines. *BRS* provides access to more than 100. These databases include indexes to articles, abstracts, and conference papers, full texts of some articles and papers, directory listings of companies, associations, or people, and corporate financial statements. Both of these vendors provide one day training sessions for individuals who want to do their own searching. The following is a list of available indexes, and their on-line equivalents, that are of particular usefulness in identifying information relating to alcohol use and abuse. Both *DIALOG* and *BRS* provide access to all but one of the databases listed below.

Abridged Index Medicus. Bethesda, MD, National Library of Medicine, 1970—. (subscription—$43/year; Superintendent of Documents, U.S. Government Printing Office, Washington, D.C. 20402 [GPO subscription code: ABIM])

This is a monthly listing of articles published in 117 English-language clinical medicine journals. It is designed for the individual practitioner and libraries of small hospitals and clinics. It cumulates annually as *Cumulated Abridged Index Medicus* (available from GPO for $43). The contents of this index are available on-line via the *MEDLINE* database.

Alcohol Awareness Service. Rockville, MD, National Clearinghouse for Alcohol and Drug Information, November 1979—. (subscription—$15/year; NCADI, Department AAS, P.O. Box 2345, Rockville, MD 20852)

This is a bimonthly list of current alcohol and drug information, complete with availability, cost, and ordering information. The references are divided into broad subject categories with an author and organization index and a cross-referenced subject index. This information is available on-line only from the NCALI.

Cumulative Index to Nursing and Allied Health Literature. Glendale, CA, Glendale Adventist Medical Center, 1977—. (subscription—$168; CINAHL, 1509 Wilson Terrace, Glendale, CA 91206)

This bimonthly index provides access to more than 300 English-language nursing publications and primary journals in more than a dozen allied health disciplines. The on-line version of this index is the *Nursing and Allied Health* database.

Hospital Literature Index. Chicago, American Hospital Association, 1957– . (subscription–$181.25; American Hospital Association, 840 N. Lake Shore Drive, Chicago, IL 60611)

This quarterly index contains references to "literature on hospital and health facility administration, including multi-institutional systems, health planning, and administrative aspects of health care delivery." Since 1978, it has been compiled with the cooperation and assistance of the National Library of Medicine. The on-line version of this index is the *Health Planning and Administration* database.

Index Medicus. Bethesda, MD, National Library of Medicine, 1960– . (subscription-$163/year; Superintendent of Documents, U.S. Government Printing Office, Washington, DC 20402 [GPO subscription code: IM])

This is a monthly listing of references to current articles from approximately 2,750 biomedical journals from around the world. Included in each issue are separate subject and author sections. It cumulates annually as *Cumulated Index Medicus* (available from GPO for $204). The contents of this index are available on-line as a part of the *MEDLINE* database.

International Nursing Index. New York, American Journal of Nursing, Co., 1966– . (subscription–$250; American Journal of Nursing Company, 555 West 57th Street, New York, NY 10019)

This is a quarterly sponsored by the American Nurses Association and the National League for Nursing and produced in cooperation with the National Library of Medicine. The contents of this index are available on-line as part of the *MEDLINE* database.

Psychological Abstracts. Washington, DC, American Psychological Association, 1927– . (subscription–$740; APA, 1400 N. Uhle Street, Arlington, VA 22201)

This is a monthly compilation of nonevaluative summaries of the literature in psychology and related fields. The references in each issue are divided into sixteen broad categories with author and brief subject indexes. A cumulated index is published at the end of each year. The contents of this service are available on-line as the *PsycINFO* database.

Sociological Abstracts. San Diego, Sociological Abstracts, Inc., 1953–. (subscription–$230; SA, P.O. Box 22206, San Diego, CA 92122-0206)

SA, issued five times per year, is "a collection of nonevaluative abstracts which reflects the world's serial literature in sociology and related disciplines." The abstracts are arranged by broad subject category with a separate bibliography of book reviews. Some issues contain supplements consisting of abstracts of conference papers. Author and subject indexes accompany each issue and cumulate at the end of the year. The on-line version of this is also *Sociological Abstracts*.

Journals

There is a growing number of journals in publication that deal with marketing in or for the health care industry. Most of these journals are indexed in *Hospital Literature Index*, as well as the business indexes. In addition, there are numerous journals relating specifically to alcohol and its consumption and abuse. These publications vary widely in audience and focus. Following is a list of these journals with brief descriptive annotations. The list is divided into five categories: (1) health care marketing journals, (2) general alcohol-related journals addressed to a broad audience interested in research or policy concerns in the alcohol field, (3) scholarly journals edited for the research and medical communities, (4) specialized population and organization journals, and (5) foreign language journals. A portion of this list is reprinted by permission from the *Alcohol Resources Directory* (December 1986).

Health Care Marketing Journals

Employee Assistance Quarterly. New York, The Haworth Press, 1985–. (subscription–$28 individuals; The Haworth Press, Inc., 10 Alice Street, Binghamton, NY 13904-1580, 607-722-5857)

This journal is published in the fall, winter, spring, and summer. Topics covered include cost management, industrial social work throughout the world, new modes of outpatient treatment for addictive problems, employee assistance programs for the post-industrial era and other related issues.

Health Marketing Quarterly. New York, The Haworth Press, 1983–. (subscription–$45 individuals; The Haworth Press, Inc., 10 Alice Street, Binghamton, NY 13904-1580, 607-722-5857)

This journal is published in the fall, winter, spring, and summer. It is the successor to *Health and Medical Care Services Review* (1978-82). Each issue is geared to a particular topic, i.e., "Marketing Ambulatory Care Services," "Marketing and Consumer Satisfaction," and "Marketing Rehabilitation Programs."

Journal of Ambulatory Care Marketing. New York, The Haworth Press, 1987–. (subscription–$32: The Haworth Press, Inc., 10 Alice Street, Binghamton, NY 13904-1580, 607-722-5857)

This journal is published biannually in the spring and fall. It promotes applied strategies, plans, approaches, programs and tactics developed by marketing professionals; and attempts to determine more accurately the professions and delivery systems that provide ambulatory health care.

Journal of Health Care Marketing. Chicago, American Marketing Association, 1980–. (subscription–$45; AMA, Subscription Department, 250 S. Wacker Dr., Chicago, IL 60606, 312-648-0536)

Issued by the Center for Management Development of the John A. Walker College of Business (Boone, NC), the journal is the official organ of the Academy of Health Services Marketing. Published quarterly, the journal includes articles related to medical care marketing.

Journal of Hospital Marketing. New York, The Haworth Press, 1987–. (subscription–$32 individuals; The Haworth Press, Inc., 10 Alice Street, Binghamton, NY 13904-1580, 607-722-5857)

This journal is published biannually in the spring/summer and fall/winter. It provides pertinent and practical material for hospital marketing professionals on new and effective ways of marketing hospital services. The journal is written by hospital marketing professionals intent on sharing current marketing applications and methodologies with their readers.

Journal of Marketing for Mental Health. New York, The Haworth Press, 1986– . (subscription–$48/year, individuals; The Haworth Press, Inc., 10 Alice Street, Binghamton, NY 13904-1580, 607-722-5857)

This journal is published twice a year in the fall and spring. The articles and editorials discuss ways in which mental health professionals can market their services.

Health Care Strategic Management: The Journal of Health Care Planning, Marketing, and Resource Allocation. Ann Arbor, MI, Chi Systems, 1983– . (subscription–$85/year, $160/2 years, $220/3 years; Chi Systems, P.O. Box 8626, Ann Arbor, MI 48107)

This journal is published monthly and attempts to present theory and practice in areas of management interest. Also included are interviews, case studies, and reviews.

Strategic Health Care Marketing. Rye, NY, Health Care Communications, 1984– . (subscription–$180/year. $330/2 years; Health Care Communications, P.O. Box 594, Rye, NY 10580, 914-967-6741)

This monthly newsletter attempts to provide "information on strategies and techniques used by marketers, advice from marketing authorities and practitioners, and actual case histories of successes and failures."

General Alcohol-Related Publications

Alcohol Health and Research World. Rockville, MD, National Institute on Alcoholism and Alcohol Abuse. (subscription–$12/year; Superintendent of Documents, U.S. Government Printing Office, Washington, DC 20402)

Wide-ranging selection of articles on research, treatment, prevention, and other topics related to alcohol consumption and abuse, addressed to a broad audience interested in the field. Occasional theme issues; e.g., alcohol and the homeless, alcohol and cancer.

Alcoholism & Addiction Magazine. Alcom, Inc. (subscription—$18.75/year; A & A, P.O. Box 31329, Seattle, WA 98103)

Glossy magazine targeted primarily at substance abuse counselors and individuals in recovery. Includes separately edited magazine on recovery, with numerous contributions from anonymous members of Al-Anon and Alateen. Feature articles tend to be light in content but provide insights into key substance abuse problems areas. Some theme issues.

The Bottom Line on Alcohol in Society. Alcohol Research Information Service. (subscription—$12/year; Alcohol Research Information Service, 1106 East Oakland Avenue, Lansing, MI 48906)

Highly readable, pro-abstinence publication describing research, events, and opinions relating to public policy in the field of alcohol use, with special emphasis on prevention of abuse.

Commission News. Texas Commission on Alcohol and Drug Abuse. (subscription—free; Texas Commission on Alcohol and Drug Abuse, 1705 Guadalupe, Austin, TX 78701)

Although technically the newsletter of a state substance abuse agency, this twelve page publication often includes articles of general interest to readers involved in alcohol abuse prevention and treatment throughout the United States.

Contemporary Drug Problems. Federal Legal Publications. (subscription—$30/year; Federal Legal Publications, Inc., 157 Chambers Street, New York, NY 10007)

Articles, averaging thirty pages in length, present the results of legal, medical, and social research on substance abuse topics. Language is particularly appropriate to lawyers and the other professionals who do not necessarily have a scientific background.

Drugs & Society: A Journal of Contemporary Issues. New York, NY, The Haworth Press. (subscription—$28/year, individuals; The Haworth Press Inc., 10 Alice Street, Binghamton, NY 13904-1580, 607-722-5857)

Provides relatively lengthy articles that critically review topical concerns in the field. Each issue is devoted to a specific topic of interest. Most suited to social scientists and policy makers.

Focus on Family and Chemical Dependency. Pompano Beach, FL, U.S. Journal of Drug and Alcohol Dependence, (subscription—$22/year; U.S. Journal of Drug and Alcohol Dependence, Inc., 1721 Blount Road, Suite #1, Pompano Beach, FL 33069)

Popularly written, forty page magazine. Content explores family relationships in households where one or more members are alcoholic or other chronic substance abusers. Other articles address results of recent sociological and biomedical research and perspectives on family participation in prevention activities.

The Globe—An International Magazine on Alcohol and Drug Problems. Osla, International Organization of Good Templars. (subscription—approximately $32/year; International Organization of Good Templars, Keysersgt. 1, 0165 Oslo, Norway)

Popularly written, twenty-five page magazine reporting public health developments affecting alcohol, narcotics, and tobacco use in Europe and the developing countries. Strictly abstinence-oriented. Many of the alcohol-related news items focus on Scandinavia but have potential interest to Americans.

The Journal. Toronto, Addiction Research Foundation. (subscription—$24; Marketing Services, *The Journal*, Department KMM, 33 Russell Street, Toronto, Canada M5S 2S1)

Unique newspaper offering news items, feature stories, and opinion pieces on drug and alcohol concerns worldwide. Lively publication emphasizes stories with Canadian bylines.

Monday Morning Report. Lansing, MI, Alcohol Research Information Service. (subscription—$18/year: Alcohol Research Information Service, 1106 East Oakland Avenue, Lansing, MI 48906)

Two page newsletter that services as companion publication to *The Bottom Line*. Provides brief coverage of late-breaking news in the alcohol, tobacco, and drug abuse fields that is often covered in greater detail in *The Bottom Line*.

NPN Network News. National Prevention Network. (subscription—free, call (202) 783-6868; NASADAD, 444 North Capital, Suite 530, Washington, DC 20001)

Four page newsletter focusing on substance abuse prevention throughout the U.S.

Prevention Pipeline. Rockville, MD, National Institute on Alcohol Abuse and Alcoholism. (subscription—free; Prevention and Public Education Branch, National Institute on Alcohol Abuse and Alcoholism, 5600 Fishers Lane, Rockville, MD 20857)

Mimeographed newsletter covering recent developments in national, state, and local alcohol programs through short news articles. Other features include brief descriptions of new publications, research reports in the prevention field, and conference notices.

Scholarly Journals

Addictive Behaviors: An International Journal. Elmsford, NY, Pergamon Press. (subscription—$55/year; Pergamon Press, Inc., Maxwell House, Fairview Park, Elmsford, NY 10523)

Often highly technical articles presenting research on a cross-section of the disciplines concerned with substance abuse.

Alcohol: An International Biomedical Journal. San Antonio, TX, ANKHO International. (subscription—$225/year institutional; ANKHO International, Inc., P.O. Box 380227, San Antonio, TX 78280)

Of interest primarily to biomedical researchers.

Alcohol and Alcoholism: International Journal of the Medical Council on Alcoholism. Medical Council on Alcoholism. (subscription—$95/year institutional; Pergamon Press, Inc., Maxwell House, Fairview Park, Elmsford, NY 10523)

Primarily of interest to health researchers and psychologists.

Alcohol and Drug Research: An International Journal for Rapid Communications in Clinical Science. Elmsford, NY, Pergamon Press. (subscription—$115/year; Pergamon Press, Inc., Maxwell House, Fairview Park, Elmsford, NY 10523)

Short, highly technical articles describing recent biomedical research.

Alcohol, Drugs and Traffic Safety. Stockholm, International Committee on Alcohol, Drugs and Traffic Safety, Documentation Center of the Swedish Council for Information on Alcohol and Other Drugs. (subscription; Prof. M. W. Perrine, Boston University School of Medicine/Public Health, Room 806, 85 East Newton Street, Boston, MA 02118)

Abstracts research appearing in 76 journals from fourteen countries. Includes articles on epidemiological, physiological and psychological effects of alcohol and other drugs, and treatment programs, in addition to research specifically devoted to drug-related traffic safety concerns.

Alcoholism. Zagreb, Center for Study and Control of Alcoholism and Addictions, and Lausanne, International Council on Alcohol and Addictions. (subscription—$10/year; Center for Study and Control of Alcoholism and Addictions, Dr. M. Stojanovic University Hospital, Zagreb, Yugoslavia)

Primarily of interest to biomedical researchers. Most articles are research reports from Eastern Europe and Italy translated into occasionally awkward English.

Alcoholism: Clinical and Experimental Research. New York, American Medical Society on Alcoholism and Other Drug Dependencies, Inc. and Research Society on Alcoholism. (subscription—membership benefit, nonmembers $60/year: 428 East Preston Street, Baltimore, MD 21202)

Primarily of interest to biomedical researchers. Includes department that reviews and critiques current psychological and biomedical research on substance abuse.

Alcoholism Treatment Quarterly. New York, NY, The Haworth Press. (subscription – $30/year individuals; The Haworth Press, Inc., 10 Alice Street, Binghamton, NY 13904-1580, 607-722-5857)

Journal presents serious analysis of issues in alcoholism treatment. Articles do not always represent original research but may instead offer observations on the philosophy of alcoholism therapy. Recent double issues devoted to treating the black alcoholic.

American Journal of Drug and Alcohol Abuse. New York, Marcel Dekker. (subscription – $97/year; Marcel Dekker, Inc., P.O. Box 11305, Church Street Station, New York, NY 10249)

Unusually readable journal presenting original research in epidemiological, psychological, and biomedical aspects of alcohol and other drug abuse.

Australian Alcohol/Drug Review. Australian Medical Society on Alcohol and Drug Related Problems. (subscription – $48/year [U.S.]; Australian Medical Society on Alcohol and Drug Related Problems (AMSAD), Marketing Division, Alcohol and Drug Foundation, G.P.O. Bos 477, Canberra, ACT 2601 Australia)

Usually a highly readable, scholarly journal covering epidemiological and sociological research in addition to specifically biomedical research. The *Review* also provides organizational communications to the AMSAD members and has offered lively debate among contributors on treatment concerns.

British Journal of Addiction. London, Society for the Study of Addiction to Alcohol and Other Drugs. (subscription – membership benefit: Society for the Study of Addiction to Alcohol and Other Drugs, Administrative Secretary of the Society, 3 Oakland Gardens, Dulwich Wood Avenue, London SE19, England)

Provides reports on biomedical and treatment research, commentaries on medical and public policy topics, and interviews with distinguished practitioners. Longest established journal in the field (founded in 1884). Currently focusing on problems of the developing countries.

Drug and Alcohol Dependence. New York, Elsevier Scientific. (subscription—$98/year; Elsevier Science Publishers, Journal Information Center, 52 Vanderbilt Avenue, New York, NY 10017)

Multidisciplinary journal covering clinical, epidemiological, psychosocial, sociocultural, educational, and legal research, with emphasis on narcotics.

International Journal of the Addictions. New York, Marcel Dekker. (subscription—$226/year; Marcel Dekker Journals, P.O. Box 11305, Church Street Station, New York, NY 10249)

Unusually readable journal, edited specifically to be comprehensible to nonprofessional audience. Most articles tend to address epidemiological, psychological, or treatment concerns.

Journal of Alcohol and Drug Education. Washington, DC, Alcohol and Drug Problems Association of North America. (subscription—membership benefit; Alcohol and Drug Problems Association, 400 North Capitol Street, Washington, DC 20001)

Provides scholarly research reports on evaluation of alcohol and other drug education activities as well as related articles on epidemiology.

Journal of Drug Education. Farmingdale, NY, Baywood Publishing. (subscription—$27/year; Baywood Publishing Company, Inc., 120 Marine Street, P.O. Box D, Farmingdale, NY 11735)

Provides research reports on treatment, prevention education, and public policy concerns, with focus on adolescent drug problems.

Journal of Drug Issues. Tallahassee, FL, Journal of Drug Issues. (subscription—$35/year; Journal of Drug Issues, Inc., P.O. Box 4021, Tallahassee, FL 32315-4021)

Forum for exchange of views on social, legal, political, economic, historical, and medical ramifications of drug policy. Many issues have a topical theme; e.g., Social Thought on Alcoholism, Adolescent Drug Use, and The Course of Drug Dependence in Youngsters: A Scandinavian Perspective.

Journal of Psychoactive Drugs. San Francisco, Haight-Ashbury Publications. (subscription – $50/year; *Journal of Psychoactive Drugs*, Haight-Ashbury Publications, 409 Clayton Street, San Francisco, CA 94117)

Publishes a wide variety of articles including critical and historical reviews, theoretical analyses, and research reports on all aspects of psychoactive substances, their use and abuse.

Journal of Studies on Alcohol. Alcohol Research Documentation. (subscription – $85/year; Alcohol Research Documentation, Inc., P.O. Box 969, Piscataway, NJ 08854)

Publishes original research reports on biomedical, behavioral, and sociocultural effects of alcohol and its use. Style of articles varies from highly technical to comprehensible to laymen with a limited knowledge of biology.

Research Communications in Substances of Abuse. Westbury, NY, PJD Publications. (subscription – $70/year; PJD Publications Ltd., P.O. Box 966, Westbury, NY 11590)

Nearly all contributions are highly technical papers in the biomedicine, pharmacology, and toxicology fields.

Specialized Population and Organization Journals

ADAMHA News. Rockville, MD, Alcohol, Drug Abuse, and Mental Health Administration, U.S. Department of Health and Human Services. (subscription – $23/year; Superintendent of Documents. U.S. Government Printing Office, Washington, DC 20402)

Provides coverage of agency-related news and research developments.

AID Bulletin. Kent, OH, Department of Sociology, Kent State University. (subscription – $6.50/year: Department of Sociology, Kent State University, Kent, OH 44242)

Nontechnical, eight page newsletter devoted to addiction intervention with the physically disabled. Includes one or two major articles – usually on intervention techniques – and departments including news briefs, resource availability, and upcoming conferences.

The Alcoholism Report. Washington, DC, Manisses Communications Group. (subscription—$87/year; Manisses Communications Group, Circulation Office, P.O. Box 3357, Wayland Square, Providence, RI 02906-0357)

Ten page newsletter for those whose jobs relate to alcoholism, focusing on reportage of Federal Government actions. Occasional job listings and seminar announcements.

The ALMACAN. Arlington, VA. Association of Labor-Management Administrators and Consultants on Alcoholism. (subscription—ALMACA membership benefit; ALMACA, Suite 907, 1800 North Kent Street, Arlington, VA 22209)

Approximately forty page professional magazine for practitioners in the field of employee assistance programs. Includes association news, notices of future meetings and seminars, and three to four feature articles on topics related to employee assistance programs.

AMA Impaired Physician Newsletter. Chicago, Department of Mental Health of the American Medical Association. (subscription—$10/year: Subscription Dept., AMA, 535 North Dearborn Street, Chicago, IL 60610)

Ten to twelve page newsletter describing treatment programs, resources, and policies affecting medical personnel impaired by substance abuse. Includes legislative updates.

Bulletin of Alcohol Policy. San Francisco, Trauma Foundation of San Francisco. (subscription—$20/year; James F. Mosher, Room 400, Building One, San Francisco General Hospital, San Francisco, CA 94110)

Nontechnical, eight to twelve page newsletter on public health and legal issues affecting alcohol use and consumption, including Industry Watch department. News items tend to have West Coast focus.

The Counselor. Arlington, VA, National Association of Alcoholism and Drug Abuse Counselors. (subscription – membership benefit; NAADAC, 951 South George Mason Drive, Arlington, VA 22204)

Twenty to thirty page magazine devoted primarily to organizational news. Up to three feature articles per issue focus on professional counseling concerns.

DISCUS Newsletter. Washington, DC, Distilled Spirits Council of the United States. (subscription – membership benefit; Communications Division, DISCUS, 1250 Eye Street, NW, Washington, DC 20005)

House organ of the distillery trade association. Devotes considerable attention to research reports and promotion of moderate drinking programs as well as trade and association news.

Dram Shop and Alcohol Reporter. SEAK. (subscription – $50/year; Ronal S. Beitman, P.O. Box 590, Falmouth, MA 02541)

Eight page newsletter describing cases in dram shop liability law and related courtroom actions. Although designed for attorneys, clearly written synopses of recent litigation are potentially of interest to other readers.

EAP Digest. Troy, MI, Performance Resource Press. (subscription – $21/year: Performance Resource Press, Inc., Suite 103, 2145 Crooks Road, Troy, MI 48084)

Eighty page magazine devoted to full range of employee assistance programs; e.g., health and child care as well as alcoholism. Not all issues include alcohol-related feature articles.

Fetal Alcohol Syndrome and Other Drugs Update. Springfield, IL, Project Prevention Resource Center. (subscription; AHTDS-Prevention Resource Center, 901 South Second Street, Springfield, IL 62703)

Nontechnical, six page newsletter devoted primarily to fetal alcohol syndrome. Includes brief research notes in laymen's language, and announcements of resource materials and program activities. Some articles have an Illinois rather than national focus.

Highway Loss Reduction Status Report. Washington, DC, Insurance Institute for Highway Safety, (subscription—free; Insurance Institute for Highway Safety, Watergate 600, Washington, DC 20037)

Eight page newsletter covering news affecting motor vehicle safety. Approximately one-third of all issues include at least one article related to alcohol.

The NACoA Network. South Laguna, CA. National Association for Children of Alcoholics. (subscription—membership benefit; NACoA, Suite 201, 31706 Coast Highway, South Laguna, CA 92677)

Eight page newsletter focusing on association news, with a calendar of events and reports on future training sessions.

NASADAD Alcohol and Drug Use Report. Washington, DC, National Association of State Alcohol and Drug Abuse Directors. (subscription—$55/year; NASADAD, 444 North Capitol Street, NW, Suite 530, Washington, DC 20001)

Eight to twelve page newsletter focusing on association news and public policy developments affecting state substance abuse programs.

Responsible Beverage Service Newsletter. Northampton, MA, Responsible Hospitality Institute. (subscription—$50/year; Center for Responsible Hospitality, 56 Main Street, Northampton, MA 01060)

Entertaining sixteen page newsletter addressed to restaurant/bar owners. Favors voluntary server intervention; opposes stricter state controls. Departments cover intervention techniques, legal concerns, research reports on effects of alcohol. Includes a regular worst ad feature.

SALIS News. Substance Abuse Librarians and Information Specialists. (subscription—free to members, nonmembers $15/year: Andrea Mitchell, Alcohol Research Group, 1816 Scenic Avenue, Berkeley, CA 94709)

Ten page newsletter devoted to professional interests of SALIS members. Includes notices of new information resources, books, and periodicals in the alcohol field.

SPAB Bulletin. Society of Psychologists in Addictive Behaviors. (subscription—membership benefit; SPAB, Indiana University Medical School, Indianapolis, IN 42223)

Bulletin provides association news and research and topical updates on aspects of addiction.

Traffic Safety. Chicago, National Safety Council. (subscription—$12.55/year members, $15.75/year nonmembers; National Safety Council, 444 N. Michigan Avenue, Chicago, IL 60611)

Approximately thirty page magazine devoted to traffic safety. Often includes one to two items related to alcohol among the seven to nine feature articles in each issue. Uses plain language to discuss research.

Foreign Language Journals

Alcool Ou Sante. Paris, Comite National de Defense Contre l'Alcoolisme. (subscription—80 francs/year; Jacques Godard, 20 rue Saint Fiacre, 750002 Paris, France)

Approximately fifty page magazine offering five to seven feature articles written in popular style, emphasizing prevention of alcoholism. Includes book review section. Does not provide English-language summaries.

Alkoholipolitikka. Helsinki, Oy Alko Ab. (subscription; P.O.B. 350, SF-00101 Helsinki, Finland)

Approximately fifty page journal on alcohol policy. Four to seven feature articles in each issue include short English summaries and offer insights applicable to other countries.

Alkohologia. Budapest, Alkoholizmus Elleni Orszagos Bizottsag. (subscription; Center for Hungarian Literature, c/o Corvin, 1590 2nd Avenue, New York, NY 10029)

Scientific journal focusing on psychological evaluation and treatment experiences among Hungarian practitioners. Very brief English-language summaries are unevenly translated.

Blutalkohol: Alcohol, Drugs and Behavior. Frankfurt/Main, International Committee on Alcohol, Drugs, and Traffic Safety. (subscription; Steintor-Veriag Hamburg GmbH, Office Lubeck, Grapengieserstr. 30, Postbox 1228, 2400 Lubeck 1, Germany)

Scholarly journal focusing on research on alcohol in forensics, including DWI cases. Articles occasionally appear in English; all articles accompanied by English-language summaries.

Bulletin de la Societe Francaise d'Alcoologie. Paris, Societe Francaise d'Alcoologie. (subscription—membership benefit; 16 rue Picot, 75116 Paris, France)

Theme issues explore biomedical and sociological aspects of specific alcohol-related topics. Recent issues include Alcohol and Suicide and Alcohol and Psychological Testing. Very brief English-language summaries accompany some articles but are generally of limited utility.

Drogalcohol—Revista Espanola de Drogodependencias. Valencia, Provincial Psychiatric Hospital of Valencia. (subscription; DROGALCOHOL, Servicio de Alcoholismo y Toxicomanias Del Hospital Psiquiatrico Provincial, Carretera Torres-Torres, s/n., Betera, Spain)

Scholarly journal covering biomedical, psychological, epidemiological, and sociological aspects of alcohol use. Most contributors are Spanish; a few are Latin American. Very brief English-language summaries included with feature articles. Journal also lists professional meetings, and includes book reviews and editorials.

Drogalkohol—Forschung und Praxis Praevention und Rehabilitation. Lausanne, IPSA-Press. (subscription; Redaktion und Administration, IPSA-Press, Postfach 1063, CH-1001 Lausanne, Switzerland)

Scholarly journal covering biomedical, epidemiological, and sociological aspects of alcohol use. Articles are accompanied by excellent English-language summaries.

Japanese Journal of Alcohol Studies and Drug Dependence. Japanese Medical Society of Alcohol Studies. (subscription—$35/year [U.S.]; K. Kuriyama, Department of Pharmacology, Kyoto Prefectual University of Medicine, Kawaramachi-Hirokoji. Kamikyu-Ku, Kyoto, 602 Japan)

Scholarly journal on biomedical aspects of alcohol consumption. Approximately half of all articles are in English.

Problemy Alkoholizmu. Pismo Spilecznega Komitetu. (subscription; Iolanta Bryszewska, ul. Lwowska 5, 00-600 Warszawa, Poland)

Twenty-four page newsletter of Christian temperance. Research reports, focusing on alcoholism incidence and prevention issues among Polish youth, are summarized in English. Most of the newsletter features organizational news.

Rivista Italiana di Alcologia. Societa Italiana di Alcologia. (subscription; Prof. C. Giulivo, Istituto di Coltivazioni Arboree, Via Gradenigo 6, 35100 Padova, Italy)

Scholarly journal reporting biomedical and psychological research on alcohol. Some full-length articles in English: all others include brief English-language abstracts.

Suchtgefahren. Neuland-Verlagsgesellschaft mbH. (subscription; Herbert Ziegler, Westring 2, Postfach 1369, 4700 Hamm, Germany)

Scholarly journal reporting biomedical and epidemiological research on substance abuse. Primarily devoted to drugs other than alcohol.

ORGANIZATIONS

There are numerous organizations, associations, and research institutions involved in the study of alcohol and the treatment of alcohol abuse. Three of them have as part of their purpose the collection and dissemination of information; Center of Alcohol Studies, National Center for Health Statistics, and National Clearinghouse for Alcohol Information. Others provide help to alcoholics in general, such as Alcoholics Anonymous, and still others provide help to specific segments of the alcoholic population, such as the American Atheist Addiction Recovery Groups. The following is a list with the names, addresses, telephone numbers, and brief descriptions of these organizations. A portion of this information is reprinted by permission from the *Alcohol Resources Directory* (August 1986). More than thirty-five additional related organizations and associations are listed in the *Encyclopedia of Associations* (1987).

Airline Pilots Association, Aeromedical Office, 12000 East 47th Avenue, Suite 117, Denver, CO 80239; (303) 371-0425.

The Aeromedical Office provides referrals to local programs for treatment of chemical dependency among the 33,000 members of the Airline Pilots Association. International, and maintains sponsoring corporate self-help and counseling programs.

Al-Anon Family Group, P.O. Box 862, Midtown Station, New York, NY 10016; (212) 302-7240.

Al-Anon Family Groups, which includes Al-Anon for adults, Al-Anon for adult children of alcoholics, and Alateen for youth, are self-help groups for family members and friends of problem drinkers and alcoholics. Local groups are listed in most telephone directories.

Alcoholics Anonymous (AA), P.O. Box 459, Grand Central Station, New York, NY 10163; (212) 686-1100.

Alcoholics Anonymous is the prototype self-help group for recovering alcoholics and alcohol abusers and by far the largest such group, with more than one million members in 114 countries. Local gropus are listed in most telephone directories. The General Service Office (listed above) can provide information about specialized AA groups.

American Atheist Addiction Recovery Groups (AAARG!), Bill Talley, Box 6120, Denver, CO 36202; (303) 758-6686.

AAARG! exists to provide a "nontheistic alternative" to mainstream rehabilitation programs. Members are part of a network of atheistic alcoholics and drug abusers and are "working to accept full personal responsibility for our individual recoveries from addiction." AAARG! also operates a speakers bureau, a library, a 24-hour "warm line," and publishes a newsletter, the *AAARG! Journal*.

American Dental Association, Advisory Committee on Chemical Dependency Issues, 211 East Chicago Avenue, Chicago, IL 50511; (800) 621-8099; in Illinois (800) 575-8309; in Alaska and Hawaii (800) 621-3291.

The Association sponsors an annual conference on the problems of alcohol and chemical dependency within the dental profession. It also maintains toll-free telephone lines for inquiries about upcoming conferences and for passing along information about local alcohol/chemical dependency activities, including peer-support groups. Such groups now exist in thirty-nine states.

American Medical Association (AMA), attn: Janice Robertson, Department of Human Behavior, 535 North Dearborn Street, Chicago, IL 60610; (312) 645-5000.

The AMA publishes the quarterly *Impaired Physician Newsletter*, which provides current information on the activities of state impaired-physician committees, programs for medical students and residents, new publications and resource materials, upcoming conferences, the activities of related groups within other health professions, and a variety of other topics.

American Public Health Association (APHA), Alcohol and Drug Section, c/o Alexander C. Wagenaar, University of Michigan, 2901 Baxter Road, Ann Arbor, MI 48901-2150.

Officially formed in 1985, this Section offers members the opportunity to share ideas and information through the annual APHA conference, the Section newsletter, and a network of professional members from all public health disciplines. Section priorities include increased federal funding for prevention research, smokeless tobacco, rotating warnings on alcohol products and advertisements, and policies affecting such issues as AIDS and drug use.

Anesthetists in Recovery (AIR), c/o Beth Visintine, CRNA, 5626 Preston Oaks Road, Unit 40D, Dallas, TX 75240; (214) 960-7296 or (913) 383-2878.

AIR is a support and advocacy group for anesthetists who have had problems with alcohol or other addicting drugs. The group's purpose is to maintain a cooperative network of anesthetists who can provide education, intervention, evaluation, referral, and reentry services to peers. Members from all health professions involved in the administration of anesthesia are welcome. AIR has contacts in most states.

Birds of a Feather, attn: Ron Donovan, 213 Glenridge Lane, Schaumburg, IL 60194; (312) 893-5706.

Birds of a Feather is a specialized group endorsed by the General Service Office of Alcoholics Anonymous, composed of active and retired members of military and civilian aircraft cockpit crews. Founded in 1976, its chapters, known as "nests," are located throughout the U.S. and seven foreign countries. Some nests accept flight attendants and air traffic controllers as members. In addition to offering the AA support program, Birds of a Feather publishes a quarterly newsletter and holds its own annual convention.

Black Women of Alcoholic Parents (B-WAP), c/o Dr. Frances Larry Brisbane, 139 D. La Boone Vie Drive West, East Patchogue, NY 11772; (516) 654-2378 or (516) 444-2138.

This small but expanding organization provides mutual support in a spiritual context for black women who have experienced the trauma of growing up in a household where one or both parents was alcoholic. Run on a club model, B-WAP is not a drop-in group, though new members are welcome.

Calix Society, R. D. Dickenson, 7601 Wayzata Boulevard, Minneapolis, MN 55426; (612) 546-0544.

The Society is primarily for Catholic members of Alcoholics Anonymous, although non-Catholic alcoholics and other interested persons are welcome. The Calix Society ("calix" is Latin for "chalice") works to sustain the abstinence and promote the spiritual development of its members in the U.S., Canada, England, and Scotland.

Center of Alcohol Studies, Rutgers, The State University, Smithers Hall, Busch Campus, Piscataway, NJ 08854; (201) 932-2190.

The Center of Alcohol Studies is involved in research, education, clinical services, and information services in alcoholism and alcohol studies. Its library maintains one of the largest and most comprehensive collections of alcohol-related literature in the world. The Center publishes a variety of material including books, pamphlets, and reprints, as well as the *Journal of Studies on Alcohol*. Components of the Center's education and training activities include the Summer School of Alcohol Studies, the New Jersey Summer School of Alcohol and Drug Studies, the Alumni Institute, and other continuing education programs.

Dentists Concerned for Dentists (DCD), attn: Diane M. Millan, 450 North Syndicate Street, Suite 117, St. Paul, MN 55104; (612) 641-0730.

DCD is a group of recovering alcoholic dentists that encourages colleagues to seek and accept help for chemical dependency problems and that provides help through education, identification, and intervention. DCD is not affiliated with any dental society and does not directly provide treatment. Telephone calls are accepted 24 hours a day.

The Emerging Women, Inc., c/o Patricia B. Heubusch, R.D. 1, Box 266, Thomasville, PA 17364; (717) 225-5472.

Emerging Women is a networking organization of women in the U.S. and Canada who are recovering from chemical dependency, or who have recovering family members. Founded in 1972, its purpose is to provide a nonthreatening, supportive climate for the personal, spiritual, and professional growth of its members. A key objective is the development of indigenous local leadership among women in recovery. Emerging Women has no local chapters, but it sponsors an annual retreat in January and an annual workshop in June. The organization publishes a quarterly newsletter and is currently considering the establishment of regional workshops.

International Advisory Council for Homosexual Men and Women in Alcoholics Anonymous (IAC), P.O. Box 492, Village Station, New York, NY 10014.

IAC is a council of Alcoholics Anonymous groups composed specifically of gay and lesbian members. Its services include general support of the gay and lesbian members of AA and information for alcoholism professionals about gay and lesbian AA groups. IAC publishes a newsletter and the annual *World Directory of Gay/Lesbian Groups of Alcoholics Anonymous*.

International Doctors in Alcoholics Anonymous (IDAA), c/o Lewis K. Reed, MD, 1950 Voiney Road, Youngstown, OH 44511; (216) 782-6216.

Founded in 1949, IDAA welcomes all doctors in the healing arts; current members include dentists, psychologists, veterinarians, and medical scientists as well as physicians in a variety of specialties. This organization sponsors an annual meeting organized each year by the regional IDAA subgroup where the meeting is to be held. The group works to assist its members to better understand their own problems, the problems of other doctors, and the problems of patient care.

International Lawyers in Alcoholics Anonymous (ILAA), c/o Igor I. Sikorsy, Jr., 39 Smith Neck Road, Old Lyme, CT 06371; (203) 434-8309.

ILAA serves as a clearinghouse in order to put attorneys in touch with local AA groups.

Lawyers Concerned for Lawyers (LCL), attn: Diane M. Miller, 450 North Syndicate Street, Suite 117, St. Paul, MN 55104; (612) 646-5590.

LCL is an independent association of lawyers and judges concerned for members of the legal profession suffering from alcohol and chemical abuse. The group provides personal and confidential help to individuals concerned about their own use of alcohol or drugs, or about that of family members of associates.

National Association of Lesbian and Gay Alcoholism Professionals (NALGAP), 1208 East State Boulevard, Fort Wayne, IN 46805; (219) 483-8280.

NALGAP is a nonprofit organization of gay and nongay members of the helping professions. AA, and Al-Anon members, drug and alcohol agencies, and gay and lesbian organizations. It exists to maintain a communication and support network for gay and lesbian alcoholism professionals, to improve treatment services for gay and lesbian clients, and to assist all alcoholism and other helping professionals to serve their gay and lesbian clients more effectively. Among other services, NALGAP publishes a quarterly newsletter and a bibliography on alcoholism and homosexuality, provides referral information about gay and lesbian AA and Al-Anon groups, and acts as a clearinghouse for resource and research information about lesbian and gay alcoholism.

National Association of Social Workers (NASW), attn: Dr. Norma Taylor, 7981 Eastern Avenue, Silver Spring, MD 20910; (301) 565-0333.

Many of NASW's state chapters now organize support groups for impaired social workers, and the national office will make referrals to these groups. NASW, also, is encouraging the remaining chapters to establish their own groups and is developing guidelines and recommendations to assist them.

National Center for Health Statistics, Department of Health and Human Services, 3700 East-West Highway, Hyattsville, MD 20782; (301) 436-8500.

The National Center for Health Statistics (NCHS) collects, analyzes, and disseminates data on the nation's health. This includes data on alcohol use and abuse. The Center has produced a list of such alcohol-related data in *An Inventory of Alcohol, Drug, and Mental Health Data Available from the National Center for Health Statistics* (Charlotte A. Schoenborn, Hyattsville, MD, U.S. Department of Health and Human Services, Public Health Service, National Center for Health Statistics, 1985). This report identifies NCHS data that contain information on clinical mental disorder, psychological well-being, psychosocial risk factors, alcohol use and abuse, and drug use and abuse, including the use of tobacco.

National Clearinghouse for Alcohol Information, P.O. Box 2345, Rockville, MD 20852; (301) 468-2600.

The National Clearinghouse for Alcohol Information (NCALI) is a service of the National Institute on Alcohol Abuse and Alcoholism (NIAAA) of the U.S. Department of Health and Human Services. The NCALI collects information from around the world on alcoholism and the use and abuse of alcohol. NCALI has developed a computerized database of more than 50,000 references to alcohol-related information from books, journals, conference proceedings, curriculum materials, and reports. Computer searches of this database are provided upon request. The NCALI distributes pamphlets, brochures, books, posters, and other materials published by the NIAAA. NCALI staff provides information in response to individual inquiries of a personal or professional nature. NCALI publishes the *Alcohol Health and Research World*, a quarterly report of research findings and practical programmatic information, and the *Alcohol Awareness Service*, a bimonthly listing of current information and how to obtain it.

National Clergy Council on Alcoholism and Related Drug Problems (NCCA), Rev. John F. X. O'Neill, CAC, 1200 Varnum Street NE. Washington, DC 20017-2796; (202) 832-3811.

NCCA exists primarily to promote adequate treatment of alcoholism and chemical dependency in Catholic clergy. The organization sponsors workshops, seminars, and a national convention to educate clergy and lay Catholics about these problems. NCCA also offers consultation and support services to interested groups and individuals.

National Self-Help Clearinghouse (NSHC), 33 West 42nd Street, City University of New York. New York, NY 10036: (212) 840-1259.

NSHC is a resource on self-help groups in general and will make referrals. The organization publishes a newsletter as well as reports, books, and brochures.

Nurses Society on Addictions, Committee on the Impaired Nurse, c/o Pat Green, 1020 Sunset Drive, Lawrence, KS 66044: (816) 254-3652 or (913) 842-3893.

The Committee keeps track of an informal network of nurses interested in the problems of impairment in the nursing profession and will make referrals to local contact people and support groups.

Psychologists Helping Psychologists (PHP), c/o Jane K. Skorina, 23439 Michigan Avenue, Dearborn, MI 48124; (313) 565-3821.

Founded in 1980, PHP currently has members throughout the United States as well as in Canada and Australia. The group exists to provide support for alcoholic and chemically dependent psychologists and to educate the professional about alcoholism. Membership is open to all doctoral-level psychologists and doctoral candidates.

Recovered Alcoholic Clergy Association (RACA), Rev. W. D. McLean III, 5615 Midnight Pass Road, Sarasota, FL 34242; (813) 349-2323.

RACA is a self-help organization for Episcopal clergy. It has three purposes: (1) mutual self-help, (2) fellowship, and (3) pastoral concern for clergy with drinking problems. RACA operates a hotline and publishes a newsletter.

Social Workers Helping Social Workers, c/o Dr. John Fitzgerald, 84 Wadsworth Street, Hartford, CT 06106; (203) 566-2186.

Social Workers Helping Social Workers is a support group for MSWs who have had a personal experience with chemical dependency. The main office serves as a clearinghouse, putting callers in touch with local or regional groups. It also publishes a newsletter and helps state chapters of the National Association of Social Workers to develop colleague assistance committees. There are four regional groups: New England, New York/New Jersey, Midwest, and Far West.

Women for Sobriety, Inc., P.O. Box 618, Quakertown, PA 18951: (215) 536-8026.

Women for Sobriety is a national organization with local units that address the specific needs of women with alcohol-related problems. The program is used in combination with other alcoholism treatment programs or as an alternative to other programs.

IV. PROMOTION NEEDS AND TECHNIQUES

The Role of Promotion in Alcoholism Treatment Marketing

Michael A. Jones
Donald R. Self
Cathleen A. Owens
Teri A. Kline

INTRODUCTION

Promotion involves the communication of information between buyer and seller in order to facilitate exchange relationships and thus the marketing process (McCarthy and Perrault, 1987). The promotion function is one of the four major variables with which a marketing manager works, and plays an important and even vital role as a component of marketing strategy. (Other major variables include price, place and product, and are discussed in other articles in this volume.) Promotion is often viewed as the "persuasive flow of information *from seller to buyer* with the objective of influencing the potential customer" (Engel et al., 1987). This includes both interpersonal communication as well as communication through a variety of other media.

A broader meaning of the term "promotion" will be assumed in this article to include the *two-way exchange* of information. Nickels (1983) states that the ideal marketing communications process is a functioning dialogue which enables an organization and consumers to achieve mutually beneficial exchange agreements. An example of such dialogue might be through a person-to-person "sales" context when listening to a potential client's concerns or questions during his search for a treatment facility.

The promotion function is not limited to communication exclusively between the buyer and the seller, but includes communication to any individual or group of significance to the welfare or success of the organization. Information is often directed at individuals who have influence in the client's decision process, such as a referral source, or referent, who may be a source of guidance or advice for the decision maker. In the case of the Alcoholism Treatment Marketer (ATM), physicians, clergy or counselors may present a channel for promotion since they possibly are important information sources for the client. (See Kline et al. earlier in this volume for a discussion of various individuals or parties in the ATM referral network.) Likewise, if a potential client's family members have significant influence over the decision, family members might be important targets for promotion. Other groups of influence may include governmental agencies (which fund or regulate public and nonprofit facilities), the press or media, or the community at large.

More Than Advertising

Promotion includes a broad range of types, or forms, of communication. Promotion management involves much more than "advertising management" because messages about a product or service are conveyed to potential customers in a variety of ways. Some messages are planned or intended, and some are not. Some are positive in context, while some are negative. Yet all information learned about the product is obviously important to the decision maker (Dommeruth, 1985). Patients, both actual and potential, form attitudes about the quality of ATM service from the physical facility, the landscaping in the parking lot, the interior decor, the behavior of various employees they encounter (both professional and non-professional staff), and the cleanliness of the bathrooms, as well as from planned advertising efforts such as brochures, signs, radio ads or the logo which appears on the ATM's stationery. One writer states for an organization marketing services, almost everything the organization does has promotion implications (Nickels, 1983). Or, as Ellis (1986) says, "many individuals not authorized to conduct marketing activities are involved in them, and may be undoing what the administration is trying to accomplish."

PROMOTION MANAGEMENT

It is the role of the person in charge of promotion to coordinate and integrate the communication flows from his/her organization in the manner which most effectively contributes toward the organization's goals. The first step is to select the image to be conveyed and then to enlist the support of the entire organization in creating and maintaining that image. However, marketing communication efforts are often not well coordinated, if coordinated at all. Academicians and practitioners agree that the promotion function is among the most mismanaged business activities not only because of its complexity, but also because of the lack of knowledge and understanding among those making promotion decisions (Lodish, 1982, Simon and Arndt, 1980). Also, it is argued that money is often misallocated to advertising in the form of overspending (Aaker and Carman, 1982).

Though it is evident that although all communication from the ATM cannot be controlled, communication can be managed to a great degree with the appropriate skills and resource commitments. Figure 1 highlights the concepts of unfocused communication versus the planned focused efforts which can be a part of the promotion plan.

ORGANIZING FOR PROMOTION MANAGEMENT: THE AD AGENCY

An issue for any smaller business organization is which personnel within the organization have the responsibility for planning and

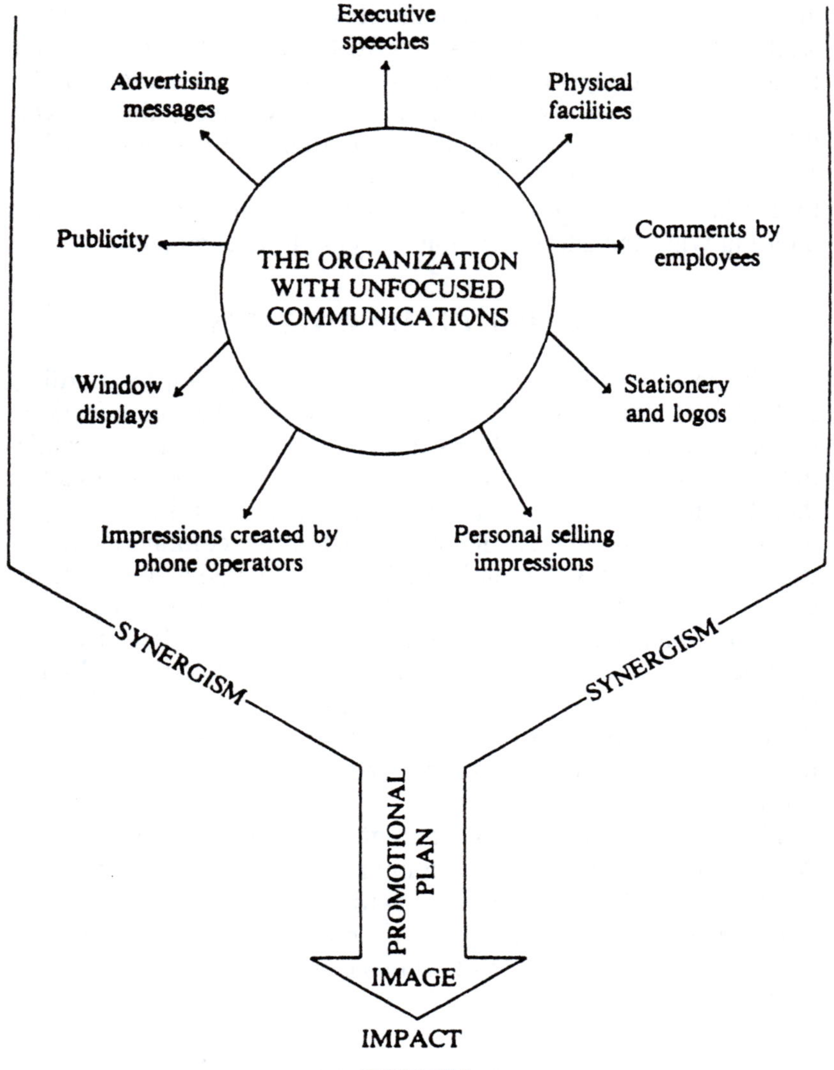
Executive speeches
Advertising messages
Physical facilities
Publicity
THE ORGANIZATION WITH UNFOCUSED COMMUNICATIONS
Comments by employees
Window displays
Stationery and logos
Impressions created by phone operators
Personal selling impressions
SYNERGISM
SYNERGISM
PROMOTIONAL PLAN
IMAGE
IMPACT

FIGURE 1

implementing promotion activities? Though large corporations have established departments which are staffed with experts in the promotion area (advertising department, public relations department, graphics and media, etc.), the small organization often has neither expertise nor manpower to effectively manage the promotion area in a comprehensive way. A common problem in health care is that many health care administrators do not have marketing or promotion expertise, and yet are increasingly faced with these types of decisions as the competitive environment changes (Schulman, 1987).

External Coordination

As with any small business lacking the resources to internally staff for a particular management area, an alternative for the ATM manager is to obtain outside help. This typically is provided by an advertising agency, which can usually provide a wide variety of promotion activities, including marketing research, consulting, public relations and publicity consulting, ad production, media buying, graphics and art work, and the subcontracting of such areas as printing or obtaining specialty advertising items. In many situations the procurement of an agency is the most effective approach to promotion problems, however special care should be exercised in selecting an agency since the control of promotion decisions and budgets are usually relinquished to the agency. No qualifying professional license exists for advertising agencies as it does for legal or accounting services, and many experts feel agencies may sometimes be biased toward recommending more services than necessary since their fees are often based upon the quantity of advertising actually conducted (Lodish, 1982). Typically only larger, more sophisticated agencies make efforts to validate the effectiveness of their advertising, therefore it is up to the ATM manager to determine if money spent through an agency is well allocated. (A useful discussion of the advantages/disadvantages of using an outside agency, and how to select and work with the right agency can be found in Engel et al., 1987, or Burnett, 1984.)

PROMOTION OBJECTIVES

The promotion function can and should be managed through an "MBO" or management by objective approach. Specific promotion objectives can be identified and prioritized based upon the specific situation or needs of the particular ATM. Once clearly focused and agreeable objectives are established, a promotion strategy can be developed to reach these objectives. Examples of objectives might be "to increase the awareness of a new facility," or "to educate or increase the knowledge of a particular benefit of a facility," or "to change attitudes about a particular aspect of the facility or its staff." Well stated, workable objectives would include (1) *who* the target audience is and (2) *what* specific message is to be communicated to this group. If it is feasible to state objectives in quantifiable terms, this might present a control device for measuring the effectiveness of implementation. (For a more complete discussion of establishing promotion objectives see Engel et al., 1987.)

Market Segmentation

Market segmentation is the process by which a relatively homogeneous population is divided into categories which provide more cohesiveness and similarity among the individual members. (A complete discussion by Judd, Self and Owens on the process and need for market segmentation, and recognized segments of the alcoholic population are contained in this volume.) It is at this point in the promotion planning process that market segments need to be developed, defined and specified in order to establish the best target markets within the alcoholic population for the ATM's promotion efforts. Obviously, the more specified the target market(s), the more effective management can be in developing communication strategies to reach the group(s) with the intended message (Govoni, 1986).

Like most organizations, the ATM would probably have a number of promotion objectives based upon the communication needs and habits of the various groups or market segments it intends to reach. Specific target audiences could be:

1. *the target client*: that segment of the alcoholic community which could best be served by the particular ATM. This segment could be based upon the nature and seriousness of the client's problem, ability to pay, socio-cultural status, geographic proximity to the facility, the type care that interests the client, the interest of the family, etc. Most facilities tailor their services to particular groups.
2. *the community at large*: the general public needing awareness or education.
3. *family members* of past, present and future clients.
4. *referent groups or individuals* (pastors, physicians, counselors, etc.).
5. *industrial or organizational buyers* (group programs).
6. *legislative bodies*, governmental agencies, or political-based groups or individuals (such as lobbyists or committee members of a legislative committee).
7. *the media*: those in the press who have power to generate communication in the form of news.

As can be seen, if objectives involved reaching multiple audiences, each target different audience might require specific communication strategies.

MARKETING ANALYSIS FOR DEVELOPING OBJECTIVES

Marketing analysis must be conducted in order to determine promotion needs and objectives in specific situations, and to then develop an effective strategy to achieve those objectives. This type of analysis is often referred to as "situation analysis," and is a standard component of marketing planning.

Analysis of Client Buying Behavior

One vital aspect of situation analysis is the evaluation of the consumer (client) purchase decision process or buying behavior. This involves understanding the nature of the decision process: the client's recognition of a need and efforts for satisfaction of that need. Included in this process is the information-seeking behavior of the potential client and his family as they search for the "best" treatment and facility. Consideration should be given to important sources and types of information for the potential client during this process. A client may have certain criteria for selecting a facility and thus need information provided which addresses those issues (Engel et al., 1987).

The media habits of a market segment can be studied to identify the most comprehensive and/or effective media vehicles for reaching that segment. For example, some demographic segments of the population obtain more information from television than from other media (e.g., radio, newspaper, etc.) (Robinson, 1978). Promotion strategies using the most effective media and messages can then be developed for each segment, based upon their particular information-processing behavior and perceived needs (see Figure 2).

Though available research on the buying process for Alcohol Treatment Centers is limited, information is available of the search process and buying process for health care services in general. For example, research indicates that in the selection of a physician, word-of-mouth referrals are by far the dominant source of information in the selection of a physician (Marketing News, 1987; George and Berry, 1981).

Signals of Quality

One important aspect of the ATM's service is that it is defined as "intangible." Because no physical properties are involved through which the buyer can evaluate the quality of the offered service, the descriptive communication of product attributes between buyer and seller is difficult (Lovelock, 1984). Perceptual differences as to true product quality are more likely to occur between buyer and seller, leading to difficulties in valuation from the buyer's standpoint. According to Kain-Candle and Marsh (1975), professionals have often cited the fact that there is no necessary connection between professional/technical quality of care and patient satisfaction. It is therefore hypothesized that consumers use whatever tangible "surrogates" available when evaluating the service quality during the shopping process. The behavior of staff, the appearance of staff members, the appearance of the facility, or the appearance of pro-

	Face-to-face	Mass media
General	Word-of-mouth influence	General content media
Marketer dominated	Personal selling	Advertising point-of-sale influence and publicity

Source: Engel, Warshaw and Kinnear, p. 75, 1987

FIGURE 2. Categories of Consumer Information Sources

motional materials, symbols or logos could all become tangible features by which the ATM's quality is evaluated. Obviously, these may have no relationship with the true quality of the service. The implication is that brochures, signs, ads, facilities, stationery, etc., play a more prominent role in the formation of beliefs and attitudes for a service, than for a tangible good like a car, clothing article, house or piece of furniture, where the consumer focuses on the physical article when evaluating quality.

K.I.S.S.

Another important implication of the intangibility factor for service promotion is the product attributes and the benefits of these attributes must be clearly stated in promotion, since they are less obvious and more difficult to grasp (George, 1981). As Unwin states, the challenge intangibility presents service advertisers is that "the service advertiser is often left with describing the invisible, articulating the imaginary and defining the indistinct" (Lovelock, 1984). Though the benefits of a leather interior or plush carpet in a center are intuitively obvious to the buyer, the benefits of a particular counseling treatment or therapy may be much less obvious and less intuitive to the buyer. Nevertheless, they must be understood.

Still another feature of the service offering is that because it is the *performance of a task by an individual*, it is by nature more variable in quality than tangible goods. Quality control is difficult resulting in uncertainty and caution for the potential client. Organizational credibility, organization image, and professional credentials are considered important by the consumer as "insurance" to reduce risk or quality variance.

Other Factors

Other important factors to evaluate in situation analysis are the competition, the competition's promotion efforts, the local economy, the local cultural environment (acceptance of alcohol treatment socially), the referent system, current knowledge or awareness levels of your facility, and current attitudes and beliefs about your facility and the treatment of alcoholism. (For a more complete discussion of "situation analysis" for promotion planning see Kincaid, 1986, or Berhardht and Kinnear, 1988.)

THE PROMOTION MIX

After analysis reveals *what* needs to be communicated to whom, *why* it needs to be communicated, and *what response(s)* might be predicted, the promotion decision maker has a variety of alternatives or methods as to *how* to communicate with its targeted audiences. These are conventionally placed into four categories:

1. advertising,
2. personal selling,
3. public relations,
4. sales promotion.

Typically two or more of these "promotion elements" are combined in promotion efforts of businesses to form the organization's "promotion mix." Because sales promotion is defined as those activities designed to induce immediate response or stimulate the consumer through incentive (coupons, discounts, special offers, contests, etc.), it is probably not appropriate or acceptable for usage by an ATM. The following discussion focuses on the other three elements, which are more appropriate and are commonly used by treatment centers. Below is a discussion of some specific promotion tools used by ATMs as revealed by a study of ATM administrators in the state of Alabama.

Promotional Tools Used by Facilities: The Alabama Study

The 1986 survey of ATM administrators in Alabama indicates the extent to which ATMs in that state employed various promotion tools. The results, reported in Table 1, were based on telephone surveys of a sample of 65 existing facilities including private, public, residential and non-residential. Respondents were asked to list promotion tools used in their facility. According to Table 1, speaker's bureaus, a public relations activity, were the most commonly used tool (57%), followed by radio advertising (52%), television

TABLE 1. Extent of Usage of Promotion Tools by Type of Facility Among Selected Alcohol Treatment Centers in Alabama, 1986.

	All Fac N=65	NR Pub N=14	NR Priv N=4	Longterm Res N=11	In Pub N=10	In Priv N=26
Speaker Bureau	57%	57%	75%	27%	90%	54%
Radio	52%	43%	50%	9%	70%	65%
T.V.	49%	43%	75%	--	50%	69%
Newspaper	45%	43%	75%	18%	40%	50%
Personal Selling	22%	21%	50%	--	10%	27%
Pamphlet	20%	29%	--	18%	20%	15%
Yellow Pages	12%	7%	--	--	10%	23%
Direct Mail	11%	--	25%	9%	10%	15%
P.S.A.	8%	14%	--	--	30%	--
Outdoor	6%	7%	--	--	--	12%

Source: The Alabama Voice, "An Analysis of the Market for Alcohol and Chemical Dependency Treatment Centers in Alabama," unpublished study, Montgomery, AL, Department of Marketing, Auburn University at Montgomery, March 1986.

advertising (49%), and newspaper advertising (45%). Outdoor media, public service announcements, direct mail and Yellow Pages were used by the fewest number of facilities, with pamphlets and personal selling reported as being moderately used.

As seen in Table 1, facilities vary in their promotional efforts significantly based upon type of facility and ownership. This can partially be explained by varying promotion budgets and promotion needs: many public facilities have very high occupancy rates and little funding available for promotional activities. For example, private facilities used advertising, which is paid media, more heavily than public facilities. Speaker's bureaus and PSAs, which are both public relations activities with lower costs associated with their usage, were used more by public facilities.

The nature of the patient's buying decision could also be an explanatory factor as to the variance in the types of promotion tools used by different types of organizations. However, there appears to be no relationship between the degree of involvement in the buying decision and the type of promotion used. Those facilities which offer services which seemingly require an extensive or involved search process do not appear to use promotional tools usually associated with a high involvement search process. For example, the decision to use expensive, private inpatient care facilities would seem to be a major decision. From a managerial standpoint, for high involvement important decisions such as the decision to use longterm private residential care, one would expect these institutions to use personal selling and more detailed print materials (e.g., brochures, pamphlets, various direct mail publications). However, as seen in Table 1, these centers use T.V. (69%) and radio (65%) advertising most frequently, and direct mail, pamphlets and personal selling to lesser extents. This seems to indicate questionable management skills in these centers in the area of promotion, especially considering the promotion needs expressed by the reference groups in the study.

APPLICATIONS OF PROMOTION TOOLS

After objectives are established, a promotion mix or strategy must be developed to reach these objectives. This involves an evaluation of the various tools or communication resources available to the ATM and the selection of those determined to be effective. The major promotional tools are briefly discussed below with respect to appropriate effective usage.

When dealing with media selection, it is important to remember marketing science has not determined the existence of one "best" medium for a given product or service. Further, advertising effectiveness is very complex and difficult to measure or evaluate (Simon and Arndt, 1980). Complicated experimentation is often needed to determine which media is most effective, or even if a single medium is used, how effective it is (Lodish, 1982).

Public Relations Tools

Public relations (PR) deals with efforts to earn and maintain the goodwill of an organization's various publics. Many scholars feel it involves formulating policies (internally) which are consistent with the interests of these publics (external) (Bertrand and Moore, 1975). Public relations efforts are associated largely with promoting the organization itself, rather than a specific product or service which the organization offers. As seen in Table 1, the major public relations tools used by ATMs in the Alabama study are public service announcements, speaker's bureaus and open houses, though a number of others are available (Moore, 1981). Because word-of-mouth is often classified as a form of publicity, and is so vital to ATMs, it is also treated in this section.

Word-of-Mouth

Evidence from research consistently indicates that word-of-mouth (people sharing with each other in day-to-day conversations) is the most dominant source of information for the purchase of professional services, particularly medical services (MacStravic, 1985). Word-of-mouth has been found to be effective in the latter stages of the buying process when the consumer is actively seeking information. Though word-of-mouth communication cannot be controlled as advertising can, it can be managed to some extent (Nickels, 1984). Though intuitively simple, one effective strategy to obtain word-of-mouth support is to provide past clients something positive to share with others. Extra satisfaction with or excitement about the service which comes from exceptional service contributes to the success of word-of-mouth communications.

In the case of the ATM, marketing research into which attributes of the service result in the greatest customer satisfaction is recommended in order to deliver the most "satisfying service" from the client's view. A number of studies are available which provide evidence into which perception attributes of the client lead to the most satisfaction for the selection of a physician (MacStravic, 1987). Among these are caring, courteous, understanding treatment; extra effort; and effective, responsive, and reliable performance of services with a clean, pleasing environment. Effective interpersonal communications with the patient has also been shown to be an important, if not the most important, attribute in the selection of a physician (Jenson and Miklovic, 1986). To generate positive word-of-mouth communication, start by interviewing current clients and referral sources regarding desired amenities and by delivering a service with these attributes.

An obvious implication for strategy for the ATM is the *internal marketing*, or the direction of marketing effort toward employees, insuring that those personnel who have patient contact will be aware of the importance of delivering quality treatment and care to the client and his/her family (Bloom, 1984; Berry, 1980). ATM employees, from janitorial staff to physicians, must understand their role in generating word-of-mouth communication, and even though they are practitioners in other areas besides marketing communications they have major impact in that area. Training programs can be implemented to inform employees of their role and increase their interpersonal communication skills. Consequently, personnel management and marketing management become interdependent and "intertwined."

Public Service Announcements

The public service announcement (PSA) is a type of publicity in which the promotion manager releases desired information to broadcast or print media for possible inclusion. Often called public service advertising, media volunteer time to non-profit organizations and worthy causes as a contribution to society. The only cost to the promotion manager is the production and distribution cost of the ad or "spot," though often a local station or ad agency will often assist in production (Lesly, 1983). The more professional the production of the spot, the better the chance of acceptance by the media. Likewise, the promotion manager must provide print PSAs to the print media.

PSAs can be very effective particularly in consideration of cost, and can be a valuable form of communication for the non-profit or government agency which has little or no budget for promotion through paid advertising or personal selling. A problem with PSAs is a lack of control, since the promotion manager has little control over if, when (time of day) or how many times the announcement will be run, unlike purchased advertising. Practitioners feel that the personal and professional relationship between the medium and the PSA sponsor impacts the extent to which the spot is run, especially on the local level. It is therefore recommended that PSAs be hand delivered if possible by a local person who has favorable relationships with the station or newspaper.

The success of a PSA campaign can be evaluated through follow-up with the station to determine when and how often the spot was carried, and if possible, the value of the air time and/or print space (some stations/newspapers provide this information). If this information is obtained, the PSA can be evaluated in terms of its communication abilities as is possible with paid advertisements.

Speaker's Bureaus

A speaker's bureau is an organized public speaking program which an organization can use as an effective communication tool. In large corporations, the public relations department would typically organize and operate the bureau, involving the recruitment, training and support of a group of volunteer employee speakers. The securement of speaking engagements could also be supported by the public relations department. Though the resources of the typical ATM are more limited, the tool can still be used effectively. Administrative staff, health care professionals or other staff members can participate as volunteer speakers. Former clients could be especially effective, serving as both communicators and role models. The target audience can be civic, professional, church, business, educational, fraternal or political organizations which might have particular significance in terms of their membership either as opinion leaders or potential clients.

The use of a speaker is a very effective form of communications when compared to mass media because it is personal and involves a two-way flow of communication. The speaker imparts information and can field questions This also "cuts through clutter" in obtaining the audiences' attention, as the speaker is the primary focus of a captive audience. The effectiveness of the communication is dependent upon the ability of the speaker to accomplish the stated objectives. Limitations include the sometime small groups of people reached, and the long time period often required to begin to reach significant numbers.

ADVERTISING

Television

Of the media available to the ATM decision maker, T.V. is to the greatest degree a "mass" media reaching more of the public in a given market than any media. It is generally felt to be effective for reaching large audiences with short messages about "low involvement" products not considered to be major purchases (Asseal, 1984). It has been found to be effective in the "awareness" stage of the buying process, and is often used for increasing awareness (top-of-mind) for a new product or service (Beal, 1968; Rogers, 1962). Television is also considered to be effective in image creation, due to the ability to create moods with sight and sound as well as through demonstration.

One caution for T.V. is its expense and tremendous "waste coverage," reaching many individuals who would probably never need or serve as a referral source for someone needing treatment services. On a cost-per-potential client contact basis it can be very expensive. Television can also involve more production costs than other media. A further limitation of television is its limitation to deliver small amounts of simple information; the shopper actively seeking an alcohol treatment center needs a good deal of detailed information. Another drawback in the use of television has to do with the "commercial" image associated with its use. Research indicates that television can create a negative image when used for the promotion of professional services, although its acceptance for this use appears to be increasing (Bloom, 1984; Traylor and Mathias, 1983).

Radio

Radio reaches more fragmented markets than television, making it more selective in reaching specific groups. It is considerably less expensive than television. For the ATM, radio could be effective in creating awareness, especially for a facility or new service, or in a reminder role. A disadvantage of radio is its limitation to sound only. Radio is often used by many as a "background listening activity," consequently the information is never "registered" with the listener.

Newspaper

Though a mass media, newspaper is more selective than T.V. or radio owing to the heavy use by specific segments of the population. For example, newspaper usage increases with income. Print induces superior retention of factual material when compared to oral presentation, and some feel print is more believable though there is no convincing research to verify this (Engel et al., 1987).

Newspaper lacks in creative qualities and thus the ability to differentiate or distinguish a product due to its limited reproductive capacity (printing quality). However, for professional services this limitation is perhaps less insignificant when promotion goals are to communicate credibility with a conservative, straightforward, informative approach versus a more creative emotional appeal often used in traditional product advertising. For example, newspaper is an accepted means for physicians or lawyers to announce a new associate or relocation, since the communication goal is factual rather than emotional.

Direct Mail

A benefit of direct mail is the ability to deliver information to very specific groups. For the ATM, these groups might include the decision maker or those important referral sources such as clergy, psychologists or physicians, current and past patients. Organizational markets could also be reached effectively with direct mail. For example, a list of personnel administrators who handle company personnel medical problems could be reached effectively through direct mail. Direct mail is also effective in communicating large amounts of detailed information that might interest a potential client, referent, or organizational buyer. This medium is especially effective when used in conjunction with speaker's bureaus, mass media and personal selling. Direct mail is also less complicated to use than other media.

PERSONAL SELLING

A final but important communication alternative for the ATM promotion manager is personal selling. Though face-to-face communication is the oldest form of promotion, and most used in terms of resource allocation by U.S. industry (Peterson et al., 1984), the use of personal selling in the conventional form has emerged only recently in medical and health care services industries (Cueny et al., 1986). No documented evidence of the extent to which personal selling is used as a part of promotion programs for ATMs exists at this writing. However, trade sources reveal a significant increase in personal selling among larger more sophisticated chain organizations (Strategic Health Care Newsletter, 1987). Hospitals have reported quite successful results from using sales representatives to call upon physicians as measured in increased patient days (Strategic Health Care Marketing Newsletter, February 1986).

Though personal selling through formally "designated" salespersons is relatively new in its application to health care, it must be remembered that providing information to potential and present patients on an *interpersonal* basis is not new in health care. This practice happens routinely at all facilities, whether or not personnel are aware of their role. For example, when a potential patient calls by phone or visits a facility for information, staff persons providing this information are involved in personal selling. Receptionists, public relations persons, administrators and/or medical staff persons may all be involved at various times with a single potential client providing different types of information. Therefore, the consideration of personal selling as a component of the promotion mix for the ATM calls for some definition of just when personal selling occurs and who might be involved. (For an excellent discussion of the role of non-sales personnel in the selling process, see Judd, Self, and Owens in this volume.)

Personal selling involves the two-way flow of communication on an interpersonal (diadic) basis. Though it is often thought of as involving direct face-to-face contact, telephone conversation is involved. Definitions vary as to the exact components of personal selling, but *providing information* to satisfy the needs and wants of the buyer is a primary universal function (Nickels, 1984). A definition of personal selling used by the American Marketing Association is:

> the personal or impersonal process of assisting and/or persuading a prospective customer to buy a commodity or service or to act favorably upon an idea that has significance to the seller.

Pederson (1984) adds that an important aspect of the selling activity is "mutual, continuous benefit of both buyer and seller." Other commonly mentioned functions of selling are prospecting, identifying decision makers (qualifying), helping customers identify (listening) and solve problems (educating, consulting), closing transactions, maintenance of customer relations, obtaining feedback from customers, providing input to the organization (marketing research), monitoring the competitive environment, and the list goes on (Young and Mondy 1982: Jackson et al., 1988).

Functions of Personal Selling for the ATM

The major functions of personal selling for the ATM include, (1) identifying important individuals or groups with which to communicate, (2) providing information, (3) obtaining patient or referent feedback, (4) following up "after sales," and (5) maintaining patient relations.

The strengths of personal selling are derived from its interpersonal nature. Since feedback concerning effectiveness of the communication from the audience is immediate and accurate in personal selling, it is far superior to the mass media in this respect; for evaluation or control the manager knows clearly who has been reached and what has been communicated. This immediate, accurate feedback allows communication to be "tailored" or customized to the needs of the audience; specific questions can be answered. The personal contact also "cuts through clutter" or noise more effectively than media, commanding the attention of the target audience and insuring exposure (Engel et al., 1983).

Though commanding in terms of its influence on the audience, personal selling has limitations. It is very expensive on a "cost per contact" basis, and is very slow in terms of reaching large numbers. With more geographically dispersed audiences it can become cost prohibitive. Personal selling is therefore effective when the consumer perceives the purchase as important (high-priced), risky or complex and is seeking information to reduce uncertainty, and when the audience is limited in numbers or geographic location. If the promotion budget is very limited a person already on staff can assume the selling function.

Personal selling could be effective for the ATM manager as a communication tool for four groups:

1. the organizational or industrial market (personnel managers of institutions or corporations seeking group coverage on employee programs),
2. third party providers (insurance providers)
3. referent groups: important referents such as physicians, clergy, counselors
4. individuals who visit or tour the facility for evaluation and are in a decision making process or "shopping" mode ("Inside Sales" as opposed to "Outside").

Selling and Public Relations

Another appropriate use of interpersonal communication is in the public relations area since direct personal contact is often involved in public relations. Calling on the press, operating speaker's bureaus, lobbying, and appearing at various events all involve personal contact, although the objective in these examples may be to sell an "idea" or cause rather than engaging in a transaction with a buyer. Nevertheless, the skills involved are very similar.

The last of the four target audiences mentioned above for which personal selling is recommended is the "on-premise shopper" who is a potential client visiting the facility prior to making a decision. Personal selling plays a crucial role in determining how "favorable" or "comfortable" a customer feels toward a facility. The staff persons meeting with the client or providing a "tour" communicate the credibility, dependability, proficiency of skills, values, compassion, philosophy, and other non-tangible attributes of the ATM organization.

An interesting characteristic of this on-premise selling process is that *several* persons might be involved in providing information to a customer visiting a facility rather than one "salesperson," which is more common when a representative makes a call on the outside. A receptionist, an administrator, a secretary, a counselor or therapist, a dietician, a nurse, or others might be involved in providing information about different aspects of the service. It becomes important then for the various staff involved to be aware of their role. One resource available to ATMs are staff psychologists already "on board" who have knowledge of behavioral and communications skills needed in convincing clients to enter the program.

SUMMARY

This article is an overview of the promotion function as a part of the ATM's marketing mix. It approaches various promotion decision areas from a managerial perspective, focusing upon some key components of promotion planning. Rather than provide specific operational or implementation details (how to write a brochure) it is more conceptual in nature and offers a framework for promotion planners.

The article addresses promotion management, promotion objectives, analysis for promotion planning, the promotion mix, and addresses the benefits and limitations of some specific promotion tools available to the ATM manager. It treats ATMs as a *service* and reveals specific implications for promotion strategy dictated by services. The article also reports promotion tools employed by Alabama ATMs citing data from the Alabama study.

Pricing Considerations for Alcoholism Treatment Facilities

Robin S. McCullin
Donald R. Self
Teri A. Kline

INTRODUCTION

Pricing of alcoholism treatment services has become more complicated as a result of such changes of prospective payment systems, the increasing intensity of competition, and the growth of preferred provider organizations and health maintenance organizations. To maintain or enhance the bottom line, it is necessary to look into the other component of profitability – volume and to examine the relationship between price and volume. It is becoming increasingly clear that there is market sensitivity to changes in prices in the health care sector (Mason, 1987). Although inflation in the economy has decreased significantly, it is still high in the health care sector. As a consequence, pressures from health care services' consumers continue, and insurers and employers are negotiating selective contracting arrangements (Mason, 1987). Pressures such as these have made the task of setting prices a critical factor in strategic planning.

When pricing services in alcoholism treatment, certain application problems persist such as what price means and where and how it can be used as a strategic tool. Specifically, third party reimbursement, regulated pricing structures such as exist in both non-profit and PPO arrangements, consumer price sensitivity/insensitivity and a lack of price awareness make pricing in this area difficult (Kotler & Clarke, 1987). In addition, the role of price varies depending on (1) whether the service is reimbursed or nonreimbursed, (2) the facility is dealing with individual medical service vs. health insurance package, and (3) the selected target market, i.e., patients, insurers, government, or employers. This paper, therefore, will explore the factors influencing pricing decisions and will discuss specific pricing strategies and tools available for use in both profit and not-for-profit treatment settings.

FACTORS INFLUENCING PRICING DECISIONS IN ALCOHOLISM TREATMENT SERVICES

The major factors influencing pricing decisions include the demand for alcoholism treatment, the role of insurance coverage, distribution of ownership of facilities, cost efficiency of treatment, and the development of Diagnosis Related Groups (DRG).

Demand for Treatment

Both the increase in population growth and the rising number of alcoholics in America contribute to the growing number of individuals seeking treatment for alcoholism and alcohol related problems. Data from a number of sources indicate that alcoholism treatment services and the number of people in treatment continue to increase; more than half a million people were reported to be in treatment in September, 1984 (Harwood et al., 1985; Noble, 1985). The State Alcohol and Drug Abuse Profile (SADAP) reports that alcohol client admissions increased by 6% from 1984 to 1985 (Butynski, Record, & Yates, 1986).

Prompted, perhaps, by the growing number of well-known individuals who have chosen to speak out about their alcohol problems and the role of treatment in their recovery, the stigma of alcoholism appears to be slowly diminishing (NIAAA, 1987). Korcok (1985) attributes the rise in treatment demand partially to the changing perceptions of alcoholism treatment from a marketing standpoint. In the rapidly changing health care marketplace, alcoholism treatment has become a dynamic and popular "product line." It is a good seller for hospitals, and a good buy for third party payers and corporate purchasers of health services.

In virtually all parts of the nation, print and broadcast messages now promote varying types of alcoholism services such as hospital inpatient programs, outpatient services, residential facilities, programs that involve the entire family, and programs designed specifically for teenagers, to name a few.

Between 1982 and 1990, the number of persons in treatment in the various types of settings is estimated to increase by 8%, on the basis of projections of the National Drug and Alcohol Treatment Utilization Survey data. Most of this increase is estimated to be accounted for by almost 22,000 men and women, 21 through 44 years old (NIAAA, 1987).

Insurance Changes

One factor involved in the above projection is the increase in involvement of third party payers; health insurers are extending their coverage of addictive illnesses. Thirty-six states (as of 1985) now require some form of alcoholism/chemical dependency coverage in health insurance policies sold in their states, either as mandatory coverage, or as an option (Korcok, 1985). More than 30 states require insurers to provide some level of outpatient benefits (Lee, 1987).

Korcok (1985) asserts that the U.S. Supreme Court's decision to uphold the right of the state of Massachusetts to require insurance companies to offer alcoholism, drug abuse and mental health policies issued in the state will solidify this trend to mandate alcoholism coverage. The availability of such insurance has had a profound effect on the fiscal health of alcoholism programs, and on their attractiveness for investors and hospital administrators seeking alternative sources of revenue (Korcok, 1985). The state of Pennsylvania also passed legislation requiring state insurers to include minimum coverage for alcoholism treatment in group health plans. Included is coverage for detoxification, residential rehabilitation, outpatient treatment and some brief inpatient stays (Super, 1986). While the legislation does not guarantee increased admissions at residential alcoholism treatment centers and detoxification programs, Super (1986) contends that it does encourage physicians to diagnose alcoholism and seek help for their patients. Various other states either have recently adopted such legislation or have impending legislation to do so.

Some industry observers, however, question whether consumers will use newly expanded coverage. Insurance policies covering alcoholism treatment programs historically are underutilized because of the stigma attached to alcoholism (Super, 1986). This trend may be changing, though, due to factors mentioned earlier such as increased public acceptance. (For an innovative PPO case study see Gomillion and Self in this volume.)

Number and Ownership of Facilities

Although the exact reasons for the rise in the demand for treatment services has not been pinpointed, it is known that the number of treatment facilities is increasing and existing facilities are expanding. The American Hospital Association survey data indicate that total alcoholism and other drug dependency treatment units increased from 465 in 1978 to 829 in 1984 (78% increase), while total in-hospital alcoholism and other drug dependency beds increased from 16,005 to 25,981 for the same-year period (62% increase). As with the hospital industry, generally the fastest growth and largest increase was in the private for-profit sector, where the number of units increased by 347% and the number of in-hospital beds increased by 392% from 1978 to 1984 (NIAAA, 1987).

Harwood, Kristiansen, and Rachal (1985) report comparative data on the ownership of services for 1978 and 1984. By 1984, state and local governments owned 20% of 25,981 beds (decrease of 20%) while investor owned, for-profit beds increased from 5% in 1978 to 15% in 1984. Non-government, non-profit control increased from 31% in 1978 to 44% in 1984. In addition, there were 1,073 hospital outpatient units for alcoholism and chemical dependency reported in 1983. In 1978 there were fewer than 800 (Korcok, 1985).

Butynski, Record, and Yates (1986) present comparative data on expenditures on alcohol and drug abuse treatment and report that states provided 52.7% of the treatment, federal sources provided 19.3%, country or local sources contributed 6.5% and other sources (for example, private health insurance, court fines, etc.) contributed 21.6%.

When seeking alcohol abuse/dependency treatment, the individual may select different treatment alternatives, the three most common being (1) inpatient or hospital treatment, (2) residential/rehabilitation, and (3) outpatient treatment. Rehabilitation/residential is an approach which provides in a hospital or non-hospital setting, a planned program of professionally directed evaluation, treatment, or rehabilitation services. Outpatient treatment is evaluation and treatment, or assistance services, provided on a short-term basis to clients who reside elsewhere (Butynski et al., 1986). The United States Department of Health and Human Services reports that as of September, 1984, 8% of the patients were in an outpatient facility, 10% were in a residential setting, and 82% were active outpatients (USDHHA, 1984).

Cost-Benefit Analysis

A question arising from analysis of alcoholism treatment concerns cost-benefit analysis. With the rising costs of providing employee benefits, purchasers of alcoholism treatment are concerned that the benefits derived from treating alcoholics balance or offset these costs. A large number of studies reviewed by Jones and Vischi (1979) prompted them to conclude that treatment benefits outweigh treatment costs. Brock and Boyaty (1978) report a 40% reduction in outpatient care utilization after alcoholism treatment while Sherman et al. (1979) found a 27% reduction in inpatient and outpatient medical care costs at Kaiser Permanente in southern California.

Hunter (1978), in a study of the Arizona Health Plan, found reductions in post-treatment care costs. With regard to dollar savings, Hayami and Freebori (1981), in the context of a health maintenance organization, estimated a savings of $0.40 for every $1.00 spent on treatment. Holder and Hallan (1978), in a study of the health benefits program of the California Public Employees Retirement system, found an annual savings of $84 per person following alcoholism treatment initiation. Holder and Hallan (1981) followed a group of 90 alcoholics and their families from the same health insurance program and reported an average annual reduction in total health care costs of $864 per person.

Holder, Blose, and Basiorowski (1985) examined the impact of alcoholism treatment on overall health care utilization and costs for individuals and families filing claims with the Aetna Life Insurance Company under the Federal Employees Health Benefit Program. On the average, families with at least one member filing a claim for alcoholism treatment during 1980-1983 used health care services and incurred costs at a rate about twice that of a comparison group consisting of a random sample of families who filed no alcoholic claims during that period. Average monthly care costs for the two groups over this period were $210 per person and $107 per person, respectively.

This study also found a gradual rise in the overall health care costs and utilization for alcoholics during the three years preceding alcoholism treatment, with the most dramatic increase occurring in the 6 months before treatment. Total monthly costs increased from about $150 per month two years prior to treatment to an average of more than $50 per month during the 6 months prior to treatment and $1,376 in the final pre-treatment month (Holder et al., 1985).

After alcoholics started treatment, their health care costs dropped significantly and eventually reached approximately the level that existed several years prior to treatment. Their total monthly costs averaged $294 during the first 6 months after treatment and declined to an average of $190 per month by two and a half to three years after treatment. The most significant drop in health care costs occurred for treated alcoholics under the age of 45 (Holder et al., 1985). In this study, 77% of all alcoholics received inpatient care, which accounted for 95% of all alcoholism treatment costs. Among the inpatient care facilities used were general hospitals (82% of all admissions), specialized alcoholism hospitals (9.5%) and hospital-affiliated inpatient/alcoholism care centers (5.6%).

The benefit cost of Aetna's alcoholism treatment coverage, i.e., the costs spread over all Aetna subscribers was $1.34 per covered individual per year. Using a variety of forecasting techniques the project estimated that the average alcoholic's treatment cost could be offset by reductions in other health care costs within two to three years following the start of treatment. That is, the average alcoholism treatment costs can be recovered within three years after initiation of treatment (Holder et al., 1985). This study found that alcoholism treatment is associated with significant reductions in total health care costs, with reductions largest for persons under 45 years of age.

Hayden and Rosenthal (1985) report that the 28-day inpatient program has been developed and accepted as the standard for the treatment of alcoholism, partly because 28 days is the time period for which most insurance companies will pay. Muszynski et al. (1983) report that only 30 plans of 300 large group insurance plans covered outpatient mental health treatment equal to any other medical outpatient coverage. The disproportionate skewing of inpatient care results from stringent restraints on outpatient psychiatric benefits (Lee, 1987). Hayden and Rosenthal (1986) contend, however, that many other types of programs constitute standard treatment today and that the cost effectiveness of these different types of programs should be examined.

Inpatient vs. Outpatient

In examining the differences in prices between inpatient versus outpatient treatment, Korcok (1986) found that alcoholics who are married, employed, socially stable, and who have experienced only a few years of drinking can be treated in a day clinic setting, with appropriate medication. There are also cost advantages to outpatient treatment. Although inpatient programs offering three- to four-week multimodal programs occupy a substantial segment of the alcoholism treatment business, various studies have shown that the great majority of alcoholics seeking treatment can be detoxified in non-hospital based units and that detoxification pharmacotherapy on an outpatient basis is a safe alternative at a small portion of the inpatient cost.

Annis (1984) concluded that in-hospital alcoholic programs of a few weeks to a few months duration show no higher success rates than periods of brief hospitalization of a few days. The great majority of alcoholics seeking treatment for alcohol withdrawal can be safely detoxified without pharmacotherapy and in non-hospital based units. Partial hospitalization (day treatment) programs have been found to have equal or superior results to inpatient hospitalization at one-half to one-third the cost. Well controlled trials have also demonstrated that outpatient programs can produce comparable results to inpatient programs for most patients. One estimate places the cost saving at $3,700 per patient compared with the typical cost of inpatient treatment (Annis, 1984). These authors and others (see for example Worden, 1982) propose that outpatient treatment programs are viable alternatives to residential care for most clients. However, some insurance companies and the federal Medicaid program are willing to pay for some treatment provided only in a hospital (Vaughn, Sherborne, & Lewis, 1985). This practice is questionable since it limits payment to the most expensive treatment option available. Treatment in a freestanding program is not as costly as in a hospital affiliated site, partially because hospitals must pay for high-cost equipment, much of which is not needed by alcohol abuse patients. Insurance, then, will play a major role in determining the types of treatment offered and entered into by the alcohol dependent person.

Diagnosis Related Groups (DRG)

Recent legislative efforts have been directed toward the development of financing strategies that will restrain the growth in health care costs. In particular, the Health Care Financing Administration (HCFA) has implemented a payment system for inpatient services delivered to Medicare beneficiaries known as diagnosis related groups (DRG) which provides hospitals with a fixed reimbursement per discharge. In terms of hospital financing (Balinsky & Starkman, 1987), this new system represents a radical shift from a multiple fee-for-service structure to a single fee-for-diagnosis structure. Based on a patient's diagnosis, the health care provider (currently limited to acute care hospitals), receives a pre-established amount for providing the needed medical care to the patient (Balinsky & Starkman, 1987). With this reimbursement procedure, the hospital cannot recover any losses from the patient but does not have to return any excess reimbursement. Therefore, hospitals are encouraged to identify costs and seeks ways to reduce or control them.

Originally the HCFA developed DRG 436 (alcohol dependence) which carried a geometric mean length stay of 8.1 days with an average payment of $2,300 for a course of detoxification and rehabilitation (Korcok, 1985). As a result, the HCFA granted alcoholism and alcoholism-units in general hospitals a temporary exemption from Medicare's prospective payment system.

The second structure release by the HCFA (June, 1985) contained five alcoholism related DRGs (Korcok, 1985). DRG 437 (substance dependence, combined rehabilitation and detoxification) called for a 14.6 geometric mean length of stay and an average payment of more than $3,900. Again, providers of treatment contested the classification structure with the common criticism being that the 14.6-day figure was too long to cover detoxification and too short for rehabilitation. HCFA extended the alcoholism treatment exemptions pending further analysis of treatment (Korcok, 1985). Included in the exemption were the same alcoholism hospitals and in-hospital alcoholism treatment units that had been operating under the previous exemption. At the time of writing, the results of the HCFA's investigation had not been determined.

A result of the implementation of DRGs is an effort to reduce costs which may swing the emphasis from inpatient care to opportunities for providing care outside the hospital, in less costly outpatient settings (Balinsky & Starkman, 1987). Further, pricing as a strategic tool may be lessened.

According to Korcok (1985), despite the perceived stringency of the DRG criteria, "both for-profit and not-for-profit programs still see great potential in the expansion of alcoholism/chemical dependency treatment" among new clients.

PRICING OBJECTIVES

Kotler and Clarke (1987) provide a useful framework for determining pricing objectives in alcoholism treatment facilities which will be followed in our discussion of pricing. When facing the pricing issue, an organization should proceed through four stages: (1) determination of pricing objectives, (2) determination of pricing strategy, (3) determination of pricing in situations such as self-pay markets and reimbursed markets, and (4) anticipation of changes in reimbursement procedures in the future.

Different pricing objectives may be selected from which to develop pricing as a strategic tool. Objectives may include (1) surplus or profit maximization, (2) maximization of net patient service revenue, (3) cost-based reimbursement, (4) usage maximization, (5) market disincentivization, and (6) cross-subsidization.

Profit Maximization

Although historically most health care organizations have not employed the profit maximization pricing objective, the continuing decline in external funds to compensate for operating losses has caused more organizations to move toward this strategy. Many non-profit organizations are now using the term profit and recognize the importance of surplus funds to build up reserves for future capital investments (Kotler & Clarke, 1987). The expansion of health care chains will make this a more commonly used strategy.

Net Patient Service Revenue

When dealing primarily in cost-based reimbursed markets, many organizations maximize net patient service revenue, what Kotler and Clarke (1987) refer to as "total revenue minus discounts, bad debts, contractual allowances, retroactive denials, and disallowed expenses" (p. 351). One outcome of this objective is to try to maximize the number of charge-based patients served by the organization since they bring in higher revenue and higher surplus per unit of service. Maximizing net patient service can be accomplished by attracting the highest possible volume of patients but by also drawing in the most financially attractive (i.e., commercially insured) patients (Kotler & Clarke, 1987). This objective, however, needs to be balanced by the ethical and often mandated considerations of serving non-reimbursed clients.

Cost Recovery

A third objective involves seeking a price per unit of service that allows the organization to recover all or a reasonable part of its costs. Cost-based reimbursement was developed with this pricing objective in mind. Organizations may choose to use either full cost recovery or partial cost recovery, depending on whether they are able to rely on external sources to compensate for unrecovered costs. This objective requires the organization to know their costs in order to set prices. DRG reimbursement is intended to be based on a cost recovery objective.

Usage Factors

Usage maximization is an alternative pricing objective where an organization seeks to maximize the total number of users of the service. This approach entails, among other activities, maximizing utilization. According to Kotler and Clarke (1987), "if variable costs are low, if there are no revenue caps, and if each user represents additional revenue to the organization, the health care organization may wish to maximize utilization" (p. 354). Additionally, organizations may *lower* their prices to maximize utilization if they feel that users and society profit from their services. In some circumstances a low price may stimulate higher usage and produce more revenue in the long run.

Market disincentivization is a pricing objective which has been observed in the insurance industry. With this objective, pricing is used as a tool to discourage as many people as possible from using or purchasing a service. Many for-profit facilities encourage indigent populations to seek services from charity or governmental based facilities.

Cross-subsidization is a major pricing objective of many health care organizations who want to balance the surpluses and losses of varying market segments and services. This is appropriate for organizations introducing new product lines or services in treatment. Currently, surpluses from alcoholism treatment are being used by many facilities to finance growth into the treatment of various addictive disorders.

SELECTION OF PRICING STRATEGY

Global or A La Carte Pricing

There are two opposite approaches to pricing medical services:

> A La Carte: considering each procedure of service or treatment as a separate, chargeable item for inpatient billing.
> Global: Combined collection of predetermined services under a single or all-inclusive or global rate. (Harry, 1987, p. 26)

Two counteracting trends tend to push ATMs in one of these two extremes. The demand for cost containment in the form of fixed-price-per discharge (Scheiderich, 1987) and the concept of "product line" and varying levels of need among potential clients (Korcok, 1985) to contain costs can become confusing.

The *Alabama Voice* (1986) study found that a per diem plus individual costs for treatment (50%), a per diem rate including most or all costs (40%), and a global price policy (10%) are all used with almost all global pricers being private inpatient facilities.

About 80% of the facilities "guarantee" their services by providing free after care, with about 10% charging for such care and 10% not providing such care. Most of the public facilities used a sliding scale based on clients' income. About one-fifth of the private inpatient facilities charge premiums, about 50% higher, for detox than for continuing treatment.

A Brief History of Hospital Pricing

> In the early 1930s, in response to the depression economy, hospitals started charging for services based on case rates. These rates varied by broad generalized diagnosis categories or length of stay. Charges had little to do with the costs of providing the services. As the economy started to improve due to the war in Europe in the late 1930s and early 1940s, hospitals returned to the more traditional a la carte charging methods that had become commonplace in the 1920s. However, at the same time, in several large urban communities such as Cleveland, Ohio, a new global pricing strategy emerged—the all-inclusive daily rate.
>
> The all-inclusive rate concept bundled routine, special care, and ancillary usage into a single daily charge that varied based on the day of stay or the clinical division. Although this global pricing approach increased in popularity during the 1940s, it also had a relatively short life. By the mid 1950s there were only a handful of hospitals still using the all-inclusive rate structures. There was a brief, but short, renewal of interest in this method of pricing during the early 1970's resulting from a federally funded research and demonstration project con-

ducted with the cooperation of hospitals in Appalachia, Denver, and Hawaii (Harry, 1987, p. 26)

Accurate cost data are an indispensable component that must be considered in the development of a pricing strategy. However, there are other factors that Mason (1987) recommends considering in the pricing process. Alcoholism treatment facilities should consider the following questions:

1. Are customers being charged for all the services provided?
2. Are the prices charged all-inclusive?
3. How would the market react to changes in the charge structure?
4. Do prices exceed cost?
5. Will market conditions allow prices to exceed cost?

Keeping these questions in mind, several different pricing strategies are appropriate for alcoholism treatment marketing, including (1) cost-oriented pricing, (2) demand-oriented pricing, (3) competition-oriented pricing, and (4) maximum reimbursement.

Cost-Oriented Pricing

Cost-oriented pricing involves setting prices largely on the basis of costs and involves different techniques such as break-even analysis. This strategy is popular because (1) there is generally less uncertainty about costs than about demand, (2) if all organizations in an industry use this strategy then prices are similar in that industry, and (3) therefore, results in perceptions of social fairness to buyers and sellers. Sensitivity analysis is a tool used by financial managers to get current prices in line with costs and determine the impact of price changes on profits (Mason, 1987). Mason adds that it is also important to be able to identify cost-behavior patterns of the various resources used to provide the facilities' services and understand their relationship to volume and profit. For the interested reader, Johnson (1987) presents an excellent procedure for developing a cost base for pricing.

Until 1982, there were basically no constraints on what hospitals could charge private patients for services. Prior to the 1980s, there were few alternative distribution systems such as HMOs and PPOs. Since Blue Cross and Blue Shield paid hospital charges with no constraints, the industry evolved a cost-oriented pricing methodology.

Demand-Oriented Pricing

In contrast, demand-oriented pricing looks at the condition of demand rather than the level of costs to set the price. Using this strategy, an organization estimates how much value individuals see in a service and price accordingly; price should reflect the buyer's perceived value. An application of this strategy is price discrimination in which a service is sold at more than one price. Using a sliding scale wherein the organization charges a poor patient less is illustrative of this concept. According to Berry (1980), price discrimination results from attempts by sellers to gain maximum profit possible in a given market by offering different prices to different customers. Price differences have been common in health services marketing.

Competition-Oriented Pricing

Competition-oriented pricing occurs when an organization sets its prices primarily on the basis of what competitors are charging. Under this strategy an organization may charge the same price as the competition, or a price higher or lower than the competition. The organization, however, does not try to maintain a rigid relationship between its price and either its own costs or demands; the price of the service does not vary with changes in cost or demand. *Going rate* pricing is an example of competition-oriented pricing and is popular with organizations where costs are difficult to measure, and also in organizations where the going rate is believed to represent the collective wisdom of the industry (Kotler & Clarke, 1987), appearing to be relatively common among similar providers. Commercial insurers and professional associations generally encourage use of this strategy. Scheiderich (1987) reports that hospitals are frequently asked to compete on price by a variety of health care purchasers including Medicaid, Blue Cross, and major commercial customers. However, at the same time, consumers (often motivated by cost-reduction bonuses) are actively beginning to shop for price.

Scheiderich contends that hospital pricing decisions based on across-the-board percentage increases or competing hospitals are ineffective and dangerous.

Maximum-Reimbursement Pricing

Maximum-reimbursement-oriented pricing occurs when organizations charge the maximum allowed by reimbursement agencies, or charge what the market will bear. According to Scheiderich (1987), increased public concern over the financial viability of Social Security and subsequent legislation by Congress has led hospitals to analyze prices in terms of cost-based activities and to maximize price increases for services that have a high percentage of charge-paying utilization in order to get the most out of price increases. Scheiderich (1987) also notes the trend toward a fixed-price-per discharge payment methodology, with Medicare, Medicaid, Blue Cross, and various major commercial accounts using this method.

Hospitals face at least two constraints as they develop pricing strategies: (1) overall hospital charges should be structured to maximize "product" contribution margins within payer-induced constraints, and (2) Part B program charges should be as high as possible so that program costs can be maximized. Services that are billed by the hospital but are not necessarily provided by the hospital are included in the Part B program charges and include alcoholism treatment and rehabilitation. Beyond the obvious constraint of not paying more than what is ultimately billed, hospitals are not allowed to make a profit on billed services (Scheiderich, 1987).

Epilogue: Developing a Client-Centered Philosophy

Donald R. Self
Teri A. Kline
Jerry J. Ingram
William I. Sauser, Jr.
Vaughan C. Judd

ORGANIZATION-ORIENTED PHILOSOPHY

Although marketing tools have been increasingly used, an anti-marketing bias on the part of many administrators and influencers exists especially in the non-profit sector. Bloom and Novelli (1981) have proposed that a major problem of *all* social marketers is that they must function in organizations where marketing functions are poorly understood, appreciated, and inappropriately located. A major cause of this is the organization-oriented philosophy.

Kotler and Andreason (1987) present characteristics of organization-oriented philosophies, inherent in the "change-agent" and "professional-client orientations" as can be seen in Table 1. The characteristics of the organization-oriented philosophy are antithetical to much of the content of traditional marketing. Since "we already know what is right," there is a lack of concern with alternate service development and client research. Although a large number of alcoholism treatment marketers are evolving away from this philosophy, many of the answers needed for an effective customer-centered orientation are still being developed.

ATM is employed by human services organizations which are involved with changing of malfunctioning individuals: the concept

The following is adapted from Self et al. (1988), and outlines the most difficult task in developing a marketing orientation.

Table 1

Organization and Client-Centered Organization

1. The organization's offering is seen as inherently desirable.	1. To whom are we planning to market?
2. Lack of organizational success is attributed to customer ignorance, absence of motivation, or both.	2. Where are they and what are they like?
3. A minor role is afforded customer research.	3. What are their current perceptions, needs, and wants?
4. Marketing is defined primarily as promotion.	4. Will these perceptions, needs and wants be different in the future when our strategy is to be implemented?
5. Marketing specialists are chosen for their product knowledge or their communication skills.	5. How satisfied are our customers with our offering?
6. One "best" marketing strategy is typically employed in approaching the market.	
7. Generic competition tends to be ignored.	

Source: Kotler, Philip and Alan R. Andreason, Strategic Marketing for Non-Profit Organizations, Englewood Cliffs, NJ: Prentice Hall, Inc., 1987, as adapted from Andreason, Alan R., "Non-Profits" Check Your Attention to Customers." Harvard Business Review, May-June 1982, pp. 105-110.

of an "exchange" which many marketing theorists perceive to be the case construct in marketing. Marketing exchanges assume, "(1) there are at least two parties; (2) each can offer something that the other perceives as valuable; (3) each is capable of communication and delivery; and (4) that each is free to accept or reject the offer" (Kotler & Clarke, 1987, pp. 46-47). Because of the intervention nature of alcoholism treatment, the inability of many organizations to limit the characteristics of "acceptable" patients and the potential clients' perceptions of "value" and "freedom" to accept the offer, the range of exchanges needs to be broadened as depicted in Figure 1.

The "moral" compliance alternative is represented by the "leap of faith" conversion experience of many AA members, while the coercive alternative is represented by various legal system variations where treatment is not on a completely voluntary basis. Persuasion and negotiation represent more central positions of the continuum. Depending upon the variables leading to the pretreatment assessment of the client, alternative strategies need to be employed.

A corollary to the need to adapt the traditional concept of exchange is the need to modify several basic marketing tenets as described below.

DIFFICULTY IN APPLYING BASIC MARKETING PRINCIPLES

Much of the traditional marketing management literature focuses on becoming a client-centered organization. As discussed above, the development of a client-oriented organization requires the information proposed in Table 1. In addition, the concept of exchange, the "marketing concept" and the development of competitor-oriented decision models also hamper the development of marketing in alcoholism treatment facilities.

Figure 1

The Exchange Process Continuum

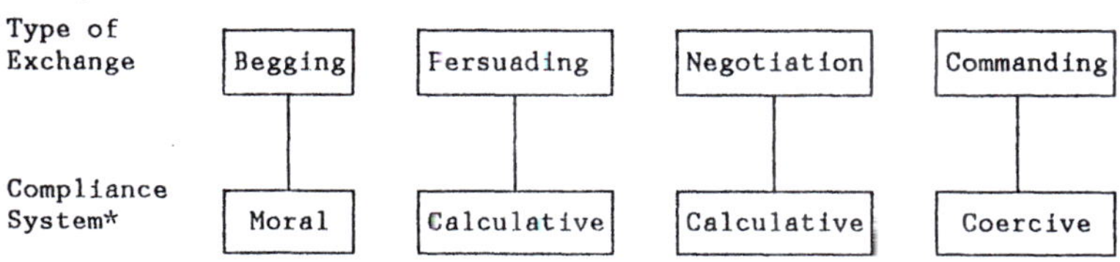

Source: Etzioni, A. A Comparative Analysis of Complex Organizations, Glencoe, Ill.: Free Press, 1969.

The "marketing concept" can be defined as a company (organization)-wide orientation in which "all facets of the organization must be involved with assessing, and then satisfying customer wants and needs" (Boone & Kurtz, 1986, p. 13). We have elsewhere (Self, Buchanan, & Ingram, 1987) proposed a "balanced approach" between the change-agent and client-orientation. This position has been defined as a *societal marketing* approach, in which "the main task of the organization is to determine the needs, wants, and interests of target markets and to adapt the organization to delivering satisfactions *that preserve and enhance the consumer's and society's well-being*" (Kotler & Clark, 1987, p. 32, emphasis added).

A further problem delineated by various ATM personnel is the lack of knowledge of how to use basic marketing concepts. This problem is common to many similar organizations as identified by a wide variety of studies.

1. Limited understanding of marketing by present organization members should be accommodated.
2. The translation of for-profit marketing to the specific non-profit context should not be done mechanically.
3. It should be granted that the organization is already doing many things that are "marketing." Marketing will be accepted more rapidly if one adopts the existing language, at least initially, rather than trying to change the organization's accustomed language to fit current marketing jargon.
4. Many non-profit managers have come to their positions from nonbusiness backgrounds and may be defensive about their naivete (although not necessarily hostile to marketing).

Bibliography

Aaker, D., and Carman, J., "Are You Overadvertising?," *Journal of Advertising Research,* 22(4), August/September, 1982.

The Alabama Voice, "An Analysis of the Market for Alcohol and Chemical Dependency Treatment Centers in Alabama," Unpublished Study, Department of Marketing, Auburn University at Montgomery, Montgomery, AL: March 1986.

Alcohol Epidemiologic Data System (AEDS), *Procedures for Assessing Alcohol Treatment Needs*, Rockville, MD: National Institute on Alcohol Abuse and Alcoholism, 1982.

Alcohol Epidemiologic Data System (AEDS), *County Alcohol Problem Indicators 1975-1977*. U.S. Alcohol Epidemiologic Data Reference Manual, Section 3. Rockville, MD: National Institute on Alcohol Abuse and Alcoholism, 1981b.

Alcohol Resources: Directory, Alcohol-Related Periodicals, Rockville, MD: National Clearinghouse For Alcohol Information, December, 1986.

Alcohol Resources: Directory, Self-Help Groups for Professionals and Special Populations, Rockville, MD: National Clearinghouse For Alcohol Information, August, 1986.

Alterman, A.I., and Tarter, R.E., "An Examination of Selected Typologies: Hyperactivity, Familial, and Antisocial Alcoholism," In: Galanter, M. (ed.), *Recent Developments in Alcoholism*, Vol. 4, New York: Plenum Press, 1986.

American Library Directory, New York: R.R. Bowker Company, 1986.

Annis, H.M., "Is Inpatient Rehabilitation of the Alcoholic Cost Effective? Con Position," *Advances in Alcohol & Substance Abuse*, 5(1-2), in press. Presented at NADAP Conference on Controversies, New York, 26 March, 1984.

Annis, H.M., and Liban, C.B., "A Follow-Up Study of Male Halfway-House Residents and Matched Nonresident Controls," *Journal of Studies on Alcohol*, 40(1): 63-69, 1979.

Armor, D.J., Polich, J.M., and Stambul, H.B., *Alcoholism and Treatment*, Rand Corp. Research Report R-1739 NIAAA, Santa Monica: The Rand Corporation, 1976.

Armor, D.J., Polich, J.M., and Stambul, H.B., *Alcoholism and Treatment*, New York: John Wiley & Sons, 1978.

Assael, H., *Consumer Behavior and Marketing Action*, Boston, MA: Kent Publishing Company, 1987.

Assael, H., *Consumer Behavior and Marketing Action*, 2nd Ed., Boston, MA: Kent Publishing Company, pp. 90-91, 1984.

Babor, T.F., and Mendelson, J.H., "Empirical Correlates of Self-Report Drinking Measures," In: Galanter, M. (ed.), *Currents in Alcoholism*, Vol. III, *Recent Advances in Research and Treatment*, New York: Grune & Stratton, pp. 161-168, 1980.

Babor, R.F., and Meyer, R.E., "Overview," In: Galanter, M. (ed.), *Recent Developments in Alcoholism*, Vol. 4, New York: Plenum Press, 1986.

Baekeland, F., and Lundwall, L., "Dropping Out of Treatment: A Critical Review," *Psychological Bulletin*, 82(5): 738-783, 1975.

Baekeland, F., "Evaluation Treatment Methods in Chronic Alcoholism," In: Kissin, B., and Begleiter, H. (eds.), *Treatment and Rehabilitation of the Chronic Alcoholic*, New York: Plenum Press, pp. 385-440, 1977.

Baekeland, F., Lundwall, L., and Kissin, B., "Methods for the Treatment of Chronic Alcoholism: A Critical Appraisal," In: Israel, Y. (ed.), *Research Advances in Alcohol and Drug Problems*, Vol. II, New York: John Wiley & Sons, Inc., 1975.

Bagozzi, R.P., *Principles of Marketing Management*, Chicago, IL: Science Research Associates, Inc., 1986.

______, "Marketing as Exchange," *Journal of Marketing*, 39: 32-39, October 1975.

Bailey, M.B., Haberman, P.W., and Alksne, H., "The Epidemiology of Alcoholism In An Urban Residential Area," *Quarterly Journal of Studies on Alcoholism*, 26: 19-40, 1965.

Bales, R.F., "Cultural Differences in Rates of Alcoholism," *Quarterly Journal of Studies on Alcoholism*, 6: 480-499, 1946.

Balinsky, W., and Starkman, J.L., "The Impact of DRGs on the Health Care Industry," *Health Care Management*, 12(3): 61-74, 1987.

Balsley, R.D., and Birsner, E.P., *Selling: Marketing Personified*, Chicago, IL: The Dryden Press, p. 353, 1987.

Bandura, A., *Principles of Behavior Modification*, New York: Holt, Rinehart, & Winston, Inc., 1969.

Battegay, R., and Ladewig, D., "Outpatient Treatment Possibilities for Alcoholics and Drug Addicts," *Therapeutische Usmachau*, 43(1): 56-62, 1986.

Baughan, D.M., "Crisis Precipitation in Alcoholism," *Western Journal of Medicine*, 145(5): 680-681, 1986.

Beal, G.M., "Information Sources In The Decision Process," *The Research Clinic On Decision Making*, Pullman, State College of Washington, pp. 36-51, 1968.

Berglas, S., "Self-Handicapping Alcohol Abuse," *Alcohol Health and Research World*, 10(2): 46-47, 54, 1986.

Berkman, H.W., and Gilson, C.C., *Consumer Behavior Concepts and Strategies*, Encino, CA: Dickenson Publishing Co., Inc., p. 418, 1978.

Bernhardt, K.L., and Kinnear, T.C., *Cases In Marketing Management*, 4th Ed., Plano, TX: Business Publications, Inc., 1988.

Berry, L., "Services Marketing Is Different," *Business*, May-June, p. 25, 1980.

Bertrand, R. Canfield, and Moore, Frazier H., *Public Relations: Principles, Cases and Problems*, 7th Ed., Homewood, IL: Irwin, 1975.

Beschner, G., "Understanding Teen-Age Drug Use," In: Beschner, G., and Friedman, A.S. (eds.), *Teen Drug Use*, Lexington, MA: Lexington Books, pp. 1-18, 1986.

Billings, A.G., and Moos, R.H., "Psychosocial Processes of Recovery Among Alcoholics and Their Families: Implications For Clinicians and Program Evaluators," *Addictive Behaviors*, 8: 205-218, 1983.

Binkoff, J.A., "Exposure and Reactivity to Alcohol Cues: Impact on Drink Refusal Skills of Problem Drinkers," *Dissertation Abstracts International*, 46(10): 3587-B, 1986.

Blane, H.T., "Issues in the Evaluation of Alcoholism Treatment," *Professional Psychology*, 8: 593-608, 1977.

Bloom, P.N., and W.D. Novelli, "Problems and Challenges in Social Marketing," *Journal of Marketing*, 45: 79-88, Spring, 1981.

Bloom, P.N., "Effective Marketing For Professional Services," *Harvard Business Review*, September-October, p. 102, 1984.

Bonoma, T.V., "Major Sales: Who Really Does the Buying?," *Harvard Business Review*, 60 (May-June), pp. 111-119, 1982.

Boone, L.E., and Kurtz, D.L., *Contemporary Marketing*, 5th Ed., Chicago: Dryden Press, 1986.

Boulding, K., "The Concept of Need for Health Services," *Millbank Memorial Fund Quarterly*, 44, Part 2, October, p. 202, 1966.

Bower, B., "Researchers Tackle The Mystery Of Alcoholism," *New Physician*, 35(3): 26-28, 42-43, 1986.

Brandsma, J.M., Maultsby, M.C., Jr., and Welsh, R.J., *Outpatient Treatment of Alcoholism*, Baltimore: University Park Press, 1980.

Braught, N.G., "Problem Drinking Among Adolescents; A Review and Analysis of Psychosocial Research," In: *U.S. National Institute On Alcohol Abuse and Alcoholism*. Special population issues. (*Alcohol and Health Monograph No. 4*.) Rockville, MD. [In press.]

Braunstein, W.B., Powell, B.J., McGowan, J.F., and Thoreson, R.W., "Employment Factors in Outpatient Recovery of Alcoholics: A Multivariate Study," *Addictive Behaviors*, 8: 345-351, 1983.

Brenman-Gibson, M., "Psychoanalysis," In: Corsini, Raymond J. (ed.), *Encyclopedia of Psychology*, 3, New York: John Wiley & Sons, pp. 86-91, 1984.

Brickman, P., Rabinowitz, V.C., Karuza, J., Coates, D., Cohn, E. et al., "Models of Helping and Coping," *American Psychology*, 37: 368-84, 1982.

Brock, C.B., and Boyaty, T.G., *Group Health Association of America Study: Alcoholism Within Prepaid Group Practice HMOs*, Report to NIAAA No. 5HAA01745, Washington, DC: Supt. of Docs., U.S. Government Printing Office, 1978.

Brody, J.A., "Aging and Alcohol Abuse," *Grassroots*, pp. 11-14, 1982.

Bromet, E., Moos, R., Bliss, F., and Wuthmann, C., "Posttreatment Functioning of Alcoholic Patients: Its Relation to Program Participation," *Journal of Consulting and Clinical Psychology*, 45(5): 829-842, 1977.

Brown, S., "Models of Alcoholism," *Treating the Alcoholic*, New York: John Wiley & Sons, 1985.

Brunning, J., Mumford, J.P., and Keaney, F.P., "Lofexidine in Alcohol Withdrawal States," *Medical Council on Alcoholism*, 21(2): 167-170, 1986.

Burian, W., "Group Therapy In The Management of Alcoholism: Theoretical and Technical Inquiry," *Wiener Zeitschrift fur Suchtforschung*, 8(1/2): 5-11, 1985.

Burnett, J.J., *Promotion Management: A Strategic Approach*, St. Paul: West Publishing, 1984.

Butynski, W., Record, N., and Yates, J., "State Resources and Services for Alcohol and Drug Abuse Problems: Fiscal Year 1985. An Analysis of State Alcohol and Drug Abuse Profile Data," National Association of State Alcohol and Drug Abuse Directors, Inc., Washington, DC, July, 1986.

Cahalan, D., "Epidemiology: Alcohol Use in American Society," In: Gomberg, E.L., White, H.R., and Carpenter, J.A. (eds.), *Alcohol Science and Society Revisited*, Ann Arbor, MI: The University of Michigan State, 1982.

Cahalan, D., and Room, R., *Problem Drinking Among American Men*, Monograph of Rutgers Center of Alcohol Studies, No. 7, New Brunswick, NJ: Rutgers Center of Alcohol Studies, 1974.

Carlson, C., "Challenges To The 'New Professionals,'" *Alcohol & Addiction*, 6(5): 15, 1986.

Carmi, A., and Schneider, S. (eds.), *Drugs and Alcohol*, New York: Springer-Verlag, 1986.

Cartwright, D.S., *Theories and Models of Personality*, Dubuque, IA: Wm. C. Brown Company, 1979.

Chafetz, M.E., *The Alcoholic Patient: Diagnosis and Management*, Oradell, NJ: Medical Economics Co., Inc., 1983.

Chafetz, M.E., and Blane, H.T., "Alcohol-Crisis Treatment Approach and Establishment of Treatment Relations with Alcoholics," *Psychol. Rep.*, 12: 862, 1963.

Cherian, R.R., "Emergence of A Day-Care Centre for Alcoholics In India: Its Referral System and Public Response," *British Journal of Addiction*, 81(1): 119-122, 1986.

Clinebell, H.J., "Pastoral Counseling of the Alcoholic and His Family," In: Catanzaro, R.J. (ed.), *Alcoholism: The Total Treatment Approach*, Springfield, IL: Thomas Books, pp. 189-207, 1968.

Cohen, S., and Callahan, J.F. (eds.), *Diagnosis and Treatment of Drug and Alcohol Abuse*, New York: The Haworth Press, Inc., 1986.

Cohen, S., *The Substance Abuse Problems*, New York: The Haworth Press, Inc., 1985.

Connors, G.J., Tarbox, A.R., and McLaughlin, E.J., "Contrasting Binge and Continuous Alcoholic Drinkers Using Demographic and Drinking History Variables," *Alcohol and Alcoholism*, 21(1): 105-110, 1986.

Cooke, D.J., "Spontaneous Recovery or Statistical Artifact?" *British Journal of Addiction*, 75: 323-324, 1980.

Cooney, N.L., Meyer, R.E., Kaplan, R.F., and Baker, L.H., "Validation Study of Four Scales Measuring Severity of Alcohol Dependence," *British Journal of Addiction*, 81(2): 223-229, 1986.

Corey, L.J. et al., "Psychiatric Ward Atmosphere," *Journal of Psychosocial Nursing*, 24(10): 10-16, 1986.

Costello, R.M., "Alcoholism Treatment and Evaluation: In Search of Methods," *International Journal of the Addictions*, 10: 251-275, 1975.

Creative Sociomedics, Inc., *The Creative Report*, 1980.

Cueny, D., Miller, K., and Eldridge, M.K., "The Healthcare Account Executive, A Sales Approach to Healthcare Marketing," *Health Care Quarterly*, 3(2/3), Winter/Spring 1986.

da Fonesca, A.F., Paiva, F.M., and Droux, A., "Aspect of Integrated Psychiatry: Application of a Structured Interview," *Revue de l'Alcoolisme*, 31(1): 9-14, 1986.

Davidson, R., and Raistrick, D., "Validity of the Short Alcohol Dependence Data (SADD) Questionnaire: A Sort Self-Report Questionnaire For The Assessment of Alcohol Dependence," *British Journal of Addiction*, 81(2): 217-222, 1986.

Davies, D.L., "Normal Drinking in Recovered Alcohol Addicts," *Q.J. Stud. Alcohol*, 23: 94-104, 1962.

Dean, J., "Multivariant Assessment and Treatment Techniques for Alcohol Problems," *International Journal of the Addictions*, 20(8): 1281-1290, 1985.

Denzin, N.K., *The Alcoholic Self*, Newbury Park, CA: Sage Publications, Inc., 1987.

Denzin, N.K., *Recovering Alcoholic*, Newbury Park, CA: Sage Publications, Inc., 1987.

Dewey, J., *How We Think*, New York: Heath Publishing Company, 1910.

Diesenhaus, H., "Current Trends in Treatment Programming For Problem Drinkers and Alcoholics," *Prevention, Intervention and Treatment: Concerns and Models,* DHHS Publication No. (ADM) 82-1192, Washington DC: U.S. Government Printing Office, pp. 219-290, 1982.

Dittrich, J.G., "Alcoholism as a Diagnosis Among Clients and Their Spouses at Outpatient Psychotherapy Clinics," PhD dissertation, Memphis State University, *Dissertation Abstracts International*, 46(10): 3589-B, 1986.

Dobson, M., "Problem Drinking," *Nursing Times*, 80(12): 57-59, 1984.

Donovan, D.M., "An Etiologic Model of Alcoholism," *American Journal of Psychiatry*, 143: 1-11, 1986.

Donovan, D.M., and Chaney, E.F., "Alcoholic Relapse Prevention and Intervention: Models and Methods," In: Marlatt, G.A., and Gordon, J.R. (eds.), *Relapse Pevention – Maintenance Strategies in the Treatment of Addictive Behaviors*, New York: Guilford Press, pp. 351-416, 1985.

Donovan, D.M., Kivlahan, D.R., and Walker, R.D., "Alcoholic Subtypes Based On Multiple Assessment Domains: Validation Against Treatment Outcome," In: Galanter, M. (ed.), *Recent Developments in Alcoholism*, Vol. 4, New York: Plenum Press, 1986.

Dubinsky, M., "Predictors of Appointment Non-Compliance in Community Mental Health Patients," *Community Mental Health Journal*, 22(2), Summer 1986.

Edwards, G., *The Treatment of Drinking Problems: A Guide for the Helping Professional*, New York: McGraw-Hill Book, Co., 1982.

Edwards, G., Duckitt, A., Oppenheimer, E., Sheehan, M., and Taylor, C., "What Happens to Alcoholics?," *The Lancet*, 2(8344): 269-270, 1983.

Elal-Lawrence, G., Slade, P.D., and Dewey, M.E., "Treatment and Follow-up Variables Discriminating Abstainers, Controlled Drinkers and Relapsers," *Journal of Studies in Alcohol*, 48(1): 39-46, 1987.

Elal-Lawrence, G., Slade, P.D., and Dewey, M.E., "Predictors of Outcome Type in Treated Problem Drinkers," *Journal of Studies in Alcohol*, 47(1): 41-47, 1986.

Ellis, W.D., "Combing Out The Snarls," *Nations Business*, December, p. 43, 1986.

Emrick, C.D., "A Review of Psychologically Oriented Treatment of Alcoholism II. The Relative Effectiveness of Different Treatment Approaches and the Effectiveness of Treatment Versus No Treatment," *Journal of Studies on Alcohol*, 36: 88-108, 1975.

Emrick, C.D., "A Review of Psychologically Oriented Treatment of Alcoholism," *Quarterly Journal of Studies on Alcohol*, 35: 523-49, 1974.

Encyclopedia of Associations 1988, Karen E. Koek and Susan B. Martin, Eds., Detroit: Gale Research Co., 1987.

Engel, J.F., Blackwell, R.W., and Miniard, P.W., *Consumer Behavior*, 5th Ed., Hinsdale, IL: Dryden Press, 1986.

Engel, J.F., Warshaw, M.R., and Kinnear, T., *Promotion Strategy*, 6th Ed., Homewood, IL: Irwin, 1987.

Estes, W.K., Koch, S., MacCorquodale, K., Meeht, P.E., Mueller, C.G., Jr., Schoenfeld, W.M., and Verplanck, W.S., *Modern Learning Theory*, New York: Appleton-Century-Crofts, 1954.

Etzioni, A., *A Comparative Analysis of Complex Organizations*, Glencoe, IL: Free Press, 1969.

Festinger, L., and Bramel, D., "The Reactions of Humans to Cognitive Dissonance," In: Bachrach, A.J., *Experimental Foundations of Clinical Psychology*, New York: Basic Books, pp. 251-62, 1962.

Fillmore, K.M., and Midanik, L., "Chronocity of Drinking Problems Among Men," *Journal of Studies on Alcohol*, 45: 228-236, 1986.

Finney, J.W., and Moos, R.H., "Characteristics and Prognoses of Alcoholics Who Become Moderate Drinkers and Abstainers After Treatment," *Journal of Studies on Alcohol*, 42(1): 94-105, 1981.

Finney, J.W., and Moos, R.H., "Treatment and Outcome For Empirical Subtypes of Alcoholic Patients," *Journal of Consulting and Clinical Psychology*, 47(1): 25-38, 1979.

Finney, J.W., Moos, R.H., and Chan, D.A., "Length of Stay and Program Component Effects in the Treatment of Alcoholism: A Comparison of Two Techniques for Process Analyses," *Journal of Consulting and Clinical Psychology*, 49(1): 120-131, 1981.

Fishbein, N., and Ajzen, I., *Belief, Attitude, Intention and Behavior: An Introduction To Theory and Research*, Reading, MA: Addison-Wesley Publishing Co., Inc., 1975.

Fitzgerald, J.L., and Mulford, H.A., "Seasonal Changes in Alcohol Consumption and Related Problems in Iowa, 1979-1980," *Journal of Studies on Alcohol*, 45(4): 363-8, 1984.

Flores, P.J., "The Efficacy of the Use of Coercion In Getting DWI Offenders Into Treatment," *Journal of Alcohol and Drug Education*, 28: 18-27, 1982.

Frank, R.W. Massy, and Wind, Y., *Market Segmentation*, Englewood Cliffs, NJ: Prentice-Hall, Inc., 1972.

French, J., Jr., and Raven, B., "The Bases of Social Power," In: Dorwin Cartwright (ed.), *Studies of Social Power*, Ann Arbor, MI: Institute for Social Research, University of Michigan, pp. 150-167, 1959.

Friedman, M., and Rosenman, R.H., *Type A Behavior and Your Heart*, New York: Knopf, 1974.

Frosch, W.A., "Analytic Overview of Addictions," In: Milkman, H.B., and Shaffer, H.J. (eds.), *Addictions: Multidisciplinary Perspectives and Treatments*, Lexington, MA: Lexington Books, pp. 29-37, 1985.

Frye, R.V., "A Multimodality Approach to the Treatment of Addiction," In: Milkman, H.B., and Shaffer, H.J. (eds.), *The Addictions: Multidisciplinary Perspectives and Treatments*, Lexington: Lexington Books, pp. 175-182, 1985.

Fuller, R.K., and Roth, H.P., "Disulfiram for the Treatment of Alcoholism: An Evaluation in 128 Men," *Annals of Internal Medicine*, 90: 901-904, 1979.

Galanter, M. (ed.), *Recent Developments in Alcoholism*, Vol. 1, New York: Plenum Press, 1983.

Gallant, D.M., "Can Some Alcoholics Become Social Drinkers?" *Alcoholism: Clinical and Experimental Research*, 10(2): 217, 1986.

Geis, G., "A Halfway House is Not A Home: Notes On The Failure Of A Narcotic Rehabilitation Project," *Drug Forum*, 4(1): 7-13, 1974.

George, W., and Berry, L.L., "Guidelines For The Advertising of Services," *Business Horizons*, July-August, pp. 52-56, 1981.

Gerard, D.L., and Saenger, G., *Outpatient Treatment of Alcoholism: A Study of Outcome and Its Determinants*, Toronto: Alcoholism and Drug Addiction Research Foundation of Ontario, University of Toronto Press, 1966.

Gharderian, A.M., "Adolescent Alcoholism: Motives and Alternatives," *Compr. Psychiatry*, 29(5): 469-474, 1979.

Gibbs, L., and Flanagan, J., "Prognostic Indicators of Alcoholism Treatment Outcome," *The International Journal of Addiction*, 12(8): 1097-1141, 1977.

Gitlow, S.E., and Peyser, H.S., *Alcoholism: A Practical Treatment Guide*, New York: Grune & Stratton, 1980.

Gomberg, E.L., White, H.R., and Carpenter, J.A. (eds.), *Alcohol Science and Society Revisited*, Ann Arbor, MI: The University of Michigan Press, 1982.

Goodwin, D.W., and Guze, S.B., "Heredity and Alcoholism," In: Kissin, B., and Begleister, H. (eds.), *The Biology of Alcoholism*, Vol. 3, *Clinical Pathology*, New York: Plenum Publishing Corporation, pp. 37-52, 1974.

Googins, B., "Avoidance of the Alcoholic Client," *Social Work*, March-April, pp. 161-166, 1984.

Gordis, L., "An Epidemiologist Views the Evaluation of Alcoholism Treatment," *Alcoholism: Clinical and Experimental Research*, 5(4): 483-488, 1981.

Gorski, T.T., "Relapse Prevention Planning: A New Recovery Tool," *Alcohol, Health and Research World*, Fall, pp. 7-11, 63, 1986.

Gorski, T.T., and Miller, M., "Staying Sober—A Guide to Relapse Prevention," Independence, MO: Herald House, 1986.

Gottheil, E., *Summaries of Alcoholism Treatment Assessment Research*, NIAAA Treatment Handbook Series I, U.S. Department of Health and Human Services, Public Health Service, 1985.

Gottheil, E., McLellan, A.T., and Druley, K.A., "Reasonable and Unreasonable Methodological Standards for the Evaluation of Alcoholism Treatment," In: Gottheil, E., McLellan, A.T., and Druley, K.A. (eds.), *Matching Patient Needs and Treatment Methods in Alcoholism and Drug Abuse*, Springfield, IL: Charles C. Thomas, pp. 371-389, 1981.

Gottlieb, N.H., and Baker, J.A., "Relative Influence of Health Beliefs," Parental and Peer Behaviors and Exercise Program Participation on Smoking, Alcohol Use and Physical Activity," *Social Science and Medicine*, 22(9): 915-927, 1986.

Govani, N. et al., *Promotion Management*, Englewood Cliffs, NJ: Prentice-Hall, Inc., 1986.

Grossman, S.P., "Physiological Needs," In *Encyclopedia of Psychology*, Vol. 3, New York: John Wiley & Sons, 1984.

Gubernick, L., "We're Filling Beds," *Forbes*, pp. 91-92, June 17, 1985.

Gulyamov, M.G., "Efficacy of Anonymous Treatment of Alcoholics In An Outpatient Addiction Center," *Zjurnal Nevropatologii i Psikhiatrii im. Korsakova*, 84(2): 254-257, 1986.

Gunby, P., "Nation's Expenditures for Alcohol, Other Drugs, in Terms of Therapy, Prevention, Now Exceed $1.6 Billion," *Journal of the American Medical Association*, 258(15): 2023, 1987.

Gurin, G. et al., *Americans View Their Mental Health*, New York: Basic Books, p. 307, 1960.

Gusfield, Jr., "Prevention: Rise, Decline and Renaissance," In: Gomberg, E.L., White, H.R., and Carpenter, J.A. (eds.), *Alcohol, Science and Society Revisited*, Ann Arbor, MI: The University of Michigan Press, 1982.

Haas, R.W., *Industrial Marketing Management*, 3rd Ed., Boston, MA: Kent Publishing Co., 1986.

Hall, C.S., and Lindzey, G., *Theories of Personality*, 2nd Ed., New York: John Wiley & Sons, 1970.

Harrell, G., *Consumer Behavior*, San Diego, CA: Harcourt Brace Jovanovich, Inc., 1986.

Harrigan, J.A., "Children of Alcoholics," *American Family Physician*, 35(1): 139-144, 1987.

Harris, J.K., et al., "Training Alcoholics In Telephone Skills For Contacting Potential Employers," *Journal of Employment Counseling*, 23(4): 146-155, 1986.

Harry, R., "Global Pricing Strategies," *Top Health Care Finance*, 14(1): 26-35, 1987.

Harwood, H.J., Kristiansen, P., and Rachal, J.V., "Social and Economic Costs of Alcohol Abuse and Alcoholism," Issue Report No. 2, Research Triangle Park, NC: Research Triangle Institute, 1985.

Hawkins, D.I., Best, R.J., and Coney, K.A., *Consumer Behavior*, Plano, TX: Business Publications, Inc., 1986.

Hayami, D.E., and Freebori, D.K., "Effect Of Coverage In The Use Of HMO Alcoholism Treatment Program, Outcome and Medical Care Utilization," *American Journal of Public Health*, 71: 1133-1144, 1981.

Hayden, J.W., and Rosenthal, M.S., "Where Are We Going Now?" *Journal of Substance Abuse Treatment*, 2(1): 1-3, 1985.

Heather, N., Robertson, I., and Davies, P. (eds.), *The Misuse of Alcohol*, New York: New York University Press, 1985.

Heather, N., and Robertson, I., *Controlled Drinking*, London: Methuen, 1981.

Hedin, C., "Native Americans and Alcoholism: Selected Program Data and Health Statistics 1983-1985," July, p. 44, 1986.

Helzer, J.G., Robins, L.N., Taylor, J.R., Carey, K., Miller, R.H. et al., "The Extent of Long-Term Moderate Drinking Among Alcoholics Discharged From Medical and Psychiatric Treatment Facilities," *North England Journal of Medicine*, 312: 1678-82, 1985.

Hesselbrook, M.N., "Alcoholic Typologies: A Review of Empirical Evaluations of Common Classification Schemes," In: Galanter, M. (ed.), *Recent Developments in Alcoholism*, Vol. 4, New York: Plenum Press, 1986.

Hewitt Associates, *Company Practices in Mental Health Coverage*, Lincolnshire, IL: Hewitt Associates, 1986.

Hilgard, E.R., and Bower, G.H., *Theories of Learning*, 4th ed., New York: Appleton-Century-Crofts, 1975.

Hill, S.Y., "A Vulnerability Model For Alcoholism In Women," *Journal of Addictions and Health*, 2(2): 68-91, 1982.

Hjelle, L., and Ziegler, D., *Personality Theories: Research and Applications*, 2nd ed., New York: McGraw-Hill, 1981.

Hodgson, R., and Stockwell, T., "The Theoretical and Empirical Basis Of The Alcohol Dependence Model: A Social Learning Perspective," In: Heather, N., Robertson, I., and Davies, P. (eds.), *The Misuse of Alcohol, Crucial Issues in Dependence Treatment and Prevention*, New York: New York University Press, pp. 17-34, 1985.

Holden, C., "Genes, Personality and Alcoholism," *Psychology Today*, 19: 38-44, 1985.

Holder, H.D., Blose, J.G., and Basiorowski, M.H., *Alcoholism Treatment Impact on Total Health Care Utilization and Costs: A Four-Year Longitudinal Analysis of the Federal Employees Health Benefit Program With AETNA Life Insurance Program*, Chapel Hill, NC: H-2, Inc., 1985.

Holder, H.D., and Hallan, J.B., *Medical Care and Alcoholism Treatment Costs and Utilization: A Five-Year Analysis of the California Pilot Project to Provide Health Insurance Coverage for Alcoholism*, Chapel Hill, NC: H-2, Inc., 1981.

Holder, H.D., and Hallan, J.B., *The California Pilot Program to Provide Health Insurance Coverage for Alcohol Treatment – One Year After*, Chapel Hill, NC: H-2, Inc., 1978.

Holmes, D.S., "Defense Mechanisms," In: Corsini, R.J. (ed.), *Encyclopedia of Psychology*, Vol. 1, New York: John Wiley & Sons, pp. 347-350, 1984.

Honig, F., and Spinner, A., "A Group Therapy Approach in the Treatment of the Spouses of Alcoholics," *Alcoholism Treatment Quarterly*, 3(3): 95-105, 1986.

Humbles, B.A.Q., "Associations Between Previous Treatments For Alcohol Addiction and Chances For Success at O'Brien Halfway House, Inc., Baton Rouge, Louisiana," Dissertation, Louisiana State University, Ann Arbor, MI: University Microfilm International, 469(9): 2819-A, 1986.

Hunt, W.A., Barnett, W., and Branch, L.G., "Relapse Rates in Addiction Programs," *Journal of Clinical Psychology*, 27: 455-456, 1971.

Hunter, H., *Arizona Health Plan Cost-Benefit Study*, Report to NIAAA No. 5H84AA01745, Washington, DC: Supt. of Docs., U.S. Government Printing Office, 1978.

Hunter, T.A., and Salomone, P.R., "Dry Drunk Symptoms & Alcoholic Relapse," *Journal of Applied Rehabilitation Counseling*, 18(1): 22-25, 1987.

Hutt, M.D., and Speh, T.W., *Industrial Marketing Management*, 2nd Ed., Chicago, IL: The Dryden Press, 1985.

Jackson, D.W., Cunningham, W.H., and Cunningham, I.S.M., *Selling*, New York: John Wiley & Sons, 1988.

Jain, S.C., *Marketing Planning and Strategy*, Cincinnati, OH: South-Western Publishing Co., p. 352, 1985.

Janke, R.J., and Young, M.H., "More Knowledge Does Not Improve Alcoholics' Compliance," *American Journal of Nursing*, 86(3): 251, 1986.

Jeffers, J. et al., "On the Demand vs. Need For Medical Services and the Concept of Shortage," *American Journal of Public Health*, 61: 46, 1971.

Jellineck, E.M., *The Disease Concept of Alcoholism*, New Brunswick, NJ: Hillhouse Press, 1960.

Jellineck, E.M., "Phases of Alcohol Addiction," *Quarterly Journal of Studies on Alcohol*, 13: 673-684, 1952.

Jellineck, E.M., "Heredity of the Alcoholic," *Quarterly Journal of Studies on Alcohol*, 6: 105, 1945.

Jenson, J., and Miklovic, N., "Consumers Cite Physicians' Interest As Most Important In Selection," *Modern Healthcare*, 16, January 17, p. 48, 1986.

Johnson, K.F., "Developing a Cost Base for Pricing," *Top Health Care Finance*, 14(1): 16-25, 1987.

Jolliffe, N., and Jellinek, E.M., "Vitamin Deficiencies and Liver Cirrhosis in Alcoholics," *Quarterly Journal of Studies on Alcohol*, 11: 544-583, 1941.

Jones, K.R., and Vischi, T.R., "Impact of Alcohol Drug Abuse, and Mental Health Treatment on Medical Care Utilization: A Review of the Research Literature," *Medical Care*, 17 (Supplement), 1979.

Jordan, K.S., Roszell, D.K., Calsyn, D.A., and Chaney, E.F., "Perceptions of Treatment Needs: Differences Between Patients and Staff of A Drug Abuse Treatment Program," *International Journal of the Addictions*, 20(2): 345-351, 1985.

Kain-Candle Marsh, P.R., and Marsh, G.N., "Patient Satisfaction in General Practice," *British Medical Journal*, 5952 (February), pp. 262-265, 1975.

Kalat, J.W., "Specific Hungers," In: *Encyclopedia of Psychology*, Vol. 3, New York: John Wiley & Sons, 1984.

Kaplan, H.B., and Meyerowitz, J.H., "Evaluation of a Half-Way House: Integrated Community Approach in the Rehabilitation of Narcotic Addicts," *The International Journal of the Addictions*, March, 4(1): 65-76, 1969.

Keenan, D.W., "A Follow-up Study on Adolescent Males and Females Who Completed Chemical Dependency Treatment During 1980," Division of Educational Psychology and Human Services, Graduate School, The University of South Dakota, May, 1984.

Kennedy, R.W., Gilbert, G.S., and Thoreson, R., "A Self-Control Program for Drinking Antecedents: The Role of Self-Monitoring and Control Orientation," *Journal of Clinical Psychology*, 34(1): 238-243, 1978.

Kincaid, W.M., *Promotion: Products, Services and Ideas*, 2nd Ed., Merrill Publishing, Columbus, OH, 1985.

Kinnear, T., and Taylor, J., *Marketing Research: An Applied Approach*, New York: McGraw-Hill Book Company, 1987.

Kirn, T.F., "Advances in Understanding of Alcoholism Initiate Evolution In Treatment Programs," *Journal of the American Medical Association*, 256(11): 1405, 1411-1412, 1986.

Kirn, T.F., "Supreme Court Case, Federal 'Initiative' Put Focus on Alcoholism," *Journal of the American Medical Association*, 258(23): 3357, December 18, 1987A.

Kirn, T.F., "Soviets Attack Problem Anew, This Time Armed With Perestrorka," *Journal of the American Medical Association*, 258(17): 2341-2348, November 6, 1987B.

Kline, T.A., Self, D.R., and Jones, M., "Power Bases As A Classification For The Referral System for Alcoholism Treatment Marketers," 1988 Proceedings of the Atlantic Marketing Association.

Kline, T.A., Self, D.R., and Ingram, J., "Deciders and Influencers in the Alcohol and Chemical Dependency Treatment Program," *Journal of Marketing for Mental Health*, Spring/Summer, 1987.

Knight, R.P., "The Dynamics and Treatment of Chronic Alcohol Addiction," Bulletin, Menninger Clinic, 1: 233-250, 1937.

Knott, D.H., *Alcohol Problems*, New York: Pergamon Press, 1986.

Knowles, P.L., "Inpatient versus Outpatient Treatment of Substance Misuse in Hospitals, 1975-1980," *Journal of Studies on Alcohol*, 44(2): 384-387, 1983.

Korcok, M., "Alcoholism Treatment A Growing 'Product Line,'" *American Medical News*, October 11, pp. 29-30, 1985.

Korcok, M., "Waging the War Against Alcohol Abuse," *Canadian Medical Association Journal*, 134(12): 1401-1404, 1986.

Kotler, P., *Marketing Management: Analysis, Planning, Implementation, and Control*, Englewood Cliffs, NJ: Prentice-Hall, 1988.

Kotler, P., and Andreason, A.R., *Strategic Marketing for Non-Profit Organizations*, Englewood Cliffs, NJ: Prentice-Hall, Inc., 1987, as adapted from Andreason, Alan R., "Non-Profits: Check Your Attention to Customers," *Harvard Business Review*, May-June, pp. 105-110, 1982.

Kotler, P., and Clarke, R.N., *Marketing for Health Care Organizations*, Englewood Cliffs, NJ: Prentice-Hall, Inc., 1987.

Kruse, W., "Questions of Addiction in Aspects of Health Care: Dealing With Alcoholics From the Viewpoint of the General Practitioner," *Munchener Medizinische Wochenschrift*, 127(12): 279-281, 1985.

Kusnetz, S., "Services for Adolescent Substance Abusers," In: Beschner, G., and Friedman, A.S. (eds.), *Teen Drug Use*, Lexington, MA: Lexington Books, pp. 123-162, 1986.

Laberg, J.C., "Alcohol and Expectancy: Subjective, Psychophysiological and Behavioral Responses to Alcohol Stimuli in Severely, Moderately and Non-Dependent Drinkers," *British Journal of Addiction*, 81(6): 797-808, 1986.

Lee, F.C., "Purchasers Address Escalating Psychiatric and Substance Abuse Utilization," *Employee Benefits Journal*, March, pp. 9-13, 1987.

Lemere, F., and Voegtlin, W.L., "An Evaluation of the Aversion Treatment of Alcoholism," *Quarterly Journal of Studies on Alcohol*, 11: 199-204, 1950.

Lesley, P., *Public Relations Handbook*, Prentice-Hall, Englewood Cliffs, NJ, p. 339, 1983.

Levitt, T., "After The Sale Is Over," *Harvard Business Review* September-October, pp. 87-93, 1983.

______, *The Third Sector: New Tactics For a Responsive Society*, New York: AMACOM, 1973.

Light, W.J.H., *Psychodynamics of Alcoholism: A Current Synthesis*, Springfield, IL: Charles C Thomas Publishers, 1986.

Lodish, L., "Advertising Budgets: Don't Leave Well Enough Alone," *Wharton Magazine*, summer, p. 27, 1982.

Loneck, R.M., "Effect of Situational Factors on the Outcome of the Alcoholism Intervention," *Dissertation Abstracts International*, 49(9): 2811-A, 1986.

Longabaugh, R., McCrady, B., Fink, E., Stout, R., McAuley, T., Doyle, C., and McNeill, D., "Cost Effectiveness of Alcoholism Treatment in Partial vs. Inpatient Settings," *Journal of Studies on Alcohol*, 44(6): 1049-1070, 1983.

Longabaugh, R., and Beattie, M., "Social Investment, Environmental Support, and Treatment Outcomes of Alcoholics," *Alcohol Health and Research World*, Vol. 10(4): 64-66, 1986.

Lovelock, C.H., *Services Marketing*, Englewood Cliffs, NJ: Prentice-Hall, Inc., 1984.

Lovelock, C.H., and Weinberg, C.B., "Public and Nonprofit Marketing Comes of Age," *Review of Marketing 1978*, Chicago, IL: American Marketing Association, pp. 413-452, 1978.

Luderer, H.J., "Drinking Style, Drinking Motives, and Relapse Among Gamma-Alcoholics and Delta-Alcoholics," 103(44): 1020-1022, 1985.

Luderer, H.J., Bocker, A., and Bocker, F.M., "Information on Personal Experience in Motivation and Rehabilitation of Alcoholics," *Suchtgefahren*, 32(3): 190-203, 1986.

Ludwig, A.M., "Pavlov's Bells and Alcohol Craving," *Addictive Behaviors*, 11(2): 87-91, 1986.

Ludwig, A., "Cognitive Processes Associated With 'Spontaneous' Recovery From Alcoholism," *Journal of Studies on Alcohol*, 46: 53-58, 1985.

MacStravic, R.S., "Manageable Evidence in Medical Care Marketing," *Journal of Health Care Marketing*, December, pp. 52-59, 1987.

MacStravic, R.S., "Word of Mouth Communications in Health Care Marketing," *Health Progress*, October, pp. 25-29, 1985.

MacStravic, R., *Determining Health Needs*, Ann Arbor, MI: Health Administration Press, 1978.

Maletta, G.J., "Alcoholism And The Aged," In: Pattison, E.M., Kaufman, E. (eds.), *Encyclopedic Handbook of Alcoholism*, New York: Gardner, pp. 779-801, 1982.

Mandell, W., "Types and Phases of Alcohol Dependence Illness," In: Glanter, M. (ed.), *Recent Developments in Alcoholism*, New York: Plenum Press, pp. 415-48, 1983.

Manello, T.A., and Seaman, F.J., *Prevalence, Cost, and Handling of Drinking Problems on Seven Railroads, Final Report*. U.S. Department of Transportation, Washington, DC: Government Printing Office, pp. 108-120, 1979.

Manning, G.L., and Reece, B.L., *Selling Today: A Personal Approach*, Dubuque, IA: Brown Publishers, 1987.

Mansfield, E., "Eating Disorders and Alcoholism: Linking Family System Dynamics," *Focus on Family and Chemical Dependency*, 7:22-28, 1984.

Marden, P., *A Procedure for Estimating the Potential Number of Alcoholism Service Program Clientele*, Rockville, MD: NIAAA, 1974.

Marketing Terms, "Referrals Top Ads As Influence On Patients Doctor Selections," American Marketing Association, January 30, p. 22, 1987.

Marlatt, G.A., "Alcohol, the Magic Elixir: Stress, Expectancy, and the Transformation of Emotional States," In: Gottheil, E., Druley, K.A., Pashko, S., Weinstein, S.P. (eds.), *Stress and Addiction*, New York: Brunner/Mazel, 1987.

Marlatt, G.A., "Psychosocial Perspectives On Alcoholism Treatment and the

Process Of Recovery," In: McCrady, B.S., Noel, N.E., and Nirenbert, T.D. (eds.), *Research Monograph 15: Future Directions in Alcohol Abuse Treatment Research*, Washington, DC: U.S. Government Printing Office, pp. 210-224, 1985.

Marlatt, G.A., Baer, J.S., Donovan, D.M., and Kivlahan, D.R., "Addictive Behaviors: Etiology and Treatment," *Annual Review of Psychology*, 39: 223-52, 1988.

Marlatt, G.A., and Gordon, J.R., "Lifestyle Modification," *Relapse Prevention*, New York: The Guilford Press, 1985.

Marlin, H., and Hartsocks, P., "Demographic Profiles of U.S. Alcohol Consumption and Use of These Profiles in Estimation of State and County Consumption Levels—An Evaluation." Paper presented at the Eleventh Annual NCA/AMSA/RSA Medical-Scientific Conference of the National Alcoholism Forum. Seattle, WA, May, 1980.

Marotta-Sims, J., "Effect Of Marital Status, Marriage Characteristics, and Demographic Variables On Alcohol Inpatient Treatment Completion," *Dissertation Abstracts International*, 46(12): 4407-B, 1986.

Marotta, J., and Rale, R., "Marital Variables and Treatment Completion," National Council on Alcoholism Forum, San Francisco, CA: 18 April-21 April, 1986.

Masi, D.A., "A Model For Evening and Weekend Treatment for Alcoholism in the Workplace," *Labor-Management Alcoholism Journal*, 12(5): 176-179, 1983.

Mason, G.R., "Evaluating Existing Rate Structures," *Top Health Care Finance*, 14(1): 36-49, 1987.

Mastrick, J.L., Jr., "Influences on the Successful Treatment of Alcoholics Referred Through Employee Assistance Programs," *Dissertation Abstracts International*, 46(9): 3251-B, 1986.

Maxwell, M.A., "Alcoholics Anonymous," In: Gomberg, E.L., White, H.R., and Carpenter J.A. (eds), *Alcohol Science and Society Revisited*, Ann Arbor, MI: The University of Michigan Press, pp. 295-305, 1982.

McCarthy, E.J., *Basic Marketing*, Homewood, IL: Richard D. Irwin, Inc., 1960.

McCarthy, E.J., and Perreault, W.D., Jr., *Basic Marketing*, 8th ed., Homewood, IL: Richard D. Irwin, Inc., 1984.

McCarthy, E.J., and Perreault, W.D., Jr., *Basic Marketing*, 9th ed., Homewood, IL: Richard D. Irwin, Inc., 1987.

McCord, W., and McCord, J.A., "A Longitudinal Study of the Personality of Alcoholics," In: Pittman, D.J., and Snyder, C.R. (eds.), *Society, Culture and Drinking Patterns*, New York: John Wiley & Sons, pp. 413-430, 1982.

McCrady, B.S. et al., "Comparative Effectiveness of Three Types of Spouse Involvement In Outpatient Behavioral Alcoholism Treatment," *Journal of Studies on Alcohol*, 47(6): 459-467, 1986.

McLachlan, J.F.C., and Stein, R.L., "Evaluation of a Day Clinic For Alcoholics," *Journal of Studies on Alcohol*, 43:251-272, 1982.

Mellott, D.W., Jr., *Consumer Behavior*, Tulsa, OK: Pennwell Publishing Company, 1983.

Menninger, K., *Man Against Himself*, New York: Harcourt Brace Jovanovich, 1938.

Milkman, H.B., and Shaffer, H.J. (eds.), *The Addictions: Multidisciplinary Perspective and Treatments*, Lexington: Lexington Books, 1985.

Milkman, H., and Sunderwirth, S.G., *Craving for Ecstasy: The Consciousness & Chemistry Of Escape*, Lexington, MA: D.C. Heath and Company, p. 222, 1987.

Miller, M.R., and Hester, R.K., "Inpatient Alcoholism Treatment: Who Benefits?" *American Psychologist*, 41(7): 794-805, 1986.

Miller, S.I., "How to Tell if Alcoholism Treatment Has Worked: Assessing Outcome Studies," *H & CP: Hospital and Community Psychiatry*, 37(6): 555-556, 1986.

Mishara, B.L., and Kastenbaum, R., "Alcohol and Old Age," In: Greenblatt, M. (ed.), *Seminars in Psychiatry*, Orlando, FL: Grune & Stratton, pp. 1-215, 1980.

Moberg, D.P., "Social Control of Deviance: Intervention With Adolescent Alcohol and Other Drug Users," *Dissertation Abstracts International*, 46(11): 3493-A, 1986.

Monteiro, R.C., "Alcohol Expectancies and Drinking Patterns in Parents and Youth," *Dissertation Abstracts International*, 47(1): 382-B-383-B, 1986.

Moore, H.F., *Public Relations*, 8th Ed., Homewood, IL: Irwin, 1981.

Moos, R.H., and Finney, J.W., "The Expanding Scope of Alcoholism Treatment Evaluation," *American Psychologist*, 38(1): 1036-1044, 1983.

Morgan, C.T., King, R.A., Robinson, N.M., *Introduction to Psychology*, 6th Ed., New York: McGraw-Hill Book Co., 1979.

Mottin, J.L., "Drug-Induced Attenuation of Alcohol Consumption: A Review and Evaluation of Claimed, Potential or Current Therapies," *Quarterly Journal of Studies on Alcohol*, 34: 444-472, 1973.

Mowbray, A., and Kessel, N., "Alcoholism and the General Practitioner," *British Journal of Psychiatry*, 148: 697-700, 1986.

Mowen, J.C., *Consumer Behavior*, New York: Macmillan Publishing Company, 1987.

Muszynski, S., Brady, J., and Sharfstein, S., *Coverage for Mental and Nervous Disorders: Summaries of 300 Private Sector Health Insurance Plans*, Washington, DC: American Psychiatric Press, p. 18, 1983.

Nakao, K., Milazzo-Sayre, L.J., Rodenstein, M.J., and Manderscheid, R.W., "Referral Patterns To and From Inpatient Psychiatric Services: A Social Network," *American Journal of Public Health*, 76(7): 755-760, 1986.

Nathan, P.E., and Lipscomb, T.R., "Behavior Therapy and Behavior Modification in the Treatment of Alcoholism," In: Mendelson, J.H., and Mello, N.K. (eds.), *The Diagnosis and Treatment of Alcoholism*, New York: McGraw-Hill, pp. 305-357, 1979.

National Institute on Alcohol Abuse and Alcoholism, *The Sixth Special Report to the U.S. Congress on Alcohol and Health*, Washington, DC: Supt. of Docs., U.S. Government Printing Office, January, 1987.

National Institute on Alcohol Abuse and Alcoholism (NIAAA), *Classification of Alcoholism Treatment Settings*, Bast, R.J. (ed.), DHHS Pub. No. (ADM) 84-1324, Rockville, MD: NIAAA, 1984.

Newbuerger, O.W., Matarazzo, J.D., Schmitz, R.E., and Pratt, H.H., "One Year Follow-Up of Total Abstinence In Chronic Alcoholic Patients Following Emetic Counter-Conditioning," *Alcoholism: Clinical and Experimental Research*, 4(3): 306-312, 1980.

Nickels, W.G., *Marketing Communications and Promotion*, 3rd Ed., New York: John Wiley & Sons, 1984.

Noble, J., "Profile of the U.S. Alcoholism Treatment Capacity, Funding and Trend Data," Paper presented at Alcohol Drug Problems Association Conference, Austin, TX, March 11, 1985.

Obinali, M.C.V., "Factors Which Characterized Alcoholics Who Successfully Completed A Residential Treatment Program," Dissertation, University of Tennessee, Ann Arbor, MI: UMI, 46(11): 4024-B, 1986.

Ojehagen, A., and Berglund, M., "Early and Late Improvement in a Two-Year Out-Patient Alcoholic Treatment Program," *Acta Psychiatrics Scandinavia*, 74(2): 129-136, 1986.

Orford, J., and Edwards, G., *Alcoholism*, Oxford: Oxford University Press, 1977.

Orford, J., and Keddie, A., "Abstinence or Controlled Drinking in Clinical Practice: A Test of the Dependence and Persuasian Hypothesis," *British Journal of Addiction*, 81(4): 495-504, 1986.

Orford, J., and Keddie, A., "Abstinence or Controlled Drinking in Clinical Practice: Indications at Initial Assessment," *Addictive Behaviors*, 11: 71-86, 1986.

Ostrum, T., "The Relationship Between the Affective, Behavioral and Cognitive Components of Attitude," *Journal of Experimental Social Psychology* (January), 5: 12-30, 1969.

Panopinto, W.C., and Simmons, L., "Treating the Illness, Not the Mandate: Techniques For Successful Referral, Engagement, and Treatment of Alcoholic Persons," *Alcoholism Treatment Quarterly*, 3(3): 37-48, 1986.

Partington, J.T., and Johnson, F.G., "Personality Types Among Alcoholics," *Quarterly Journal of Studies on Alcohol*, 30: 21-34, 1969.

Pattison, E.M., "The Selection of Treatment Modalities for the Alcoholic Patient," In: Mendelson, J.H., and Mello, N.K. (eds.), *The Diagnosis and Treatment of Alcoholism*, New York: McGraw-Hill, pp. 126-227, 1979.

Pattison, E.M., "A Critique of Alcoholism Treatment Concepts, With Special Reference to Abstinence," *Quarterly Journal of Studies on Alcoholism*, 27: 49-71, 1966.

Pattison, E.M., Sobell, M.B., and Sobell, L.C., *Emerging Concepts of Alcohol Dependence*, New York: Springer, 1977.

Peacey, J.E., and Kapur, B.M., "Monitoring Drinking Behavior with the Alcohol Dipsticks During Treatment," *Clinical and Experimental Research*, 10(b): 663-666, 1986.

Pederson, C.A., Wright, M., and Weitz, B., *Selling Principles and Methods*, Homewood, IL: Irwin, 1984.

Pendery, M.L., Maltzman, I.M., and West, L.J., "Controlled Drinking By Alcoholics? New Findings and a Re-Evaluation of a Major Affirmative Study," *Science*, 217(4555): 169-175, 1982.

Penk, W.E., Charles, H.L., and Van-Hoose, T.A., "Comparative Effectiveness of Day Hospital and Inpatient Psychiatric Treatment," *Journal of Consulting and Clinical Psychology*, 46(1): 94-101, 1978.

Pettinati, H.M., Sugerman, A.A., Di Donato, N., and Maurer, H.S., "The Natural History of Alcoholism Over Four Years After Treatment," *Journal of Studies on Alcohol*, 43(3): 201-215, 1982.

Pfrang, H., and Schenk, J., "Controlled Drinkers in Comparison to Abstinents and Relapsed Drinkers With Regard to Attitudes and Social Adjustment," *International Journal of the Addictions*, 20(11/12): 1793-1802, 1986.

Pickens, R.W., Hatsukami, D.K., Spicer, J.W., and Srikis, D.S., "Relapse by Alcohol Abusers," *Alcoholism: Clinical and Experimental Research*, 9(3): 244-247, 1985.

Plaut, T.F., *Alcohol Problems: A Report to the Nation by the Cooperative Commission on the Study of Alcoholism*, New York: Oxford University Press, 1967.

Pokorny, L.J., "Estimating Psychiatric Bed and Other Mental Health Service Needs: A Challenge to Evaluators," May, 1984.

Polich, J.M., Armor, D.J., and Braiker, H.B., *The Course of Alcoholism*, New York: John Wiley & Sons, 1981.

Polich, J., Armor, D., and Braiker, H., *The Course of Alcoholism: Four Years After Treatment*, Santa Monica, CA: The Rand Corporation, 1980.

Potamianos, G. et al., "Randomized Trial of Community-Based Center Versus Conventional Hospital Management in Treatment of Alcoholism," *Lancet*, 2(8510): 797-799, 1986.

Pride, W.M., and Ferrell, D.C., *Marketing: Basic Concepts and Decisions*, Boston: Houghton Mifflin Company, 1987.

Pronko, N.H., "Physiological Psychology (Nonreductionism)," In: *Encyclopedia of Psychology*, Vol. 3, New York: John Wiley & Sons, 1984.

Prugh, T., "Recovery Without Treatment," *Alcohol, Health & Research World*, 11(1): 24, 71, 1986.

Public Law 93-641, Sections 1521 (d), 1523.

Rados, D.L., *Marketing for Non-Profit Organizations*, Boston, MA: Auburn House Publishing Co., 1981.

Reeder, R., and Reeder, B., "The Quasi-Industrial (Resellers) Market, An Important Element in Industrial Marketing Policy," *Marketing: Issues and Trends*, Springfield, MO: Atlantic Marketing Association, 1987.

Regan, J.M. et al., "Services for the Families of Alcoholics," *Journal of Studies on Alcohol*, 44(6): 1072-1081, 1983.

Reichard, C.J., "Industrial Selling Beyond Price and Persistance," *Harvard Business Review*, March-April, pp. 127-33, 1985.

Revell, A., Wesnes, K., and Warburton, D.M., "Self-Medication with Alcohol as a Coping Strategy," *Advanced Concepts in Alcoholism*, Oxford, England: Pergam Press Ltd., 1984.

Ricardo-Campbell, R., "Economics and Health," *Vital Speeches of the Day*, LII (11), March 15, pp. 345-349, 1986.

Richter, C.P., "Biology of Drives," *Journal of Comparative and Physiological Psychology*, 40: 129-134, 1947.

Richter, C.P., "The Self-Selection of Diets," In: *Essays in Biology in Honor of Herbert M. Evans*, Berkley, CA: University of California Press, 1943.

Roberts, S.J., "Relationship of Alcoholic Subtypes to Treatment Outcome," Dissertation, Texas Tech University, Ann Arbor, MI: University Microfilms International, 46(8): 2822B, 1986.

Robertson, I., Heather, N., Dzialdowski, A., Crawford, J., and Winton, M., "Comparison of Minimal Versus Intensive Controlled Drinking Treatment Interventions for Problem Drinkers," *British Journal of Clinical Psychology*, 25: 185-194, 1986.

Robinson, J.P., "Daily News Habits of the American Public," ANAP News Research Report No. 15, September 22, American Newspaper Publishers Association, Washington, DC, 1978.

Robinson, P.J., Faris, C.W., and Wind, Y., *Understanding The Industrial Buyer*, Vol. 3, Cambridge, MA: Marketing Science Institute, 1967.

Rogers, E.M., *Diffusion of Innovation*, New York: The Free Press of Glencoe, 1962.

Rudy, D.R., *Becoming Alcoholic*, Carbondale and Edwardsville: Southern Illinois University Press, 1986.

Ruga, W., "Environmental Design Can Strengthen a Hospital's Marketing Campaign," In W.J. Winston (ed.), *Innovations in Hospital Marketing*, New York: The Haworth Press, Inc., 1984.

Rush, B.R., and Ogborne, A.C., "Acceptability of Nonabstinence Treatment Goals Among Alcoholism Treatment Programs," *Journal of Studies on Alcohol*, 47(2): 146-150, 1986.

Ryan, K., "Facts For Planning 10. Assessment of Need For Alcoholism Treatment Services: Planning Procedures," *Alcohol, Health and Research World*, 9(2): 37-44, 1984/85.

Saulter, S., and League, V.C. (eds.), *Prevention Action Manual*, Oakland, CA: A.H. Training and Development Systems, Inc., 1986.

Saunders, B., "The Case for Controlling Alcohol Consumption," In: Heather, N. et al. (eds.), *The Misuse of Alcohol*. New York: New York University Press, 1985.

Saunders, W.M., and Kershaw, P.W., "Spontaneous Remission From Alcoholism – A Community Study," *British Journal of Addiction*, 74: 251-65, 1979.

Scheiderich, W.A., "Pricing Constraints," *Top Health Care Finance*, 14(1): 5-15, 1987.

Schmidt, W., and de Lint, W., "Estimating the Prevalence of Alcoholism From Alcohol Consumption and Mortality Data," *Quarterly Journal Stud. Alc.*, 31: 957-964, 1970.

Schmittdiel, C.J., and Ford, W.E., Department of Public Institutions, Lincoln, NE, "Predicting Alcoholism Service Needs from a National Treatment Utilization Survey," *International Journal of the Addictions*, 1983.

Schulman, J., "The Transition from Clinician to Administrator to Marketer," *Journal of Health Care Marketing*, December, p. 45, 1987.

Self, D.R., "The Third Party Administrator As A Channel Member In The Employee Insurance Services Distribution System," accepted for publication by *Journal of Professional Services Marketing*, 3(4) Spring/Summer, 1988.

Self, D.R., Buchanan, W., and Ingram, J., "Non-Profit Services: Adoption or Adaptation of Marketing," accepted for publication by *Journal of Professional Services Marketing*, 2(4) Spring, 1987.

Self, D.R., Ingram, J., McKinney, R., and Buchanan, W., "The Evolution of Marketing Thought In A Change-Agent Discipline," accepted for publication by *Journal of Professional Services marketing*, 2(4) Spring, 1987.

Self, D.R., Kline, T.A., Ingram, J.J., Sauser, W.I., and Judd, V.C., "Alcoholism Treatment Marketing: Controversies and Evolving Knowledge," (invited editorial) accepted for publication by *Health Marketing Quarterly*, IV (2), Winter 1987-88.

Selzer, M.L., "The Michigan Alcoholism Screening Test: The Quest For A New Diagnostic Instrument," *The American Journal of Psychiatry*, 127(12): 1653-1658, 1971.

Sereny, G., Sharma, V., Holt, J., and Gordis, F., "Mandatory Supervised Antabuse Therapy in an Outpatient Alcoholism Program: A Pilot Study," *Alcoholism: Clinical and Experimental Research*, 10(3): 290-292, 1986.

Shelley-McIntyre, B., "Perceptual Differentiation, Level Of Aspiration, and Degree Of Alcohol Dependence Among Alcoholics," *Dissertation Abstracts International*, 47(7): 3126-B, 1987.

Sherif, M., and Cantril, H., "The Psychology of 'Attitudes,'" *Psychological Review*, 52: 295-313, 1945.

Sherman, R.M., Reiff, S., and Forsythe, A.B., "Utilization of Medical Services By Alcoholics Participating in an Outpatient Treatment Program," *Alcoholism: Clinical and Experimental Research*, 3(115), 1979.

Simmermacher, D.G., *Self-Image Modification Training*, Hollywood, FL: Health Communications, Inc., 1981.

Simon, J.L., and Arndt, J., "The Shape of the Advertising Response Function," *Journal of Advertising Research*, 20(4): 11, August, 1980.

Simon, R. et al., "1985 Annual Statistical Report On Outpatient Counseling and Treatment Facilities for Addicts in the Federal Republic of Germany: January 1 to December 31, 1985," p. 41, 1986.

Skinner, H.A., "Assessment of Alcohol Problems: Basic Principles, Critical Issues, and Future Trends," In: Isarel, Y., Glash, F.B., Klant, H., Popham,

R.E., Schmidt, W., and Smart, R.C. (eds.), *Research Advances in Alcohol and Drug Problems*, Vol. 6, New York: Plenum Press, pp. 319-369, 1981.

Skinner, H.A., "Different Strokes for Different Folks: Different Treatment for Alcohol Abuse," In: Meyer, R.E. et al. (eds.), *Evaluation of the Alcoholic: Implications for Research, Theory and Treatment*, NIAAA Research Monograph No. 5, Washington DC: Superintendent of Documents, U.S. Government Printing Office, pp. 349-367, 1981.

Smart, R.G., "Do Some Alcoholics Do Better In Some Types of Treatment Than Others?" *Drug and Alcohol Dependence*, 3:65-75, 1978.

Smart, R.G., "Spontaneous Recovery in Alcoholics: A Review and Analysis of the Available Research," *Drug and Alcohol Dependence*, 1: 277-285, 1975/76.

Smith, D.E., Milkman, H., and Sunderwith, S., "Addictive Disease: Concept and Controversy," In: Milkman and Shaffer (eds.), *The Addiction: Multidisciplinary Perspective and Treatment*, Lexington, MA: Lexington Books, pp. 145-159, 1985.

Sobell, M.B., and Sobell, L.C., "Alcoholics Treated by Individualized Behavior Therapy: One-Year Treatment Outcome," *Behavior Research and Therapy*, 11: 599-618, 1973.

Sobell, M.B., and Sobell, L.C., *Behavioral Treatment of Alcohol Problems*, New York: Plenum Press, 1978.

Sobell, M.B., and Sobell, L.C., "Individualized Behavior Therapy for Alcoholics: Rationale, Procedures, Preliminary Results, and Appendix," *California Mental Health Research Monograph No. 13*, Department of Mental Health, Hygiene, Sacramento, California, 1972.

Solomon, M., "Differences Between Alcoholic Drunk Drivers Who Abstain, Control Their Drinking or Relapse After Treatment," PhD dissertation, University of Windsor, Windsor, Ontario, Canada, *Dissertation Abstractions International*, 46(9): 3231-B, 1986.

Stabenau, J., Dolinsky, Z., and Fischer, B., "Alcohol Consumption: Effect Of Gender And Psychopathology," *Alcoholism: Clinical and Experimental Research*, 10(3): 335-336, 1986.

Stall, R., "An Examination of Spontaneous Remission From Problem Drinking in the Bluegrass Region of Kentucky," *Journal of Drug Issues*, 13: 191-206, 1983.

Stanhope, J.M., Gehlharr, P., and Florio, T., "Halfway to Where? A Halfway House for Employed Alcoholics," *Community Health Studies*, 10(1): 68-76, 1986.

Stanton, W.J., and Futrell, C., *Fundamentals of Marketing*. New York: McGraw-Hill Book Company, 1987.

Stimmel, B., *Controversies in Alcoholism and Substance Abuse*, New York: The Haworth Press, Inc., 1986.

Stockman, S.J., "Eliciting Help-Seeking In Hospitalized Alcoholics," *Dissertation Abstracts International*, 47(7): 3128-B, 3129-B, 1987.

Strategic Health Care Marketing Newsletter, Health Care Communications, Rye, New York: 3(6), June, 1987.

Strategic Health Care Marketing Newsletter, Health Care Communications, Rye, New York: February, 1986.

Strug, D.L., Priyadarsini, S., and Hyman, M.M. (eds.), *Alcohol Interventions: Historical and Sociocultural Approaches*, New York: The Haworth Press, Inc., 1986.

Sugerman, A.A., "Alcoholism: An Overview of Treatment Models and Methods," In: Gomberg, E.L., White, H.R., and Carpenter, J.A. (eds.), *Alcohol Science and Society Revisited*, Ann Arbor, MI: The University of Michigan Press, pp. 262-278, 1982.

Super, K.E., "Joint Ventures Alcoholism Center May Benefit from State Insurance Law," *Modern Healthcare*, August 1, pp. 40-41, 1985.

Talbott, G.D., and Beson, E.B., "Impaired Physicians – The Dilemma Of Identification," *Postgrad Med*, 66(6): 56-64, 1980.

Tarter, R., and Edwards, K., "Antecedents to Alcoholism: Implications for Prevention and Treatment," *Behavior Therapy*, 17(4): 346-361, 1986.

______, "Neurobehavioral Correlates Of Alcoholism Vulnerability" In: Norman, C.C., and Chao, H.M. (eds.), *Research Monograph No. 17: Early Identification of Alcohol Abuse*, Washington, DC, U.S. Government Printing Office, p. 354 (pp. 149-167), 1985.

Taylor, J.W., "The Role of Risk in Consumer Behavior," *Journal of Marketing*, Vol. 38, April, 1974.

Thom, B., "Sex Differences In Help-Seeking For Alcohol Problems: 1. The Barriers to Help-Seeking," *British Journal of Addiction*, 81(6): 777-788, 1986.

Thrower, J.H., and Tyler, "Edwards Personal Preference Schedule Correlates of Addiction Counselor Effectiveness," *International Journal of the Addictions*, 21(2): 191-193, 1986.

Topolnicki, D.M., "Where To Take a Drug or Drinking Problem," *Money*, 15(1): 120-122, 124, 126-128, 1986.

Traylor, M.B., and Mathias, A.M., "The Impact of T.V. vs. Word of Mouth on the Image of Lawyers," *Journal of Advertising*, 12(4): 42, 1983.

Trice, H.M., "Alcoholism: Group Factors in Etiology and Therapy," *Human Organization*, 15: 33-40, 1956.

Tuchfeld, B.S., "Spontaneous Remission in Alcoholics: Empirical Observations and Theoretical Implications," *Journal of Studies on Alcohol*, 42(7): 626-641, 1981.

United States Department of Commerce, *An Overview of the 1982 Economic Censuses*, Washington, DC: Government Printing Office, 1984.

United States Department of Commerce, *1982 Census of Manufactures – General Summary, Part 2 – Industry Statistics By Employment Size of Establishment*, Washington, DC: Government Printing Office, 1985A.

United States Department of Commerce, *1982 Census of Manufacturers – Industry Series, Household Furniture*, Washington, DC: Government Printing Office, 1985B.

United States Department of Commerce, *1982 Census of Retail Trade – Industry Series, Establishment and Firm Size*, Washington, DC: Government Printing Office, 1985C.

United States Department of Commerce, *County Business Patterns, 1985 – Illinois*, Washington, DC: Government Printing Office, 1987.

United States Department of Health and Human Services Fifth Special Report to the U.S. Congress on Alcohol and Health, DHHS Pub. No. (ADM) 84-1291, Washington, DC: Supt. of Docs., U.S. Government Printing Office, 1984.

United States Executive Office of the President, *Standard Industrial Classification Manual, 1987*, Washington, DC: Government Printing Office, 1987.

United States Office of the Public Printer, *Federal Depository Libraries*, Washington, DC: Government Printing Office, 1983.

Vaillant, G., *The Natural History of Alcoholism: Causes, Patterns, and Paths to Recovery*, Harvard University Press, p. 315, 1983.

Valle, S.K., *Drunk Driving in America: Strategies and Approaches to Treatment*, New York: The Haworth Press, Inc., 1986.

Varadaraj, R., and Mendonca, J.D., "Blood Alcohol Survey in Patients With Self-Poisoning," *British Journal of Psychiatry*, 148: 615, May, 1986.

Vaughn, R., Sherborne, R., and Lewis, D., "Drug Treatment Arduous, Costly," *Nashville Tennesseean*, 16, September, 1985.

Vestal, R.E. et al., "Aging and Ethanol Metabolism," *Clin Pharmacol Ther*, 21(3): 343-354, 1977.

Volger, R.E., Weissbach, T.A., and Compton, J.V., "Learning Techniques For Alcohol Abuse," *Behaviour Research and Therapy*, 15: 31-8, 1977.

Walker, R.D., "Length of Stay, Neuropsychological Performance, and Aftercare: Influences on Alcohol Treatment Outcome," *Journal of Consulting and Clinical Psychology*, 51(6): 900-911, 1983.

Walsh, D.A., "Effects of Family Treatment and the Psychological Functioning of Chemically Dependent and Co-Dependent Adults," *Dissertation Abstracts International*, 47(1): 393-B, 1986.

Wegscheider, D., "Day Treatment," *Alcohol & Addiction*, 6(5): 20, 1986.

Weighill, V.E., Hodge, G., and Peck, D.F., "Keeping Appointments With Clinical Psychologists," *British Journal of Clinical Psychology*, 143-144, 1983.

Westermeyer, J., "Role of Ethnicity In Substance Abuse," In: Stimmel, B. (ed.), *Cultural and Sociological Aspects of Alcoholism and Substance Abuse*, New York: The Haworth Press, Inc., pp. 9-18, 1984.

Whitley, M.J., and Zankowski, G.L., "Family Therapy In A Hospital Setting: A Model For Time-Limited Treatment," *Journal of Psychoactive Drugs*, 18(1): 61-64, 1986.

Wilkie, W.L., *Consumer Behavior*, New York: John Wiley & Sons, Inc., 1986.

Williams, F., "Psychological, Demographic, and Supportive System Variables Associated With Recovery of Hospitalized Alcoholics," Dissertation, United States International University, Ann Arbor, MI: UMI, 46(2): 668B, 1985.

Williams, R.J., "The Etiology of Alcoholism: A Working Hypothesis Involving the Interplay of Hereditary and Environmental Factors," *Quarterly Journal of Studies on Alcohol*, 7: 567-587, 1947.

Williams, R.J., *Alcoholism: The Nutritional Approach*, Austin: University of Texas Press, 1959.

Winston, W., *How to Write A Marketing Plan for Health Care Organizations*, New York: The Haworth Press, Inc., 1985.

Young, J.R., and Mondy, W., *Personal Selling*, Chicago: The Dryden Press, 1982.

Zepeda, R., "Hispanic Program: Careunit Hospital of Los Angeles. Los Angeles, California," *Journal of Substance Abuse Treatment*, 3(2): 135-137, 1986.

Ziegler, D.J., "Psychoanalytic Stages," In: Corsini, R.J. (ed.), *Encyclopedia of Psychology*, Vol. 3, New York: John Wiley & Sons, pp. 91-92, 1984.

For Product Safety Concerns and Information please contact our EU representative GPSR@taylorandfrancis.com Taylor & Francis Verlag GmbH, Kaufingerstraße 24, 80331 München, Germany

Batch number: 10725881

Printed by Printforce, the Netherlands

Electroceramics for High Performance Supercapacitors

Scrivener Publishing
100 Cummings Center, Suite 541J
Beverly, MA 01915-6106

Publishers at Scrivener
Martin Scrivener (martin@scrivenerpublishing.com)
Phillip Carmical (pcarmical@scrivenerpublishing.com)

Electroceramics for High Performance Supercapacitors

Edited by
Inamuddin
Tariq Altalhi
and
Sayed Mohammed Adnan

Scrivener Publishing

WILEY

This edition first published 2024 by John Wiley & Sons, Inc., 111 River Street, Hoboken, NJ 07030, USA
and Scrivener Publishing LLC, 100 Cummings Center, Suite 541J, Beverly, MA 01915, USA

For more information about Scrivener publications please visit www.scrivenerpublishing.com.

Wiley Global Headquarters
111 River Street, Hoboken, NJ 07030, USA

For details of our global editorial offices, customer services, and more information about Wiley products visit us at www.wiley.com.

Library of Congress Cataloging-in-Publication Data

ISBN 978-1-394-16625-1

Cover image: Pixabay.Com
Cover design by Russell Richardson

Set in size of 11pt and Minion Pro by Manila Typesetting Company, Makati, Philippines

Printed in the USA

10 9 8 7 6 5 4 3 2 1

Contents

Preface

In the near future, high-energy density materials will be required to accommodate the increased demand for gadgets, hybrid cars, and massive electrical energy storage systems. Fuel cells, supercapacitors, and batteries have the highest energy densities, but traditional capacitors have gained attention for intermittent energy harvesting owing to their high energy transfer rate and quick charging/discharging capability. The large amount of electric breakdown strength and modest remnant polarization are keys to the high energy density in dielectric capacitors. Above 100°C or 212°F, polymer dielectric capacitors become unstable and begin to suffer a dielectric breakdown. Hence, dielectric ceramics are the sole viable option for high-temperature applications. When it comes to consumer electronics, where most capacitors are made without using lead, Pb-based ceramics materials like lanthanum-doped Pb zirconate-titanate have tremendous energy harvesting capabilities. Due to this, lead-free materials with a higher energy transfer rate capability are needed.

This book provides a basic understandings of dielectric-based energy harvesting. After a detailed analysis of the state of the art, it proceeds to explain the specific strategies to enhance energy storage features, including managing the local structure and phases assembly, raising the dielectric width, and enhancing microstructure and electrical uniformity. Also discussed is the need for novel materials with applications in high-density supercapacitors.

Chapter 1 discusses lead-free electrical energy storage systems. The characteristic features, energy storage efficiency, advantages, limitations, and outlook of various kinds of lead-free dielectric materials—such as ferroelectric ceramics, relaxor ferroelectric ceramics, antiferroelectric ceramics, glass ceramics, films, and polymer-based nanocomposites—are all covered.

Chapter 2 explores various ceramic materials, especially metal-based oxides, mixed ceramics, single- and multi-element-based ceramics, and spinal ceramics. The principle and characteristics of various types of electro-ceramics are also discussed. The development of ceramic materials for supercapacitor application and their key characteristics are highlighted, as well.

Chapter 3 is designed to be the source for ceramic materials and their applications as supercapacitors for energy storage applications. It includes the principles of energy storage devices and factors affecting the performance of supercapacitors. This section details various oxide-based ceramic materials used in supercapacitor applications with suitable examples. The primary focus is on understanding the metal oxide behavior and their performance as supercapacitor electrodes.

Chapter 4 discusses the multilayer ceramic capacitors using ferroelectric ceramics, $BaTiO_2$, lead-based and lead-free materials. The chapter also provides information about quick charging/discharging rates and high energy density, plus other characteristics like fatigue resistance, temperature/frequency stability, lifetime dependability, production cost, and equivalent series resistance, which are all crucial for practical applications.

Chapter 5 summarizes various low- and high-temperature superconducting materials that are utilized for their magnetic energy storage applications. The magnetic storage properties have been discussed with an emphasis on their role in recent energy storage projects. The future potential is also considered, by highlighting the flaws of the current scenarios.

Chapter 6 explores the main key factors for the maximum optimization of supercapacitors for energy storage. Types of supercapacitors, such as electric double-layer capacitors and pseudo capacitors, are discussed briefly. Capacitance, specific capacitance, and energy density as key factors are discussed, as well. Optimization of energy density via pre-size, grain size, bandgap, surface, and the functional group is explained. Optimization of voltage is outlined, with positive and negative electrode materials, asymmetric supercapacitors, and battery supercapacitor hybrid devices.

Chapter 7 discusses energy storage properties, and lead-based and lead-free antiferroelectric materials that can be used for energy storage. Factors to optimize the performance of these anti-ferroelectrics are provided. Challenges faced by antiferroelectric, such as energy conversion efficiency are given thorough attention. Optimization factors, from phase engineering and grain size engineering to domain engineering, and doping, are all deliberated.

Chapter 8 examines the last decade's research about the development of mixed ternary iron/cobalt ferromagnetic oxides and their polymer nanocomposites for use as electrode materials in the fabrication of supercapacitors. The role of the main components of supercapacitors is thoroughly discussed. The remarkable effect of the architectural morphology of electrode material on the performance of supercapacitors is highlighted.

Chapter 9 discusses the importance of transition metal oxides (TMOs) as electrode materials for energy storage devices. The chapter explains how TMOs can be used in supercapacitors as electrode materials. by focusing on their morphology-dependent improvements in electrochemical capacitive properties for supercapacitors, which occurs by broadening the operating potential window to increase the energy density of the devices.

Chapter 10 summarizes the most recent developments related to supercapacitors and gives an overview of aqua-based electrolytes.

Chapter 11 outlines the latest advanced materials used for supercapacitors, batteries, pumped-hydro storage, flywheel energy storage, and superconducting magnetic energy storage.

Chapter 12 explores various the new cutting edge electroceramics that are being used for energy storage. Among these new materials are lead-based ceramics that include relaxor ferroelectric and antiferroelectric ceramics. Lead-based materials such as PLZT, PLZ, and PLZST are discussed in the lead-based ceramics category. Lead-free ceramics are covered as well, such as barium titanate-based, strontium titanate, bismuth ferrite-based, niobate-based, and bismuth-based ceramics. Furthermore, applications of ceramic multilayers and films are deliberated. This chapter provides a wide overview of various new materials that are currently being explored in the energy storage field.

Finally, chapter 13 discusses ceramics and their potential applications. Additional, different types of ceramics, like metal oxide and spinel oxide for high-performance supercapacitors, are given thorough attention. Moreover, the chapter provides a comparison of Pb-based ceramics and Pb-free ceramics.

Our thanks go to Wiley and Scrivener Publishing for their continuous support and guidance.

Inamuddin
Department of Applied Chemistry, Zakir Husain College of Engineering and Technology, Aligarh Muslim University, Aligarh, India
Tariq Altalhi
Department of Chemistry, College of Science, Taif University, Taif, Saudi Arabia
Sayed Mohammed Adnan
Department of Chemical Engineering, Zakir Husain College of Engineering and Technology, Aligarh Muslim University, Aligarh, India

1

Lead-Free Energy Storage Ceramics

Sahidul Islam[1,2], Arindam Das[2] and Ujjwal Mandal[2*]

[1]*Department of Chemistry, Krishnath College, Berhampore, Murshidabad, West Bengal, India*

[2]*Department of Chemistry, The University of Burdwan, Golapbag, Burdwan, West Bengal, India*

Abstract

With the technological advancement in various fields, there is a growing demand for electronic materials having a high power density that has provoked the fabrication of capacitors with high-energy storage capacity and features like high voltage, high frequency, high-energy density, high capacitance density, high-temperature tolerance, light-weight and non-polluting to environment. For storage of electrical energy, dielectric capacitors are regarded as a promising device as their charging–discharging process is fast and has very high-power density. The development of multilayer ceramic capacitors satisfies such demands well as compared to the electrolytic and film counterpart. In a multilayer ceramic capacitor, the equivalent series resistance is extremely low, the current handling capability is high, and is stable in high temperatures. These features are essential for the generation of clean energy, designing smart grids, 5G base stations, etc. However, the main limitation in lead-free energy capacitors arises due to low energy density. Lead is present in most of the high-energy density capacitors, thus limiting their widescale application due to environmental concerns as lead is a toxic heavy metal. The power density of dielectric capacitors is higher than fuel cells, Li-ion batteries, and supercapacitors. However, their lower-energy density hinders their commercialization. The energy storage density can largely be enhanced in the dielectric/ferroelectric capacitors.

Keywords: Dielectric capacitors, ferroelectric capacitors, lead-free energy storage

**Corresponding author*: umandal@chem.buruniv.ac.in

Inamuddin, Tariq Altalhi and Sayed Mohammed Adnan (eds.) Electroceramics for High Performance Supercapacitors, (1–24) © 2024 Scrivener Publishing LLC

1.1 Introduction

With the evolution of economic society, the crisis of fossil energy resources is emerging along with the increase of environmental pollution and climate change [1, 2]. This leads to the emphasis on the essence of renewable and clean energy sources like water, wind, thermal and solar energy [3, 4]. Thus, an increasing demand is there on devices capable of storing energy like fuel cells, batteries, electrochemical supercapacitors, supercapacitors made of dielectric parallel plates, etc. [5–8]. Among these energy storage systems, the devices having high-energy density are batteries and fuel cells (10–300 W-h/kg and 200–1000 W-h/kg, respectively) but the power density of these storage systems is low (below 500 W/kg). The slow movement of charge carriers in these systems creates a limitation in their applications in high-power systems [9, 10]. In supercapacitors, the energy density is moderate (0.04 to 30 W-h/kg) and the power density is quite high (10^1 to 10^6 W/kg) but the long charge-discharge process (order of seconds) sets the main limitation in these storage systems [11, 12]. Contrarily in dielectric capacitors, the charge–discharge process is fast (~ns) and power density is reasonably high (~10^8 W/kg), which is sufficient to meet the required criteria in high-power electronic components in devices like space crafts, satellites, defibrillators used for medical purpose, hybrid electric vehicles, electronic weapons, etc. [13, 14]. However, in dielectric capacitors, the major limitation is attributed to the low-energy density as compared to batteries, fuel cells, and electrochemical capacitors [15, 16]. In pulsed power systems and power electronics, dielectric capacitors occupy almost one-fourth of the size and mass [17]. Hence, in dielectric capacitors, the development of novel dielectric material is necessary to increase the power density significantly. To obtain this, researchers have given many efforts with the materials like lead magnesium niobate-lead titanate, lead lanthanum zirconate titanate, lead lanthanum zirconate stannate titanate, etc. as these materials have higher-energy density as compared to other dielectrics [18–20]. However, the use of lead in these materials sets the major drawbacks in their application as lead is a toxic heavy metal that pollutes the environment and endangers the health of living creatures, including human beings [21]. This drives the search for materials capable to store energy and free of lead.

In recent times, progress in the development of ceramics and dielectric materials free of lead, polymer-based composites, and various films happened to a considerable extent [22, 23]. In the sustainable energy program, energy storage plays an important role as this can enhance the more efficient use of energy from renewable energy sources, stabilize the energy market, and take the matter of environmental impact into account [24]. Designing capacitors renders such quality greatly as their power density is high and the charge/discharge process is fast as compared to the batteries [25]. Although the energy-storing capacity of dielectrics is less as compared to Li batteries, fuel cells, and supercapacitors, their use is proposed in high-power applications, such as defibrillators, power electronics, detonators, etc [26–28]. Recently, a great effort is given by researchers across the globe for developing materials having a dielectric constant very high and an energy storage capacity very large. In recent times, for lead-free antiferroelectric films, the reported recoverable energy density (50 J cm^{-3}) is found to be very high at room temperature [29, 30]. Moreover, the energy density (39 J cm^{-3}) and thermal stability of some lead-based materials are good even though the temperature increases up to 200°C [30, 31]. However, lead-based material is harmful to human beings and the environment at large. Thus, there is a limitation on the applicability of lead-based materials for energy storage. The research on lead-free materials is extremely important and is done on so many materials and found promising results for some materials like $Hf_{0.3}Zr_{0.7}O_3$ thin film (η_{reco}=40 Joule cm^{-3} and η=50% at room temperature) [32, 33]. A very high value of η (=81%) and η_{reco} (=37 J cm^{-3}) is obtained for $0.88BaTiO_3$–$0.12Bi(MgTiO_3)$ film at room temperature [34]. Although there is considerable progress in the research of lead-free materials for the storage of energy, it was found that the performance of lead-free materials is much poor as compared to that of lead-based materials. Hence, the achievement of high performance on lead-free materials is the main aim of the researchers to meet the requirement for large-scale applications in power converters, portable power electronics, and DC link capacitors [35]. Previously it was reported that materials having high piezoelectric coefficient and dielectric constant are suitable for good energy storage capacitors [36]. The performance of ferroelectric or dielectric multilayer capacitors is higher as compared to single-layer capacitors [37, 38].

1.2 Dielectric Capacitor and Energy Storage

A typical dielectric capacitor is made of two parallelly placed electrodes sandwiching the dielectric material between them. The energy storage capacity is quantified by the capacitance, as represented mathematically,

$$C = \varepsilon_0 \varepsilon_r \frac{A}{d} \tag{1.1}$$

C, ε_0, ε_r here represents capacitance, permittivity in a vacuum and relative permittivity (also known as dielectric constant), respectively. *A* and *d* represent overlapping areas and distance between the two parallelly placed plates [39, 40]. On applying the electric field between the two plates, the orientation of the dipoles of the dielectric material occurs in the direction of the applied electric field, thus in the two plates, the charge is induced and charging happens. The process of charging is stopped when the generated potential difference between the two plates due to the accumulation of charge (±Q) becomes equal to the voltage applied externally and the storing of the electric field occurs. Another way of mathematical representation of capacitance (C) is,

$$C = \frac{dQ}{dV} \tag{1.2}$$

While charging, the total stored energy W can be expressed as [39, 40],

$$W = \int_0^Q V\,dq \tag{1.3}$$

Hence, the energy storage in unit volume i.e., the energy density of the dielectric material can be expressed as,

$$J = \frac{W}{Ad} = \frac{\int_0^{Q_{max}} Vdq}{Ad} = \frac{\int_0^{\delta_{max}} Vd\delta}{d} = \int_0^{D_{max}} EdD \tag{1.4}$$

where $E = \frac{V}{d}$ is the externally applied electric field, δ represents the charge density on the surface and *D* represents electrical displacement. The dielectric constant for linear dielectric materials (such as glass, and mica) remains unchanged with the change of electric field applied externally. hence the calculation of energy storage density (*J*) could be done as,

$$J = \int_{0}^{D_{max}} E\,dD = \int_{0}^{E_{max}} \varepsilon_0 \varepsilon_r E dE = \frac{1}{2}\varepsilon_0 \varepsilon_r E^2 \tag{1.5}$$

It is clear from equation (1.5), the density of energy storage linearly varies as a function of the square of the applied electric field and direly to the relative permittivity of the medium. However, the dielectric constant for non-linear dielectric materials is changed with the applied electric field, hence equation (1.5) is not applicable. The extent of electrical displacement in the dielectric materials having large dielectric constant becomes almost near to the polarization. Equation (1.4) in these cases takes the form:

$$J = \int_{0}^{P_{max}} E\,dP \tag{1.6}$$

Here, spontaneous polarization and maximum polarization of dielectric material are represented by *P* and P_{max} [39–42]. It is evident from equation (1.6), the confined area between vertical axes and hysteresis loop in the process of charging represents the energy density (J). In Figure 1.1 (3), Polarization-Electric field diagrams i.e. hysteresis loops (represented by *P-E* diagrams) have been shown in the cases of linear dielectric materials (like, Al_2O_3), ferroelectric (FE) materials (like, $PbZr_xTi_{1-x}O_3$), relaxor

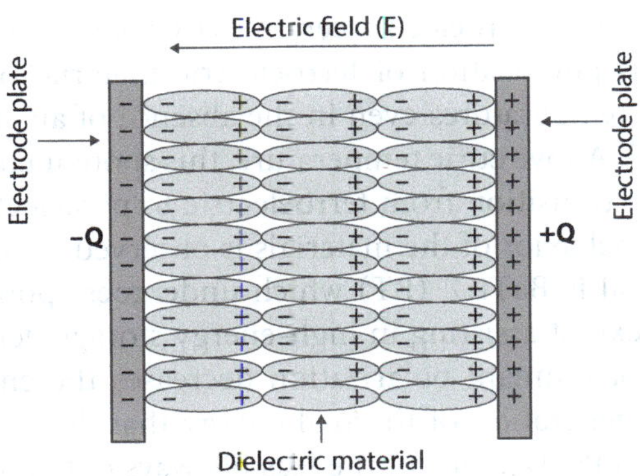

Figure 1.1 Polarization of the dielectric material during the process of charging.

ferroelectric (RFE) materials (like, $xPb(Mg_{1/3}Nb_{2/3})O_3$-$(1-x)PbTiO_3$) and antiferroelectric (AFE) materials (like, $PbZrO_3$). The releasing of all the stored energy is not possible as there is energy loss (J_{loss}) due to electric hysteresis in the process of charging. The enclosed area between vertical axes and hysteresis loops during the process of discharging represents the recoverable energy storage density (J_{rec}) [43].

$$J_{rec} = -\int_{P_{max}}^{P_r} E\,dP \tag{1.7}$$

The mathematical representation of energy efficiency (η) is,

$$\eta = \frac{J_{rec}}{J_{rec} + J_{loss}} \tag{1.8}$$

From equation (1.7) and diagram (1.3), it is clear that a high value of electric field breakdown strength (BDS), the large value of maximum polarization, small remnant polarization, and slim *P-E* hysteresis loops imply the high value of J_{rec} and η. In linear dielectrics, the BDS and energy loss for the materials are low but as their maximum polarization is small, their application in the high-energy storage system is not suitable [40].

1.3 Energy Storage of Dielectric Ceramics Free of Lead

(i) Energy storage and ferroelectric ceramics free of lead (Figure 1.2)
The spontaneous polarization of ferroelectric material occurs within a certain range of temperatures even in the absence of an applied external electric field [44]. Above curie temperature, this spontaneous polarization disappears and a transition from ferroelectric to paraelectric occurs and linear dielectric behavior of the materials is observed [45]. One such ferroelectric material is $BaTiO_3$ (BT) which undergoes spontaneous polarization to large extent assisting in high-energy storage density. However, its large extent of remnant polarization decreases the energy efficiency resulting in the generation of thermal energy that decreases the service life of the device [46, 47]. One of the feasible ways of tailoring the energy storage performance in ferroelectric material is doping [48]. The property

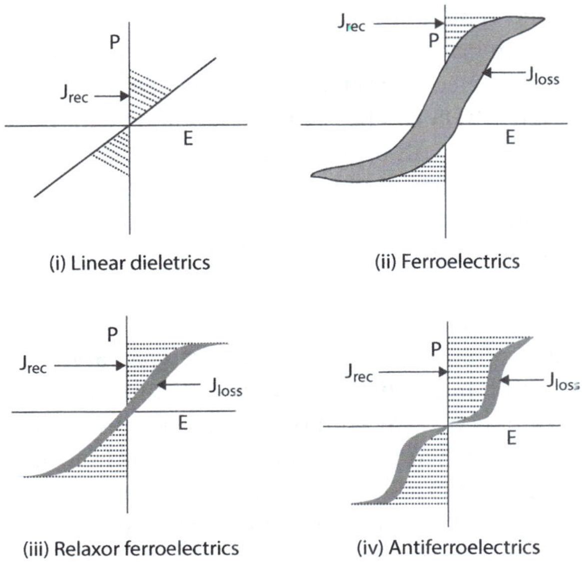

Figure 1.2 P-E hysteresis loops and characteristic parameters of (i) linear dielectric (ii) ferroelectric (iii) relaxor ferroelectric and (iv) antiferroelectric materials for energy storage.

of storage of energy of $BaTiO_3$ ceramics is significantly increased if Ba^{2+} and Ti^{4+} ions are substituted with equivalent ions (that may be even hetero valent) [49]. The substitution of Ba^{2+} with Ca^{2+} or Sr^{2+} and the substitution of Ti^{4+} with Zr^{4+} decreases the remnant polarization, thus energy density and efficiency increase [50]. One such example is $Ba_{0.70}Ca_{0.3}0TiO_3$ (BCT), having moderate energy efficiency of 60% (density of energy is 1.41 J cm^3 which is convertible) and it is 40% higher as compared to $BaTiO_3$ [51]. The remnant polarization and energy loss in the case of BCT are less and have a slimmer *P-E* hysteresis loop as compared to $BaTiO_3$. It is because Zr^{4+} has a fixed valence state whereas Ti is multivalent (Ti^{3+} and Ti^{4+}). The electron conduction between Ti^{3+} and Ti^{4+} can be decreased by doping Zr^{4+}, hence there is a decrease in energy loss [52–55]. In Zr^{4+} doped $BaTiO_3$ ceramics ($BaZr_{0.1}Ti_{0.9}O_3$), Zhang *et al.* have shown that at the appropriate sintering temperature, the quality of dielectric material becomes good and the capacity of energy storage become high (Dielectric constant: 2998, energy density: 0.5 J cm^3, dielectric loss: 0.007) [56]. By sol-gel method, Scott *et al.* synthesized the ceramics $[(BaZr_{0.2}Ti_{0.8})O_3]_{1-x}$- $[(Ba_{0.7}Ca_{0.3})TiO_3]_x$ (BZT-BCT, x = 0.10, 0.15, 0.20) doped with ca^{2+} and Zr^{2+} which has improved energy storage capacity (when x=0.10, the reported energy density is 0.6 J cm^3 which is dischargeable). The reason for this improvement is the increased P_{max} and reduced P_r [57]. Apart from low rampant polarization and high maximum polarization, the other parameter which plays a crucial role to achieve dielectric material with excellent energy storage is high BDS [58]. The large BDS can be obtained by improving the quality of *FE* ceramics i.e., ceramics with uniform and fine particle grain size and low porosity [59]. From the study of Jin *et al.*, it was established that the grain size of $Ba_{0.4}Sr_{0.6}TiO_3$ ceramics is reduced to 0.44 μm when the ceramics are sintered in the O_2 atmosphere as the lack of oxygen vacancies inhibits the growth in grain size. In this ceramic material, a large value of BDS and energy storage density (16.72 kV/mm and 1.081 J cm^3, respectively) and a moderate value of energy storage efficiency (73.78%) was found [60]. Surface modification in ceramics is another promising method of increasing BDS. An example of such kind of surface modification is to be found in resulting ceramics when $BaTiO_3$ is modified by Al_2O_3 (i.e., A@BT) and $BaTiO_3$ modified by B_2O_3–SiO_2 (i.e., G@BT) [61, 62]. BDS in these two modified ceramics is found to increase by 69% and 117% on going from unmodified to modified $BaTiO_3$ ceramics. The enhancement of BDS in G@BT as compared to that of $BaTiO_3$ is due to a decrease in pore defect concentration. The voltage endurance in A@BT ceramics is increased as the Al_2O_3 coating layer act as an insulator which decreases the thermally caused breakdown that occurs due to avalanche and electron accumulation. For these ceramic materials, the density of energy storage was reported, at 2.5 and 3.2 J cm^3 which are quite high compared to the density of energy (0.88 J cm^3) for pure $BaTiO_3$ [62].

(ii) Energy storage and relaxor ferroelectric ceramics free of lead (Table 1.1)

The relaxor ferroelectric ceramics are dipolar glasses lacking a well-ordered long-range structure. Example of these type of relaxor ferroelectrics are $PbMg_{1/3}Nb_{2/3}O_3$, $PbSc_{1/2}Nb_{1/2}O_3$, and $PbZn_{1/3}Nb_{2/3}O_3$ [68, 69]. The remnant polarization in relaxor ferroelectric materials is near zero and the *P-E* hysteresis loop is slim as compared to that of the ferroelectric materials, hence the energy efficiency becomes high [70]. In relaxor ferroelectrics, the diffuse phase transition can occur around dielectric maxima which renders good temperature stability [71]. Among many lead-free energy storage materials, BT-based materials have caught increasing attention as the BT materials can be converted into other ferroelectric-relaxor materials by introducing other elements in A- or B- site of it [72, 73]. The addition of $Bi(Mg_{2/3}Nb_{1/3})O_3$ (BMN) in BT leads to the conversion into the material where relaxor-like behavior was observed and high maximum energy density (1.13 J cm^3) was found [74]. The introduction of $Bi(Zn_{0.5}Ti_{0.5})O_3$ (BZT) in BT as reported by Dong *et al.*, increases the relaxor feature along with thermal stability and energy storage properties (Table 1.2) [75].

Table 1.1 Performance of energy storage of some lead-free ferroelectric ceramics.

Lead-free ferroelectric ceramics	E(kV/cm)	J_{rec}(J cm³)	η(%)	Reference
$(Ba_{0.4}Sr_{0.6})TiO_3$	180	1.15	82	53
$0.85(K_{0.5}Na_{0.5})NbO_3$–$0.15SrTiO_3$	400	4.03	52	54
$0.85BaTiO$–$0.15Bi(Mg_{2/3}Nb_{1/3})O_3$	140	1.13	90	55
$Ba_{0.4}Sr_{0.6}TiO_3$–5vol%(BaO–SiO_2–B_2O_3)	175	0.89	76	56
$0.92(0.92Bi_{0.5}Na_{0.5}TiO_3$–$0.08BaTiO_3)$–$0.1NaNbO_3$	70	0.71	66	57

Table 1.2 Performance of energy storage of some lead-free relaxor ferroelectric ceramics.

Lead-free relaxor ferroelectric ceramics	E(kV/cm)	J_{rec}(J/cm³)	η(%)	Reference
$0.8BaTiO_3$–$0.2BiNbO_4$	117	0.31	99.7	76
$0.88BaTiO_3$–$0.12Bi(Zn_{1/2}Zr_{1/2})O_3$	100	0.758	98	77
$0.88BaTiO_3$–$0.12Bi(Mg_{1/2}Ti_{1/2})O_3$	150	1.6	99.6	78
$0.86BaTiO_3$–$0.14Bi(Zn_{1/2}Ti_{1/2})O_3$	120	0.81	94	79
$0.875BaTiO_3$–$0.125Bi(Mg_{2/3}Nb_{1/3})O_3$	240	1.89	83	80

(iii) Energy storage and antiferroelectric ceramics free of lead

While spontaneous polarization occurs in ferroelectrics, the presence of antiparallel dipoles in almost equal proportion leads to the net polarization zero [81]. In presence of an appropriately high electric field, known as the field (E_F) for AFE-FE phase transition, the dipoles that are anti-parallelly oriented in the AFE phase, reorient to parallel dipoles, thus AFE-FE phase transition occurs and macroscopic polarization is induced [82]. On application of electric field E_A lesser than E_F, FE materials are converted back into AFE materials. Hence, for antiferroelectric materials, unique double *P-E* loops are found leading to the large value of J_{rec} and η. From the *I-E* curve, the values of E_F and E_A can be found.

The positive-current peak relevant to E_F and negative peak-current relevant to E_A is obtained by applying the positive and negative electric field, respectively [83]. The discharge rate in antiferroelectric is faster (~ns) as compared to ferroelectric as in the switching electric field E_A, the FE phase is suddenly disappeared in antiferroelectric. Ferroelectrics and relaxor ferroelectrics have higher J_{rec} and η than antiferroelectrics [84, 85]. In the past few years, researchers have shown some interest in $PbZrO_3$-based antiferroelectrics because of high J_{rec} and η. But as lead is a toxic element in its various states, the shifting of research interest to lead-free antiferroelectric materials such as $AgNbO_3$ and $(Bi_{0.5}Nb_{0.5})TiO_3$ was very normal. Ding *et al.* reported 0.9 J cm³ (quite high) energy density for antiferroelectric ceramics $0.89Bi_{0.5}Na_{0.5}TiO_3$–$0.06BaTiO_3$–$0.05K_{0.5}Na_{0.5}NbO_3$ where low remnant polarization (5.4 μC/cm²) is the favorable factor [86]. From the study of Wang *et al.*, it was found that Zr containing in the ceramics $[(Bi_{0.5}Na_{0.5})_{0.94}Ba_{0.06}]\ La_{(1-x)}\ Zr_xTiO_3$ lead to a slimmer hysteresis loop and *AFE* behavior and the combination of these two features lead to high recoverable energy density 1.58 J cm³ [87]. While emphasizing lead-free materials, $AgNbO_3$-based materials attracted the attention of researchers recently as AFE materials have high J_{rec} and η. The AFE fabrics of $AgNbO_3$ were prepared by Wei *et al.* by sintering at solid state with the flow of oxygen, thus achieving the dielectrics with high recoverable energy density (2.1 J cm³) but due to the poor stability of the AFE phase of $AgNbO_3$, they have not found the double *P-E* loops [88]. To increase the value of J_{rec}, the AFE phase should be stable and E_A should be high. In perovskite structure (ABO_3), the phase stability can be assumed in terms of tolerance factor, *t*. The mathematical definition of t is [89],

$$t = \frac{(r_A + r_O)}{\sqrt{2}(r_B + r_O)}$$

Here r_A and r_B represent the ionic radii of cations present in A- and B-sites, respectively, r_O represents, the ionic radii of the anionic oxygen atom. The stability of FE phase is seen when t>1 and the stability of AFE phase is seen when t<1. The replacement of cation (Ag^+) of A site with cations having smaller size enhances the stability of AFE phase. One such example is the doping of Bi^{3+} ions in $AgNbO_3$ by Tian *et al.* As the size of the Bi^{3+} ion (1.17 Å) is lesser than Ag^+ ion (1.28 Å) the tolerance factor is decreased and the stability of AFE phase in the $Ag_{0.91}Bi_{0.03}NbO_3$ ceramic is increased, hence, they found high J_{rec} value (2.6 J cm³) and η (86%) [90, 91].

So far, the largest J_{rec} value reported for the lead-free ceramic $Ag(Nb_{0.85}Ta_{0.15})O_3$ is 4.2 J cm³ (Table 1.3) [92].

Table 1.3 Performance of energy storage of some lead-free antiferroelectric ceramics.

Lead-free antiferroelectric ceramics	E(kV/cm)	J_{loss} (J/cm³)	J_{rec} (J/cm³)	η(%)	Reference
$AgNbO_3$	175	3.15	2.10	40	93
$Ag(Nb_{0.85}Ta_{0.15})O_3$	230	1.90	4.20	69	94
$(Ag_{0.97}Bi_{0.01})NbO_3$	175	2.45	3.0	55	95
$AgNbO_3$ –0.1wt%MnO_2	150	2.30	2.50	52	96
$0.84(Bi_{0.5}Na_{0.5})TiO_3$–$0.16(K_{0.5}Na_{0.5})NbO_3$	100	0.10	1.20	92	97

(iv) Energy storage and glass ceramics free of lead

To achieve large J_{rec}, the high value of BDS is important. But BDS is insufficient in lead-free ceramics due to high defect density, hence it set the limitation in their application in ceramic-based capacitors. Several factors on which BDS depends are (i) porosity, (ii) grain size, (iii) interfacial polarization, (iv) secondary phase, and (v) charge transport [98]. In the ceramic matrix, the embedding of glass increases density and reduces grain size, and the electric field is decreased across the grain boundaries, thus there is an increase in BDS. The electrical durability and wettability of B_2O_3–SiO_2–based glass are quite good. Hence, it may be effectively added to the ceramics to increase the energy density [99]. One such example is, Wang *et al.* achieved higher-energy density (0.72 J cm³) at a higher electric field of 280.5 kV/cm by adding BaO–B_2O_3–SiO_2–Na_2CO_3–K_2CO_3 into $Ba_{0.4}Sr_{0.6}TiO_3$ [100]. Zhang *et al.* established by their research work, the introduction of 20 vol% glass (BaO–SiO_2–B_2O_3) in $Ba_{0.4}Sr_{0.6}TiO_3$ ceramic increased the BDS value to 23.9 kV/mm from 12.1 kV/mm for pure $Ba_{0.4}Sr_{0.6}TiO_3$ ceramic, thus there is an enhancement of BDS by 1.9 times. The reason behind the increase of BDS is the decrease in grain size, pore size, and porosity, thus the energy density is increased [101]. From the investigation of Wang *et al.*, it was found that the grain size and BDS of $BaTiO_3$ are largely affected by the addition of the glass BaO–SrO–TiO_2–Al_2O_3–SiO_2–BaF_2. They found that BDS is related to grain size as well as charge transport across the grain boundaries and has an inversely proportional relationship with average field strength, E_{GB}. The electric field E_{GB} can be defined as,

$$E_{GB} = E\left(\frac{d_B}{d_{GB}}\right)$$

Here E is the electric field applied externally, d_B represents grain size and d_{GB} represents grain-boundary space-charge layer width. Due to the addition of glass material, d_B is decreased and d_{GB} is increased, so, the average electric field is decreased in the grain boundary space charge layer and BDS is increased [102]. Recently, upon the addition of 9 wt% Bi_2O_3–B_2O_3–SiO_2 (BBS) glass with lead-free ceramics, $Ba_{0.4}Sr_{0.6}TiO_3$ (BST), a higher-energy density (1.98 J cm³) and efficiency 90.57% is achieved. The BDS is increased with the increase of BBS glass content in the ceramic composition (Table 1.4) [103].

Table 1.4 Performance of energy storage of lead-free glass ceramics.

Lead-free glass ceramics	E(kV/cm)	J_{rec} (J cm³)	η(%)	Reference
5% B_2O_3-Al_2O_3-SiO_2 glass doped $Ba_{0.85}Ca_{0.15}Zr_{0.1}Ti_{0.9}O_3$	--	1.153	75	104

(v) Storage of energy and lead-free films
The concentration of internal defects is high and BDS is low in lead-free bulk materials. Hence, there are limitations in their energy storage capacity. The defects in thin and thick films are very less as compared to bulk materials, thus BDS becomes higher, and consequently, energy density becomes higher [105]. One such example is Mn doped relaxor thin film of 0.7 $(Na_{0.5}Bi_{0.5})TiO_3$–0.3$SrTiO_3$ developed on Pt/Ti/SiO_2/Si substrate by the sol-gel method has high BDS (1894 kV/cm) and J_{rec} (27 J/cm³) [106]. The thin films grown by the physical method have better crystalline quality compared to the films developed by the chemical method; hence the BDS and energy storage capacity of the former are higher [107]. Using radio frequency magnetron sputtering, a high-quality thin film of epitaxial $BaZr_{0.2}Ti_{0.8}O_3$ was prepared by Jia *et al.* by doping Nb on $SrTiO_3$ substrate. The resulting material shows high-energy storage density (81.7%) and J_{rec} (30.4 J cm³) when 3MV/cm external electric field is applied. So far the largest J_{rec} (154 J cm³) is reported for the epitaxial lead-free relaxor thin films $(Bi_{1/2}Na_{1/2)}0.9118La_{0.02}Ba_{0.0582}(Ti_{0.97}Zr_{0.03})O_3$ (prepared by pulsed laser

deposition, applying electric field 3500 kV/cm) [108]. The energy storage capacity of these films is high because of (i) the high value of BDS (ii) epitaxially, the structure is good (iii) the excellent relaxor, and (iv) the two phases, FE and AFE coexist at the vicinity of morphotropic phase boundary (MPB). Although the density of energy is high in lead-free thin films, their overall energy-storing capacity is very limited and it is because of the limited thickness. The comparatively thick films (>1 μm) can be useful for energy storage (Table 1.5) [109].

Table 1.5 Performance of energy storage of some lead-free films.

Lead-free films	*E*(kV/cm)	J_{rec} (J cm^3)	η(%)	Reference
0.95($Na_{0.5}Bi_{0.5}$)TiO_3–0.05$SrTiO_3$ (Thick film)	1965	36.1	40.80	110
($Bi_{1/2}Na_{1/2}$)0.9118$La_{0.02}Ba_{0.0582}$($Ti_{0.97}Zr_{0.03}$)O_3 (Epitaxical thin film)	3500	154	97.00	111

(vi) Energy storage and polymer-based nanocomposites free of lead

The ferroelectric polymers having high machinability and BDS can be useful as dielectric capacitors. An example of such a polymer is poly(vinylidene fluoride) (PVDF). However, the main limitation of these types of polymers is very low energy density due to small P_{max} [112]. This problem can be overcome by proposing ceramic-polymer-based nanocomposites where the high value of maximum polarization and high value of BDS of ceramic fillers and polymer matrix, respectively get combined. But again, limitations in energy storage properties arise for two reasons (i) interfacial compatibility of an organic matrix with inorganic filler is poor, and (ii) ceramic fillers are agglomerated in the matrix of the polymer [113]. When the surface of ceramic fillers is modified, the interfacial compatibility issue is reduced. Gao *et al.* worked on the hydroxylation of the surface of BT with H_2O_2 and then they modified it with titanate coupling agent DN-101, hence the formation of nanocomposites PVDF/H_2O_2–DN-101–$BaTiO_3$ (D-h-BT) occur where P_{max} and BDS are larger as compared to the nanocomposites PVDF/DN-101–$BaTiO_3$(D-B-T). In this case, an increase (3.01–4.31 J cm^3) in the density of discharge energy was found [114]. An improvement in energy storage can also be done by using the core-shell structure of polymer-based nanocomposites. One example of such type is $BaTiO_3$–SiO_2 core-shell (BT@SO) filled novel PVDF-based nanocomposites where the particle size is less than 10 nm. The interface of the ultrafine nanostructure is larger than conventional 100 nm fillers, hence the polarization becomes high [115]. Apart from this, BDS also becomes high due to the presence of a strongly insulating SiO_2 layer. The maximum energy density and efficiency in the case of nanocomposite with BT@SO (3 vol%) were found to be 11.5 J cm^3 64%, respectively [116]. Recently, the fabrication of sandwich-structure nanocomposites and embedding them with a high BDS layer increase the electric displacement and BDS [117]. Luo *et al.* fabricated such type of sandwich-structured nanocomposites with the central layer of pure P(VDF-HPF) and two neighboring layers of $BaTiO_3$-(VDF-HPF). In the sandwich-structured nanocomposites, BDS and effective electric displacement (P_{max}–P_r) was found to be increased so also the density of discharge energy from 2.32 to 5.22 J cm^3 Table (1.6) [118].

Table 1.6 Performance of energy storage of some lead-free nanocomposites.

Lead-free nanocomposites	*E*(kV/cm)	J_{rec} (J cm^3)	η(%)	Reference
3vol% $BaTiO_3$@TiO_2 nanofibers/(PVDF-HFP)	7977	31.2	78	119
TiO_2 nanorod arrays/PVDF	3400	10.62	70	120
10 vol% H_2O_2–DN-101–$BaTiO_3$/PVDF	2600	4.31	47.83	121

1.4 Conclusion and Outlooks

For the practical application of lead-free dielectric capacitors, the criteria that need to be fulfilled are (i) recoverable energy density needs to be large, (ii) energy efficiency should be high, (iii) the charging and discharging process should be fast, and (iv) life span should be long. The energy efficiency and recoverable energy density of lead-free ceramics are very low as their P_r is large and BDS is low. The high-energy efficiency in the case of lead-free relaxor ceramics (ferroelectric and antiferroelectric) is because of their slim hysteresis loops, but due to small BDS, their recoverable energy density is not sufficient to be utilized practically. The recoverable energy density and energy efficiency of the lead-free thin film are quite high but due to their low volume, storing efficiency of energy become low. Similarly, the recoverable energy density is high in the case of thick films and various composites (polymer-based) but because of low efficiency in the ceramic matrix, the main limitations arise in their energy efficiency. These are the facts that good energy storage properties in lead-free materials can be achieved by increasing the BDS in lead-free ferroelectric or antiferroelectric materials, increasing the volume of thin films without affecting the BDS value, and increasing the energy efficiency in nanocomposites and thick films. In Bulk ceramics, BDS is related to the microstructure of the material which in turn is related to the grain size density of the materials. The appropriate microstructure can be achieved by monitoring the preparation and processing techniques (of ceramic powder) such as co-precipitation, spark plasma sintering, sol-gel method, etc. One important scope of improvement in overall low energy density in thin films and small BDS in bulk ceramics is the embedding of an alternating layer of conductive metal electrodes parallelly. In polymer-based nanocomposites, the energy efficiency and discharge energy density are high at room temperature, but in gentle conditions like that in embedded capacitors and harsh conditions like that in hybrid electric vehicles, the dissipation of energy can increase the temperature and as the melting point of polymer is low, the appropriate cooling system is required where extra energy is consumed. Thus, the development of an appropriate polymer-based capacitor is required which can function in a wide range of temperatures [122–124].

Acknowledgments

The financial support for the research along with this work was received from UGC-BSR and SERB-DST. SI is serving in the Department of Chemistry, Krishnath College with the capacity of Assistant Professor, and pursuing his research in the Chemistry Department, Burdwan University as a Ph.D. student. He thanks his colleagues and the Principal of the college for their support and encouragement in the best possible ways. UM is an Assistant Professor, serving in Chemistry Department, Burdwan University. All the authors acknowledge the Department of Chemistry, The University of Burdwan on the academic aspect.

References

1. George, J., Sreekala, M.S., Thomas, S.A., A review on interface modification and characterization of natural fiber reinforced plastic composites. *Polym. Eng. Sci.*, 41, 1471, 2001.

2. Perera, F., Pollution from fossil-fuel combustion is the leading environmental threat to global pediatric health and equity: Solutions exist. *Int. J. Environ. Res. Public Health*, 15, 16, 2017.
3. Kreps, B.H., The rising costs of fossil-fuel extraction: An energy crisis that will not go away. *Am. J. Econ. Sociol.*, *79*, 695, 2020.
4. Gielen, D., Boshell, F., Saygin, D., Bazilian, M.D., Wagner, N., Gorini, R., The role of renewable energy in the global energy transformation. *Energy Strategy Rev.*, 24, 38, 2019.
5. Jurasz, J., Canales, F.A., Kies, A., Guezgouz, M., Beluco, A., A review on the complementarity of renewable energy sources: Concept, metrics, application and future research directions. *Sol. Energy*, 195, 703, 2020.
6. Trahey, L., Brushett, F.R., Balsara, N.P., Ceder, G., Cheng, L., Chiang, Y.M., Hahn, N.T., Ingram, B.J., Minteer, S.D., Moore, J.S., Mueller, K.T., Nazar, L.F., Persson, K.A., Siegel, D.J., Xu, K., Zavadil, K.R., Srinivasan, V., Crabtree, G.W., Energy storage emerging: A perspective from the Joint Center for Energy Storage Research. *Proc. Natl. Acad. Sci.*, 117, 12550, 2020.
7. Smith, W., The role of fuel cells in energy storage. *J. Power Sources*, 86, 74, 2000.
8. Raza, W., Ali, F., Raza, N., Luo, Y., Kwon, E.E., Yang, J., Kumar, S., Mehmood, A., Kim, K.H., Recent advancements in supercapacitor technology. *Nano Energy*, 52, 441, 2018.
9. Sung, J. and Shin, C., Recent studies on supercapacitors with next-generation structures. *Micromachines*, 11, 1125, 2020.
10. Haisheng, C., Thang, N.C., Wei, Y., Chunqing, T., Yongliang, L., Yulong, D., Progress in electrical energy storage system: A critical review. *Prog. Nat. Sci.*, 19, 291, 2009.
11. Gröger, O., Gasteiger, H.A., Suchsland, J.P., Review—Electromobility: Batteries or fuel cells? *J. Electrochem. Soc.*, 162, A2605, 2015.
12. Poonam, Sharma, K., Arora, A., Tripathi, S.K., Review of supercapacitors: Materials and devices. *J. Energy Storage*, 21, 801, 2019.
13. González, A., Goikolea, E., Barrena, J.A., Mysyk, R., Review on supercapacitors: Technologies and materials. *Renew. Sustain. Energy Rev.*, 58, 1189, 2016.
14. Dongxu, L., Xiaojun, Z., Zhipeng, L., Yang, S.Z., Hua, H., Wenqin, L., Xingcai, W., Fusheng, S., Zhumei, W., Yueming, L., Progress and perspectives in dielectric energy storage ceramics. *J. Adv. Ceram.*, 10, 675, 2021.
15. Phillips, J., Toward an improved understanding of the role of dielectrics in capacitors. *Materials*, 11, 1519, 2018.
16. Zhang, T., Chen, X., Thakur, Y., Lu, B., Zhang, Q., Runt, J., Zhang, Q.M., A highly scalable dielectric metamaterial with superior capacitor performance over a broad temperature. *Sci. Adv.*, 6, 6622, 2020.
17. Praharaj, S. and Rout, D., Lead-free dielectrics: A state-of-the-art for green energy storage, in: *Advances in Nanostructured Materials*, B.P. Swain (Ed.), pp. 978–981, Springer, Singapore, 2022.

18. Liu, S., Ma, B., Narayanan, M., Tong, S., Koritala, R.E., Hu, Z., Balachandran, U., Dielectric properties of lead lanthanum zirconate titanate thin films with and without ZrO_2 insertion layers. *J. Appl. Phys.*, 113, 174107, 2013.
19. Giuseppe, G., Federico, C., Danilo, D.R., Giovanni, L., Augusto, M., Dielectric constant enhancement in a silicone elastomer filled with lead magnesium niobate–lead titanate. *Mater. Sci. Eng. C*, 27, 110, 2007.
20. Kelley, M., Eek, P.S., Shoko, Y., Eric, C., Effect of compositional variations in the lead lanthanum zirconate stannate titanate system on electrical properties. *J. Am. Ceram. Soc.*, 79, 3297, 1996.
21. Wani, A.L., Ara, A., Usmani, J.A., Lead toxicity: A review. *Interdiscip. Toxicol.*, 8, 55, 2015.
22. Zetian, Y., Hongliang, D., Li, J., Dirk, P., High-performance lead-free bulk ceramics for electrical energy storage applications: Design strategies and challenges. *J. Mater. Chem. A*, 9, 18026, 2021.
23. Siwal, S.S., Zhang, Q., Devi, N., Thakur, V.K., Carbon-based polymer nanocomposite for high-performance energy storage applications. *Polymers*, 12, 505, 2020.
24. Blanco, H. and Faaij, A., A review at the role of storage in energy systems with a focus on Power to Gas and long-term storage. *Renew. Sustain. Energy Rev.*, 81, 1049, 2018.
25. Wu, Z., Li, L., Yan, J.M., Zhang, X.B., Materials design and system construction for conventional and new-concept supercapacitors. *Adv. Sci.*, 4, 1600382, 2017.
26. Winter, M. and Brodd, R.J., What are batteries, fuel cells, and supercapacitors? *Chem. Rev.*, 104, 4245, 2004.
27. Feng, M., Feng, Y., Zhang, T., Li, J., Chen, Q., Chi, Q., Lei, Q., Recent advances in multilayer-structure dielectrics for energy storage application. *Adv. Sci.*, 8, 2102221, 2021.
28. Wang, K., Zhu, P., Xu, C., Zhang, Q., Yang, Z., Shen, R., Firing performance of microchip exploding foil initiator triggered by metal-oxide-semiconductor controlled thyristor. *Micromachines*, 11, 550, 2020.
29. Han, K., Li, Q., Chanthad, C., Gadinski, M.R., Zhang, G.Z., Wang, Q., A hybrid material approach toward solution-processable dielectrics exhibiting enhanced breakdown strength and high energy density. *Adv. Funct. Mater.*, 25, 3505, 2015.
30. Peng, B., Zhang, Q., Li, X., Sun, T., Fan, H.Q., Ke, S.M., Ye, M., Wang, Y., Lu, W., Niu, H.B., Zeng, X.R., Huang, H.T., Large energy storage density and high thermal stability in a highly textured (111)-Oriented $Pb_{0.8}Ba_{0.2}ZrO_3$ relaxor thin film with the coexistence of antiferroelectric and ferroelectric phases. *ACS Appl. Mater. Interfaces*, 7, 13512, 2015.
31. Xie, Z.K., Yue, Z.X., Peng, B., Zhang, J., Zhao, C., Zhang, X.H., Ruehl, G., Li, L.T., Large enhancement of the recoverable energy storage density and piezoelectric response in relaxor-ferroelectric capacitors by utilizing the seeding layers engineering. *Appl. Phys. Lett.*, 106, 202901, 2015.

32. Park, M.H., Kim, H.J., Kim, Y.J., Moon, T., Kim, T.D., Hwang, C.S., Effect of the annealing temperature of thin $Hf_{0.3}Zr_{0.7}O_2$ films on their energy storage behavior. *Phys. Status Solidi RRL*, 8, 857, 2014.
33. Park, M.H., Kim, H.J., Kim, Y.J., Moon, T., Kim, K.D., Hwang, C.S., Thin $Hf_xZr_{1-x}O_2$ films: A new lead-free system for electrostatic supercapacitors with large energy storage density and robust thermal stability. *Adv. Energy Mater.*, 4, 1400610, 2014.
34. Kwon, D.K. and Lee, M.H., Temperature-stable high-energy-density capacitors using complex perovskite thin films. *Ultrason. Ferroelectr. Freq. Control*, 59, 1894, 2012.
35. Tan, D., Zhang, L., Chen, Q., Irwin, P., High-temperature capacitor polymer films. *J. Electron. Mater.*, 43, 4569, 2014.
36. Liu, W.F. and Ren, X.B., Large piezoelectric effect in Pb-free ceramics. *Phys. Rev. Lett.*, 103, 257602, 2009.
37. Lee, H.N., Christen, H.M., Chisholm, M.F., Rouleau, C.M., Lowndes, D.H., Strong polarization enhancement in asymmetric three-component ferroelectric superlattices. *Nature*, 433, 395, 2005.
38. Liu, M., Ma, C.R., Collins, G., Liu, J., Chen, C.L., Dai, C., Lin, Y., Shui, L., Xiang, F., Wang, H., He, J., Jiang, J.C., Meletis, E.I., Cole, M.W., Interface engineered $BaTiO_3/SrTiO_3$ heterostructures with optimized high-frequency dielectric properties. *ACS Appl. Mater. Interfaces*, 4, 5761, 2012.
39. Yao, Z.H., Song, Z., Hao, H., Yu, Z.Y., Cao, M.H., Zhang, S.J., Lanagan, M.T., Liu, H.X., Homogeneous/inhomogeneous-structured dielectrics and their energy-storage performances. *Adv. Mater.*, 29, 1601727, 2017.
40. Hao, X.H., A review on the dielectric materials for high energy-storage application. *J. Adv. Dielectr.*, 3, 1330001, 2013.
41. Wang, F., Xu, M., Tang, Y., Wang, T., Shi, W., Leung, C.M., Large strain response in the ternary $Bi_{0.5}Na_{0.5}TiO_3$-$BaTiO_3$-$SrTiO_3$ solid solutions. *J. Am. Ceram. Soc.*, 95, 1955, 2012.
42. Kosec, M., Bobner, V., Hrovat, M., Bernard, J., Malic, B., Holc, J., New lead-free relaxors based on the $K_{0.5}Na_{0.5}NbO_3$-$SrTiO_3$ solid solution. *J. Mater. Res.*, 19, 1854, 2004.
43. Dan, Y., Xu, H.J., Zou, K.L., Zhang, Q.F., Lu, Y.M., Chang, G., Huang, H.T., He, Y.B., Energy storage characteristics of $(Pb,La)(Zr,Sn,Ti)O_3$ antiferroelectric ceramics with high Sn content. *Appl. Phys. Lett.*, 113, 063902, 2016.
44. Liu, G., Zhang, S., Jiang, W., Cao, W., Losses in ferroelectric materials. *Mater. Sci. Eng. R Rep.*, 89, 1, 2015.
45. Hafner, J., Benaglia, S., Richheimer, F., Teuschel, M., Franz, J., Maier, F.J., Werner, A., Sebastian, W., Platz, D., Schneider, M., Hradil, K., Fernando, A., Castro, F.A., Garcia, R., Schmid, U., Multi-scale characterisation of a ferroelectric polymer reveals the emergence of a morphological phase transition driven by temperature. *Nat. Commun.*, 12, 152, 2021.

46. Acosta, M., Novak, N., Rojas, V., Patel, S., Vaish, R., Koruza, J., Rossetti, G.A., Rödel, J., $BaTiO_3$-based piezoelectrics: Fundamentals, current status, and perspectives. *Appl. Phys. Rev.*, 4, 041305, 2017.
47. Wang, Y., Zhang, L., Wang, J., Li, Q., Wang, H., Gu, L., Chen, J., Deng, J., Kun Lin, K., Huang, L., Xing, X., Chemical-pressure-modulated $BaTiO_3$-thin films with large spontaneous polarization and high curie temperature. *J. Am. Chem. Soc.*, 143, 6491, 2021.
48. Huo, Z., Xie, H., Xu, J., Yang, L., Qiu, W., Zhang, X., Zhou, C., Wang, H., Tailoring the structure, energy storage, strain, and dielectric properties of $Bi_{0.5}(Na_{0.82}K_{0.18})0.5TiO_3$ ceramics by $(Fe_{1/4}Sc_{1/4}Nb_{1/2})^{4+}$ multiple complex ions. *Front. Mater.*, 7, 8, 2020.
49. Mahajan, S., Thakur, O.P., Sreenivas, K., Prakash, C., Effect of Nd doping on structural, dielectric and ferroelectric properties of $Ba(Zr_{0.05}Ti_{0.95})O_3$ ceramic. *Integr. Ferroelectr.*, 122, 83, 2010.
50. Chao, C., Hourong, Z., Xiaona, Z., Dou, Z., Kechao, Z., Haixue, Y., Effect of Ca substitution sites on dielectric properties and relaxor behavior of Ca doped barium strontium titanate ceramics. *J. Mater. Sci.: Mater. Electron.*, 26, 2486, 2015.
51. Puli, V.S., Pradhan, D.K., Riggs, B.C., Chrisey, D.B., Katiyar, R.S., Structure, ferroelectric, dielectric and energy storage studies of $BaCaTiO_3$ Ba(ZrTi)O ceramic capacitors. *Integr. Ferroelectr.*, 157, 139, 2014.
52. Chen, Z., Li, G.Z., Sun, X.J., Liu, L.J., Fang, L., La_2O_3 modified $0.4(Ba_{0.8}Ca_{0.2})TiO_3$-$0.6Bi(Mg_{0.5}Ti_{0.5})O_3$ ceramics for high-temperature capacitor applications. *Ceram. Int.*, 41, 11057, 2015.
53. Eoh, Y.J. and Kim, E.S., Dependence of dielectric properties on microstructural characteristics of $(Ba_{0.7}Sr_{0.25}Ca_{0.05})(Ti_{0.9}Zr_{0.1})O_3$ ceramics. *Ceram. Int.*, 41, S2, 2015.
54. Wu, T., Pu, Y.P., Chen, K., Dielectric relaxation behavior and energy storage properties in $Ba_{0.4}Sr_{0.6}Zr_{0.15}Ti_{0.85}O_3$ ceramics with glass additives. *Ceram. Int.*, 39, 6787, 2013.
55. Xiao, S., Xiu, S.M., Zhang, W.Q., Shen, B., Zhai, J.W., Zhang, Y., Effects of $Ba_xSr_{1-x}TiO_3$ ceramics additives on structure and energy storage properties of $Ba_{0.4}Sr_{0.6}TiO_3$-BaO-B_2O_3-Al_2O_3-SiO_2 glass-ceramic. *J. Alloys Compd.*, 675, 15, 2016.
56. Zhang, Y., Li, Y.Y., Zhu, H.K., Fu, Z.X., Zhang, Q.T., Sintering temperature dependence of dielectric properties and energy-storage properties in $(Ba,Zr)TiO_3$ ceramics. *J. Mater. Sci.: Mater. Electron.*, 28, 514, 2017.
57. Puli, V.S., Kumar, A., Chrisey, D.B., Tomozawa, M., Scott, J.F., Katiyar, R.S., Barium zirconate-titanate/barium calcium-titanate ceramics via sol-gel process: Novel high-energy-density capacitors. *J. Phys. D: Appl. Phys.*, 44, 395403, 2011.
58. Feng, M., Feng, Y., Zhang, T., Li, J., Chen, Q., Chi, Q., Lei, Q., Recent advances in multilayer-structure dielectrics for energy storage application. *Adv. Sci.*, 8, 2102221, 2021.

59. Wang, G., Lu, Z., Li, Y., Li, L., Ji, H., Feteira, A., Zhou, D., Wang, D., Zhang, S., Reaney, I.M., Electroceramics for high-energy density capacitors: Current status and future perspectives. *Chem. Rev.*, 121, 6124, 2021.
60. Jin, Q., Pu, Y.P., Wang, C., Gao, Z.Y., Zheng, H.Y., Enhanced energy storage performance of $Ba_{0.4}Sr_{0.6}TiO_3$ ceramics: Influence of sintering atmosphere. *Ceram. Int.*, 43, 232, 2017.
61. Wang, G., Lu, Z., Li, Y., Li, L., Ji, H., Feteira, A., Zhou, D., Wang, D., Zhang, S., Reaney, I.M., Electroceramics for high-energy density capacitors: Current status and future perspectives. *Chem. Rev.*, 121, 6124, 2021.
62. Liu, Z.F., Zhang, Z.Q., Zhang, F.Q., Li, Y.X., Enhanced energy storage properties of barium titanate ceramics made from surface modified particles. *J. Adv. Dielectr.*, 3, 1350023, 2013.
63. Song, Z., Zhang, S.J., Liu, H.X., Hao, H., Cao, M.H., Li, Q., Wang, Q., Yao, Z.H., Wang, Z.J., Lanagan, M.T., Improved energy storage properties accompanied by enhanced interface polarization in annealed microwave-sintered BST. *J. Am. Ceram. Soc.*, 98, 3212, 2015.
64. Yang, Z.T., Du, H.L., Qu, S.B., Hou, Y.D., Ma, H., Wang, J.F., Wang, J., Wei, X.Y., Xu, Z., Significantly enhanced recoverable energy storage density in potassium-sodium niobate-based lead-free ceramics. *J. Mater. Chem. A*, 4, 13778, 2016.
65. Wang, T., Jin, L., Li, C.C., Hu, Q.Y., Wei, X.Y., Relaxor ferroelectric $BaTiO_3$-$Bi(Mg_{2/3}Nb_{1/3})O_3$ ceramics for energy storage application. *J. Am. Ceram. Soc.*, 98, 559,2015.
66. Zhang, Q.M., Wang, L., Luo, J., Tang, Q., Du, J., Improved energy storage density in barium strontium titanate by addition of BaO-SiO_2-B_2O_3 glass. *J. Am. Ceram. Soc.*, 92, 1871, 2009.
67. Xu, Q., Li, T.M., Hao, H., Zhang, S.J., Wang, Z.J., Cao, M.H., Yao, Z.H., Liu, H.X., Enhanced energy storage properties of $NaNbO_3$ modified $Bi_{0.5}Na_{0.5}TiO_3$ based ceramics. *J. Eur. Ceram. Soc.*, 35, 545, 2015.
68. Rainer, W., Ulrich, B., Stephan, T., Relaxor ferroelectrics - from random field models to glassy relaxation and domain states, in: *Polar Oxides: Properties, Characterization, and Imaging*, R. Waser, U. Bottger, S. Tiedke (Eds.), pp. 275–301, 2004.
69. Shvartsman, V.V., Dkhil, B., Kholkin, A.L., Mesoscale domains and nature of the relaxor state by piezoresponse force microscopy. *Annu. Rev. Mater. Res.*, 43, 423, 2013.
70. Yang, L., Ting, L., Aziguli, H., Wenhan, X., Yao, Z., Li, L., Seong, H.K., Qing, W., Relaxor ferroelectric polymers: Insight into high electrical energy storage properties from a molecular perspective. *Small Sci.*, 1, 2000061, 2021.
71. Raddaoui, Z., El Kossi, S., Dhahri, J., Abdelmoula, N., Taibi, K., Study of diffuse phase transition and relaxor ferroelectric behavior of $Ba_{0.97}Bi_{0.02}Ti_{0.9}Zr_{0.05}Nb_{0.04}O_3$ ceramic. *RSC Adv.*, 9, 2412, 2019.
72. Lin, Y., Li, D., Zhang, M., Zhan, S., Yang, Y., Yang, H., Yuan, Q., Excellent energy storage properties achieved in $BaTiO_3$-based lead-free relaxor

ferroelectric ceramics via domain engineering on the nanoscale. *ACS Appl. Mater. Interfaces*, 11, 36824, 2019.
73. Triamnak, N., Yimnirun, R., Pokorny, J., Cann, D.P., Relaxor characteristics of the phase transformation in (1-x)$BaTiO_3$-xBi$(Zn_{1/2}Ti_{1/2})O_3$ perovskite ceramics. *J. Am. Ceram. Soc.*, 96, 3176, 2013.
74. Qiu, Y., Lin, Y., Liu, X., Yang, H., $Bi(Mg_{2/3}Nb_{1/3})O_3$ addition inducing high recoverable energy storage density in lead-free 0.65$BaTiO_3$-0.35$Bi_{0.5}Na_{0.5}TiO_3$ bulk ceramics. *J. Alloys Compd.*, 797, 348, 2019.
75. Zhao, X.B., Zhou, Z.Y., Liang, R.H., Liu, F.H., Dong, X.L., High-energy storage performance in lead-free (1-x)$BaTiO_3$-xBi$(Zn_{0.5}Ti_{0.5})O_3$ relaxor ceramics for temperature stability applications. *Ceram. Int.*, 43, 9066, 2017.
76. Huang, J., Zhang, J., Yu, H., Wei, M., Chen, H., Yang, C., Improvement of dielectric and energy storage properties in $BaTiO_3$ ceramics with $BiNbO_4$ modified. *Ferroelectrics*, 510, 8, 2017.
77. Si, F., Tang, B., Fang, Z., Zhang, S., Structural and dielectric relaxor properties of $(1-x)BaTiO_3-xBi(Zn_{1/2}Zr_{1/2})O_3$ ceramics for energy storage applications. *J. Mater. Sci. Mater. Electron.*, 30, 2772, 2019.
78. Hu, Q., Wang, T., Zhao, L., Jin, L., Xu, Z., Wei, X., Dielectric and energy storage properties of $BaTiO_3$–$Bi(Mg_{1/2}Ti_{1/2})O_3$ ceramic: Influence of glass addition and biasing electric field. *Ceram. Int.*, 43, 35, 2017.
79. Si, F., Tang, B., Fang, Z., Li, H., Zhang, S., Enhanced energy storage and fast charge-discharge properties of (1-x)$BaTiO_3$-xBi$(Ni_{1/2}Sn_{1/2})O_3$ relaxor ferroelectric ceramics. *Ceram. Int.*, 45, 17580, 2019.
80. Liu, G., Li, Y., Shi, M., Yu, L., Chen, P., Yu, K., Yan, Y., Jin, L., Wang, D., Gao, J., An investigation of the dielectric energy storage performance of $Bi(Mg_{2/3}Nb_{1/3})O_3$-modifed $BaTiO_3$ Pb-free bulk ceramics with improved temperature/frequency stability. *Ceram. Int.*, 45, 19189, 2019.
81. Genenko, Y.A., Glaum, J., Hoffmann, M.J., Albe, K., Mechanisms of aging and fatigue in ferroelectrics. *Mater. Sci. Eng. B*, 192, 52, 2015.
82. Tolédano, P. and Guennou, M., Theory of antiferroelectric phase transitions. *Phys. Rev. B*, 94, 014107, 2016.
83. Jin, L., Li, F., Zhang, S.J., Decoding the fingerprint of ferroelectric loops: Comprehension of the material properties and structures. *J. Am. Ceram. Soc.*, 97, 27, 2014.
84. Pan, W.Y., Dam, C.Q., Zhang, Q.M., Cross, L.E., Large displacement transducers based on electric field forced phase transitions in the tetragonal $(Pb_{0.97}La_{0.02})(Ti,Zr,Sn)O_3$ family of ceramics. *J. Appl. Phys.*, 66, 6014, 1989.
85. Xu, R., Xu, Z., Feng, Y.J., Wei, X.Y., Tian, J.J., Nonlinear dielectric and discharge properties of $Pb_{0.94}La_{0.04}[(Zr_{0.56}Sn_{0.44})0.84Ti_{0.16}]O_3$ antiferroelectric ceramics. *J. Appl. Phys.*, 120, 144102, 2016.
86. Ding, J.X., Liu, Y.F., Lu, Y.N., Qian, H., Gao, H., Chen, H., Ma, C.J., Enhanced energy-storage properties of 0.89$Bi_{0.5}Na_{0.5}TiO_3$-0.06$BaTiO_3$-0.05$K_{0.5}Na_{0.5}NbO_3$ lead-free anti-ferroelectric ceramics by two-step sintering method. *Mater. Lett.*, 114, 107, 2014.

87. Wang, Y.F., Lv, Z.L., Xie, H., Cao, J., High energy-storage properties of $[(Bi_{1/2}Na_{1/2})0.94Ba_{0.06}]La_{(1-x)}Zr_xTiO_3$ lead-free anti-ferroelectric ceramics. *Ceram. Int.*, 40, 4323, 2014.
88. Tian, Y., Jin, L., Zhang, H.F., Xu, Z., Wei, X.Y., Politova, E.D., Stefanovich, S.Y., Tarakina, N.V., Abrahams, I., Yan, H.X., High energy density in silver niobate ceramics. *J. Mater. Chem. A*, 4, 17279, 2016.
89. Zhang, Q.F., Tong, H.F., C.J., Lu, Y.M., Yang, T.Q., Yao, X., He, Y.B., High recoverable energy density over a wide temperature range in Sr modified $(Pb,La)(Zr,Sn,Ti)O_3$ antiferroelectric ceramics with an orthorhombic phase. *Appl. Phys. Lett.*, 109, 262901, 2016.
90. Tian, Y., Jin, L., Zhang, H.F., Xu, Z., Wei, X.Y., Viola, G., Abrahams, I., Yan, H.X., Phase transitions in bismuth-modified silver niobate ceramics for high power energy storage. *J. Mater. Chem. A*, 5, 17525, 2017.
91. Shannon, R.D., Revised effective ionic radii and systematic studies of interatomic distances in halides and chalcogenides. *Acta Crystallogr. A*, 32, 751, 1976.
92. Zhao, L., Liu, Q., Gao, J., Zhang, S., Li, J.F., Lead-free antiferroelectric silver niobate tantalate with high energy storage performance. *Adv. Mater.*, 29, 1701824, 2017.
93. Tian, Y., Jin, L., Zhang, H.F., Xu, Z., Wei, X.Y., Politova, E.D., Stefanovich, S.Y., Tarakina, N.V., Abrahamsc, I., Yan, H.X., High energy density in silver niobate ceramics. *J. Mater. Chem. A*, 4, 17279, 2016.
94. Zhao, L., Liu, Q., Gao, J., Zhang, S.J., Li, J.F., Lead-free antiferroelectric silver niobate tantalate with high energy storage performance. *Adv. Mater.*, 29, 1701824, 2017.
95. Tian, Y., Jin, L., Zhang, H.F., Xu, Z., Wei, X.Y., Viola, G., Abrahams, I., Yan, H.X., Phase transitions in bismuth-modified silver niobate ceramics for high power energy storage. *J. Mater. Chem. A*, 5, 17525, 2017.
96. Zhao, L., Liu, Q., Zhang, S.J., Li, J.F., Lead-free $AgNbO_3$ antiferroelectric ceramics with an enhanced energy storage performance using mno_2 modification. *J. Mater. Chem. C*, 4, 8380, 2016.
97. Hao, J.G., Xu, Z.J., Chu, R.Q., Li, W., Du, J., Fu, P., Enhanced energy-storage properties of $(1\text{-}x)[(1\text{-}y)(Bi_{0.5}Na_{0.5})TiO_3\text{-}y(Bi_{0.5}K_{0.5})TiO_3]\text{-}x(K_{0.5}Na_{0.5})NbO_3$ lead-free ceramics. *Solid State Commun.*, 204, 19, 2015.
98. Wu, Z.H., Liu, H.X., Cao, M.H., Shen, Z.Y., Yao, Z.H., Hao, H., Luo, D.B., Effect of $BaO\text{-}Al_2O_3\text{-}B_2O_3\text{-}SiO_2$ glass additive on densification and dielectric properties of $Ba_{0.3}Sr_{0.7}TiO_3$ ceramics. *J. Ceram. Soc. Jpn.*, 116, 345, 2008.
99. Divya, P.V. and Kumar, V., Crystallization studies and properties of $(Ba_{1-x}Sr_x)TiO_3$ in borosilicate glass. *J. Am. Ceram. Soc.*, 90, 472, 2007.
100. Wang, T., Jin, L., Shu, L., Hu, Q., Wei, X., Energy storage properties in $Ba_{0.4}Sr_{0.6}TiO_3$ ceramics with addition of semi-conductive $BaO\text{-}B_2O_3\text{-}SiO_2\text{-}Na_2CO_3\text{-}K_2CO_3$ glass. *J. Alloys Compd.*, 617, 399, 2014.

101. Zhang, Q.M., Wang, L., Luo, J., Tang, Q., Du, J., Improved energy storage density in barium strontium titanate by addition of $BaO-SiO_2-B_2O_3$ glass. *J. Am. Ceram. Soc.*, 92, 1871, 2009.
102. Wang, X.R., Zhang, Y., Song, X.Z. Yuan, Z.B., Ma, T., Zhang, Q. Deng, C.S., Liang, T.X., Glass additive in barium titanate ceramics and its influence on electrical breakdown strength in relation with energy storage properties. *J. Eur. Ceram. Soc.*, 32, 559, 2012.
103. Yang, H.B., Yan, F., Lin, Y., Wang, T., Enhanced energy storage properties of $Ba_{0.4}Sr_{0.6}TiO_3$ lead-free ceramics with $Bi_2O_3-B_2O_3-SiO_2$ glass addition. *J. Eur. Ceram. Soc.*, 38, 1367, 2018.
104. Yang, H.B., Yan, F., Zhang, G., Lin, Y., Wang, F., Dielectric behavior and impedance spectroscopy of lead-free $Ba_{0.85}Ca_{0.15}Zr_{0.1}Ti_{0.9}O_3$ ceramics with $B_2O_3-Al_2O_3-SiO_2$ glass-ceramics addition for enhanced energy storage. *J. Alloys Compd.*, 720, 116, 2017.
105. Vignaswaran, V., Federica, B., Theresa, G., Marco, D., Strategies to improve the energy storage properties of perovskite lead-free relaxor ferroelectrics: A review. *Materials*, 13, 5742, 2020.
106. Zhang, Y.L., Li, W.L., Cao, W.P., Feng, Y., Qiao, Y.L., Zhang, T.D., Fei, W.D., Mn doping to enhance energy storage performance of lead-free 0.7NBT-0.3ST thin films with weak oxygen vacancies. *Appl. Phys. Lett.*, 110, 243901, 2017.
107. Dang, C.N., Viet, C.L., Dinh, T.B., Duc, T.P., Xuan, D.L., Ngoc, H.V., Duc, Q.N., Effect of crystallization temperature on energy-storage density and efficiency of lead-free $Bi_{0.5}(Na_{0.8}K_{0.2})0.5TiO_3$ thin films prepared by sol-gel method. *J. Sci.: Adv. Mater. Devices*, 4, 370, 2019.
108. Sun, Z.X., Ma, C.R., Wang, X., Liu, M., Lu, L., Wu, M., Lou, X.J., Wang, H., Jia, C.L., Large energy density, excellent thermal stability, and high cycling endurance of lead-free $BaZr_{0.2}Ti_{0.8}O_3$ film capacitors. *ACS Appl. Mater. Interfaces*, 9, 17096, 2017.
109. Yang, B.B., Guo, M.Y., Jin, L.H., Tang, X.W., Wei, R.H., Hu, L., Yang, J., Song, W.H., Dai, J.M., Lou, X.J., Zhu, X.B., Sun, Y.P., Ultrahigh energy storage in lead-free $BiFeO_3Bi_{3.25}$ $L_{0.75}Ti_3O_{12}$ thin film capacitors by solution processing. *Appl. Phys. Lett.*, 112, 033904, 2018.
110. Xu, Z.S., Hao, X.H., An, S.L., Dielectric properties and energy-storage performance of $(Na_{0.5}Bi_{0.5})TiO_3-SrTiO_3$ thick films derived from polyvinylpyrrolidone-modified chemical solution. *J. Alloys Compd.*, 639, 387, 2015.
111. Peng, B.L., Zhang, Q., Li, X., Sun, T.Y., Fan, H.Q., Ke, S.M., Ye, M., Wang, Y., Lu, W., Niu, H.B., Scott, J.F., Zeng, X.R., Huang, H.T., Giant electric energy density in epitaxial lead-free thin films with coexistence of ferroelectrics and antiferroelectrics. *Adv. Electron. Mater.*, 1, 1500052, 2015.
112. Meng, N., Ren, X., Santagiuliana, G., Ventura, L., Zhang, H., Wu, J., Yan, H., Reece, M.J., Bilotti, E., Ultrahigh β-phase content poly(vinylidene fluoride) with relaxor-like ferroelectricity for high energy density capacitors. *Nat. Commun.*, 10, 4535, 2019.

113. Dias, C.J., Igreja, R., Mendes, R., Inacio, P., Mendes, J.N., Gupta, D.K., Recent advances in ceramic-polymer composite electrets. *IEEE Trans. Dielectr. Electr. Insul.*, 11, 35, 2004.
114. Gao, L., He, J.L., Hu, J., Li, Y., Large enhancement in polarization response and energy storage properties of poly(vinylidene fluoride) by improving the interface effect in nanocomposites. *J. Phys. Chem. C*, 118, 831, 2014.
115. Ke, B., Meihua, B., Yanan., H., Wei, L., Ziming, C., Xiaohui, W., Huang, Y., Ultrafine core-shell $BaTiO_3$@SiO_2 structures for nanocomposite capacitors with high energy density. *Nano Energy*, 51, 513, 2018.
116. Bi., K., Bi, M.H., Hao, Y.N., Luo, W., Cai, Z.M., Wang, X.H., Huang, Y.H., Ultrafine core-shell $BaTiO_3$@SiO_2 structures for nanocomposite capacitors with high energy density. *Nano Energy*, 51, 523, 2018.
117. Hu, P., Wang, J., Shen, Y., Guan, Y., Lin, Y., Nan, C.W., Highly enhanced energy density induced by hetero-interface in sandwich-structured polymer nanocomposites. *J. Mater. Chem. A*, 1, 12321, 2013.
118. Luo, H., Zhang, D., Wang, L., Chen, C., Zhou, J., Zhou, K.C., Highly enhanced dielectric strength and energy storage density in Hydantoin@$BaTiO_3$-P(VDF-HFP) composites by a sandwich-structure. *RSC Adv.*, 5, 52809, 2015.
119. Zhang, X., Shen, Y., Xu, B., Zhang, Q.H., Gu, L., Jiang, J.Y., Ma, J., Lin, Y.H., Nan, C.W., Giant energy density and improved discharge efficiency of solution-processed polymer nanocomposites for dielectric energy storage. *Adv. Mater.*, 28, 2055, 2016.
120. Yao, L.M., Pan, Z.B., Liu, S.H., Zhai, J.W., Haydn, H.D., Significantly enhanced energy density in nanocomposite capacitors combining the TiO_2 nanorod array with poly(vinylidene fluoride). *ACS Appl. Mater. Interfaces*, 8, 26343, 2016.
121. Gao, L., He, J.L., Hu, J., Li, Y., Large enhancement in polarization response and energy storage properties of poly(vinylidene fluoride) by improving the interface effect in nanocomposites. *J. Phys. Chem. C*, 118, 831, 2014.
122. Chen, L.M., Sun, N.N., Li, Y., Zhang, Q.W., Zhang, L.W., Hao, X.H., Multifunctional antiferroelectric MLCC with high-energy-storage properties and large field-induced strain. *J. Am. Ceram. Soc.*, 101, 2313, 2018.
123. Wang, D.W., Fan, Z.M., Zhou, D., Khesro, A., Murakami, S., Feteira, A., Zhao, Q.L., Tan, X.L., Reaney, I.M., Bismuth ferrite-based lead-free ceramics and multilayers with high recoverable energy density. *J. Mater. Chem. A*, 6, 4144, 2018.
124. Chen, X.F., Zhang, H.L., Cao, F., Wang, G.S., Dong, X.L., Gu, Y., He, H.L., Liu, Y.S., Charge-discharge properties of lead zirconate stannate titanate ceramics. *J. Appl. Phys.*, 106, 034105, 2009.

2

Lead-Based Ceramics for High-Performance Supercapacitors

Muneer Hussain[1], Muhammad Tahir Khan[1*], Ata-ur-Rehman[2†] and Syed Mustansar Abbas[3‡]

[1]*Department of Physics, Riphah International University, Islamabad, Pakistan*
[2]*Department of Chemistry, Govt. Graduate College, Asghar Mall, Rawalpindi, Pakistan*
[3]*Nanoscience & Technology Department, National Centre for Physics, Islamabad, Pakistan*

Abstract

Nowadays, supercapacitors are extensively used in energy storage devices owing to their rapid diffusion of charge, large cyclic life, huge power density, and non-toxicity. There is a lot of research on nanomaterials to obtain cheap, efficient, and stable electrode materials. In this regard, ceramic-based materials have highlighted new options for supercapacitor electrodes, but the lower specific surface area impedes the performance characteristics, thereby hampering their use on a large scale. Thus, there is a dire need to understand the basics of these ceramics, the optimization techniques, and the research development to improve electrical conductivity, cycling life, power density, and ion transferability. Here, in this study, various ceramic materials are overviewed especially metal-based oxides, mixed ceramics, single-element and multi-element-based ceramics, hydro-oxide ceramics, and other binary metallic oxides (spinal ceramics). Each composition has its own merits and demerits, which greatly rely on the synthesis technique and additives concentration. Other factors like temperature and the sintering environment also affect key parameters like particle size. Moreover, the principle and characteristics of various types of electroceramics have also been discussed in detail. Our focus is to highlight the development of ceramic materials for supercapacitor application and their key factors, and characteristics, lead-based ferroelectric, relaxor, and

**Corresponding author*: qau_abbas@yahoo.com
†*Corresponding author*: ata.qau@gmail.com
‡*Corresponding author*: mtahir.khan@riphah.edu.pk

Inamuddin, Tariq Altalhi and Sayed Mohammed Adnan (eds.) Electroceramics for High Performance Supercapacitors, (25–52) © 2024 Scrivener Publishing LLC

anti-ferroelectric materials. Additionally, the conclusion and futuristic approach have also been discussed.

***Keywords*:** Lead-based ceramics, supercapacitors, lead-based ferroelectric, carbon nanotubes, piezoelectric

2.1 Introduction

Attempts to unveil electrical energy-storing systems for diverse materials and applications have been rising day by day due to their extensive use in many fields of science and technology. To meet energy demands, several renewable energy resources have been developed. For example, solar technology, geothermal energy, wind energy, tidal energy, and biofuel are the main energy generation techniques used for decades. Besides energy production, there is a need to store energy in an efficient manner [1, 2]. There are many energy storage technologies to store electrical energy, including fuel cells (chemical storage and conversion), thermal and thermochemical energy storage devices, flywheel (mechanical storage), electrical devices (ordinary physical capacitors, dual-layered capacitors), and electrochemical devices (batteries). Nowadays, capacitors and batteries are the two major devices that can store electrical energy very efficiently. These two devices offer a unique charge/discharge mechanism, and their utilization depends upon the kind of device that is to be employed [3]. For long-lasting with stable performance requirements, batteries are being used with slow discharging phenomena for hours, while capacitors have been extensively utilized for a rapid charge-discharge pre-requisite. The time for discharging electrochemical capacitors is approximately 10 seconds, while electrostatic discharge is very rapid within a few microseconds. If this short discharging time is combined with the large power density, then these capacitors are very favorable for energy storage applications in many applications, especially pulsed power applications [4]. Supercapacitors are electrochemical capacitors that can store charge rapidly with discharging time of 1-10 seconds, brilliant reversibility, huge cycling stability (>30,000 hours, 10^5 cycles approximately), easy operational mode, nontoxic, large energy and power densities (10 KW Kg^{-1}) [5–7]. These special properties lead supercapacitors to fill the gap of large energy and power densities in fuel cells and batteries [8]. Moreover, a charge storage phenomenon is very simple which produces lower thermochemical heat [9]. These ultra-capacitors have created a wider space in consumer electronics, backup storage, memory technologies, and commercialized power systems [10, 11]. There are several materials used for supercapacitor electrodes i.e., carbon, carbon nanotubes (CNTs), graphene oxide (GO), conducting polymers [12], oxides and hydroxides [13, 14], sulfides [15, 16], nitrates [17] and metal-organic frameworks (MOFs) [18]. Usually, capacitance (ability to store charge), resistance (series equivalent), and operating potential are the significant features to check out the capacitor's performance [19]. One of the important features which determine the capacitor's performance is cyclic stability [20]. Other factors which are also to be considered are the material from which the electrode has been fabricated, the electrolyte being used as well as potential window [21, 22]. Moreover, current development in an investigation on the structural sketch and fabrication of electrodes is to create a huge specific area of surface, a larger abundant porous surface, and better conductivity. This enables better electron and ion diffusion capabilities [23]. Nowadays, several metals, polymeric materials, and ceramics MOFs have been searched for supercapacitor electrodes. Ceramics are frequently ignored due to their small surface area and surface activity, but on the other hand, their excellent corrosion ability, great thermal resistance, stability, and shock resistance make these materials favorable for the supercapacitor electrode materials [24–27].

2.2 General Idea of Ceramics for Supercapacitors

Ceramics are a kind of nonmetallic, non-organic, and water-insoluble materials that may be crystal or glassy, or they may contain both structures. These materials can offer ion involvement in their respective chemical bonding. These materials have various applications in different electronic devices, and their application is not ignorable [28]. A revolution in the development of ferroelectric ceramics had been started during World War II due to their large dielectric constant, better piezo-electrical constants, and coefficients. In those days, the composite $BaTiO_3$ had been used for small plates and tube capacitors. Since the 1970s, monolithic multilayered capacitors (MLCs) have been frequently engaged in extensive applications. Currently, the yearly estimated production level of MLCs has roughly increased to a hundred billion. Furthermore, microwave ceramics has been extensively common for wireless communications using resonators, filters, and other devices. The type of ceramics composed of lead, tin, and zirconia oxide composite is generally referred to as piezoelectric ceramics that have extensive applications in ultrasound cleaners, alarm systems, sound navigation and ranging systems (SONAR), accelerometer, echo sounders system, acoustic wave system, filters, acoustic delay line system and other applications. The excellent performance of ceramics has made ceramics a favorable material that has large mechanical strength, better thermal strength, and excellent optical, magnetic, and electrical characteristics [29, 30].

2.2.1 Metallic Oxide Ceramics for Supercapacitors

Metallic oxide materials are extensively utilized because of their availability, cheapness, easy synthesis, environmental friendliness, and large valences [31–33]. Metal oxides are used in supercapacitor electrodes [34–37], lithium-ion batteries (LIBs) [38–40], and fuel cells. Transition metal oxides are commonly investigated because these materials are cheap and non-toxic. [41–43]. Recently, metal oxide ceramics are introduced as supercapacitor electrodes i.e., Co_3O_4, MnO_2, Mn_3O_4. To achieve high energy density, surface redox chemistry is adopted by utilizing transition metal oxides. Lang's group worked on MnO_2 electrode with V_2O_3 and obtained higher electrical power up to 422 W cm^{-3} [44]. The conductivity, pseudo-capacitance, and rate capability improved a lot due to electronic correlation and efficient charge transfer of MnO_2 constituents. Transition metal oxide ceramics (TMOCs) can also be synthesized by electro-spinning, a less hazardous technique that can yield a smaller diameter, highly crystalline structure. For instance, Co_3O_4 with nano-wire has been fabricated by using electro-spinning, and it produces highly crystalline structured material [45]. The supercapacitor was fabricated by using as-prepared Co_3O_4 anode while carbon is being used as a cathode material and this can produce a capacity of the power density of around 1400 W kg^{-1} with an energy density of 48 Wh kg^{-1}. Likewise, nickel oxide (NiO) nanowires were synthesized by using the electrospinning technique and it produces greater crystallinity and cycling stability as well as better columbic efficiency [46]. Table 2.1 shows the different metal oxide ceramic materials for the application of the supercapacitors.

2.2.2 Binary Metal Oxides

2.2.2.1 Ceramics of Spinal Oxide Material

Spinal oxides consist of binary metals, which enhance oxidation-reduction reactions more than a single oxide component [62]. Binary coupled metal oxides represent enhanced conductivity and better electrochemical activity than single-constituted metal oxide. A study of MFe_2O_4 reveals that this composition is better for supercapacitors use as an electrode.

Table 2.1 Metal oxide ceramic materials for the application of the supercapacitor.

Materials	Methods	Shape	Capacitance	Reference
$SnO_2/CaSnO_3$-Ba	Spray pyrolysis	Core-shell	-	[47]
Al_2O_3	Laser etching process	Micropillars	5.5 $mFcm^{-2}$ at 5 mVs^{-1}	[48]
V_2O_5	Sol gel process	Scaffold's lamellar	-	[49]
NiO/ZrO_2	Template process	Membranes	342 Fg^{-1} at 2 Ag^{-1}	[50]
NiO/Ni	Colloidal technique	Core-shell structure	755 Fg^{-1} at 2 Ag^{-1}	[51]
Nickle oxide	Precipitation	Nanostructured platelets	1000 Fg^{-1} at 2 Ag^{-1}	[52]
Nickle oxide	Electrospinning	Nanowire	670 Fg^{-1} at 5 Ag^{-1}	[53]
CuO Co_3O_4	Electrospinning	Nanowire	1277 Fg^{-1} at 2 Ag^{-1}	[54]
Co_3O_4	Electrospinning	Nanowire in thin form	1110 Fg^{-1} at 1 Ag^{-1}	[55]
Co_3O_4	Hydrothermal process	Urchin type nanoparticles	-	[56]
V_2O_3/MnO_2	Pulsed electrodeposited method	Corundum like crystals	1172 F cm^{-3} at 10 mV s^{-1}	[57]
(Fe, Zn)OOH-PNT	Chemical precipitation	Composite	4 Fcm^{-2} at 2 mVs^{-1}	[58]

(Continued)

Table 2.1 Metal oxide ceramic materials for the application of the supercapacitor. *(Continued)*

Materials	**Methods**	**Shape**	**Capacitance**	**Reference**
Mn_3O_4-carbon nanotube (CNT)	Chemical precipitation technique	Flakes	5 Fcm^{-2} at 2 mVs^{-1}	[58]
MnO_2-foamed Ni	Spray pyrolysis process	Thin film	45 Fg^{-1}	[59]
Mn_3O_4-multiwalled CNT	Liquid-liquid extraction method	Nanostructured	3 Fcm^{-2} at 2 mVs^{-1}	[60]
MnO_2-multiwalled CNT	Liquid-liquid extraction method	Nanostructured	5.7 Fcm^{-2} at 2 mVs^{-1}	[60]
MnO_x	Mild template and hydrothermal processes	Cellular foamed shape	-	[61]

$NiFe_2O_4$ presented a better choice, fabricated by different processes that significantly influence the properties like specific capacity and porosity. Anwar *et al.* fabricated $NiFe_2O_4$ by a sol-gel technique which has shown a specific capacity of 98 F g^{-1} [63]. On the other hand, $CoZnFe_2O_4$ prepared by the co-precipitation method showed promisingly enhanced capacitance of up to 380 F g^{-1} at the scan rate of about 10 millivolts per second. Zinc manganese oxide has also been investigated, which shows this composition consists of four band gaps and also furnishes a suitably larger surface area just after calcination and has been concluded that this composition can be a superior choice as an electrode material [64]. Kovalenko and coworkers studied Ni-Co_2O_4 and reported that the valence of nickel and cobalt greatly enhances the conductivity of the supercapacitor electrode [65].

2.2.2.2 Barium Titanate Ceramics

These ceramics refer to polymers with some alkaline earth metal titanates, which are used as polymeric separators in energy storage applications. For instance, $BaTiO_3$ film was fabricated by solvent precipitation method and porosity increased by adding lithium chloride with heating. This technique dramatically increases the rate of charge transfer. $BaTiO_3$ composition enhances the dielectric constant to be used as a separator. Polymeric $BaTiO_3$ presents small electrochemical resistance with higher specific capacitance. Gu *et al.* worked on $BaTiO_3$ by combining the roll coating method with the thermal curing method and suggested that particle size affects the dielectric properties of the prepared sample. It will affect the electrochemical performance of $BaTiO_3$ ceramics [66]. The reaction mechanism also affects the performance of the material. Under the hydrothermal reaction mechanism, the morphology of $BaTiO_3$ has been observed to vary from cubic to starfish and snowflake type. Moreover, compatibility can also be improved by altering $BaTiO_3$ with amine groups. The core-shell matrix was investigated by Chung *et al.* and concluded that this structure comprises $Ba_2TiSi2O_8$ second phase with improved electrochemical properties. [67]. In another study, $BaTiO_3$ coated with a silica shell was prepared by sintering at a reduced temperature. In such a reaction, at the temperature of 850°C and 1000°C, Ba diffused into a silica shell with fresnoite crystallite growth on the surface of the $BaTiO_3$ [68]. The permittivity of around 2000 can be obtained by microwave and spark plasma sintering, stabilizing the dielectric losses. This technique can also be applied to the core-shell structure of silica shell mixed $BaTiO_3$, reducing dielectric losses that produce rapid sintering and cooling rate. It will lead to re-oxidation and dielectric barrier resulting in supercapacitor behavior. Thus, $BaTiO_3$ with a silica shell is a potential ceramic-based electrode ceramic in supercapacitors [69].

2.2.3 Multimetal Oxidized Ceramics

Recently, some studies on rare earth elements incorporated in ceramics have been reported due to their better dielectric characteristics [70]. Table 2.2 shows the multi-metal oxidized ceramics materials for the application of the supercapacitors. Variable oxidation states provided by the transition metal can offer high electrical conductivity with a reduction in activation energy for charge diffusion, leading to increased specific capacitance. For instance, Marity *et al.* prepared $CaCu_3Ti_4O_{12}$ (CCTO) with molten salt and revealed that this composition could lead to high permittivity [71]. Furthermore, A^{+3} acceptor dopant and B^{+5} donor dopant furnish better performance in supercapacitor applications. Acceptor dopants include, Yb, Ga, Sc, Bi, Sm, In, etc and donor dopants include Sb, Nb, Ta, etc [72]. The multi-elemental oxidized ceramics represent huge dielectric permittivity due to the electronic defect dipole process. A study by Shire *et al.* reported the yttrium aluminum garnet electrode by pulsed voltage process and deduced a specific capacitance of 250 F g^{-1} [73]. The same type of composition is prepared by an electro-polymerization mechanism with cyclic voltammetry (CV). This technique enhances specific capacitance with an improvement in cyclic stability due to a better charge diffusion mechanism. Yttrium oxide has also been used to prepare the separator of the ultracapacitors [74]. In another study, $Li_{0.33}La_{0.56}TiO_3$ composition is suitable for solid-state ultra-capacitors with a capacitive ability of 0.28 MF g^{-1} under 2 V potential at a temperature of 300 Kelvin [75]. Temperature, Ceramic grain, and ceramic grain boundary are three factors that affect ion diffusion. Moreover, the structure could be changed by altering Li^+ ion concentration. For example, a tetragonal structure can be converted into cubic by increasing Li^+ ion concentration, which increases conductivity in the crystal grains with no effect on the conductivity of the grain boundaries. Liu *et al.* coated copper oxide layer on the composition $La_{1-x}Sr_xCo_{-}O_{3-\delta}$ and deduced that high conductive CuO makes electrode ideal for capacitive applications [76].

2.2.4 Metal Hydroxide-Type Ceramics

Metal hydroxide (MHC) is a potential source for supercapacitor application due to its higher capacity and the material's mechanical strength. $Cu(OH)_2$ prepared with a three-dimensional printing method leads to high columbic efficiency with better reversibility [92]. Furthermore, Cu $(OH)_2$ supercapacitor resulted in a large capacitance (volumetric) of around 6.28 F cm^{-3} with 60% capacity retention. The synthesized sample shows a rate of energy transfer (power density) of 315 W kg^{-1} and density per unit mass (specific density) of 25 Wh kg^{-1}, which is suitable for supercapacitor

Table 2.2 Reported multi-metal oxidized ceramics materials for the application of the supercapacitor.

Materials	Methods	Structure	Capacitance	Ref
$LiM_2(PO_4)_3$	Heating process	Bulk	-	[77]
$Li_{1.4}Al_{0.4}Ti_{1.6}(PO_4)_3$ single-walled CNT	Sol-gel technique	Nanostructured	3.2 m Fg^{-1} at 5 mV s^{-1}	[78]
$Li_{1.4}Al_{0.4}Ti_{1.6}(PO_4)_3$	Sol-gel technique	Pallet	55 μ Fg^{-1} at 50 mV s^{-1}	[79]
$Li_{1.3}Al_{0.3}Ti_{1.7}P_3O_{12}$	Solid state process	3 D Bulky structure	0.1 F cm^{-1} at 2 mV s^{-1}	[80]
$Li_3V_2(PO_4)_3$	Heating process	Nanostructure	116 Fg^{-1} at 0.50 Ag^{-1}	[81]
$0.3Ca_8H_2(PO_4)_6.5H_2O$	Solution precipitation	Plate type structure	6 m Ahg^{-1}	[82]
$La_{0.7}Sr_{0.3}CoO_{3-\delta}$/Nio	Solid state process	Porous Substrate technique	1064 Fg^{-1} at 20 mA cm^{-2}	[83]
$La_{1-x}Sr_xCoO_{3-\delta}$-CuO	Solid-state process	Porous Substrate technique	545 Fg^{-1} at 1 mA cm^{-2}	[84]
$Li_{3x}La_{2/3-x}TiO_3$	Solid-state method	Cubic	0.3 m Fg^{-1}at 10 mV s^{-1}	[85]
$Li_{3x}La_{2/3-x}TiO_3$	Solid-state method	Cubic	-	[86]
$Li_{0.5}La_{0.5}TiO_3$	Solid-state method	Tetragonal	-	[87]
$Na_{0.5}Bi_{0.5}TiO_3$	Solid-state method	Thin Film and nanostructure	-	[88]
$CaCu_3Ti_4O_{12}$	Molton salt Process	Nanocubic shape	1185 mF cm^{-2} at 10 mV s^{-1}	[89]
$CaCu_3Ti_4O_{12}$	Solid state technique	Particles in a spherical shape	-	[90]
$CaCu_3Ti_4O_{12}$	Ball milling process	Grains	-	[91]

applications. This wonderful performance is due to three dimensional and large surface area of the material with better ion diffusion. A study by Gonzalez *et al.* indicates that nickel oxide film also can be used for supercapacitor application. $\beta - Ni(OH_2)$ Core-shell structure provides the ions diffusion pathway to produce 100 % capacitance retention after every thousand rounds (cycles) with a specific capacitance of around 399 F g^{-1}. In another technique, octyl gallate has been used as an extractor in FeOOH ceramic particles, which thereby shows a capacitive ability of 2.4 F cm^{-2} at a rated potential of 2 milli-Volts per second [93].

2.3 Principle Involved in Electroceramics

2.3.1 Electrostatic Capacitor

The most common dielectric-based capacitor comprises binary plates at some distance apart and can polarize when a certain amount of electric field has been applied. Polarization is the primary behavior in dielectric materials. An ideal capacitor has a capacitance that is equal to the proportion of actual charge say "Q" to the externally applied potential as shown in the following equation.

$$C(F) = \frac{Q}{V} \tag{2.1}$$

Practically, equation 2.1a has the following form,

$$D = \epsilon_0 E + P \tag{2.1a}$$

where "D" is displacement, "E" is the electric field and "P" is polarization. The polarization phenomena in the electrostatic capacitor is shown in the Figure 2.1.

From Gauss's law, we can write,

$$V = \frac{Q\,d}{\epsilon\,d} \tag{2.2}$$

Comparing equations 2.1 and 2.2 we get,

$$C = \frac{A}{\epsilon\,d} \tag{2.3}$$

The above equation indicates that the ability of a capacitor depends on the dielectric constant "ϵ".

Energy storage in the dielectric related to potential is given by the following equation,

$$W = \int_0^{Q_{Max}} V\,dq \tag{2.4}$$

Here "Q_{max}" shows the maximum value of charge obtained at the last cycle, "dq" is the increase in the charge.

The energy density (U_{vol}) is the most important factor for supercapacitors. Energy stored in a unit volume (U_{vol}) can be represented by the following equation,

$$U_{vol} = \frac{W}{Ad} = \frac{\int_0^{Q_{Max}} V\,dq}{Ad} = \int_0^{D_{Max}} E\,dD\left(\frac{Joul}{m^3}\right) \tag{2.5}$$

Here "D_{max}" and "E" are the electric displacement and electric fields, Therefore we can write:

$$D = \epsilon_0 E + P \tag{2.6}$$

Where "P" refers to polarization. In the case of a large value, displacement "D" is identical to the polarization "P". Hence $D = \epsilon_0\epsilon_r E$ where ϵ_0 refers to the permittivity of vacuum and ϵ_r shows the relative permittivity of the medium.

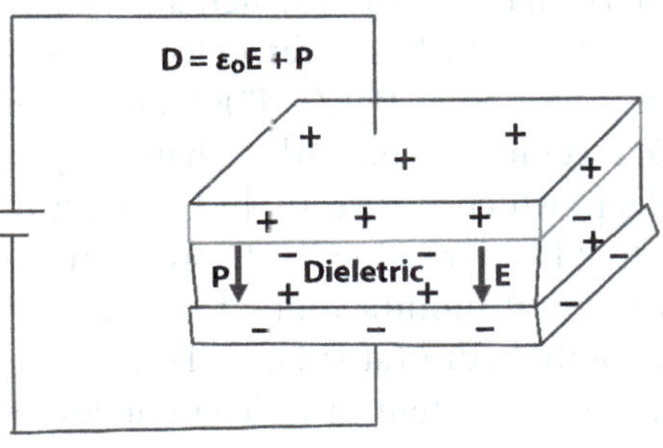

Figure 2.1 Representation of the electrostatic capacitor.

Energy density can be written as follows,

$$U_{vol} = \int_0^{P_{Max}} E\,dP\left(\frac{Joul}{m^3}\right) = \int_0^{E_{Max}} \epsilon_0\,\epsilon_r\,E\,dE\left(\frac{Joul}{m^3}\right) \tag{2.7}$$

Here "P_{max}" represents the maximum value of polarization. By integrating the polarization and electric field intensity hysteresis loop, we can calculate the energy density of the material.

2.4 Lead-Based Ceramics

Lead-based ceramics are the most widely applicable piezoelectric materials which were discovered in era of the 1950s. Lead-based ceramics are industrially used due to their high energy density and efficiency [94]. There are various examples of lead-based ceramics in which the most famous lead zirconate titanate (PZT) was discovered first and this composition has been mostly used as ferroelectrics. Another example of lead-based ferrite is related to the composition $Pb(B'B'')O_3$ where B' indicates Zn^{2+}, Ni^{2+}, Mg^{2+} etc while B'' shows Ta^{5+}, W^{6+}, Nb^{5+} etc. This composition is used as a relaxor ferroelectric. Other compositions include lead lanthanum zirconium Titanium Oxide (Pb, La) (Zr, Ti) O_3, lead lanthanum zirconium tin titanium oxide (Pb, La) (Zr, Sn, Ti) O_3, and lead lanthanum zirconium tin-based oxide (Pb, La) (Zr, Sn) O_3 which can be used as an anti-ferroelectric (AFE).

2.4.1 Lead-Based Ferroelectrics

Ferro electricity is a natural property of a material in which material is polarized due to the influence of the field intensity E and this property is reversible just like ferromagnetism in which a substance has a permanent dipole moment [95, 96]. Lead-based ferroelectrics is a perovskite system whose composition is written as $Pb(Zr, Ti)O_3$ and abbreviated as PZT. An investigation of PZT ceramics concluded that the proportion of Zr and Ti influences bandgap, which is directly linked with dielectric properties [97]. It is observed that by increasing Zr/Ti proportion, the bandgap tends to increase with structural modifications from tetragonal (at larger titanium content) to rhombohedra (at smaller Ti content). In another study, it is concluded that La/Ca content in PZT enhances dielectric properties, which ultimately enhances ferroelectric characteristics [98]. Thin-film orientation and substrate also influence ferroelectric properties. In a study of

$Pb(Zr_{0.53}Ti_{0.47})O_3$ thin film, this fact has been observed by various researchers [99, 100].

2.4.2 Lead-Based Relaxor Ferroelectrics

A kind of ferroelectric substance that has very large electrostriction is known as relaxor ferroelectrics. There are various kinds of relaxor ferroelectrics that have not been studied yet, but lead-based relaxor ferroelectrics have a unique perovskite shape, and it is mostly used in manifold layered capacitors and other piezoelectric devices (actuator, transducers, etc.). These materials have excellent piezoelectric and dielectric characteristics, which are due to their perovskite structure [101–103]. Lead-based perovskites can be written using the chemical equation $Pb(B'B'')O_3$. The first letter B' indicates Zn^{2+}, Ni^{2+}, Mg^{2+} etc while B'' shows Ta^{5+}, W^{6+}, Nb^{5+} [104, 105]. Relaxors are similar to ferroelectric materials except for their property of more than one atom's randomness in a unit cell. $A(B'B'')O_3$ Perovskite structure is accompanied by two kinds of heterovalent cations occupied at B sites. Most relaxor has such kind of chemical non-homogeneity. To maintain the stability of perovskite with improved electrical properties, lead titanate oxide has been put into relaxor ferroelectric PNM [105]. Except for PNM, other relaxors have a very high piezoelectric constant in a solution of solids (1-x) PNM–X PT. When $x>0.32$, such kinds of materials consist of a normal ferroelectric phase which is kept at a low temperature [106] and is very suitable for military and various industrial applications.

2.4.3 Lead-Based Anti-Ferroelectrics

A property of a material to form a dipole under an electric field just like ferroelectric materials but adjacent dipoles arranged in opposite directions are known as antiferroelectric materials [107]. In this type, spontaneous polarization tends to zero due to the cancellation of each dipole by its adjacent dipole. Various factors affect the properties of anti-ferroelectric materials, such as temperature, and electric field. The growth method of these materials also affects their properties of these types of materials. The temperature at which its properties vanish is termed Neel or Curie temperature. Lead zirconium oxide ($PbZrO_3$) was the 1st ever known anti-ferroelectric (AFE), which creates double hysteresis below a critical temperature (T_c). Furthermore, at room temperature, a larger field is required for anti-ferroelectric (AFE) to ferroelectric transition (FE) phase transition which hinders its applications for energy storage devices, i.e., capacitors. To overcome this, chemical doping is required, which can reduce the switching field. In this regard, three main compositions have been tried:

i. Lead lanthanum zirconium titanium oxide (Pb, La)(Zr, Ti)O_3 [108]
ii. Lead lanthanum zirconium tin titanium oxide (Pb, La)(Zr, Sn, Ti)O_3 [109]
iii. Lead lanthanum zirconium tin oxide (Pb, La)(Zr, Sn)O_3 [110]

i. Lead lanthanum zirconium titanium oxide (Pb, La)(Zr, Ti)O_3
A study on the (Pb, La)(Zr, Ti)O_3 indicates that when lead ions are replaced by La-ions (less than 30%) at "A site" orthorhombic ant ferroelectric equivalent to lead zirconium ($PbZrO_3$) structure appeared which is rich in Zr. Furthermore, in the case of 10% La has been used for energy storage [111]. It is suggested that larger composition leads to smaller polarization, and therefore has lower energy density. According to Li and its co-experimentalists, increasing La in the composition (Pb, La)(Zr, Ti)O_3 resulted in an increase in energy density with slim hysterics. Furthermore, after 105 cycles there is no degradation in the performance of the ceramics material [112]. Another successful method to improve PLZrT ceramics is to adjust Zr/Ti composition ratio. Qiao *et al.* investigated that altering Zr/Ti ratio results in a dropped tolerance and therefore upsurges in the anti-ferroelectricity [113]. It is also assumed that Mn doping can also enhance anti-ferroelectric properties [114].

ii. Lead lanthanum zirconium tin titanium oxide (Pb, La)(Zr, Sn, Ti)O_3
To improve energy-storing characteristics, tin is introduced on the B site of the PLZT-type ceramics. It is evident that by enhancing tin content decrease in the switching field has been observed which ultimately decreases antiferoelectricity [115]. If the proportion of zirconium tin titanium oxide is kept at 0.5: 0.45: 0.05 then the highest stability of ceramics has been obtained [109]. The ability of the (Pb, La)(Zr, Sn, Ti)O_3 ceramics is also affected by the lead/lanthanum proportion [116,117]. As Pb content increases, it leads to more stable AFE ceramics. Adding Ba and Sr content on the A site upgrades the fatigue resistance as well as temperature stability with a decrease in internal stress. This will finally lead to an improvement in energy density [118–120].

iii. Lead lanthanum zirconium tin oxide (Pb, La)(Zr, Sn)O_3
This composition is tried by Wang and his co-scientists who reported that this structure has special electric field-induced ultra-phase AFE-FE

transitions, with an improvement in the polarization [110]. It is reported that the proportion of the composition leads to changes in the characteristics of the energy applications. For instant, the doping of Sr content in the ($Pb_{0.98-x}$, $La_{0.02}$, $Sr_x(Zr_{0.9}$, $Sn_{0.1})O_3$ highly improves the energy storage capacity [110].

2.5 Characteristics of Lead-Based Ceramics

2.5.1 Characteristics of Lead Zirconate Titanate

The relative permittivity of lead-based ceramics lies between 300 and 20,000, which greatly depends on the doping as well as the orientation of the constituents. These materials refer to as pyroelectric, which means that they create a potential difference across their two terminals as their temperature changes; ultimately, they can be applied as a sensor application [121]. Lead ceramics are also ferroelectric, meaning that they have natural polarization under an electric field, and these properties can be reversed just like ferromagnetic materials [96]. One of the main features of lead-based ceramics is its large relative permittivity [122]. In some combinations, current increases exponentially with the field until avalanche breakdown occurs, and the dielectric strength of lead-based ceramics relies on the time of dielectric breakdown, which is a function of voltage and temperature.

2.5.2 Characteristics of Lead Magnesium Niobate

These materials have the property of electrostrictions which means that their shape changes under an applied electric field. This property arises due to the displacement of all positive ions toward the electric field and negative ions on the opposite side of the applied external electric field. This behavior continues throughout the bulk material, creating strain along the field. The thickness decreases in the perpendicular direction according to the poisons ratio equation.

2.5.3 Characteristics of Lead Zinc Niobate

The Curie temperature of the lead-zinc niobate (PZN) material is relatively very high (140°C), which means that at this temperature, the phase of the ceramic materials changes. At room temperature, this system is rhombohedral, while at Curie temperature, it becomes cubic. This ceramic is widely used in capacitors and actuators due to its large dielectric constant and electrostrictive characteristics. However, the structural properties of the PZN remain poor due to the mixture of the perovskite and pyrochlore phases [123].

2.6 Conclusion and Perspectives

Ceramic materials consist of hydroxide ceramics, single and multi-elemental oxide ceramics, and spinal-type ceramics. To explain each type, some famous examples with composition and structural skeleton with an extraordinary emphasis on the electrochemical activity have been provided. The main techniques are to optimize the required material and control the size, shape, structure, and elemental content, which significantly influence the surface area, porosity, and electron or ions diffusion mechanism. Despite an extensive range of supercapacitor uses of nanoceramics and mixed nanoceramics, there is a dire need to focus on many areas. Herein some areas on which the study should focus are discussed below:

2.6.1 Up-to-Date Sintering and Molding Process

Huge temperatures and long sintering and shaping time during sintering result in severe energy utilization, a barrier to clean energy. Moreover, grain restriction during large sintering temperatures of ceramic materials is tough to control by ordinary sintering methods, which makes the material uncontrollable. More importantly, large sintering temperature ceramic will result in minor surface area and porosity, which limits ion transfer capability. It will make difficulties in supercapacitor performance. Thus, there is a need to use up-to-date and smart molding techniques to produce complex shapes and small shrinkage ceramics in a very small time [124, 125].

2.6.2 Microscopical and Flexible Ceramics Electrode Materials

The microscopic ability and flexibility of ceramic electrodes make it possible to obtain more smart electronic materials which can apply to all devices. Furthermore, this will produce a supercapacitor that can charge in a few seconds with better power density. On the other hand, the main problems are the brittleness and hardness of ceramic materials, which limits their progress. It is because hard and tough material is challenging to operate, especially for making flexible and lighter materials. Nowadays, there are many techniques to produce more tough ceramics, such as adding nanosheets, wires, and any other particles which have significant thermal coefficients [126, 127], and building a complex network-like structure to improve the fracture defects [128, 129]. Furthermore, a lot of effort is required in the development of supercapacitors microscopically and flexible ceramics electrode materials.

2.6.3 Improvement of Efficiency of the Ceramic Electrode Materials

The electrochemical characteristics, for example, capacitance, power, energy densities, cycling life, etc., of supercapacitors need to be improved. These factors affect the reliability of the electrode, electrolytic substance, and device skeleton [130, 131]. There are many techniques to mitigate these problems, such as nanostructured design, alteration in the interface, defect production, and doping, that could have been applied to improve the efficiency of the electrode. The futuristic approach will be self-supported, binder-free, and large-area ceramic materials, making device fabrication very simple and smart. Moreover, another technique would be the activation of the electrode surface, which removes the inactive layer, thereby improving the charge diffusion path mechanism. As long as the electrolyte is concerned, the potential transfer has been limited when hydrogen and oxygen are evolved in the electrolyte [35]. On the other hand, a liquid ion medium would provide the possibility of a larger output potential [132]. In response to safer and leak-free voltage, gel/solid electrolyte would be a better choice. Device assembly is also a crucial task that relies on the current collector's selection, a gap between both electrodes (positive and negative) during the process of assembling [133].

References

1. Chen, H., Cong, T.N., Yang, W., Tan, C., Li, Y., Ding, Y., Progress in electrical energy storage system: A critical review. *Prog. Nat. Sci.*, 19, 291, 2009.
2. Noori, A., El-Kady, M.F., Rahmanifar, M.S., Kaner, R.B., Mousavi, M.F., Towards establishing standard performance metrics for batteries, supercapacitors and beyond. *Chem. Soc. Rev.*, 48, 1272, 2019.
3. Kötz, R. and Carlen, M., Principles and applications of electrochemical capacitors. *Electrochim. Acta*, 45, 2483, 2000.
4. Macdougall, F., Ennis, J., Cooper, R., Bates, J., Seal, K., High energy density pulsed power capacitors, in: *Digest of Technical Papers, 14th IEEE*

International Pulsed Power Conference (IEEE Cat. No. 03CH37472), IEEE, 2003.

5. Zhang, S. and Pan, N., Supercapacitors performance evaluation. *Adv. Energy Mater.*, 5, 1401401, 2015.
6. Zhang, L.L. and Zhao, X., Carbon-based materials as supercapacitor electrodes. *Chem. Soc. Rev.*, 38, 2520, 2009.
7. Zeng, X., Yang, B., Li, X., Yu, R., Three-dimensional hollow CoS_2 nanoframes fabricated by anion replacement and their enhanced pseudocapacitive performances. *Electrochim. Acta*, 240, 341, 2017.
8. Zhai, S., Karahan, H.E., Wang, C., Pei, Z., Wei, L., Chen, Y., 1d supercapacitors for emerging electronics: Current status and future directions. *Adv. Mater.*, 32, 1902387, 2020.
9. Kurzweil, P. and Chwistek, M., Electrochemical stability of organic electrolytes in supercapacitors: Spectroscopy and gas analysis of decomposition products. *J. Power Sources*, 176, 555, 2008.
10. Winter, M. and Brodd, R.J., What are batteries, fuel cells, and supercapacitors? *Chem. Rev.*, 104, 4245, 2004.
11. Xue, Q., Sun, J., Huang, Y., Zhu, M., Pei, Z., Li, H., Wang, Y., Li, N., Zhang, H., Zhi, C., Recent progress on flexible and wearable supercapacitors. *Small*, 13, 1701827, 2017.
12. Najib, S. and Erdem, E., Current progress achieved in novel materials for supercapacitor electrodes: Mini review. *Nanoscale Adv.*, 1, 2817, 2019.
13. Abdah, M.A.A.M., Azman, N.H.N., Kulandaivalu, S., Sulaiman, Y., Review of the use of transition-metal-oxide and conducting polymer-based fibres for high-performance supercapacitors. *Mater. Des.*, 186, 108199, 2020.
14. Gonçalves, J.M., Da Silva, M.I., Toma, H.E., Angnes, L., Martins, P.R., Araki, K., Trimetallic oxides/hydroxides as hybrid supercapacitor electrode materials: A review. *J. Mater. Chem. A*, 8, 10534, 2020.
15. Zhao, Y., Shi, Z., Li, H., Wang, C.-A., Designing pinecone-like and hierarchical manganese cobalt sulfides for advanced supercapacitor electrodes. *J. Mater. Chem. A*, 6, 12782, 2018.
16. Zhao, Y., Shi, Z., Lin, T., Suo, L., Wang, C., Luo, J., Ruan, Z., Wang, C.-A., Li, J., Brownian-snowball-mechanism-induced hierarchical cobalt sulfide for supercapacitors. *J. Power Sources*, 412, 321, 2019.
17. Chen, T., Li, M., Song, S., Kim, P., Bae, J., Biotemplate preparation of multilayered TiC nanoflakes for high performance symmetric supercapacitor. *Nano Energy*, 71, 104549, 2020.
18. Wang, H., Li, J., Li, K., Lin, Y., Chen, J., Gao, L., Nicolosi, V., Xiao, X., Lee, J., Transition metal nitrides for electrochemical energy applications. *Chem. Soc. Rev.*, 50, 1354, 2021.
19. Allagui, A., Freeborn, T.J., Elwakil, A.S., Fouda, M.E., Maundy, B.J., Radwan, A.G., Said, Z., Abdelkareem, M.A., Review of fractional-order electrical characterization of supercapacitors. *J. Power Sources*, 400, 457, 2018.

20. Mohanty, A., Jaihindh, D., Fu, Y.-F., Senanayak, S.P., Mende, L.S. Ramadoss, A., An extensive review on three dimension architectural metal-organic frameworks towards supercapacitor application. *J. Power Sources*, 488, 229444, 2021.
21. González, A., Goikolea, E., Barrena, J.A., Mysyk, R., Review on supercapacitors: Technologies and materials. *Renew. Sustain. Energy Rev.*, 58, 1189, 2016.
22. Zhao, H., Liu, L., Vellacheri, R., Lei, Y., Recent advances in designing and fabricating self-supported nanoelectrodes for supercapacitors. *Adv. Sci.*, 4, 1700188, 2017.
23. Wang, F., Wu, X., Yuan, X., Liu, Z., Zhang, Y., Fu, L., Zhu, Y., Zhou, Q., Wu, Y., Huang, W., Latest advances in supercapacitors: From new electrode materials to novel device designs. *Chem. Soc. Rev.*, 46, 6816, 2017.
24. Gibbons, J.H., Nichols, R.W., Bowman, J.M., Buffenbarger, R., Clark, J., Goldberg, S., Lambert, S., McLean, A.F., Congress, U., *New structural materials technologies: Opportunities for the use of advanced ceramics and composites a technical memorandum*, U.S. Government Printing Office, Washington, DC, 1986.
25. Shen, Z.-Y., Wang, Y., Tang, Y., Yu, Y., Luo, W.-Q., Wang, X., Li, Y., Wang, Z., Song, F., Glass modified barium strontium titanate ceramics for energy storage capacitor at elevated temperatures. *J. Materiomics*, 5, 641, 2019.
26. Colombo, P., Conventional and novel processing methods for cellular ceramics. *Philos. Trans. R. Soc. A, Math. Phys. Eng. Sci.*, 364, 109, 2006.
27. Studart, A.R., Gonzenbach, U.T., Tervoort, E., Gauckler, L.J., Processing routes to macroporous ceramics: A review. *J. Am. Ceram. Soc.*, 89, 1771, 2006.
28. Setter, N. and Waser, R., Electroceramic materials. *Acta Mater.*, 48, 151, 2000.
29. Harrati, A., Manni, A., El Bouari, A., El Hassani, I.-E.E.A., Sadik, C., Elaboration and thermomechanical characterization of ceramic-based on moroccan geomaterials: Application in construction. *Mater. Today: Proc.*, 30, 876, 2020.
30. Faseeva, G., Nafikov, R., Lapuk, S., Zakharov, Y.A., Novik, A., Vjuginova, A., Kabirov, R., Garipov, L., Ultrasound-assisted extrusion of construction ceramic samples. *Ceram. Int.*, 43, 7202, 2017.
31. Kuang, M., Han, P., Huang, L., Cao, N., Qian, L., Zheng, G., Electronic tuning of Co, Ni-based nanostructured (hydr) oxides for aqueous electrocatalysis. *Adv. Funct. Mater.*, 28, 1804886, 2018.
32. Kwon, H.J., Shin, K., Soh, M., Chang, H., Kim, J., Lee, J., Ko, G., Kim, B.H., Kim, D., Hyeon, T., Large-scale synthesis and medical applications of uniform-sized metal oxide nanoparticles. *Adv. Mater.*, 30, 1704290, 2018.
33. Hu, M., Yang, W., Tan, H., Jin, L., Zhang, L., Kerns, P., Dang, Y. Dissanayake, S., Schaefer, S., Liu, B.J.M., Template-free synthesis of mesoporous and crystalline transition metal oxide nanoplates with abundant surface defects. *Matter*, 2, 1244, 2020.

34. Nguyen, T. and Montemor, M.D.F., Metal oxide and hydroxide–based aqueous supercapacitors: From charge storage mechanisms and functional electrode engineering to need-tailored devices. *Adv. Sci.*, 6, 1801797, 2019.
35. Yin, X., Li, H., Yuan, R., Jiao, Y., Lu, J., Templated synthesis of spinel cobaltite MCo_2O_4 (M= ni, co and mn) hierarchical nanofibers for high performance supercapacitors. *J. Materiomics*, 7, 858, 2021.
36. Sekhar, S.C., Nagaraju, G., Yu, J.S., High-performance pouch-type hybrid supercapacitor based on hierarchical NiO-Co_3O_4-NiO composite nanoarchitectures as an advanced electrode material. *Nano Energy*, 48, 81, 2018.
37. Zeng, Y., Yu, M., Meng, Y., Fang, P., Lu, X., Tong, Y., Iron-based supercapacitor electrodes: Advances and challenges. *Adv. Energy Mater.*, 6, 1601053, 2016.
38. Jiang, T., Bu, F., Feng, X., Shakir, I., Hao, G., Xu, Y., Porous Fe_2O_3 nanoframeworks encapsulated within three-dimensional graphene as high-performance flexible anode for lithium-ion battery. *ACS Nano*, 11, 5140, 2017.
39. Wang, S., Yang, Y., Dong, Y., Zhang, Z., Tang, Z., Recent progress in Ti-based nanocomposite anodes for lithium ion batteries. *J. Adv. Ceram.*, 8, 1, 2019.
40. Osgood, H., Devaguptapu, S.V., Xu, H., Cho, J., Wu, G., Transition metal (Fe, Co, Ni, and Mn) oxides for oxygen reduction and evolution bifunctional catalysts in alkaline media. *Nano Today*, 11, 601, 2016.
41. Liu, Y., Tian, D., Biswas, A.N., Xie, Z., Hwang, S., Lee, J.H., Meng, H., Chen, J.G., Transition metal nitrides as promising catalyst supports for tuning Co/H_2 syngas production from electrochemical CO_2 reduction. *Angew. Chem.*, 59, 11345, 2020.
42. Wang, C., Zeng, X., Jiang, G., Chen, M., Zhu, L., Yu, R., General self-template synthesis of transition-metal oxide microspheres and their excellent charge storage properties. *Electrochim. Acta*, 283, 190, 2018.
43. Liu, Y., Li, X., Shen, W., Dai, Y., Kou, W., Zheng, W., Jiang, X., He, G., Multishelled transition metal-based microspheres: Synthesis and applications for batteries and supercapacitors. *Small*, 15, 1804737, 2019.
44. Lang, X.Y., Liu, B.T., Shi, X.M., Li, Y.Q., Wen, Z., Jiang, Q., Ultrahigh-power pseudocapacitors based on ordered porous heterostructures of electron-correlated oxides. *Adv. Sci.*, 3, 1500319, 2016.
45. Vidyadharan, B., Abd Aziz, R., Misnon, I.I., Kumar, G.M.A., Ismail, J., Yusoff, M.M., Jose, R., High energy and power density asymmetric supercapacitors using electrospun cobalt oxide nanowire anode. *J. Power Sources*, 270, 526, 2014.
46. Krishnan, S.G., Reddy, M., Harilal, M., Vidyadharan, B., Misnon, I.I., Ab Rahim, M.H., Ismail, J., Jose, R., Characterization of $MgCo_2O_4$ as an electrode for high performance supercapacitors. *Electrochim. Acta*, 161, 312, 2015.
47. Tennakone, K., Apsonsu, G., Ariyasinghe, Y., Buchanan, R., Perera, V., Tennakone, H., Wijayarathna, T., Dye-sensitized solar cells based on nanostructured semiconductor oxide ceramics with ultra-thin barrier layers. *Integr. Ferroelectr.*, 115, 120, 2010.

48. Li, T., Cao, Y., Xue, W., Sun, B., Zhu, D., Self-assembly of graphene-based planar micro-supercapacitor with selective laser etching-induced superhydrophobic/superhydrophilic pattern. *Appl. Sci.*, 2, 1, 2020.
49. KnöLler, A., Kilper, S., Diem, A.M., Widenmeyer, M., RunčEvski, T.E., Dinnebier, R.E., Bill, J., Burghard, Z., Ultrahigh damping capacities in lightweight structural materials. *Nano Lett.*, 18, 2519, 2018.
50. Pang, Z., Duan, J., Zhao, Y., Tang, Q., He, B., Yu, L., A ceramic NiO/ZrO_2 separator for high-temperature supercapacitor up to 140° C. *J. Power Sources*, 400, 126, 2018.
51. Yus, J., Ferrari, B., Herencia, A.J., Caballero, A., Morales, J., Gonzalez, Z.J.C., *In situ* synthesis and electrophoretic deposition of Nio/Ni core-shell nanoparticles and its application as pseudocapacitor. *Coatings*, 7, 193, 2017.
52. Yus, J., Ferrari, B., Sanchez-Herencia, A.J., Gonzalez, Z., Understanding the effects of different microstructural contributions in the electrochemical response of nickel-based semiconductor electrodes with 3d hierarchical networks shapes. *Electrochim. Acta*, 335, 135629, 2020.
53. Vidhyadharan, B., Zain, N.K.M., Misnon, I.I., Abd Aziz, R., Ismail, J., Yusoff, M.M., Jose, R.J., Compounds, High performance supercapacitor electrodes from electrospun nickel oxide nanowires. *J. Alloys Compd.*, 610, 143, 2014.
54. Jose, R., Krishnan, S., Vidyadharan, B., Misnon, I., Harilal, M., Aziz, R., Ismail, J., Yusoff, M., Supercapacitor electrodes delivering high energy and power densities. *Mater. Today Proc.*, 3, S48, 2016.
55. Vidyadharan, B., Abd Aziz, R., Misnon, I.I., Kumar, G.M.A., Ismail, J., Yusoff, M.M., Jose, R.J., High energy and power density asymmetric supercapacitors using electrospun cobalt oxide nanowire anode. *J. Power Sources*, 270, 526, 2014.
56. Shen, S.F., Xu, M.L., Lin, D.B., Pan, H.B., Ultrahigh-power pseudocapacitors based on ordered porous heterostructures of electron-correlated oxides. *Adv. Sci.*, 396, 327, 2017.
57. Lang, X.Y., Liu, B.T., Shi, X.M., Li, Y.Q., Wen, Z., Jiang, Q.J., Ultrahigh-power pseudocapacitors based on ordered porous heterostructures of electron-correlated oxides. *Adv. Sci.*, 3, 1500319, 2016.
58. Poon, R., Liang, W., Zhitomirsky, I.J.M., A, M.T., Mn_3O_4 and (ZnFe)OOH composites for supercapacitors with high active mass. *Metall. Mater. Trans. A*, 51, 855, 2020.
59. Gorokhovsky, A., Saunina, S., Maximova, L., Tretyachenko, E., Goffman, V., Escalante-Garcia, J.I., Vikulova, M., Synthesis and electric properties of the high-k ceramic composites based on potassium polytitanate modified by manganese. *Res. Chem. Intermed.*, 48, 1227, 2022.
60. Milne, J., Silva, R.M., Zhitomirsky, I., Surface modification and dispersion of ceramic particles using liquid-liquid extraction method for application in supercapacitor electrodes. *J. Eur. Chem. Soc.*, 39, 3450, 2019.

61. Xing, Y., Guo, X., Wu, D., Liu, Z., Fang, S., Suib, S., Compounds, Construction of macroscopic 3d foams of metastable manganese oxides via a mild templating route: Effects of atmosphere and calcination. *J. Alloys Compd.*, 719, 22, 2017.
62. Zhang, Y., Guo, Z., Han, Z., Xiao, X., Effect of rare earth oxides doping on $MgAl_2O_4$ spinel obtained by sintering of secondary aluminium dross. *J. Alloys Compd.*, 735, 2597, 2018.
63. Anwar, S., Muthu, K.S., Ganesh, V., Lakshminarasimhan, N., A comparative study of electrochemical capacitive behavior of $NiFe_2O_4$ synthesized by different routes. *J. Electrochem. Soc.*, 158, A976, 2011.
64. Shamitha, C., Senthil, T., Wu, L., Kumar, B.S., Anandhan, S., Sol–gel electrospun mesoporous $ZnMn_2O_4$ nanofibers with superior specific surface area. *J. Mater. Sci.: Mater. Electron.*, 28, 15846, 2017.
65. Kovalenko, A., Shilova, O., Morozova, L., Kalinina, M., Drozdova, I., Arsent'ev, M.Y., Features of the synthesis and the study of nanocrystalline cobalt-nickel spinel. *Glass Phys. Chem.*, 40, 106, 2014.
66. Gu, L., Li, T., Xu, Y., Sun, C., Yang, Z., Zhu, D., Chen, D., Effects of the particle size of $BaTiO_3$ fillers on fabrication and dielectric properties of $BaTiO_3$/polymer/al films for capacitor energy-storage application. *Mater.*, 12, 439, 2019.
67. Chung, U.C., Elissalde, C., Mompiou, F., Majimel, J., Gomez, S., Estournès, C., Marinel, S., Klein, A., Weill, F., Michau, D., Interface investigation in nanostructured $BaTiO_3$/silica composite ceramics. *J. Am. Ceram. Soc.*, 93, 865, 2010.
68. Maglione, M., Elissalde, C., Chung, U.-C., Interface control in $BaTiO_3$ based supercapacitors, in: *Oxide-Based Materials and Devices*, The International Society for Optics and Photonics, SPIE, U.S., 2010.
69. Chung, U., Elissalde, C., Mornet, S., Maglione, M., Estournès, C., Controlling internal barrier in low loss $BaTiO_3$ supercapacitors. *Appl. Phys. Lett.*, 94, 072903, 2009.
70. Bhattacharya, D., Ghoshal, D., Mondal, D., Paul, B.K., Pal, J., Gupta, B., Bose, N., Nandy, P., Basu, M., Das, S., Delafossite type $CuCo_{0.5}Ti_{0.5}O_2$ composite structure: A futuristic ceramics for supercapacitor and emi shielding application. *Ceram. Int.*, 47, 9907, 2021.
71. Maity, S., Samanta, M., Sen, A., Chattopadhyay, K.K., Investigation of electrochemical performances of ceramic oxide $CaCu_3Ti_4O_{12}$ nanostructures. *J. Solid State Chem.*, 269, 600, 2019.
72. Xia, W., Liu, Y., Wang, G., Li, J., Cao, C., Hu, Q., Chen, Y., Lu, Z., Wang, D., Frequency and temperature independent $(Nb_{0.5}Ga_{0.5})_x(Ti_{0.9}Zr_{0.1})_{1-x}O_2$ ceramics with giant dielectric permittivity and low loss. *Ceram. Int.*, 46, 2954, 2020.
73. Shiri, H.M., Ehsani, A., Shayeh, J.S., Synthesis and highly efficient supercapacitor behavior of a novel poly pyrrole/ceramic oxide nanocomposite film. *RSC Adv.*, 5, 91062, 2015.

74. Zhang, X., He, B., Zhao, Y., Tang, Q., A porous ceramic membrane tailored high-temperature supercapacitor. *J. Power Sources*, 379, 60, 2018.
75. Lu, D.-L., Zhao, R.-R., Wu, J.-L., Ma, J.-M., Huang, M.-L., Yao, Y.-B., Tao, T., Liang, B., Zhai, J.-W., Lu, S.-G., Investigations on the properties of $Li_{3x}La_{2/3-x}$ TiO_3 based all-solid-state supercapacitor: Relationships between the capacitance, ionic conductivity, and temperature. *J. Eur. Ceram. Soc.*, 40, 2396, 2020.
76. Liu, P., Weng, X., Liu, Z., Zhang, Y., Qiu, Q., Wang, W., Zhou, M., Cai, W., Ni, M., Liu, M., High-performance quasi-solid-state supercapacitor based on CuO nanoparticles with commercial-level mass loading on ceramic material $La_{1-x}Sr_xCOO_{3-\delta}$ as cathode. *ACS Appl. Energy Mater.*, 2, 1480, 2019.
77. Chowdari, B., Rao, G.S., Lee, G.J., XPS and ionic conductivity studies on Li_2O–Al_2O_3–(TiO_2 or GeO_2)–P_2O_5 glass–ceramics. *Ind. Acad. Sci.*, 136, 1067, Elsevier, 2000.
78. Liao, G., Geier, S., Mahrholz, T., Wierach, P., Wiedemann, M., Temperature influence on electrical properties of carbon nanotubes modified solid electrolyte-based structural supercapacitor, in: *Conference on Smart Materials, Adaptive Structures and Intelligent Systems*, American Society of Mechanical Engineers, 2017.
79. Liao, G., Geier, S., Mahrholz, T., Wierach, P., Wiedemann, M., Li1.4Al0.4Ti1.6(PO4)3 used as solid electrolyte for structural supercapacitors, in: *Conference on Smart Materials, Adaptive Structures and Intelligent Systems*, American Society of Mechanical Engineers, 2015.
80. Hu, X., Chen, Y., Hu, Z., Li, Y., Ling, Z.J., All-solid-state supercapacitors based on a carbon-filled porous/dense/porous layered ceramic electrolyte. *J. Electrochem. Soc.*, 165, A1269, 2018.
81. El-Desoky, M., Al-Syadi, A., Al-Assiri, M., Hassan, H., El Enany, G., Electrochemical performance of novel $Li_3V_2(PO_4)_3$ glass-ceramic nanocomposites as electrodes for energy storage devices. *J. Electrochem Soc.*, 20, 2663, 2016.
82. Tuncer, M., Bakan, F., Gocmez, H., Erdem, E.J.N., Capacitive behaviour of nanocrystalline octacalcium phosphate (OCP)($Ca_8H_2(PO_4)_6$ $5H_2O$ as an electrode material for supercapacitors: Biosupercaps. *Nanoscale*, 11, 18375, 2019.
83. Liu, P., Liu, Z., Wu, P., Ou, X., Zhang, Y., Cai, W., Yu, F., Ni, M., Cheng, S., Liu, M.J., Enhanced capacitive performance of nickel oxide on porous $La_{0.7}Sr0_3COO_{3-\delta}$ ceramic substrate for electrochemical capacitors. *Int. J. Hydrog. Energy*, 43, 19589, 2018.
84. Liu, P., Weng, X., Liu, Z., Zhang, Y., Qiu, Q., Wang, W., Zhou, M., Cai, W., Ni, M., Liu, M.J., High-performance quasi-solid-state supercapacitor based on CuO nanoparticles with commercial-level mass loading on ceramic material $La_{1-x}Sr_xCOO_{3-\delta}$ as cathode. *ACS Appl. Energy Mater.*, 2, 1480, 2019.
85. Lu, D.-L., Zhao, R.-R., Wu, J.-L., Ma, J.-M., Huang, M.-L., Yao, Y.-B., Tao, T., Liang, B., Zhai, J.-W., Lu, S.-G., Investigations on the properties of

$Li_{3x}La_{2/3-x}TiO_3$ based all-solid-state supercapacitor: Relationships between the capacitance, ionic conductivity, and temperature. *J. Am. Chem. Soc.*, 40, 2396, 2020.

86. Bohnke, O., The fast lithium-ion conducting oxides $Li_{3x}La_{2/3-x}TiO_3$ from fundamentals to application. *Solid State Ion.*, 179, 9, 2008.
87. Gu, R., Yu, K., Wu, L., Ma, R., Sun, H., Jin, L., Xu, Y., Xu, Z., Wei, X., Dielectric properties and iv characteristics of $Li_{0.5}La_{0.5}TiO_3$ solid electrolyte for ceramic supercapacitors. *Ceram. Int.*, 45, 8243, 2019.
88. Lahmar, A., Belhadi, J., El Marssi, M., Zannen, M., Khemakhem, H., Al-Dahoudi, N., Energy storage property of lead-free $Na_{0.5}Bi_{0.5}TiO_3$ ceramic and thin film, in: *2017 International Conference in Energy and Sustainability in Small Developing Economies (ES2DE)*, IEEE, 2017.
89. Maity, S., Samanta, M., Sen, A., Chattopadhyay, K.K., Investigation of electrochemical performances of ceramic oxide $CaCu_3Ti_4O_{12}$ nanostructures. *J. Solid State Chem.*, 269, 600, 2019.
90. Shao, S., Zhang, J., Zheng, P., Zhong, W., Wang, C.J., Microstructure and electrical properties of $CaCu_3Ti_4O_{12}$ ceramics. *J. Appl. Phys.*, 99, 084106, 2006.
91. Lee, J.-W. and Koh, J.-H.J.C.I., Grain size effects on the dielectric properties of $CaCu_3Ti_4O_{12}$ ceramics for supercapacitor applications. *Ceram. Int.*, 41, 10442, 2015.
92. Chang, P., Mei, H., Zhao, Y., Huang, W., Zhou, S., Cheng, L., 3d structural strengthening urchin-like $Cu(OH)_2$-based symmetric supercapacitors with adjustable capacitance. *Adv. Funct. Mater.*, 29, 1903588, 2019.
93. Gonzalez, Z., Ferrari, B., Sanchez-Herencia, A., Caballero, A., Morales, J., Use of polyelectrolytes for the fabrication of porous nio films by electrophoretic deposition for supercapacitor electrodes. *Electrochim. Acta*, 211, 110, 2016.
94. Wang, X., Zhai, H., Qie, B., Cheng, Q., Li, A., Borovilas, J., Xu, B., Shi, C., Jin, T., Liao, X., Rechargeable solid-state lithium metal batteries with vertically aligned ceramic nanoparticle/polymer composite electrolyte. *Nano Energy*, 60, 205, 2019.
95. Känzig, W., Ferroelectrics and antiferroeletrics. *Solid State Phys.*, Elsevier, 4, 1–97, 1957.
96. Lines, M.E. and Glass, A.M., *Principles and applications of ferroelectrics and related materials*, Oxford University Press, Clarendon, UK, 2001.
97. Samanta, S., Sankaranarayanan, V., Sethupathi, K., Band gap, piezoelectricity and temperature dependence of differential permittivity and energy storage density of PZT with different Zr/Ti ratios. *Vacuum*, 156, 456, 2018.
98. Zhu, H., Ma, H., Zhao, Y., Enhanced energy storage and pyroelectric properties of highly (100)-oriented $(Pb_{1-x-y}La_xCa_y)Ti_{1-x/4}O_3$ thin films derived at low temperature. *Phys. Lett. A*, 382, 1409, 2018.
99. Nguyen, M.D., Houwman, E.P., Dekkers, M., Nguyen, C.T., Vu, H.N., Rijnders, G., Research update: Enhanced energy storage density and energy

efficiency of epitaxial $Pb_{0.9}La_{0.1}(Zr_{0.52}Ti_{0.48})O_3$ relaxor-ferroelectric thin-films deposited on silicon by pulsed laser deposition. *APL Mater.*, 4, 080701, 2016.

100. Zhang, T., Li, W., Hou, Y., Yu, Y., Song, R., Cao, W., Fei, W., High-energy storage density and excellent temperature stability in antiferroelectric/ferroelectric bilayer thin films. *J. Am. Ceram. Soc.*, 100, 3080, 2017.
101. Kutnjak, Z., Petzelt, J., Blinc, R., The giant electromechanical response in ferroelectric relaxors as a critical phenomenon. *Nature*, 441, 956, 2006.
102. Zhang, S., Jiang, W., Meyer Jr., R.J., Li, F., Luo, J., Cao, W., Measurements of face shear properties in relaxor-$PbTiO_3$ single crystals. *J. Appl. Phys.*, 110, 064106, 2011.
103. Zhang, Y., Gao, G., Chan, H.L., Dai, J., Wang, Y., Hao, J., Piezo-phototronic effect-induced dual-mode light and ultrasound emissions from ZnS:Mn/PMN–PT thin-film structures. *Adv. Mater.*, 24, 1729, 2012.
104. Jaffe, B., Cook, W., Jaffe, H., *Piezoelectric ceramics*, Academic Press, Elsevier, 1971.
105. Luo, N., Li, Y., Xia, Z., Li, Q.J.C., Progress in lead-based ferroelectric and antiferroelectric single crystals: Composition modification, crystal growth and properties. *CrystEngComm*, 14, 4547, 2012.
106. Cowley, R., Gvasaliya, S., Lushnikov, S., Roessli, B., Rotaru, G., Relaxing with relaxors: A review of relaxor ferroelectrics. *Adv. Phys.*, 60, 229, 2011.
107. Brears, R.C., *Nature-based solutions to 21st century challenges*, Routledge, Abingdon, Oxfordshire, England, 2020.
108. Jo, H.R. and Lynch, C.S., A high energy density relaxor antiferroelectric pulsed capacitor dielectric. *J. Appl. Phys.*, 119, 024104, 2016.
109. Chen, S., Wang, X., Yang, T., Wang, J., Composition-dependent dielectric properties and energy storage performance of (Pb, La)(Zr, Sn, Ti)O_3 antiferroelectric ceramics. *J. Electroceram.*, 32, 307, 2014.
110. Liu, X., Li, Y., Hao, X., Ultra-high energy-storage density and fast discharge speed of $(Pb_{0.98-x}La_{0.02}Sr_x)(Zr_{0.9}Sn_{0.1})_{0.995}O_3$ antiferroelectric ceramics prepared via the tape-casting method. *J. Mater. Chem. A*, 7, 11858, 2019.
111. Li, B., Liu, Q.-X., Tang, X.-G., Zhang, T.-F., Jiang, Y.-P., Li, W.-H., Luo, J., Antiferroelectric to relaxor ferroelectric phase transition in PbO modified $(Pb_{0.97}La_{0.02})(Zr_{0.95}Ti_{0.05})O_3$ ceramics with a large energy-density for dielectric energy storage. *RSC Adv.*, 7, 43327, 2017.
112. Li, B., Liu, Q., Tang, X., Zhang, T., Jiang, Y., Li, W., Luo, J., High energy storage density and impedance response of PLZT2/95/5 antiferroelectric ceramics. *Mater.*, 10, 143, 2017.
113. Qiao, P., Zhang, Y., Chen, X., Zhou, M., Yan, S., Dong, X., Wang, G., Enhanced energy storage properties and stability in $(Pb_{0.895}La_{0.07})(Zr_xTi_{1-x})O_3$ antiferroelectric ceramics. *Ceram. Int.*, 45, 15898, 2019.
114. Samanta, S., Sankaranarayanan, V., Sethupathi, K., Effect of Nb and Fe Co-doping on microstructure, dielectric response, ferroelectricity and energy storage density of plzt. *J. Mater. Sci.: Mater. Electron.*, 29, 20383, 2018.

115. Bersuker, I.B., Pseudo Jahn-Teller origin of perovskite multiferroics, magnetic-ferroelectric crossover, and magnetoelectric effects: The d_0–d_{10} problem. *Phys. Rev. Lett.*, 108, 137202, 2012.
116. Zhuo, F., Li, Q., Li, Y., Gao, J., Yan, Q., Zhang, Y., Chu, X., Cao, W., Effect of a-site La^{3+} modified on dielectric and energy storage properties in lead zirconate stannate titanate ceramics. *Mater. Res. Express*, 1, 045501, 2014.
117. Xu, R., Tian, J., Zhu, Q., Zhao, T., Feng, Y., Wei, X., Xu, Z., Effects of La-induced phase transition on energy storage and discharge properties of PLZST ferroelectric/antiferroelectric ceramics. *Ceram. Int.*, 43, 13918, 2017.
118. Jiang, S., Zhang, L., Zhang, G., Liu, S., Yi, J., Xiong, X., Yu, Y., He, J., Zeng, Y., Effect of Zr:Sn ratio in the lead lanthanum zirconate stannate titanate anti-ferroelectric ceramics on energy storage properties. *Ceram. Int.*, 39, 5571, 2013.
119. Wang, X., Shen, J., Yang, T., Xiao, Z., Dong, Y., Phase transition and energy storage performance in Ba-doped PLZST antiferroelectric ceramics. *J. Mater. Sci.: Mater. Electron.*, 26, 9200, 2015.
120. Zhang, G., Zhu, D., Zhang, X., Zhang, L., Yi, J., Xie, B., Zeng, Y., Li, Q., Wang, Q., Jiang, S., High-energy storage performance of $(Pb_{0.87}Ba_{0.1}La_{0.02})(Zr_{0.68}Sn_{0.24}Ti_{0.08})O_3$ antiferroelectric ceramics fabricated by the hot-press sintering method. *J. Am. Ceram. Soc.*, 98, 1175, 2015.
121. Ashcroft, N.W. and Mermin, N.D., *Solid state physics*, p. 10, Brooks Cole, Cengage Learning, Boston, Massachusetts, United States, 1976.
122. Rouquette, J., Haines, J., Bornand, V., Pintard, M., Papet, P., Bousquet, C., Konczewicz, L., Gorelli, F., Hull, S., Pressure tuning of the morphotropic phase boundary in piezoelectric lead zirconate titanate. *Phys. Rev. B*, 70, 014108, 2004.
123. Halliyal, A. and Safari, A., Synthesis and properties of lead zinc niobate: $Pb(Zn_{1/3}Nb_{2/3})O_3$ based relaxor ferroelectrics. *Ferroelectrics*, 158, 295, 1994.
124. Chen, Z., Li, Z., Li, J., Liu, C., Lao, C., Fu, Y., Liu, C., Li, Y., Wang, P., He, Y., 3d printing of ceramics: A review. *J. Eur. Ceram. Soc.*, 39, 661, 2019.
125. Yang, L., Zeng, X., Zhang, Y., 3d printing of alumina ceramic parts by heat-induced solidification with carrageenan. *Mater. Lett.*, 255, 126564, 2019.
126. Verma, A.S., Kumar, D., Dubey, A.K., A review of an innovative concept to increase the toughness of the ceramics by piezoelectric secondary phases. *Ceram. Int.*, 44, 16119, 2018.
127. Nan, B., Liu, Y., You, Q., Wan, J., Shen, Z., Li, H., Yuan, B., Cheng, L., Wang, G., Microstructure and properties of porous SiC ceramics modified by CVI-SiC nanowires. *Adv. Eng. Mater.*, 21, 1800653, 2019.
128. Moriana, A.D. and Zhang, S., Lead-free textured piezoceramics using tape casting: A review. *J. Materiomics*, 4, 277, 2018.
129. Sun, M., Bai, Y., Li, M., Fan, S., Cheng, L., Improved toughness and electromagnetic shielding-effectiveness for graphite-doped SiC ceramics with a net-like structure. *J. Eur. Ceram. Soc.*, 38, 5271, 2018.

130. Zhao, H. and Lei, Y., 3d nanostructures for the next generation of high-performance nanodevices for electrochemical energy conversion and storage. *Adv. Energy Mater.*, 10, 2001460, 2020.
131. Simon, P. and Gogotsi, Y., Perspectives for electrochemical capacitors and related devices. *Nat. Mater.*, 19, 1151, 2020.
132. Djire, A., Ishimwe, J.Y., Choi, S., Thompson, L.T., Enhanced performance for early transition metal nitrides via pseudocapacitance in protic ionic liquid electrolytes. *Electrochem. Communi.*, 77, 19, 2017.
133. Kitazawa, Y., Iwata, K., Kido, R., Imaizumi, S., Tsuzuki, S., Shinoda, W., Ueno, K., Mandai, T., Kokubo, H., Dokko, K., Polymer electrolytes containing solvate ionic liquids: A new approach to achieve high ionic conductivity, thermal stability, and a wide potential window. *Chem. Mater.*, 30, 252, 2018.

3

Ceramic Films for High-Performance Supercapacitors

Santhosh G.[1*] **and Nayaka G. P.**[2]

[1]*Department of Mechanical Engineering, NMAM Institute of Technology, Nitte Deemed to University, Nitte, Karkala, Karnataka, India*
[2]*Physical and Materials Chemistry Division, CSIR-National Chemistry Laboratory, Pune, Maharashtra, India*

Abstract
Supercapacitors are the most appraised devised for energy storage applications as it exhibits fast storage capabilities, high-energy density, and long cycle stability. Ceramic materials are considered promising candidates for high-performance supercapacitors (SCs). Yet, their low specific area and surface activity make them unacceptable for the supercapacitor's applications. Hence, it is very much essential to understand the basic behavior of ceramic materials to enhance their electrical conductivity and electron transfer capabilities. In this chapter, we present the fundamental aspects to improve the energy storage capabilities with enhanced electrical homogeneity, and the prospects for new hybrid materials with high-energy density are also discussed.

Keywords: Supercapacitors, ceramic, high-energy density, electrical homogeneity

3.1 Introduction

In recent years, as the world population is increasing the demand for the consumption of energy is also increasing and the continuous depletion of fossil fuels is creating an alternative way to find an innovative and alternative energy storage device to meet the energy demand [1]. It is very

Corresponding author: drsanthug@gmail.com

Inamuddin, Tariq Altalhi and Sayed Mohammed Adnan (eds.) Electroceramics for High Performance Supercapacitors, (53–72) © 2024 Scrivener Publishing LLC

shocking to know that, by 2035 total worldwide, the demand for fossil fuels will reach approximately 18 billion tons of oil equivalent [2]. With the increase in demand for the usage of fossil fuels, CO_2 emissions also increase to 37 billion tons [3]. Hence, the need for clean and sustainable energy sources such as wind, solar, geothermal, and biofuel also increasing day by day [4, 5]. Further, it is also true that the need for energy generation, storage, and conversation technologies is very much essential to meet the energy demand. So far, a huge number of electrical energy storage devices were manufactured, such as fuel cells, thermal and thermochemical energy storage systems, electrical energy storage devices, and electrochemical energy storage devices [6, 7].

The supercapacitor is one such energy device that is widely appreciated and considered to be the best among other energy devices like batteries and dielectric capacitors [8]. The application of energy storage capacitors is presented in Figure 3.1. Based on the storage method, the SCs are categorized into (i) Electric double layer capacitors, and (ii) Pseudo-capacitors [9, 10]. In double-layer capacitors, energy storage is due to double-layer charge separation at the electrode-electrolyte interface, and in pseudo-capacitors, it is due to the faradic reaction, where the charge transfer between electrode and electrolyte takes place by reversible redox reactions. Pseudo-capacitors perform better compared to Electric double layer capacitors as they exhibit higher specific capacitance and energy density [11]. It is well-known that to fabricate supercapacitors with high capacitance, the electrodes must have a higher/large surface area with a very thin dielectric layer and higher dielectric constant.

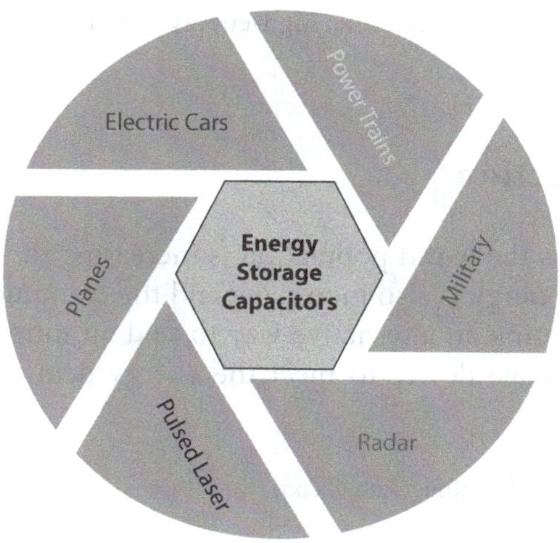

Figure 3.1 Application of energy storage capacitors.

The idea of using ceramic capacitors as energy devices can be dated back to the 1960s, lead researchers like Jaffe, Burn, and Smyth have evaluated the effete of $SrTiO_3$ (ST) and BT with the applied electric field to understand the nature and behavior of the ceramics for supercapacitor applications [12, 13]. The researchers emphasized about the energy density of the material prepared, it was found that to have maximum energy density supercapacitors must have thinner dielectric layers with lesser defect sites. Later in the year 1990 Love and group investigated energy storage ability in ceramic-based supercapacitors and emphasized design strategies to enhance the storage capacity of the capacitor [14]. The team manufactured commercial C0 G-type capacitors with a higher energy storage density of 1 J/cm^3. Fletcher and team [15] have developed capacitors with high-energy density by adjusting the curie temperature of the FE materials used.

Several carbon-based materials such as carbon nanotubes (CNTs), graphene oxide (GO), metal oxides (MO), sulfides, and conducting polymers have been used as supercapacitor electrodes [16–20]. Generally, to understand the performance and characteristics of supercapacitors are evaluated by the energy density and power density of the electrodes and are calculated by using capacitance, equivalent series resistance, and operating voltage [21]. Further, the cycling stability of the prepared electrode is the key parameter to assess the performance of the supercapacitor electrodes [22]. However, the electrochemical performance of the supercapacitors depends primarily on the electrode material, and electrolyte used [23, 24]. The current research trend indicates the focus on materials structure and design of the electrodes resulting in porous structures with good surface area, and conductivity [25]. In the present decade, a huge variety of materials like metals, ceramics, polymers, metal-organic, and covalent organic frameworks have been used as supercapacitor electrodes [26–28]. Although ceramic electrodes have failed to impress as electrodes due to low specific surface area and low surface activity, their corrosion resistance, and high thermal and radiation resistance still make them potential candidates in supercapacitor applications [29–32]. Further, ceramic materials exhibit excellent mechanical, thermal, optical, electrical, and magnetic properties, which makes them unique and widely used materials in various fields such as construction, energy, electronics, and biomedical engineering [33–44]. Although the basic characteristics of ceramic materials make them prominent candidates in various fields, they are equally important in energy device applications. the reason for considering ceramics in energy-related applications is the over-exploitation of various conventional energy sources. Therefore, it is very much essential to develop new and advanced electrode materials to meet new energy demands. Among various electrode materials, the use of ceramics as electrodes in supercapacitor applications is no exception. Lang *et al.*, have developed V_2O_3/MnO_2-based ceramic hybrid electrodes with very high performance due to improved interfacial electron transfer [45]. Liu and co-workers have synthesized CuO-loaded multi-metal ceramic electrode, the prepared electrode exhibited rapid electron transfer and diffusion of ions with very high specific capacitance values [46]. This chapter aims to provide insight into various ceramic electrodes with selected examples to highlight the electrochemical behavior of the materials for supercapacitors.

3.2 Energy Storage Principles

The basic dielectric capacitors system has two parallel metal plates separated by an insulating material and become polarized once an electric field is applied, this behavior is the fundamental nature of dielectric materials. The charge storage capacity of ideal dielectric materials under the influence of an electric field is the ratio of the charge stored to the applied voltage, the equation is shown below. Figure 3.2 illustrates the real device which is used to calculate the capacitance of the electrostatic system using Gauss's law.

$$C = \frac{Q}{V} = \frac{A}{\varepsilon d} \quad F \tag{3.1}$$

Where C is the capacitance, Q is the charge and V is the voltage applied.

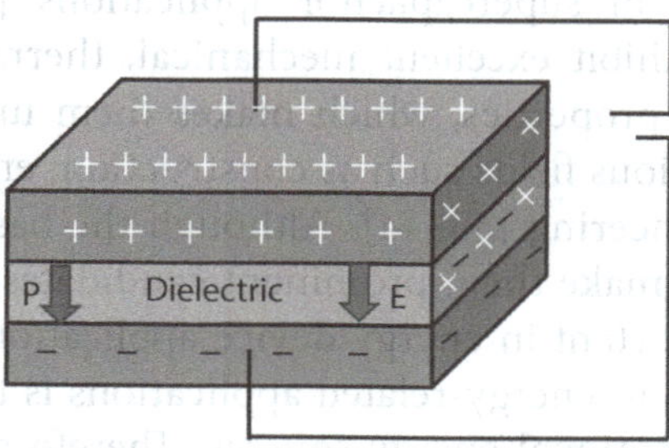

Figure 3.2 Schematic of an electrostatic capacitor.

The energy storage capabilities of the dielectric materials are assessed by estimating the electrostatic capacity with the applied voltage. The electrostatic energy of the dielectric material is evaluated by the following equation.

$$w = \int_0^{Q_{max}} V\,dq \quad J \tag{3.2}$$

Where "Q_{max}" is the Maximum charge achieved and "dq" is the incremental charge.

The performance of the dielectric material is analyzed by volumetric energy density (W_{st}). Volumetric energy density is the energy stored in the dielectric materials per unit volume which signifies the performance of the dielectric, the below equation is used to calculate the energy stored per unit volume.

$$W_{st} = \frac{W}{Ad} = \frac{\int_0^{Q_{max}} V\,dq}{Ad} \tag{3.3}$$

3.3 Factors Optimizing Energy Density

Electro ceramics with high-energy density are preferred in high-performance supercapacitors to meet the needs of currently increasing energy demand. However, the microstructural features, band gap, distributive conductivity, and resistivity of the electroceramics become critical factors in optimizing energy density.

3.3.1 The Intrinsic Band Gap (E_g)

E_g is described as "the energy between the valence band and conduction band", the intrinsic electrical response along with distributive conductive and resistive elements the energy density can be evaluated or optimized. The bandgap in materials is used to define insulators, semiconductors, and conductors. The bandgap for insulators is greater than 4 eV, for semiconductors it is between 0 to 4 eV and for conductors, it is 0 eV. The ceramic material with a wider bandgap offers better breakdown strength and thermal stability to enhance the energy storage of the capacitor.

3.3.2 Electrical Microstructure

The electrical microstructure is the most important parameter of the electroceramic material, wherein the different regions of the electroceramic material will have different conductivity and electrical permittivity [47]. In many cases, ceramic materials have a heterogeneous distribution which leads to the localization of electrical field strength with low relative permittivity, as a result, interconnected conducting regions are formed. However, with the third end member, the electrical heterogeneity can be eliminated [48].

3.3.3 Density and Grain Size

Density, porosity, and grain size play a very important role in deciding the electrical behavior of ceramic materials, particularly the breakdown strength. The high-density ceramic materials at higher electric field exhibit properties close to intrinsic breakdown strength. Low-density ceramics have conductive paths comprised of voids resulting in the short circuit even with a moderate electric field [49, 50]. However, densifying ceramic material is difficult with conventional techniques. The densification of ceramics is usually done by sintering, during the sintering process sintering conditions are optimized to increase the density of the ceramics [51–54]. The grain size of the ceramic materials also plays a crucial role in energy storage, ceramic materials having high density and fine grain size are used to optimize energy storage [55, 56]. The grain size of the ceramic materials can be altered by chemical doping and film coating on primary particles before the sintering process is required to enhance the performance of capacitors [57–60].

3.4 Ceramics for Supercapacitors

The overwhelming performance of ceramics makes them unique and strong contenders used in various energy devices. Ceramics materials with high mechanical, thermal, electrical, optical, and good chemical stability are widely preferred [61–70]. Further, the anticorrosive, temperature resistance, and radiation resistance nature of ceramics make them more suitable electrodes for supercapacitors. Accordingly, the metal oxides/hydroxide, multi-element oxide, ceramic electrodes, and carbon/carbide/nitride ceramics electrodes were developed for supercapacitor applications.

3.4.1 Metal Oxide Ceramics

Metal oxides are the most important class of materials used in the field of energy storage as they are abundantly available, cheap, and exhibit high performance [71–75]. Among various metal oxides, transition metal oxides are widely preferred due to their eco-friendly nature and low cost [76–79]. The wide acceptance of metal oxides is primarily attributed to the charge storage and electrochemical performance. The energy storage and electrochemical behavior of metal oxides are based on valence change through proton intercalation/deintercalation, surface absorption/desorption, and redox reaction with anions [80–82]. In the last few years, the use of metal oxide ceramics as electrodes for supercapacitors is gradually increasing. Transition metal oxide ceramics such as MnO_2, Mn_3O_4, Co_3O_4 and Al_2O_3 are widely studied as electrode materials for supercapacitors as they can store high-density energy. The details of a few metal oxide ceramic materials are tabulated in Table 3.1.

Lang *et al.*, have prepared MnO_2/V_2O_3 electrodes and their study reveals that the prepared electrode can deliver ultra-high capacity up to 422 W/cm^3 [83] (Figure 3.3). The electrical conductivity of the electrode was significantly enhanced with improved pseudocapacitive nature of MnO_2. Vidyadharan *et al.*, synthesized Co_3O_4 and NiO nanowires via electrospinning technique has high crystallinity and capacitance, and the Co_3O_4 electrode delivered 47.6 Wh/kg of energy density at 1400 W/kg [84]. NiO nanowires also exhibited 670 F/g capacitance at 1000 cycles with 100% retention of cycle stability [85].

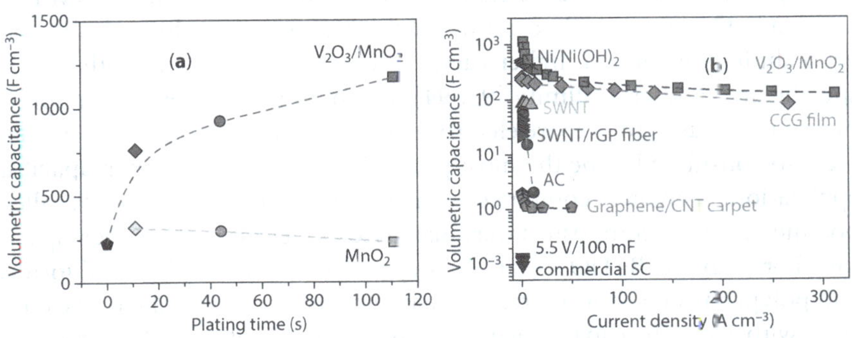

Figure 3.3 Volumetric capacitance of NP V_2O_3/MnO_2 electrodes (a) as a function of planting time (b) current density [83].

Table 3.1 Metal oxide ceramic electrodes.

Sl. no.	Metal oxides	Capacitance	Shape of materials	References
1	MnO_2	0.34 (F/cm^2)	Film	[106]
2	$KxMnO_2.y(H_2O)z$	353 (F/g)		[107]
3	MnO_2-foamed nickel	45 (F/g)		[108]

3.4.2 Multielemental Oxides

Multielemental oxide ceramics containing two or more two metals are considered to be more efficient than single-metal oxide ceramics as multi-elemental-oxide ceramics offer rich redox reactions [86–90]. The multielement oxides exhibit better electrical conductivity and electrochemical behavior. These multi-elemental oxides can be prepared by various such as combustion and sol-gel methods. Binary metal oxide electrodes like MFe_2O_4 and $NiFe_2O_4$ ceramic materials were prepared and have been used for supercapacitor applications [91]. $NiFe_2O_4$ ceramic electrode behavior is similar to electrical double-layer capacitors prepared by the sol-gel technique have the highest capacitance of 97.5 F/g after 100 CV cycles [91]. Further, cobalt-doped zinc ferrite ceramic electrodes were prepared by the co-precipitation method [92]. The doping of cobalt increased the capacitance of the electrode. The capacitance of cobalt-based electrodes exhibits better capacitance compared to other ceramic electrodes. Many spinel oxide electrodes have been prepared and studied for their potential application in supercapacitors. The spinel materials, such as $ZnMn_2O_4$ and $NiCo_2O_4$ spinel oxide ceramic electrodes, prepared through the sol-gel technique exhibited higher capacitance and conductivity with higher specific area and crystallinity [93, 94]. Further, not only binary or spinel materials are used to prepare electrodes but also polymer-based electrodes are also considered to be the most promising materials for supercapacitor applications. Polymers combined with various alkaline earth metals called polymer-ceramic composites were also used as electrodes for supercapacitors. For example, $BaTiO_3$ ceramics prepared with polyvinylidene fluoride, and polypropylene show increased charge transfer rate and dielectric constant with a specific capacitance of 305.6 F/g [95]. Santhosh *et al.* prepared $NiCoO_4/CeO_2$ mixed metal oxide materials by sol-gel technique for supercapacitor applications. The prepared materials are analyzed by scanning electron microscopic technique and transmission electron microscopic

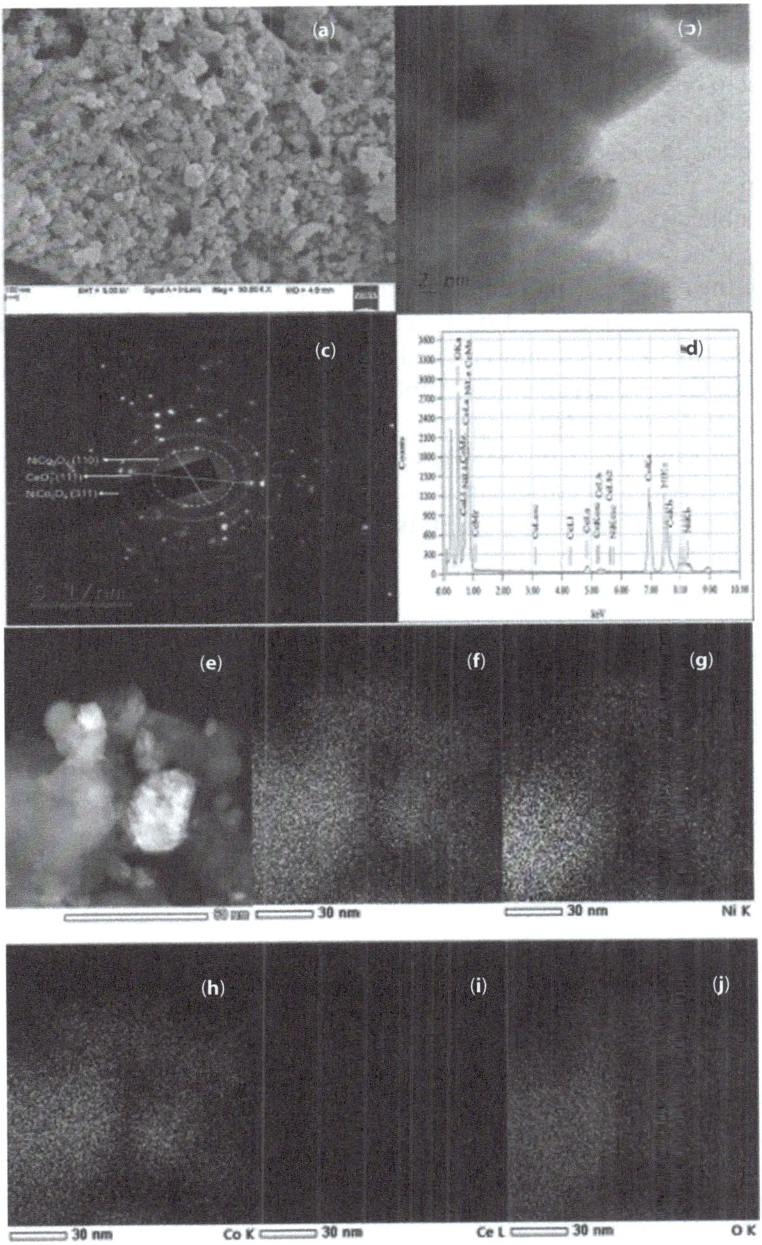

Figure 3.4 (a) Scanning electron and (b) Transmission micrographs of $NiCo_2O_4$ sample with 0.2 moles of Ce (c) SAED pattern of $NiCo_2O_4$ sample with 0.2 moles of Ce (d) EDS mapping with 0.2 moles of Ce (e) STEM image with 0.2 moles of Ce and (f) corresponding EDS mapping of (g) Ni (h) Co (i) Ce (j) O elements [96].

technique (Figure 3.4). The particle size with elemental mapping is presented in Figure 3.4. The synthesized mixed metal oxide material was found to be 52.56 nm in size. The authors varied the CeO_2 content to study the performance of the electrode, the variation of CeO_2 has created a huge impact on the electrochemical performance of the electrode. The electrochemical performance of the mixed metal oxide electrodes was done by reversible cyclic voltammetric technique. Figure 3.5 shows the variation of CeO_2, which exhibits a remarkable behavior of the electrode. The practical use of the electrodes prepared is decided on their cyclic performance, and the stability of the $NiCoO_4/CeO_2$ electrode was done by charge-discharge studies. The electrode showed excellent electrochemical performance with the least CeO_2 (0.2, 0.4, 0.6, 0.8 moles of Ce) content [96].

Figure 3.6 shows $NiCoO_4/CeO_2$ electrodes with 0.2 moles of Ce exhibit a specific capacitance of 1355 Fg^{-1} at 5 Ag^{-1} after 6000 cycles. This behavior of $NiCoO_4/CeO_2$ electrodes is unique and rare in high-performance supercapacitors. To validate these results, the specific capacitance of CeO_2 prepared by Zeng *et al.* has 779 Fg^{-1} at 1 Ag^{-1} [97]. Sheng *et al.* also prepared

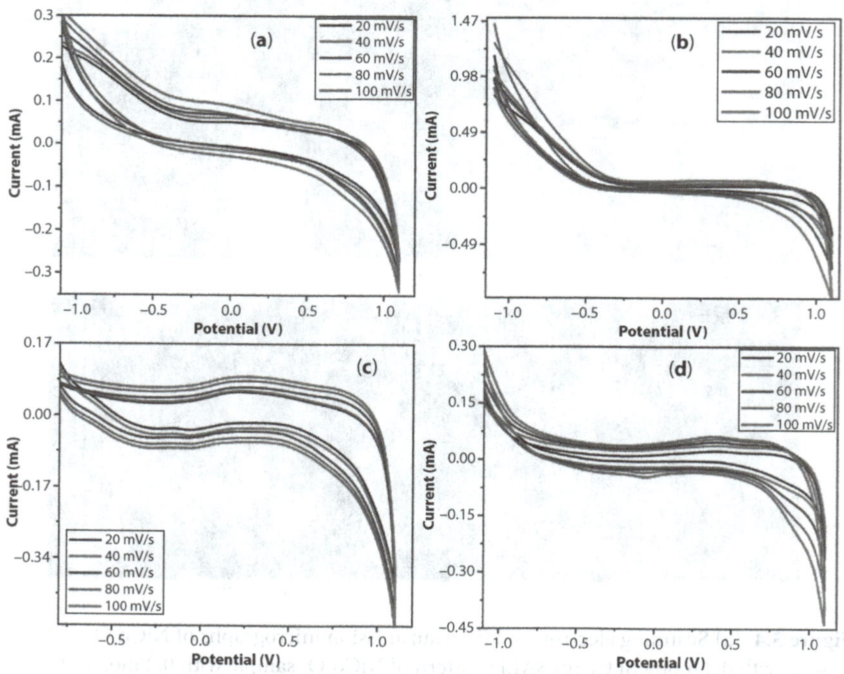

Figure 3.5 CV curves of $NiCo_2O_4$ with (a) 0.2 moles of Ce (b) 0.4 moles of Ce (c) 0.6 moles of Ce (d) 0.8 moles of Ce [96].

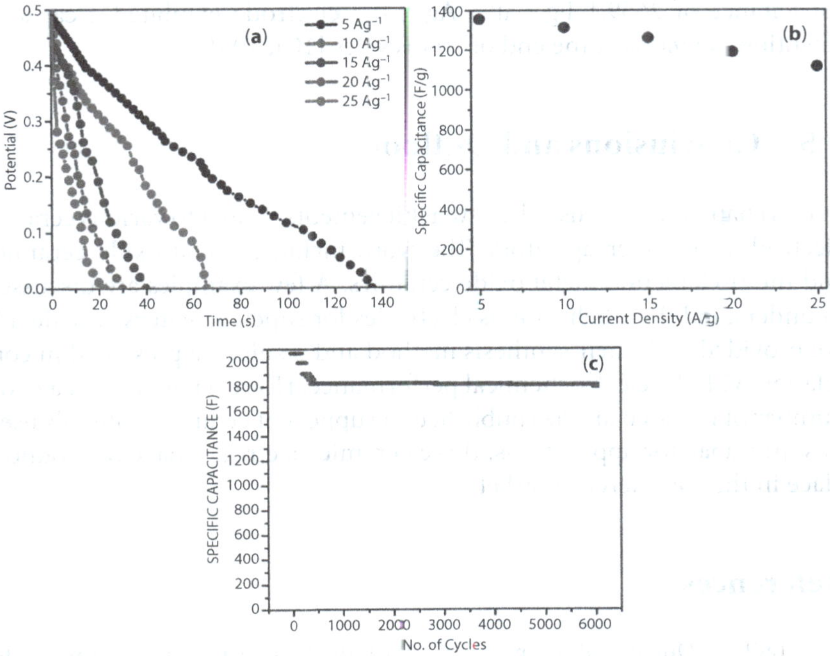

Figure 3.6 (a) Charge/discharge voltage profile (b) calculated specific capacitance (c) specific capacitance cycling performance for $NiCo_2O_4$ sample with 0.2 moles of Ce electrode.

$NiCo_2O_4$ electrodes that exhibit the capacitance of 965 Fg^{-1} at 5 Ag^{-1} at the end of 4000 cycles [98]. Wang *et al.* fabricated a $NiCo_2O_4$ electrode that exhibited a capacitance retention of 95.3 % at 30 Ag^{-1} at the end of 1000 cycles [49].

From the literature it is found that mixed metal oxides like $FeCo_2O_4$, $MnCo_2O_4$, and $ZnCo_2O_4$ were also used as electrodes, the specific capacitance of these electrodes was measured at the current density of 2 Ag^{-1} [99]. Further, several $NiCo_2O_4$-based hybrid metal oxide electrodes were fabricated and studied.

Co_3O_4 with $NiCo_2O_4$ revealed a capacitance of 770 F/g at 1 A/g [100] and MnO_2 mixed with $NiCo_2O_4$ have 1485.24 F/g of specific capacitance at 2 F/g [101] after 3000 cycles with the cycling stability of 87.5 %. A similar result was noticed for NiO-based $NiCo_2O_4$ electrodes exhibiting 85.2 % of capacity retention e at the end of 2000 cycles [102]. The nanostructures such as Mn_3O_4/$NiCo_2O_4$/NiO electrodes have a specific capacitance of 1905 F/g at 1 F/g with 92% capacity retention at the end of 10000 cycles [103]. Wei *et al.* prepared a $NiCo_2O_4$/CeO_2 electrode which exhibits a specific capacitance of 2659.1 Fg^{-1} at 5 Ag^{-1}, the electrode exhibited a capacity retention of 99.6 % at the end of 5000 cycles [104, 105].

3.5 Conclusions and Outlook

In this chapter, we discussed, a few achievements related to various ceramic electrodes for supercapacitors. The work includes metal oxide ceramics and multi-elemental metal oxide ceramics. A few examples are discussed to understand their behavior as electrodes for supercapacitors. The details are provided with their synthesis method and results are presented in correlation with the electrochemical performance. However, with such a good number of research articles published in support of ceramic materials used in supercapacitor applications, these ceramic electrodes have not found a place in the commercial market.

References

1. Tajik, S., Dubal, D.P., Romero, P.G., Rashidi, A., Yadegari, A., Nasernejad, B., Inamuddin, Asiri, A.M., Nanostructured mixed transition metal oxides for high performance asymmetric supercapacitors: Facile synthetic strategy. *Int. J. Hydrog. Energy*, 42, 12384–12395, 2017.
2. Singh, S., Jain, S., Venkateswaran, P.V., Tiwari, A.K., Nouni, M.R., Pandey, J.K., Goel, S., Hydrogen: A sustainable fuel for future of the transport sector. *Renew. Sustain. Energy Rev.*, 51, 623–633, 2015.
3. Ritchie, H. and Roser, M., CO_2 and greenhouse gas emissions, 2017, https://ourworldindata.org/co2-and-other-greenhouse-gas-emissions.
4. Azcarate, C., Mallor, F., Mateo, P., Tactical and operational management of wind energy systems with storage using a probabilistic forecast of the energy resource. *Renew. Energy*, 102, 445–456, 2017.
5. McKone, J.R., DiSalvo, F.J., Abruna, H.D., Solar energy conversion, storage, and release using an integrated solar-driven redox flow battery. *J. Mater. Chem. A*, 5, 5362–5372, 2017.
6. Chen, H.S., Cong, T.N., Yang, W., Tan, C.Q., Li, Y.L., Ding, Y.L., Progress in electrical energy storage system: A critical review. *Prog. Nat. Sci.*, 19, 291–312, 2009.
7. Noori, A., El-Kady, M.F., Rahmanifar, M.S., Kaner, R.B., Mousavi, M.F., Towards establishing standard performance metrics for batteries, supercapacitors and beyond. *Chem. Soc. Rev.*, 48, 1272–1341, 2019.
8. Dubal, D.P., Ayyad, O., Ruiz, V., Romero, G.P., Hybrid energy storage: The merging of battery and supercapacitor chemistries. *Chem. Soc. Rev.*, 44, 1777–1790, 2015.

9. Kima, D.K., Hwanga, M., Koa, D., Kanga, J., Seonga, K., Piaoa, Y., Electrochemical performance of 3D porous Ni-Co oxide with electrochemically exfoliated graphene for asymmetric supercapacitor applications. *Electrochim. Acta*, 246, 680–688, 2017.
10. Wang, Y., Guo, J., Wang, T., Shao, J., Wang, D., Yang, Y.W., Mesoporous transition metal oxides for supercapacitors. *Nanomaterials*, 5, 1667–1689, 2015.
11. Li, J., Huang, X., Cui, L., Chenn, N., Qu, L., Preparation and supercapacitor performance of assembled graphene fiber and foam. *Prog. Nat. Sci.: Mater. Int.*, 26, 212–220, 2016.
12. Jaffe, B., Antiferroelectric ceramics with field-enforced transitions: A new nonlinear circuit element. *Proc. IRE*, 49, 1264–1267, 1961.
13. Burn, I. and Smyth, D.M., Energy storage in ceramic dielectrics. *J. Mater. Sci.*, 7, 339–343, 1972.
14. Love, G.R., Energy storage in ceramic dielectrics. *J. Am. Ceram. Soc.*, 73, 323–328, 1990.
15. Fletcher, N.H., Hilton, A.D., Ricketts, B.W., Optimization of energy storage density in ceramic capacitors. *J. Phys. D: Appl. Phys.*, 29, 253–258, 1996.
16. Miller, E.E., Hua, Y., Tezel, F.H., Materials for energy storage: Review of electrode materials and methods of increasing capacitance for supercapacitors. *J. Energy Storage*, 20, 30–40, 2018.
17. Najib, S. and Erdem, E., Current progress achieved in novel materials for supercapacitor electrodes: Mini review. *Nanoscale Adv.*, 1, 2817–27, 2019.
18. Abdah, M.A.A., Azman, N.H., Kulandaivalu, S., Sulaiman, Y., Review of the use of transition-metal-oxide and conducting polymer-based fibres for high-performance supercapacitors. *Mater. Des.*, 186, 108199, 2020.
19. Zhao, Y.C., Shi, Z., Lin, T.Q., Suo, L.M., Wang, C., Luo, J., Ruan, Z.S., Wang, C.A., Li, J., Brownian-snowball-mechanism-induced hierarchical cobalt sulfide for supercapacitors. *J. Power Sources*, 412, 321–330, 2019.
20. Zhao, Y.C., Shi, Z., Li, H.Y., Wang, C.A., Designing pinecone-like and hierarchical manganese cobalt sulfides for advanced supercapacitor electrodes. *J. Mater. Chem. A*, 6, 12782–12793, 2018.
21. Allagui, A., Freebornc, T.J., Elwakil, A.S., Fouda, M.E., Maundy, B.J., Radwan, A.G., Said, Z., Abdelkareem, M., Review of fractional-order electrical characterization of supercapacitors. *J. Power Sources*, 400, 457–467 2018.
22. Mohanty, A., Jaihindh, D., Fu, Y.P., Senanayak, S.P., Mende, L.S., Ramadoss, A., An extensive review on three dimension architectural metal-organic frameworks towards supercapacitor application. *J. Power Sources*, 488, 229444, 2021.
23. Gonzalez, A., Goikolea, E., Barrena, J.A., Mysyk, R., Review on supercapacitors: Technologies and materials. *Renew. Sustain. Energy Rev.*, 58, 1189–1206, 2016.
24. Zhao, H.P., Liu, L., Vellacheri, R., Lei, Y., Recent advances in designing and fabricating self-supported nanoelectrodes for supercapacitors. *Adv. Sci.*, 4, 1700188, 2017.

25. Wang, F.X., Wu, X.W., Yuan, X.H., Liu, Z.C., Zhang, Y., Fu, L.J., Zhu, Y.S., Zhou, Q.M., Wu, Y.P., Huang, W., Latest advances in supercapacitors: From new electrode materials to novel device designs. *Chem. Soc. Rev.*, 46, 6816–6854, 2017.
26. Zhang, Y.Z., Wang, Y., Cheng, T., Yao, L.Q., Li, X.C., La, W.Y., Huang, W., Printed supercapacitors: Materials, printing and applications. *Chem. Soc. Rev.*, 48, 3229–64, 2019.
27. Zhou, J.W. and Wang, B., Emerging crystalline porous materials as a multifunctional platform for electrochemical energy storage. *Chem. Soc. Rev.*, 46, 6927–45, 2017.
28. Choudhary, N., Li, C., Moore, J., Nagaiah, N., Zhai, L., Jung, Y., Thomas, J., Asymmetric supercapacitor electrodes and devices. *Adv. Mater.*, 29, 1605336, 2017.
29. U.S. Congress, *New structural materials technologies: Opportunities for the use of advanced ceramics and composites-a technical memorandum*, Office of Technology Assessment. OTA-TM-E-32, US Government Printing Office, Washington DC, USA, 1986.
30. Shen, Z.Y., Wang, Y., Tang, Y.X., Yu, Y.Y., Luo, W.Q., Wang, X.C., Li, Y.M., Wang, Z.M., Song, F.S., Glass modified barium strontium titanate ceramics for energy storage capacitor at elevated temperatures. *J. Materiomics*, 5, 641–648, 2019.
31. Colombo, P., Conventional and novel processing methods for cellular ceramics. *Philos. Trans. R. Soc. A*, 364, 109–124, 2006.
32. Studart, A.R., Gonzenbach, U.T., Tervoort, E., Gauckler, L.J., Processing routes to macroporous ceramics: A review. *J. Am. Ceram. Soc.*, 89, 1771–1789, 2006.
33. Harrati, A., Manni, A., Bouari, A.E., Hassani, I.E.E.A., Sadik, C., Elaboration and thermomechanical characterization of ceramic-based on Moroccan geomaterials: Application in construction. *Mater. Today: SAVE Proc.*, 30, 876–882, 2020.
34. Faseeva, G.R., Nafikov, R.M., Lapuk, S.E., Zakharov, Y.A., Novik, A.A., Vjuginova, A.A., Kabirov, R.R., Garipov, L.N., Ultrasound-assisted extrusion of construction ceramic samples. *Ceram. Int.*, 43, 7202–7210, 2017.
35. Li, D.X., Shen, Z.Y., Li, Z.P., Luo, W.Q., Song, F.S., Wang, X.C., Wang, Z.M., Li, Y.M., Optimization of polarization behavior in (1-x)BSBNT-xNN ceramics for pulsed power capacitors. *J. Mater. Chem. C*, 8, 7650–7657, 2020.
36. Dutta, P., Sikdar, A., Majumdar, A., Borah, M., Padma, N., Ghosh, S., Mait, U.N., Graphene aided gelation of MXene with oxidation protected surface for supercapacitor electrodes with excellent gravimetric performance. *Carbon*, 169, 225–234, 2020.
37. Wang, X., Zhai, H.W., Qie, B.Y., Cheng, Q., Li, A.J., Borovilas, J., Xu, B.Q., Shi, C.M., Jin, T.W., Liao, X.B., Li, Y.B., He, X.D., Du, S.Y., Fu, Y.K., Dontigny, M., Zaghib, K., Yang, Y., Rechargeable solid-state lithium metal batteries with

vertically aligned ceramic nanoparticle/polymer composite electrolyte. *Nano Energy*, 60, 205–212, 2019.

38. Zhao, Y., Yan, J.H., Cai, W.P., Lai, Y.M., Song, J., Yu, J.Y., Ding, B., Elastic and well-aligned ceramic LLZO nanofiber based electrolytes for solid-state lithium batteries. *Energy Storage Mater.*, 23, 306–13, 2019.
39. Chen, G., Chen, J., Pei, W.J., Lu, Y.M., Zhang, Q.F., Zhang, Q., He, Y.B., Bismuth ferrite materials for solar cells: Current status and prospects. *Mater. Res. Bull.*, 110, 39–49, 2019.
40. Li, D.X., Shen, Z.Y., Li, Z.P., Luo, W.Q., Wang, X.C., Wang, Z.M., Song, F.S., Li, Y.M., P-E hysteresis loop going slim in $Ba_{0.3}Sr_{0.7}TiO_3$-modified $Bi_{0.5}Na_{0.5}TiO_3$ ceramics for energy storage applications. *J. Adv. Ceram.*, 9, 183–192, 2020.
41. Bae, K., Kim, D.H., Choi, H.J., Son, J.W., Shim, J.H., High-performance protonic ceramic fuel cells with 1 mm thick Y: $Ba(Ce,Zr)O_3$ electrolytes. *Adv. Energy Mater.*, 8, 1801315, 2018.
42. Zeng, X.J., Shui, J.L., Liu, X.F., Liu, Q.T., Li, Y.C., Shang, J.X., Zheng, L.R., Yu, R.H., Single-atom to single-atom grafting of Pt1 onto Fe-N_4 center: Pt1@ Fe-N-C multifunctional electrocatalyst with significantly enhanced properties. *Adv. Energy Mater.*, 8, 1701345, 2018.
43. Jiang, C.S., Dunlap, N., Li, Y.J., Guthrey, H., Liu, P., Lee, S.H., Al-Jassim, M.M., Nonuniform ionic and electronic transport of ceramic and polymer/ceramic hybrid electrolyte by nanometer-sale operando imaging for solid-state battery. *Adv. Energy Mater.*, 10, 2070097, 2020.
44. Shu, L.L., Liang, R.H., Rao, Z.G., Fei, L.F., Ke, S.M., Wang, Y., Flexoelectric materials and their related applications: A focused review. *J. Adv. Ceram.*, 8, 153–73, 2019.
45. Lang, X.Y., Liu, B.T., Shi, X.M., Li, Y.Q., Wen, Z., Jiang, Q., Ultrahigh-power pseudocapacitors based on ordered porous heterostructures of electron-correlated oxides. *Adv. Sci.*, 3, 1500319, 2016.
46. Liu, P.P., Weng, X.L., Liu, Z.J., Zhang, Y.P., Qiu, Q.Y., Wang, W, Zhou, M.Y., Cai, W.Z., Ni, M., Liu, M.L., Liu, J., High-performance quasi-solid-state supercapacitor based on CuO nanoparticles with commercial-level mass loading on ceramic material $La_{1-x}Sr_xCoO_{3-\delta}$ as cathode. *ACS Appl. Energy Mater.*, 2, 1480–1488, 2019.
47. Irvine, J.T.S., Sinclair, D.C., West, A.R., Electroceramics: Characterization by impedance spectroscopy. *Adv. Mater.*, 2, 132–138, 1990.
48. Wang, G., Li, J., Zhang, X., Fan, Z., Yang, F., Feteira, A., Zhou, D., Sinclair, D.C., Ma, T., Tan, X., Ultrahigh energy storage density lead-free multilayers by controlled electrical homogeneity. *Energy Environ. Sci.*, 12, 582–588, 2019.
49. Ray, S., *An introduction to high voltage engineering*, Prentice-Hall of India, New Delhi, 2004.
50. Frohlich, H., On the theory of dielectric breakdown in solids. *Proc. R. Soc. Lond. A*, 188, 521–532, 1947.

51. Wang, J., Chen, X., Wang, J., Wang, G., Nie, H., Cao, F., Dong, X., Improved dielectric break down strength of $Pb_{0.99}(Zr_{0.95}Ti_{0.05})_{0.98}Nb_{0.02}O_3$ ferroelectric ceramics with the addition of CuO. *J. Mater. Sci.: Mater. Electron.*, 26, 8207–8211,2015.
52. Pu, Y., Yao, M., Zhang, L., Chen, M., Enhanced energy storage density of $0.55Bi_{0.5}Na_{0.5}TiO_3$-$0.45Ba_{0.85}Ca_{0.15}Ti_{0.85}Zr_{0.1}Sn_{0.05}O_3$ with MgO addition. *J. Alloys Compd.*, 702, 171–177, 2017.
53. Diao, C., Liu, H., Hao, H., Cao, M., Yao, Z., Effect of SiO_2 additive on dielectric response and energy storage performance of $Ba_{0.4}Sr_{0.6}TiO_3$ ceramics. *Ceram. Int.*, 42, 12639–12643, 2016.
54. Qi, J., Cao, M., Heath, J.P., Dean, J.S., Hao, H., Yao, Z., Yu, Z., Liu, H., Improved breakdown strength and energy storage density of a Ce doped strontium titanate core by silica shell coating. *J. Mater. Chem. C*, 6, 9130–9139, 2018.
55. Yang, L., Kong, X., Cheng, Z., Zhang, S., Enhanced energy storage performance of sodium niobate-based relax or dielectrics by a ramp-to-spike sintering profile. *ACS Appl. Mater. Interfaces*, 12, 32834–32841, 2020.
56. Xie, J., Yao, M., Gao, W., Su, Z., Yao, X., Ultrahigh breakdown strength and energy density in PLZST@ PBSAZM antiferroelectric ceramics based on core-shell structure. *J. Eur. Ceram. Soc.*, 39, 1050–1056, 2019.
57. Lu, X., Zhang, L., Talebinezhad, H., Tong, Y., Cheng, Z.Y., Effects of Cuo additive on the dielectric property and energy-storage performance of BaTiO3-SiO2 ceramic-glass composite. *Ceram. Int.*, 44, 16977–16983, 2018.
58. Bian, F., Yan, S., Xu, C., Liu, Z., Chen, X., Mao, C., Cao, F., Bian, J., Wang, G., Dong, X., Enhanced breakdown strength and energy density of antiferroelectric $Pb,La(Zr,Sn,Ti)O_3$ Ceramic by forming core-shell structure. *J. Eur. Ceram. Soc.*, 38, 3170–3176, 2018.
59. Xu, C., Su, R., Wang, Z., Wang, Y., Zhang, D., Wang, J., Bian, J., Wu, C., Lou, X., Yang, Y., Tuning the microstructure of $BaTiO_3$@SiO_2 core-shell nanoparticles for high energy storage composite ceramics. *J. Alloys Compd.*, 784, 173–181, 2019.
60. Zhao, P., Cai, Z., Chen, L., Wu, L., Huan, Y., Guo, L., Li, L., Wang, H., Wang, X., Ultra-high energy storage performance in lead-free multilayer ceramic capacitors via a multiscale optimization strategy. *Energy Environ. Sci.*, 13, 4882–4890, 2020.
61. Harrati, A., Manni, A., Bouari, A.E., Ei Hassani, I.E.E.A., Sadik, C., Elaboration, and thermomechanical characterization of ceramic-based on Moroccan geomaterials: Application in construction. *Mater. Today SAVE Proc.*, 30, 876–882, 2020.
62. Faseeva, G.R., Nafikov, R.M., Lapuk, S.E., Zakharov, Y.A., Novik, A.A., Vjuginova, A.A., Kabirov, R.R., Garipov, L.N., Ultrasound-assisted extrusion of construction ceramic samples. *Ceram. Int.*, 43, 7202–7210, 2017.
63. Li, D.X., Shen, Z.Y., Li, Z.P., Luo, W.Q., Song, F.S., Wang, X.C., Wang, Z.M., Li, Y.M., Optimization of polarization behavior in (1-x) BSBNT-xNN ceramics for pulsed power capacitors. *J. Mater. Chem. C*, 8, 7650–7657, 2020.

64. Dutta, P., Sikdar, A., Majumdar, A., Borah, M., Padma, N., Ghosh, S., Mait, U.N., Graphene aided gelation of MXene with oxidation protected surface for supercapacitor electrodes with excellent gravimetric performance. *Carbon*, 169, 225–234, 2020.
65. Wang, X., Zhai, H.W., Qie, B.Y., Cheng, Q., Li, A.J., Borovilas, J., Xu, B.Q., Shi, C.M., Jin, T.W., Liao, X.B., Li, Y.B., He, X.D., Du, S.Y., Fu, Y.K., Dontigny, M., Zaghib, K., Yang, Y., Rechargeable solid-state lithium metal batteries with vertically aligned ceramic nanoparticle/polymer composite electrolyte. *Nano Energy*, 60, 205–212, 2019.
66. Zhao, Y., Yan, J.H., Cai, W.P., Lai, Y.M., Song, J., Yu, J.Y., Ding, B., Elastic and well-aligned ceramic LLZO nanofiber based electrolytes for solid-state lithium batteries. *Energy Storage Mater.*, 23, 306–313, 2019.
67. Chen, G., Chen, J., Pei, W.J., Lu, Y.M., Zhang, Q.F., Zhang, Q., He, Y.B., Bismuth ferrite materials for solar cells: Current status and prospects. *Mater. Res. Bull.*, 110, 39–49, 2019.
68. Li, D.X., Shen, Z.Y., Li, Z.P., Luo, W.Q., Wang, X.C., Wang, Z.M., Song, F.S., Li, Y.M., P-E hysteresis loop going slim in $Ba_{0.3}Sr_{0.7}TiO_3$-modified $Bi_{0.5}Na_{0.5}TiO_3$ ceramics for energy storage applications. *J. Adv. Ceram.*, 9, 183–92, 2020.
69. Bae, K., Kim, D.H., Choi, H.J., Son, J.W., Shim, J.H., High-performance protonic ceramic fuel cells with 1 mm thick Y:Ba(Ce, Zr)O_3 electrolytes. *Adv. Energy Mater.*, 8, 1801315, 2018.
70. Zeng, X.J., Shui, J.L., Liu, X.F., Liu, Q.T., Li, Y.C., Shang, J.X., Zheng, L.R., Yu, R.H., Single-atom to single-atom grafting of Pt1 onto Fe-N4 center: Pt1@Fe-N-C multifunctional electrocatalyst with significantly enhanced properties. *Adv. Energy Mater.*, 8, 1701345, 2018.
71. Kuang, M., Han, P., Huang, L.S., Cao, N., Qian, L.P., Zheng, G.F., Electronic tuning of Co, Ni-based nanostructured (hydr) oxides for aqueous electrocatalysis. *Adv. Funct. Mater.*, 28, 1804886, 2018.
72. Kwon, H.J., Shin, K., Soh, M., Chang, H., Kim, J., Lee, J., Ko, G., Kim, B.H., Kim, D., Hyeon, T., Large-scale synthesis and medical applications of uniform-sized metal oxide nanoparticles. *Adv. Mater*, 30, 1704290, 2018.
73. Hu, M.Z., Yang, W.J., Tan, H.Y., Jin, L., Zhang, L., Kerns, P., Dang, Y.L., Dissanayake, S., Schaefer, S., Liu, B., Zhu, Y.Y., Suib, S.L., He, J., Template-free synthesis of mesoporous and crystalline transition metal oxide nanoplates with abundant surface defects. *Matter*, 2, 1244–1259, 2020.
74. Guan, B.Y., Yu, L., Lou, X.W., General synthesis of multishell mixed-metal oxyphosphide particles with enhanced electrocatalytic activity in the oxygen evolution reaction. *Angew. Chem. Int. Ed.*, 56, 2386–2389, 2017.
75. Zeng, X.J., Yang, B., Li, X.P., Li, R.F., Yu, R.H., Solvothermal synthesis of hollow Fe_3O_4 sub-micron spheres and their enhanced electrochemical properties for supercapacitors. *Mater. Des.*, 101, 35–43, 2016.
76. Osgood, H., Devaguptapu, S.V., Xu, H., Cho, J., Wu, G., Transition metal (Fe, Co, Ni, and Mn) oxides for oxygen reduction and evolution bifunctional catalysts in alkaline media. *Nano Today*, 11, 601–625, 2016.

77. Liu, Y.M., Tian, D., Biswas, A.N., Xie, Z.H., Hwang, S., Lee, J.H., Meng, H., Chen, J.G.G., Transition metal nitrides as promising catalyst supports for tuning CO/H_2 syngas production from electrochemical CO_2 reduction. *Angew. Chem. Int. Ed.*, 59, 11345–11348, 2020.
78. Wang, C.Y., Zeng, X.J., Jiang, G.M., Chen, M., Zhu, L.Y., Yu, R.G., General self-template synthesis of transition-metal oxide microspheres and their excellent charge storage properties. *Electrochim. Acta*, 283, 190–196, 2018.
79. Liu, Y., Li, X.C., Shen, W.M., Dai, Y., Kou, W., Zheng, W.J., Jiang, X.B., He, G.H., Multishelled transition metal-based microspheres: Synthesis and applications for batteries and supercapacitors. *Small*, 15, 1804737, 2019.
80. Li, J.F., Chen, D., Wu, Q.S., A Fe_2O_3 cased carbon composite as pure negative electrode for application as supercapacitor. *Eur. J. Inorg. Chem.*, 2019, 1301–1312, 2019.
81. Sugimoto, W., Yokoshima, K., Murakami, Y., Takasu, Y., Charge storage mechanism of nanostructured anhydrous and hydrous ruthenium-based oxides. *Electrochim. Acta*, 52, 1742–1748, 2006.
82. Casella, I.G. and Gatta, M., Study of the electrochemical deposition and properties of cobalt oxide species in citrate alkaline solutions. *J. Electroanal. Chem.*, 534, 31–38, 2002.
83. Lang, X.Y., Liu, B.T., Shi, X.M., Li, Y.Q., Wen, Z., Jiang, Q., Ultrahigh-power pseudocapacitors based on ordered porous heterostructures of electron-correlated oxides. *Adv. Sci.*, 3, 1500319, 2016.
84. Vidyadharan, B., Aziz, R.A., Misnon, I.I., Kumar, G.M.A., Ismail, J., Yusoff, M.M., Jose, R., High energy and power density asymmetric supercapacitors using electrospun cobalt oxide nanowire anode. *J. Power Sources*, 270, 526–535, 2014.
85. Vidhyadharan, B., Zain, N.K.M., Misnon, I.I., Aziz, R.A., Ismail, J., Yusoff, M.M., Jose, R., A novel supercapacitor electrode material with superior charge storage capacity. *J. Alloys Compd.*, 610, 143–150, 2014.
86. Zhang, Y., Guo, Z.H., Han, Z.Y., Xiao, X.Y., Effect of rare earth oxides doping on $MgAl_2O_4$ spinel obtained by sintering of secondary aluminium dross. *J. Alloys Compd.*, 735, 2597–603, 2018.
87. Zheng, X.Y., Liu, W.J., Qu, Q.T., Zheng, H.H., Huang, Y.H., Bi-functions of titanium and lanthanum co-doping to enhance the electrochemical performance of spinel $LiNi_{0.5}Mn_{1.5}O_4$ cathode. *J. Materiomics*, 5, 156–63, 2019.
88. Liu, Y., Ying, Y.R., Fei, L.F., Liu, Y., Hu, Q.Z., Zhang, G.G., Pang, S.Y., Lu, W., Mak, C.L., Luo, X., Zhou, L.M., Wei, M.D., Huang, H.T., Valence engineering via selective atomic substitution on tetrahedral sites in spinel oxide for highly enhanced oxygen evolution catalysis. *J. Am. Chem. Soc.*, 141, 8136–45, 2019.
89. Zhou, Y., Sun, S.N., Wei, C., Sun, Y.M., Xi, P.X., Feng, Z.X., Xu, Z.C.J., Significance of engineering the octahedral units to promote the oxygen evolution reaction of spinel oxides. *Adv. Mater.*, 31, 902509, 2019.
90. Hirakawa, T., Shimokawa, Y., Tokuzumi, W., Sato, T., Tsushida, M., Yoshida, H., Hinokuma, S., Ohyama, J., Machida, M., Multicomponent spinel oxide

solid solutions: A possible alternative to platinum group metal three-way catalysts. *ACS Catal.*, 9, 11763–11773, 2019.

91. Anwar, S., Muthu, K.S., Ganesh, V., Lakshminarasimhan, N., A comparative study of electrochemical capacitive behavior of $NiFe_2O_4$ synthesized by different routes. *J. Electrochem. Soc.*, 58, A976–81, 2011.
92. Rani, B.J., Ravi, G., Yuvakkumar, R., Ganesh, V., Ravichandran, S., Thambidurai, M., Rajalakshmi, A.P., Sakunthala, A., Pure and cobalt-substituted zinc-ferrite magnetic ceramics for supercapacitor applications. *Appl. Phys. A*, 124, 511, 2018.
93. Shamitha, C., Senthil, T., Wu, L.X., Kumar, B.S., Anandhan, S., Sol-gel electrospun mesoporous $ZnMn_2O_4$ nanofibers with superior specific surface area. *J. Mater. Sci.: Mater. Electron.*, 28, 15846–15860, 2017.
94. Kovalenko, A.S., Shilova, O.A., Morozova, L.V., Kalinina, M.V., Drozdova, I.A., Arsentev, M.Y., Features of the synthesis and the study of nanocrystalline cobalt-nickel spinel. *Glass Phys. Chem.*, 40, 106–113, 2014.
95. Sanchez, C.O., Ramírez, J.A., Quiles, E.O., Ferret, R., Nicolau, E., Polymer-$MTiO_3$ (M.Ca,Sr,Ba) composites as facile and scalable supercapacitor separators. *Energy Sci. Eng.*, 7, 730–740, 2019.
96. Santhosh, G., Nayaka, G.P., Bhatt, S., Ultrahigh capacitance of $NiCo_2O_4$/CeO_2mixed metal oxide material for supercapacitor applications. *J. Alloys Compd.*, 899, 163312, 2022.
97. Zeng, G.J., Chen, Y., Chen, L., Xiong, P.X., Wei, M.D., Hierarchical cerium oxide derived from metal-organic frameworks for high performance supercapacitor electrodes. *Electrochim. Acta*, 222, 773780, 2016.
98. Shen, L.F., Yu, L., Yu, X.Y., Zhang, X.G., Lou, X.W., Self-templated formation of uniform $NiCo_2O_4$ hollow spheres with complex interior structures for lithium-ion batteries and supercapacitors. *Angew. Chem. Int. Ed.*, 54, 18681872, 2015.
99. Tajik, S., Dubal, D.P., Romero, P.G., Yadegari, A., Rashidi, A., Nasernejad, B., Asiri, A.M., Nanostructured mixed transition metal oxides for high performance asymmetric supercapacitors: Facile synthetic strategy. *Int. J. Hydrogen Energy*, 42, 12384–12395, 2017.
100. Rashti, A., Lu, X., Dobson, A., Hassani, E., Nejad, F.F.K., He, K., Oh, T.S., Tuning MOF-derived Co_3O_4/$NiCo_2O_4$ nanostructures for high-performance energy storage. *ACS Appl. Energy Mater.*, 4, 15371547, 2021.
101. Taoa, B., Hea, J., Miao, F., Zhang, Y., MnO_2/$NiCo_2O_4$ loaded on nickel foam as a high-performance electrode for advanced asymmetric supercapacitor. *Vacuum*, 195, 110668, 2022.
102. Jin, J., Dai, Y., Lu, J., Dai, X., Tie, N., Ma, F., Wang, W., Pu, L., Zhang, H., Hydrothermal synthesis of NiO/NiCo2O4 nanomaterials for applications in electrochemical energy storage. *J. Mater. Sci. Mater. Electron.*, 33, 354–366, 2021.
103. Wu, C., Cai, J., Zhu, Y., Zhang, K., Hybrid reduced graphene oxide nanosheet supported Mn-Ni-Co ternary oxides for aqueous asymmetric supercapacitors. *ACS Appl. Mater. Interfaces*, 9, 1911419123, 2017.

104. Wei, C., Zhang, R., Zheng, X., Ru, Q., Chen, Q., Cui, C., Li, G., Zhang, D., Hierarchical porous $NiCo_2O_4/CeO_2$ hybrid materials for high performance supercapacitors. *Inorg. Chem. Front.*, 5, 31263134, 2018.
105. Wei, C., Zheng, X., Li, R., Wang, X., Xaio, Z., Wang, L., Mesoporous hybrid NiCo2O4/CeO2 hierarchical hollow spheres for enhanced supercapacitors. *ChemistrySelect*, 4, 1114911155, 2019.
106. Liu, Y., Ata, M.S., Shi, K., Zhu, G.Z., Botton, G.A., Zhitomirsky, I., Surface modification and cathodic electrophoretic deposition of ceramic materials and composites using celestine blue dye. *RSC Adv.*, 4, 29652, 2014.
107. Wei, J., Nagarajan, N., Zhitomirsky, I., Manganese oxide films for electrochemical supercapacitors. *J. Mater. Process. Technol.*, 186, 356–361, 2007.
108. Shilova, O.A., Antipov, V.N., Tikhonov, P.A., Kruchinina, I.Y., Arsentev, M.Y., Panova, T.I., Morozova, L.V., Moskovskaya, V.V., Kalinina, M.V., Tsvetkova, I.N., Ceramic nanocomposites based on oxides of transition metals of ionistors. *Glass Phys. Chem.*, 39, 570–578, 2013.

4

Ceramic Multilayers and Films for High-Performance Supercapacitors

Dulal Chandra Patra[1], Nitumoni Deka[1] and Pinku Chandra Nath[2]*

[1]*Department of Physics, National Institute of Technology Agartala, Jirania, Tripura, India*

[2]*Department of Applied Biology, University of Science & Technology, Meghalaya, Techno City, Ri-Bhoi, Meghalaya, India*

Abstract

Supercapacitors (SCs) are one of the greatest attractive electrical energy stored devices because of their rapid storage capacity; extended cycle stability, high-power density, and non-poisonous. The development of nanomaterials to generate affordable, extremely effective, and stable anodes has been the subject of significant research. Electroceramic materials are potential candidates for SCs electrodes. Therefore, enabling good electrical conductivity and excellent electron transport capabilities, as well as realizing commercially viable electroceramic electrodes, requires a basic understanding of electroceramic materials, an optimization strategy, and advancements in electroceramic electrode research. Lead-contained ceramics, like La-based lead zirconate titanate, have excellent energy storage capacities, but the poisonousness raises concerns about their utilization in commercial applications in that case lead-free capacitors are the most effective opportunity solution. Thus, Pb-free ceramics with higher power densities are needed. The regulation of local assembly, segment assembly, dielectric coating thickness, morphology, electrical homogeneousness, and conductivity through the selection of alloying, dopants, and base systems are some of the main elements covered to progress energy storage qualities. Furthermore, also discussed are the technological problems, applications, and prospects of electroceramic electrodes.

Keywords: electroceramics, supercapacitors, nanomaterials, lead-based ceramics, lead-free ceramics

**Corresponding author*: nathpinku005@gmail.com

Inamuddin, Tariq Altalhi and Sayed Mohammed Adnan (eds.) Electroceramics for High Performance Supercapacitors, (73–94) © 2024 Scrivener Publishing LLC

4.1 Introduction

Energy storage is thus becoming a crucial facilitator for environmentally friendly sustainable technologies, in more specialized applications like heart defibrillators and active armor, but also for the electrification of transportation [1]. Electrostatic capacitors, electrochemical supercapacitors, and Batteries are a few examples of existing energy storage technologies [2–4]. The prototype ferroelectric (FE) ceramics, $BaTiO_3$ (BT), is used to make multilayer ceramic capacitors (MLCCs) [5, 6]. The dielectric capacitors or nonpolarized electrostatics have more power density (~104–105 W/kg) in comparison to fuel cells or Li-ion batteries because of their quicker charging/discharging properties, which is useful for power electronics impulse power applications and electrical vehicles (EVs), which are shown in Figure 4.1(a) [7–9]. Due to high-power density and energy, electrostatic capacitors are therefore developing as potential options used for energy storage devices. It is explained by the exponential growth of papers dedicated to energy storage using electrostatic ceramic capacitors [10]. In addition to having a quick charging/discharging rate and a high-energy density, other characteristics like fatigue resistance, temperature/frequency stability, lifetime dependability, production cost, and equivalent series resistance are all correspondingly

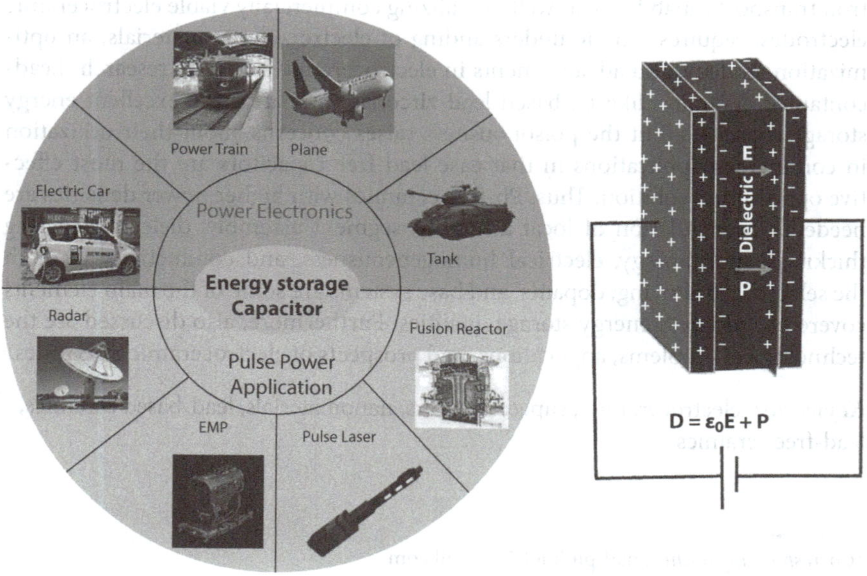

Figure 4.1 (a) Applications for energy storage capacitors for power electronics and pulse power application. (b) Diagram illustration of an electrostatic capacitor.

crucial for dielectric capacitors are utilized in practical applications [11–13]. In direction to change these requirements, the electroceramics essential (i) provide conversion efficiencies (>90%) and highly dense of energy (W_{rec}> 10 J/cm^3); (ii) withstand a broader frequency range (1–1000 Hz) and range of temperatures (–50°C to 250°C); (iii) show fatigue resistance and greater reliability (>105 cycles); and (iv) be well suited with affordable inner electrodes and be simple. Electrostatic capacitors have historically been made from an extensive variety of dielectric materials, including paper, plastic, and ceramics [14]. Slurry preparation, tape-casting, screen printing, laminating, considering, and termination are among the production techniques used to create ceramic MLs [15, 16]. This fabrication method, which is based on powder, allows for scaling up from laboratory research to industrial manufacturing. The market for ceramic MLs for electronic applications, such as but not limited to mobile phones, computers, and automobiles, was $5.3 billion in 2017 and would increase to $7.8 billion by 2024 [17]. Nowadays, capacitors are made of ceramics because they provide the optimum functionality in terms of breakdown strength(BDS), thermal stability, dielectric loss, and capacitance. Nowadays, emphasis is placed on obtaining the highest energy density possible for ceramics with thinner dielectric layers due to the decreased likelihood of defects (voids, like pores or microcracks), which are familiar causes of dielectric breakdown. Enhanced energy storage in capacitors through the use of empirical design principles in electroceramic capacitors, as shown in Table 4.1.

4.2 Fundamentals of Energy Storage in Electroceramics

4.2.1 Electrostatic Capacitors

The easy form of dielectric capacitors is made up of two parallel metal substrates that are separated by an insulating material. This insulator polarises in response to the utilization of a magnetic or acoustic field. A perfect capacitor has the charge "Q" reserved on each of its metal plates, and the voltage "V" that is implemented to the capacitor is what determines its real capacitors "C" (also known as its capacity to reserve charge), as shown by the following equation:

$$C = \frac{Q}{V} \tag{4.1}$$

The real device which is demonstrated in Figure 4.1 (b).

Table 4.1 Overall features of commercial category ceramic materials applicable for energy storage using Electronic Industries Alliance (EIA) arrangements.

Dielectric type	Dielectric BDS ($V\ \mu m^{-1}$)	Relative permittivity, ε_r	t (μm)	Energy at 1 kV ($J\ cm^{-3}$)	Reference
X7R	40	2000	30	1.34	[28]
X7R	30	2000	38	1.40	[64]
X7T	16	2800	70	0.71	[34]
Z5U	13.2	7500	95	0.02	[47]
C0G	65	75	18.5	0.88	[23]
X7R	90	1800	20	4.82	[55]

Gauss's law can be used to calculate the field strength induced in a dielectric by a voltage "V" across a separation distance between parallel plates of area "A."

$$V = Qd/\varepsilon A \tag{4.2}$$

'ε' is the dielectric's permittivity, which can also be thought of as a measurement of its polarizability. The following relationship can be derived from Eqns. (4.1) and (4.2).

4.2.2 Important Factors Designed for Assessing Energy Storage Characteristics

Electrostatic energy stored in the dielectric, W, through the application of a V, is calculated within the following equation:

$$W = \int_0^{Q_{max}} V.dq \tag{4.3}$$

In which, dq = incremental charge growth throughout the charging cycle.
Q_{max} = highest charge attained at the end of the cycle.
W_{st}, = energy stored per volume unit Ad.

$$W_{st} = \frac{W}{Ad} = \frac{\int_0^{Q_{max}} V\,dq}{Ad} = \int_0^{D} E \tag{4.4}$$

In the above Eqns. (4.4), D represents the electric displacement and E represents the electric field in the material. D represents electrical displacement and is calculated by the equation $D = \varepsilon_0 E + P$, (P = Polarisation). This calculation makes it possible to explain the results of stored energy density (W_{st}) about the parameter P.

$$W_{st} = \int_0^{P_{max}} E\,dP = \int_0^{E_{max}} \varepsilon_0 \varepsilon_r E\,dE \tag{4.5}$$

where P_{max} is the highest level of polarisation attained at E_{max}. Figure 4.2 shown in four different forms of polarisation response, to find the area of

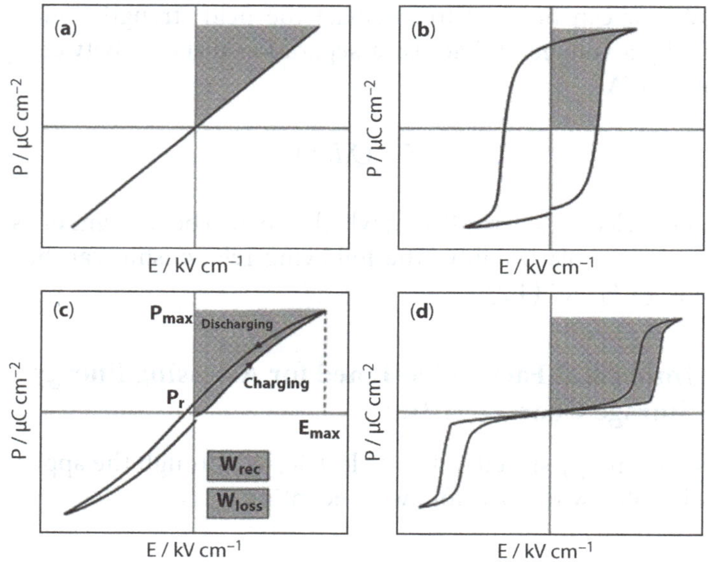

Figure 4.2 Four individual P–E hysteresis loops and their energy storage characteristics: (a) linear, (b) FE, (c) relaxor-ferroelectric (with the representation of energy storage calculation), and (d) antiferroelectric materials. *W_{loss} is loss energy density.

the polarization–electric (P–E) loop, mathematical integration essentially yields an approximation of W_{rec} [18].

The formula for calculating W_{rec} illustrated in Figure 4.2 (a) from the P–E response is

$$W_{rec} = \frac{1}{2}\varepsilon_0 \varepsilon_r E^2 \tag{4.6}$$

It unmistakably demonstrates how W_{rec} is reliant on E and. Figure 4.2 (b) and (d) illustrates instances where polarization responses diverge from linearity, necessitating the use of Eqn. (4.6) to compute W_{rec}.

From the above, it is clear that energy dissipation (W_{loss}) occurs in non-linear dielectric materials like AFEs, RFEs, and FEs; as a result, W_{rec} is essentially the utmost crucial parameter, as shown in Figure 4.2(c) (red mark area) and W_{rec} then converts

$$W_{rec} = \int_{P_r}^{P_{max}} E.dP$$

The capacitors energy alteration efficiency can then be computed as

$$\eta = \frac{W_{rec}}{W_{rec} + W_{loss}}$$

where W_{loss}, which corresponds to the region the P–E loop encloses, is the energy loss during discharge (Figure 4.2(c) green area).

4.3 Important Factors for Maximizing Energy Density

Electroceramics' microstructural characteristics are grain size, density, core-shell structures, and secondary phases, which show a significant impact on their ability to store energy. The distributions of resistive and conductive elements in the electrical microstructure as well as the inherent electrical response, such as the band gap, are both crucial elements for the maximization of energy density. The segment that follows covers these elements and provides scenarios for when and in what way they could be enhanced.

4.3.1 Intrinsic Band Gap

The energy gap between the upper of the valence band (VB) and the lowest of the conduction band (CB) is called a band gap (E_g). The terms insulator metal ($E_g = 0$ eV), semiconductor (0 E_v to E_g 4 eV), and insulator ($E_g > 4$ eV) are frequently used to describe materials. The inherent BDS for semiconductors can be described as

$$BDS = 1.36 \times 10^7 \times \left(\frac{E_g}{4.0}\right)^3 (V/cm)$$

where E_g and BDS are directly proportional [19]. The intrinsic BDS of semiconductors with wider E_g is higher as a result. With the use of experimental techniques like diffuse reflectance spectroscopy and absorbance spectroscopy, as well as theoretical methods like linear discriminant analysis, it is possible to study the band gaps and electronic structure of semiconductors [20]. A good instruction of thumb remains that conduction-activated energy (E_a) is about equal to E_g. Together can be enhanced by creating solid solutions or by doping, which frequently results in higher W_{rec} and BDS W_{rec} [21, 22].

4.3.2 Electrical Microstructure

The so-called electrical microstructure of electroceramics includes significant components such as the distribution of regions with various levels of $_r$and conductivity [23]. In many cases, the distributions are noticeably mixed and result in localization of the electric-field intensity in minor$_r$ areas/paths for collapse throughout interrelated conducting areas, such as the grain boundary response or core-shell microstructure of BT-based ceramics.

Impedance-spectroscopy (IS) is successful to display numerous responses for substances through multiple bulk regions, such as phase mixes, surface layers, or core-shell microstructures. The resistance and capacitance can be retrieved from these materials. Energy storage capacity is influenced by both the volume proportion and variance in the magnitude of capacitance and resistance for various electric responses. Specifying the significance of electrical microstructure, a full summary of the function of impedance spectroscopy is provided, and it has benefited over direct current techniques are highlighted [24].

4.4 Different Types of Electroceramics Capacitors for Energy Storage

4.4.1 Pb-Doped Ceramics

Due to their superior W_{rec} and η, lead-doped ceramics are employed industrially as energy storage components for high-powered pulsed capacitors [25–27].

4.4.1.1 Pb-Doped RFEs

There have been numerous reports of lead-based RFEs as prospective candidates for energy storage capacitors, including $Pb(Zn_{0.33}Nb_{0.67})\ O_3$–$PbTiO_3$(PZN-PT), $Pb(Mg_{0.33}Nb_{0.67})\ O_3$–$PbTiO_3$(PMN-PT), and (Sr, Pb, Bi)–TiO_3(SPBT)–based materials [28–30]. The (1-x) PMN-xPT ceramics relaxation behavior and energy storage capabilities, with W_{rec}~0.47 J cm^{-3} at ambient temperature. Figure 4.3 shows the impact of domain assembly on W_{rec} and thermal constancy of 0.2PMN–0.8 $Pb(Sn_xTi_{1-x})\ O_3$(PMN-PS_xT_{1-x})

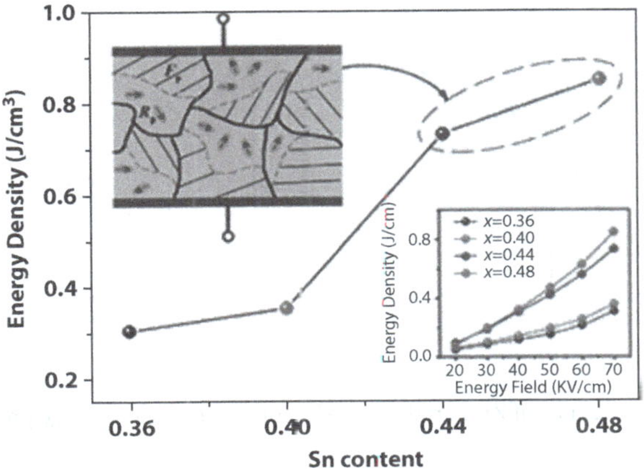

Figure 4.3 W_{rec} of 0.2PMN–0.8PS_xT_{1-x} ceramics with different Sn (x) contents at 70 kV cm^{-1}. The insets display the mechanism of improved energy storage due to existent-phase structure and the W_{rec} for PMN–PS_xT_{1-x} ceramics under different electric fields.

ceramics. W_{rec}~0.85 J cm^{-3} and high thermal constancy were found in 0.2PMN–0.8PST ceramics, which were accredited to the existence of ferroelectric domains [31–33].

4.4.1.2 Lead-Doped Antiferroelectrics

The initial identified AFE is $PbZrO_3$(PZ), which displays a cyclic P–E hysteresis loop under T_C. Though, applications for energy storage are inhibited by the highly serious switching field essential for an Antiferroelectrics-FE phase change at ambient temperature. A successful approach to solve the issue is the chemical replacement, and three eminent $PbZrO_3$-based structures are examined: (Pb, La)(Zr, Sn)O_3(PLZS) [34]; (Pb, La)(Zr, Sn)O_3(PLZST) [35]; and (Pb, La)(Zr, Ti)O_3(PLZT) [36]. Although, for energy storage applications, only PLZT with less than 10 mol% La is commonly used [37, 38]. Since weaker polarization and hence lower W_{rec} are associated with higher concentrations. A solid-state reaction method has been created $(La_{0.02}Pb_{0.97})$–$(Ti_{0.05}Zr_{0.95})O_3$ ceramics, producing W_{rec} values of 0.83 J cm^{-3} and 70% below a 55-kV cm^{-1} electric field [39]. The substitution of La and extra PbO in PLZT can both produce AFE and RFE behavior, which improves W_{rec} by encouraging a thin and slanted hysteresis loop. After 10^5 cycles, it is possible to get a high W_{rec} of 3.04 J cm^{-3} and 92% with minimal performance loss [36]. The W_{rec} of PLZT ceramics has also been confirmed to be effectively improved by fine-tuning the Ti/Zr ratio. In $(La_{0.07}Pb_{0.895})(Zr_xTi1_x)O_3$ ceramics, slimmer P–E loops have been

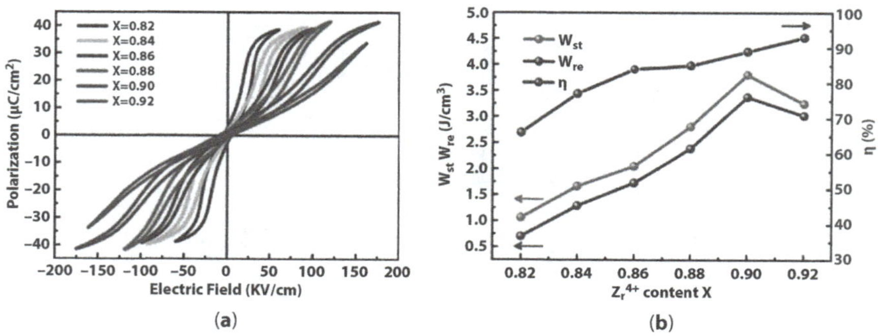

Figure 4.4 Consequence of Zr/Ti ratio on P–E loops and energy storage properties of PLZT.

given a W_{rec} = 3.48 J/cm³, It was blamed on the tolerance factor going down and "enhancing of antiferroelectricity" (Figure 4.4). It is also projected that Mn doping will rise the W_{rec} of PLZT by "growing antiferroelectricity" [38, 40].

4.4.2 Pb-Free Ceramics

Because of worries about the harmfulness of lead-doped compounds, the substantial investigation has concentrated on Pb-free electroceramics in the previous few decades [41, 42]. To replace current lead-based materials, there has been a fixed but continual development in their power storage recital [43, 44]. For power storage applications, several lead-free ceramic systems, together with those based on ST, BT, BF, NBT, NN, and $AgNbO_3$ (AN), are being studied as potential replacements for PLZT.

4.4.2.1 $BaTiO_3$-Based Ceramics

Since they were first developed, BT-doped dielectric ceramics have dominated the ceramic capacitor industry. Numerous investigations have documented enhancements in the power storage capacity of $BaTiO_3$-doped ceramics by (i) replacing oxides are MgO, SiO_2, Al_2O_3, and La_2O_3 [45–48] to improve BDS; (ii) using various techniques are cold sintering (CS), citrate precursor (CP), and SPS, to improve control grain growth or ceramic density [49–51]; (iii) addition of sintering assistances are $NiNd(Zn_{0.5}Ti_{0.5})O_3$, $ZnNb_2O_6$, $Bi(Zn_{0.67}Nb_{0.33})$-O_3, Bi-$(Zn_{0.5}Ti_{0.5})O_3$, $Bi(Zn_{0.5}Zr_{0.5})O_3$, $Bi(Li_{0.5}Nb_{0.5})O_3$, $BiYbO_3$, Bi-$(Mg_{0.5}Ti_{0.5})O_3$, BMN, $BiYbO_4$, $BiYbO_3$, Bi-$(Zn_{0.5}Ti_{0.5})O$ and $Bi_{0.9}Na_{0.1}In_{0.8}Zr_{0.2}O_3$ [51–61]. The outline of a Bi-doped perovskite with a multi-cation B-site, however, is the most successful strategy. By doping the Ba-site with a Bi ion that has an electrical $6s^2$ single pair structure, P_{max} is increased. By establishing a situation known as a "weakly coupled relaxor," in which numerous B-site ions from Ti with different valences and ionic radii obstruct long-range polar coupling, P_r is decreased. By applying this theory, it was possible to create BMT-BT that was temperature steady at 170°C and had a high W_{rec} of 4.49 J cm^{-3} with an of 93% (variation W_{rec} 5% and 4%). Higher commercial potential, because of the existence of 4 mol% Bi on the A-site, $BT_{0.06}B_{0.67}MN$ ($BT_{0.06}B_{0.67}MN$) has attributes similar to those of $BT_{0.06}$ even though $BT_{0.06}B_{0.67}MN$ is not electrically homogenous, Figure 4.5(c) and (d) shows that BDS and W_{rec} were nevertheless optimized by minimizing, albeit not removing, the discrepancy between grain boundary and the bulk responses concerning undoped $BT.Bi_{0.67}(Mg_{0.33}Nb_{0.67})O_3$($BT_{0.06}B_{0.67}MN$), but in arrangements appropriate with Pd/Ag electrodes. For $BT_{0.06}B_{0.67}MN$ ceramics, which also

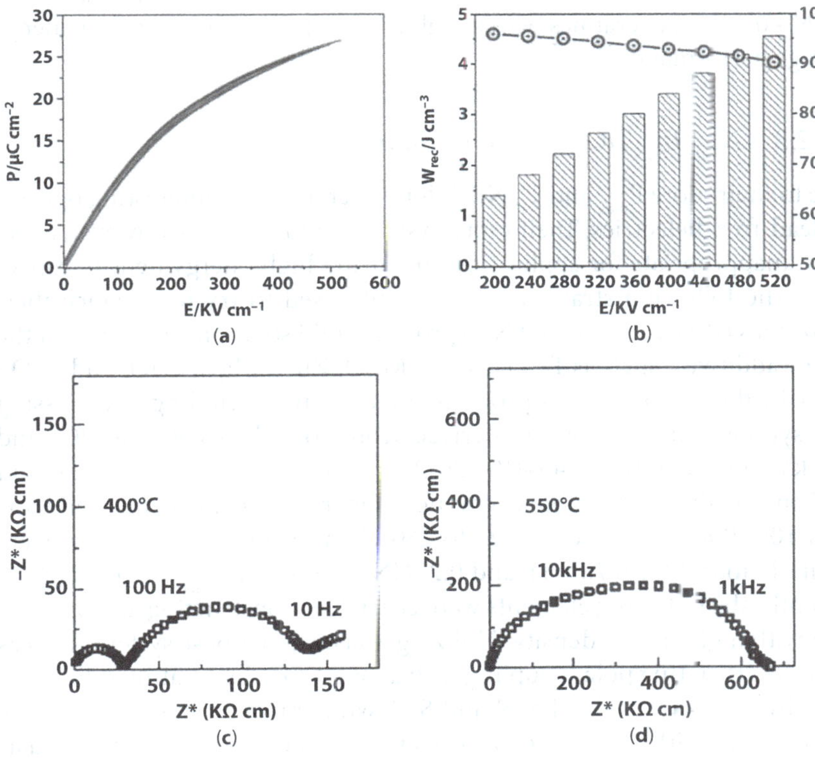

Figure 4.5 (a) Unipolar P–E loops under E_{max} and (b) calculated W_{rec} and η at different electric field for BT–0.06$B_{2/3}$MN ceramics. (c) Z* plots of (c) BT at 400°C and (d) BT–0.06$B_{2/3}$MN at 550°C.

promoted from the high breakdown strength, 520 kV cm^{-1}, among all published BT-doped arrangements, like power storage qualities, W_{rec} = 4.5 J/cm^3 and 92% (Figure 4.5(a),(b)) to BTBMT, were found [62].

4.4.2.2 $K_{0.5}Na_{0.5}NbO_3$-Doped Ceramics

When KNN (Na, Bi) HfO_3 solid solutions energy storage capabilities were initially studied in 2016, W_{rec} 0.55 J cm^{-3} was attained at 130 kV/cm. By reducing porosity and limiting grain formation, CuO and ZnO were added as sintering supports to improve W_{rec} in KNN-based ceramics. The 0.8KNN–0.2Sr($Nb_{0.5}Sc_{0.5}$)O_3 ceramic with 0.5 mol% CuO and ZnO increased the density of 0.1BMN–0.9KNN ceramics and decreased the sintering temperature. It was determined that this material has a BDS of 400 kV cm^{-1}. Additionally, it has been shown that a third perovskite final member, such as BMN, BF, or ST, can improve energy storage capabilities [54–56]. W_{rec} of 4.04 J cm^{-3} at 400 kV cm^{-1} was achieved in 0.15ST –0.85KNN bulk ceramics, and 0.10 BMN –0.90KNN ceramics with a high P_{max} (41 μC cm^{-2}) realized in energy storage performance.

4.4.2.3 $Na_{0.5}Bi_{0.5}TiO_3$–Doped Ceramics

Due to their more P_{max} and T_c, NBT-doped ceramics are interesting options for lead-free dielectrics. Their more hysteresis and low BDS, however, make them inappropriate for applications requiring high-energy density capacitors. The following strategies are typically used to try to enhance their properties (i) SBT, NN, and AN to produce solid solutions [63–71]; (ii) the use of additives, such as Fe_2O_3, SnO_2, MnO, ZnO, MgO, CaO, and ZrO_2; and (iii) the use of various processing techniques including hot-pressing and synthesis using powders derived from sol-gel. Notably, at 200 and 720 kV cm^{-1}, 0.55NBT0.45–($Bi_{0.2}Sr_{0.7}$)TiO_3(SBT) produced W_{rec} ~ 2.6 and 9.6 J cm^{-3} with > 90% for bulk ceramic. Higher W_{rec} of 7.02 J cm^{-3} and 85%, with 10% fluctuation from 25°C to 250°C and from 0.1 to 100 Hz, were similarly found for 0.78NBT and 0.22NN ceramics at E_{max} of 360 kV/cm. Recently, the following elements were crucial for constructing an optimum RFE with high-energy density: Utilizing a vastly polar base system, such as NBT, (i) disrupting polar coupling with a long-range by creating solid solutions by compounds like BMN and SBT while maintaining average ionic polarizability, (ii) simultaneously causing or maintaining electrical equality with an extremely resistive single element in IS (260 kV/cm^2 at 650°C). Wrec = 7.5 J/cm^3, E_{max} = 470 kV/cm, and = 92% for 0.62NBT–0.08BMN–0.30SBT are the results of these factors together.

4.4.2.4 *$AgNbO_3$-Based Ceramics*

Because of their high P_{max} and low P_r, AFEs have been regarded as the best possible choice for energy storage capacitors. Only a few lead-free AFE systems exist; one in particular, AN, which has a significant saturation polarization of 52 μC cm^{-2} below an E_{max} of 220 kV cm^{-1}, shows great potential. Recent studies on AN ceramic have concentrated on stabilizing the AFE segment to shift the switching field to higher fields while also improving P_{max}. Numerous studies on AN have recently concentrated on (i) substituting isovalent B-site oxides like WO_3 and MnO_2 [72, 73] (ii) doping Bi, Sr, Ba, La, Sm, Gd, and Ca on the A site frequently with isovalent Ta coating on the B site [74–78] (iii) making solid solutions with end-members like $Bi(Zn_{0.66}Nb_{0.33})O_3$ and $BiMnO_3$. Table 4.2 has been shown an outline of the power storage capabilities of lead-free materials.

4.5 Application of Electroceramics Supercapacitor

More than 20 years ago, there has been discussion on even if lead-free electroceramics can completely change their lead-doped equivalents. On most criteria, lead-based compositions perform better than their lead-free

Table 4.2 Summary of energy storage properties for lead-free ceramics.

Compounds	E (kV cm^{-1})	P (μC cm^{-2})	W_{rec} (J cm^{-3})	η (%)	Reference
0.9NN–0.10BMN	300	23	2.8	82	[35]
0.8NN–0.2ST	323	34.5	3.02	80.7	[45]
$Na_{0.7}Bi_{0.1}NbO_3$	250	30	4.03	85.4	[55]
NN–0.09Bi$(Zn_{0.5}Ti_{0.5})O_3$	200	29	2.1	76	[27]
0.92NN–0.08Bi $(Mg_{0.5}Ti_{0.5})O_3$	480	38	5.57	71	[28]
$(Na_{0.9}1La_{0.09})(Nb_{0.82}Ti_{0.18})O_3$	550	42	6.5	65.9	[54]
$Ag_{0.96}Ba_{0.02}NbO_3$	180	34	2.3	46	[49]
0.6 mol % $BiMnO_3$–AN	175	36	2.4	54	[33]
$Ag_{0.91}Bi_{0.03}NbO$	200	30	2.6	86	[31]
$Ag_{0.92}Ca_{0.04}NbO_3$	220	37.6	3.55	63	[29]
$Ag_{0.90}Ca_{0.05}Nb_{0.95}Ta_{0.05}O_3$	210	37	3.36	58	[26]

counterparts. In addition, many other formulations would be needed to address the features of basically doped PZT in lead-free compositions. However, it is extremely expected that Pb-free electroceramics will start to change their Pb-doped equivalents and achieve extensive manufacture in the next years as a result of environmental regulations, provided that the performance, dependability, and price of Pb-free are comparable with PZT. Among other applications, lead-free capacitors have the best chance of being manufactured on a large scale because (i) the Performance of Pb-free configurations approaches that of Pb-doped configurations; (ii) a decrease in inherent electrical characteristics can be made up for by an increase in BDS, frequently by reducing film thickness; and (iii) the lead-free BT-based MLCCs dominate the capacitor market, so it is anticipated that the associated price will In the case of piezoelectric ceramics, which are conquered by PZT and its by-products, this second claim is false. Figure 4.6 summarizes and plots the energy storage performances for lead-doped and lead-free ceramics, including Emax, P, W_{rec}, and (note: glass ceramics are excluded). Figure 4.6(a) shows a relationship between W_{rec} and E_{max} for various lead-free/doped bulk ceramics. In comparison to lead-free options, lead-doped bulk ceramics offer the advantages of more E_{max} (up to 400 kV cm^{-1}) and W_{rec} (up to 15 J cm^{-3}). For lead-free compositions, NN-doped ceramics presently give the maximum W_{rec} under more E (>350 kV cm^{-1}), followed by NBC-, AN-, KNN-, and BF- based materials. ST and BT-doped ceramics, which are the current foundation for MLCC manufacture, have the lowest W_{rec} despite having a more E_{max} of 450 kV cm^{-1}. However, they are also among the greatest commercially attractive dielectrics. Figure 4.6(b) compares P and W_{rec}. BF-, Lead-, and NBT- doped materials have extremely high P values (up to 60 μC/cm^2), followed by AN-and AFE NN- doped materials (40 μC/cm^2) and KNN-doped materials (35 μC/cm^2), with BT- and ST-doped materials having the lowermost P values (up to 25 μC/cm^2). Due to their high polarization, containing electroceramics such as NBT and BF have recently received a lot of attention as potential lead-free electroceramic materials. By lowering the P_r throughout chemical replacement by perovskite end members to construct a relaxor through an incredibly thin P–E loop, a more P (60 μC cm^{-1}) is attained in BF and NBT-doped materials. Therefore, the benefit of an end member with a strong intrinsic polarisation, like BF, is somewhat diminished. For AFEs like NN- and AN-doped materials, intermediate P 40 μC cm^{-2} values are recorded, although P_{max} is frequently constrained because compositions show polarisation saturation as a purpose of the applied field. Used for a variety of compositions, W_{rec} vs. is contrasted in Figure 4.6(c). The best (90%) is revealed by ST-based

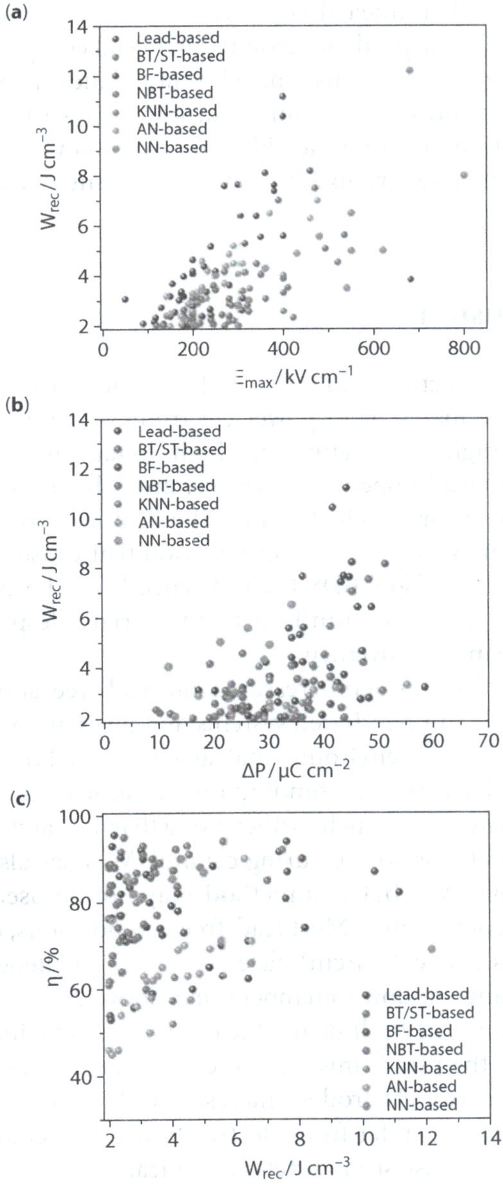

Figure 4.6 Comparison of (a) E_{max} vs W_{rec}; (b) ΔP vs W_{rec}; and (c) W_{rec} vs η for lead-based/lead-free bulk ceramics.

materials since of their linear-like dielectric property. Since it depends on several variables, changes depend on the material composition for NBT-, BT-, and lead-doped materials. The ST + Li_2O_3 and the NBT0.06BT layers' breakdown routes were minimized, improving BDS, and electrical field redistribution and interface blocking were key factors. The difference in ε_r and thickness ratio between the adjacent layers has an impact on BDS as well [78, 80].

4.6 Conclusion

In modern microelectronics, lead-doped ceramics have a lot of potential as energy storage materials in power electronic and pulsed power applications, where high temperature and high voltage are required. Energy density is high in lead-doped AFE-type ceramics, but optimizing BDS and lowering electro strains is challenging. The lead/lead oxide volatilization causes lead-vacancy ($VPb^{\cdot\cdot}$) and VO. Creation that causes present leakage is a common cause of low BDS (300 kV/cm). It has been challenging to achieve the BDS values seen in lead-free materials, despite possible processing and dopant improvements.

This chapter does in-depth research on lead-free applicants like ST, NBT, BF, AN, BT, and NN-based systems and gives an overview of them. Because of how possible environmental laws about making and using lead-based products have affected funding organizations and prizes, research into lead-free materials is much further along than research into lead-based materials. Current work on texturing ceramic MLs has also shown that it can help improve W_{rec}, but this method may not be used commercially because it is so complicated. Most lead-free compositions, especially those with W_{rec} values above 10 J/cm^3, face two major challenges: (i) expanding their operating window to temperatures above 200°C and frequencies above 100 Hz, and (ii) finding an efficient inexpensive interior electrode system to enable their trade misuse. Presently, nearly the entire ML records are cited by Pt interior electrodes. Interestingly, lead-free AFEs, RFEs, and RFEs typically do not suffer from electro strains, a foremost flaw in lead-doped material, because strain levels are typically noticeably lesser (0.5%) at high fields. Similar to lead-based ceramics, the high field *in situ* experiments are needed to fully understand the energy storage mechanisms. The W_{rec}, cyclic reliability, and thermal stability can all be improved by teaching more about the role that defects chemistry, alloying, and doping play in these characteristics.

References

1. Yao, Z., Song, Z., Hao, H., Yu, Z., Cao, M., Zhang, S., Lanagan, M.T., Liu, H., Homogeneous/inhomogeneous-structured dielectrics and their energy-storage performances. *Adv. Mater.*, 29, 1601727, 2017.
2. Sherrill, S.A., Banerjee, P., Rubloff, G.W., Lee, S.B., High to ultra-high power electrical energy storage. *Phys. Chem. Chem. Phys.*, 13, 20714, 2011.
3. Liu, C., Li, F., Ma, L.-P., Cheng, H.-M., Advanced materials for energy storage. *Adv. Mater.*, 22, E28–E62, 2010.
4. Liu, C., Yu, Z., Neff, D., Zhamu, A., Jang, B.Z., Graphene-based supercapacitor with an ultrahigh energy density. *Nano Lett.*, 10, 4863–4868, 2010.
5. Wang, D., Zhou, D., Song, K., Feteira, A., Randall, C.A., Reaney, I.M., Cold-sintered C0G multilayer ceramic capacitors. *Adv. Electron. Mater.*, 5, 1900025, 2019.
6. Pan, M.-J. and Randall, C.A., A brief introduction to ceramic capacitors. *IEEE Electr. Insul. Mag.*, 26, 44–50, 2010.
7. Li, Q., Liu, F., Yang, T., Wang, Q., Sandwich-structured polymer nanocomposites with high energy density and great charge–discharge efficiency at elevated temperatures. *Proc. Natl. Acad. Sci. U.S.A.*, 113, 9995–10000, 2016.
8. Whittingham, M.S., Materials challenges facing electrical energy storage. *MRS Bull.*, 33, 411–419, 2008.
9. Sun, H., Wang, W., Yu, Z., Yuan, Y., Wang, S., Jiao, S., A new aluminium-ion battery with high voltage, high safety and low cost. *Chem. Commun.*, 51, 11892–11895, 2015.
10. Feng, M., Zahang, T., Li, J., Chen, Q., Chi, Q., Lei, Q., Recent advances in multilayer-structure dielectrics for energy storage application. *Adv. Sci.*, 8, 2102221, 2021.
11. Li, W.B., Zhou, D., Xu, R., Wang, D.W., Su, J.Z., Pang, L.X., Liu, W.F., Chen, G.H., $BaTiO_3$ -Based multilayers with outstanding energy storage performance for high temperature capacitor applications. *ACS Appl. Energy Mater.*, 2, 5499–5506, 2019.
12. Wang, G., Lu, Z., Li, Y., Li, L., Ji, H., Feteira, A., Zhou, D., Wang, D., Zahang, S., Reaney, I.M., Electroceramics for high-energy density capacitors: Current status and future perspectives. *Chem. Rev.*, 121, 6124–6172, 2021.
13. Zhao, P., Chi, Z., Wu, L., Zhu, C., Li, L., Wang, X., Perspectives and challenges for lead-free energy-storage multilayer ceramic capacitors. *J. Adv. Ceram.*, 10, 1153–1193, 2021.
14. Yadav, A.K., Fan, H., Yan, B., Wang, C., Ma, J., Zhang, M., Wang, W., Dong, W., Wang, S., Enhanced storage energy density and fatigue free properties for $0.94Bi_{0.50}(Na_{0.78}K_{0.22})_{0.50}Ti_{1-x}(Al_{0.50}Nb_{0.50})_XO_3$-$0.06BaZrO_3$ceramics. *Ceram. Int.*, 46, 17044–17052, 2020.

15. Wang, D., Wang, G., Murakami, S., Fan, Z., Feteira, A., Zhou, D., Sun, S., Zhao, Q., Reaney, I.M., $BiFeO_3$-$BaTiO_3$: A new generation of lead-free electroceramics. *J. Adv. Dielectr.*, 08, 1830004, 2018.
16. Murakami, S., Wang, D., Mostaed, A., Khesro, A., Feteira, A., Sinclair, D.C., Fan, Z., Tan, X., Reaney, I.M., High strain (0.4%) $Bi(Mg_{2/3}Nb_{1/3})O_3$-$BaTiO_3$-$BiFeO_3$ lead-free piezoelectric ceramics and multilayers. *J. Am. Ceram. Soc.*, 101, 5428–5442, 2018.
17. Sakabe, Y., Multilayer ceramic capacitors. *Curr. Opin. Solid State Mater. Sci.*, 2, 584–587, 1997.
18. Jaffe, B., Antiferroelectric ceramics with field-enforced transitions: A new nonlinear circuit element. *Proc. IRE*, 49, 1264–1267, 1961.
19. Wang, L.M., Relationship between intrinsic breakdown field and bandgap of materials, in: *2006 25th International Conference on Microelectronics*, IEEE, pp. 576–579, 2006.
20. Wang, D., Wang, G., Lu, Z., Al-Jlaihawi, Z., Feteira, A., Crystal structure, phase transitions and photoferroelectric properties of $KNbO_3$-based lead-free ferroelectric ceramics: A brief review. *Front. Mater.*, 7, 91, 2020.
21. Neudeck, P.G., Okojie, R.S., Chen, L.Y., High-temperature electronics - a role for wide bandgap semiconductors? *Proc. IEEE*, 90, 1065–1076, 2002.
22. Qi, H., Xie, A., Tian, A., Zuo, R., Superior energy-storage capacitors with simultaneously giant energy density and efficiency using nanodomain engineered $BiFeO_3$-$BaTiO_3$-$NaNbO_3$ lead-free bulk ferroelectrics. *Adv. Energy Mater.*, 10, 1903338, 2020.
23. Yu, X., Chai, S., Kuang, X., Su, C., Pan, F., Fang, L., Su, Q., Conductivity, dielectric loss, and electrical heterogeneous microstructure of eight-layer twinned hexagonal perovskite ceramics $Ba_8CuTa_6O_{24-\delta}$. *J. Am. Ceram. Soc.*, 96, 2510–2514, 2013.
24. Wang, G., Li, J., Zhang, X., Fan, Z., Yang, F., Feteira, A., Zhou, D., Sinclair, D.C., Ma, T., Tan, X., Wang, D., Reaney, I.M., Ultrahigh energy storage density lead-free multilayers by controlled electrical homogeneity. *Energy Environ. Sci.*, 12, 582–588, 2019.
25. Yuan, J., Wang, D.W., Lin, H.B., Zhao, Q.L., Zhang, D.Q., Cao, M.S., Effect of ZnO whisker content on sinterability and fracture behaviour of PZT piezoelectric composites. *J. Alloys Compd.*, 504, 123–128, 2010.
26. Wang, D.W., Cao, M.S., Yuan, J., Zhao, Q.L., Li, H.B., Zhang, D.Q., Agathopoulos, S., Enhanced piezoelectric and ferroelectric properties of Nb_2O_5 modified lead zirconate titanate-based composites: Rapid communications of the American Ceramic Society. *J. Am. Ceram. Soc.*, 94, 647–650, 2011.
27. Zhao, Q.L., Cao, M.S., Yuan, J., Lu, R., Wang, D.W., Zhang, D.Q., Thickness effect on electrical properties of $Pb(Zr_{0.52}Ti_{0.48})O_3$ thick films embedded with ZnO nanowhiskers prepared by a hybrid sol–gel route. *Mater. Lett.*, 64, 632–635, 2010.
28. Zhang, T.F., Tang, X.G., Liu, Q.X., Jiang, Y.P., Huang, X.X., Zhou, Q.F., Energy-storage properties and high-temperature dielectric relaxation behaviors of

relaxor ferroelectric $Pb(Mg_{1/3}Nb_{2/3})O_3$–$PbTiO_3$ ceramics. *J. Phys. D: Appl. Phys.*, 49, 095302, 2016.

29. Chao, M., Liu, J., Zeng, M., Wang, D., Yu, H., Yuan, Y., Zhang, S., High discharge efficiency of (Sr, Pb, Bi) TiO_3 relaxor ceramics for energy-storage application. *Appl. Phys. Lett.*, 112, 203903, 2018.
30. Liu, Z., Lu, T., Ye, J., Wang, G., Dong, X., Withers, R., Liu, Y., Antiferroelectrics for energy storage applications: A review. *Adv. Mater. Technol.*, 3, 1800111, 2018.
31. Li, Y., Sun, N., Li, X., Du, J., Chen, L., Gao, H., Hao, X., Cao, M., Multiple electrical response and enhanced energy storage induced by unusual coexistent-phase structure in relaxor ferroelectric ceramics. *Acta Mater.*, 146, 202–210, 2018.
32. Shkuratov, S.I., Baird, J., Antipov, V.G., Hackenberger, W., Luo, J., Zhang, S., Lynch, C.S., Chase, J.B., Jo, H.R., Roberts, C.C., Complete stress-induced depolarization of relaxor ferroelectric crystals without transition through a non-polar phase. *Appl. Phys. Lett.*, 112, 122903, 2018.
33. Qi, X., Zhao, Y., Sun, E., Du, J., Li, K., Sun, Y., Yang, B., Zhang, R., Cao, W., Large electrostrictive effect and high energy storage performance of Pr^{3+}-doped PIN-PMN-PT multifunctional ceramics in the ergodic relaxor phase. *J. Eur. Ceram. Soc.*, 39, 4060–4069, 2019.
34. Liu, X., Li, Y., Hao, X., Ultra-high energy-storage density and fast discharge speed of $(Pb_{0.98-x}La_{0.02}Sr_x)(Zr_{0.9}Sn_{0.1})_{0.995}O_3$ antiferroelectric ceramics prepared *via* the tape-casting method. *J. Mater. Chem. A*, 7, 11858–11866, 2019.
35. Zhao, Q., Lei, H., He, G., Di, J., Wang, D., Tan, P., Jin, H., Cao, M., Effects of thickness on energy storage of (Pb, La)(Zr, Sn, Ti)O_3 antiferroelectric films deposited on $LaNiO_3$ electrodes. *Ceram. Int.*, 42, 1314–1317, 2016.
36. Jo, H.R. and Lynch, C.S., A high energy density relaxor antiferroelectric pulsed capacitor dielectric. *J. Appl. Phys.*, 119, 024104, 2016.
37. Li, B., Liu, Q.X., Tang, X.G., Zhang, T.F., Jiang, Y.P., Li, W.H., Luo, J., Antiferroelectric to relaxor ferroelectric phase transition in PbO modified $(Pb_{0.97}La_{0.02})(Zr_{0.95}Ti_{0.05})O_3$ ceramics with a large energy-density for dielectric energy storage. *RSC Adv.*, 7, 43327–43333, 2017.
38. Qiao, P., Zhang, Y., Chen, X., Zhou, M., Wang, G., Dong, X., Effect of Mn-doping on dielectric and energy storage properties of $(Pb_{0.91}La_{0.06})(Zr_{0.96}Ti_{0.04})O_3$ antiferroelectric ceramics. *J. Alloys Compd.*, 780, 581–587, 2019.
39. Li, B., Liu, Q., Tang, X., Zhang, T., Jiang, Y., Li, W., Luo, J., High energy storage density and impedance response of PLZT2/95/5 antiferroelectric ceramics. *Materials*, 10, 143, 2017.
40. Samanta, S., Sankaranarayanan, V., Sethupathi, K., Effect of Nb and Fe co-doping on microstructure, dielectric response, ferroelectricity and energy storage density of PLZT. *J. Mater. Sci.: Mater. Electron.*, 29, 20383–20394, 2018.
41. Mohammed, T.I., Kog, S.C.L., Reaney, I.M., Sinclair, D.C., Mustapha, K.B., Acquaye, A., Are lead-free piezoelectrics more environmentally friendly? *MRS Commun.*, 7, 1–7, 2017.

42. Mohammed, T.I., Kog, S.C.L., Reaney, I.M., Acquaye, A., Wang, D., Taylor, S., Genovese, A., Integrated hybrid life cycle assessment and supply chain environmental profile evaluations of lead-based (lead zirconate titanate) versus lead-free (potassium sodium niobate) piezoelectric ceramics. *Energy Environ. Sci.*, 9, 3495–3520, 2016.
43. Hao, X., A review on the dielectric materials for high energy-storage application. *J. Adv. Dielectr.*, 03, 1330001, 2013.
44. Sun, Z., Wang, Z., Tian, Y., Wang, G., Wang, W., Yang, M., Wang, X., Zhang, F., Pu, Y., Progress, outlook, and challenges in lead-free energy-storage ferroelectrics. *Adv. Electron. Mater.*, 6, 1900698, 2020.
45. Yang, H., Yan, F., Zhang, G., Lin, Y., Wang, F., Dielectric behavior and impedance spectroscopy of lead-free $Ba_{0.85}Ca_{0.15}Zr_{0.1}Ti_{0.9}O_3$ ceramics with B_2O_3-Al_2O_3-SiO_2 glass-ceramics addition for enhanced energy storage. *J. Alloys Compd.*, 720, 116–125, 2017.
46. Ren, P., Wang, Q., Li, S., Zhao, G., Energy storage density and tunable dielectric properties of $BaTi_{0.85}Sn_{0.15}O_3$/MgO composite ceramics prepared by SPS. *J. Eur. Ceram. Soc.*, 37, 1501–1507, 2017.
47. Ma, R., Cui., B., Shanggun, M., Wang, S., Wang, Y., Chang, Z., Wang, Y., A novel double-coating approach to prepare fine-grained BaTiO3@La2O3@SiO2 dielectric ceramics for energy storage application. *J. Alloys Compd.*, 690, 438–445, 2017.
48. Zhao, Q., Wang, X., Gong, H., Liu, B., Luo, B., Li, L., The properties of Al_2O_3 coated fine-grain temperature stable $BaTiO_3$-based ceramics sintered in reducing atmosphere. *J. Am. Ceram. Soc.*, 101, 1245–1254, 2018.
49. Zhan, D., Xu, Q., Huang, D.P., Liu, H.X., Chen, W., Zhang, F., Contributions of intrinsic and extrinsic polarization species to energy storage properties of $Ba_{0.95}Ca_{0.05}Zr_{0.2}Ti_{0.8}O_3$ ceramics. *J. Phys. Chem. Solids*, 114, 220–227, 2018.
50. Ma, J.P., Chen, X.M., Quyang, W.Q., Wang, J., Li, H., Fang, J.L., Microstructure, dielectric, and energy storage properties of $BaTiO_3$ ceramics prepared via cold sintering. *Ceram. Int.*, 44, 4436–4441, 2018.
51. Liu, B., Wu, Y., Huang, Y.H., Song, K.X., Wu, Y.J., Enhanced dielectric strength and energy storage density in $BaTi_{0.7}Zr_{0.3}O_3$ ceramics via spark plasma sintering. *J. Mater. Sci.*, 54, 4511–4517, 2019.
52. Yuan, Q., Yao, F., Wang, Y., Ma, R., Wang, H., Relaxor ferroelectric $0.9BaTiO_3$-$0.1Bi(Zn_{0.5}Zr_{0.5})O_3$ ceramic capacitors with high energy density and temperature stable energy storage properties. *J. Mater. Chem. C*, 5, 9552–9558, 2017.
53. Cui, C., Pu, Y., Shi, R., High-energy storage performance in lead-free (0.8-x) $SrTiO_3$-$0.2Na_{0.5}Bi_{0.5}TiO_3$-$xBaTiO_3$ relaxor ferroelectric ceramics. *J. Alloys Compd.*, 740, 1180–1187, 2018.
54. Dong, X., Chen, H., Wei, M., Wu, K., Zhang, J., Structure, dielectric and energy storage properties of $BaTiO_3$ ceramics doped with $YNbO_4$. *J. Alloys Compd.*, 744, 721–727, 2018.

55. Wang, T., Jin, L., Li, C., Hu, Q., Wei, X., Relaxor ferroelectric $BaTiO_3$-Bi($Mg_{2/3}$ $Nb_{1/3}$)O_3 ceramics for energy storage application. *J. Am. Ceram. Soc.*, 98, 559–566, 2015.
56. Li, W.-B., Zhou, D., Pang, L.-X., Enhanced energy storage density by inducing defect dipoles in lead free relaxor ferroelectric $BaTiO_3$-based ceramics. *Appl. Phys. Lett.*, 110, 132902, 2017.
57. Wu, L., Wang, X., Li, L., Lead-free $BaTiO_3$–Bi($Zn_{2/3}$ $Nb_{1/3}$)O_3 weakly coupled relaxor ferroelectric materials for energy storage. *RSC Adv.*, 6, 14273–14282, 2016.
58. Li, W.-B., Zhou, D., Pang, L.-X., Xu, R., Guo, H.-H., Novel barium titanate based capacitors with high energy density and fast discharge performance. *J. Mater. Chem. A*, 5, 19607–19612, 2017.
59. Zhang, Q. and Li, Z., Weakly coupled relaxor behavior of $BaTiO_3$-Bi($Mg_{1/2}Ti_{1/2}$)O_3 lead-free ceramics. *J. Adv. Dielectr.*, 03, 1320001, 2013.
60. Li, W.-B., Zhou, D., Xu, R., Pang, L.-X., Reaney, I.M., $BaTiO_3$–Bi($Li_{0.5}$ $Ta_{0.5}$) O_3, Lead-free ceramics, and multilayers with high energy storage density and efficiency. *ACS Appl. Energy Mater.*, 1, 5016–5023, 2018.
61. Yuan, Q., Li, G., Yao, F.Z., Cheng, S.D., Wang, Y., Ma, R., Mi, S.B., Gu, M., Wang, K., Li, J.F., Wang, H., Simultaneously achieved temperature-insensitive high energy density and efficiency in domain engineered $BaTiO_3$-Bi(Mg0.5$Zr_{0.5}$)O_3 lead-free relaxor ferroelectrics. *Nano Energy*, 52, 203–210, 2018.
62. Yang, H., Lu, Z., Li, L., Bao, W., Ji, H., Li, J., Feteira, A., Xu, F., Zhang, Y., Sun, H., Huang, Z., Lou, W., Song, K., Sun, S., Wang, G., Wang, D., Reaney, I.M., Novel $BaTiO_3$-based, Ag/Pd-compatible lead-free relaxors with superior energy storage performance. *ACS Appl. Mater. Interfaces*, 12, 43942–43949, 2020.
63. Yang, Z., Gao, F., Du, H., Jin, L., Yan, L., Hu, Q., Yu, Y., Qu, S., Wei, X., Xu, Z., Wang, Y.Z., Grain size engineered lead-free ceramics with both large energy storage density and ultrahigh mechanical properties. *Nano Energy*, 58, 768–777, 2019.
64. Yang, Z., Du, H., Qu, S., Hou, Y., Ma, H., Wang, J., Wang, J., Wei, X., Xu, Z., Significantly enhanced recoverable energy storage density in potassium–sodium niobate-based lead free ceramics. *J. Mater. Chem. A*, 4, 13778–13785, 2016.
65. Shao, T., Du, H., Ma, H., Qu, S., Wang, J., Wang, J., Wei, X., Xu, Z., Potassium–sodium niobate based lead-free ceramics: Novel electrical energy storage materials. *J. Mater. Chem. A*, 5, 554–563, 2017.
66. Pan, Z., Hu, D., Zhang, Y., Liu, J., Shen, B., Zhai, J., Achieving high discharge energy density and efficiency with NBT-based ceramics for application in capacitors. *J. Mater. Chem. C*, 7, 4072–4078, 2019.
67. Huang, Y., Li, F., Hao, H., Xia, F., Liu, H., Zhang, S., ($Bi_{0.51}Na_{0.47}$)TiO_3 based lead free ceramics with high energy density and efficiency. *J. Materiomics*, 5, 385–393, 2019.

68. Qiu, Y., Lin, Y., Liu, X., Yang, H., $Bi(Mg_{2/3}Nb_{1/3})O_3$ addition inducing high recoverable energy storage density in lead-free $_{0.65}BaTiO_3$-$_{0.35}Bi_{0.5}Na_{0.5}TiO_3$ bulk ceramics. *J. Alloys Compd.*, 797, 348–355, 2019.
69. Ren, P., Liu, Z., Wang, X., Duan, Z., Wan, Y., Yan, F., Zhao, G., Dielectric and energy storage properties of $SrTiO_3$ and $SrZrO_3$ modified $Bi_{0.5}Na_{0.5}TiO_3$-$Sr_{0.8}Bi_{0.10.1}TiO_{3f}$ based ceramics. *J. Alloys Compd.*, 742, 683–689, 2018.
70. Liu, X., Yang, H., Yan, F., Qin, Y., Lin, Y., Wang, T., Enhanced energy storage properties of $BaTiO_3$-$Bi_{0.5}Na_{0.5}TiO_3$ lead-free ceramics modified by $SrY_{0.5}Nb_{0.5}O_3$. *J. Alloys Compd.*, 778, 97–104, 2019.
71. Bin, H.U., Huiqing, F., Li, N., Shang, G., Zhaojun, Y., Li, Q., Enhanced energy-storage performance and dielectric temperature stability of (1-x)($0.65Bi_{0.5}Na_{0.5}TiO_3$-$0.35Bi_{0.1}Sr_{0.85}TiO_3$)-$xKNbO_3$ ceramics. *Ceram. Int.*, 44, 10968–10974, 2018.
72. Zhao, L., Liu, Q., Zhang, S., Li, J.-F., Lead-free $AgNbO_3$ anti-ferroelectric ceramics with an enhanced energy storage performance using MnO_2 modification. *J. Mater. Chem. C*, 4, 8380–8384, 2016.
73. Zhao, L., Gao, J., Liu, Q., Zhang, S., Li, J.-F., Silver niobate lead-free antiferroelectric ceramics: Enhancing energy storage density by B-site doping. *ACS Appl. Mater. Interfaces*, 10, 819–826, 2018.
74. Luo, N.N., Han, K., Zhuo, F.P., Xu, C., Zhang, G.Z., Liu, L.J., Chen, X., Hu, C., Zhou, H., Wei, Y., Aliovalent A-site engineered $AgNbO_3$ lead-free antiferroelectric ceramics toward superior energy storage density. *J. Mater. Chem. A*, 7, 14118–14128, 2019.
75. Luo, N., Han, K., Zhuo, F., Liu, L., Chen, X., Peng, B., Wang, X., Feng, Q., Wei, Y., Design for high energy storage density and temperature-insensitive lead-free antiferroelectric ceramics. *J. Mater. Chem. C*, 7, 4999–5008, 2019.
76. Gao, J., Zhang, Y., Zaho, L., Lee, K., Liu, Q., Studer, A., Hinterstein, M., Zhang, S., Li, J.F., Enhanced antiferroelectric phase stability in La-doped $AgNbO_3$: P;erspectives from the microstructure to energy storage properties. *J. Mater. Chem. A*, 7, 2225–2232, 2019.
77. Xu, C., Fu, Z., Liu, Z., Wang, L., Yan, S., Chen, X., Cao, F., Dong, X., Wang, G., La/Mn/Co doped $AgNbO_3$ lead-free antiferroelectric ceramics with large energy density and power density. *ACS Sustain. Chem. Eng.*, 6, 16151–16159, 2018.
78. Tian, Y., Jin, L., Zhang, H., Xu, Z., Wei, X., Viola, G., Abrahams, I., Yan, H., Phase transitions in bismuth-modified silver niobate ceramics for high power energy storage. *J. Mater. Chem. A*, 5, 17525–17531, 2017.
79. Yan, F., Yang, H., Ying, L., Wang, T., Enhanced energy storage properties of a novel lead-free ceramic with a multilayer structure. *J. Mater. Chem. C*, 6, 7905–7912, 2018.
80. Heath, J.P., Harding, J.H., Sinclair, D.C., Dean, J.S., Electric field enhancement in ceramic capacitors due to interface amplitude roughness. *J. Eur. Ceram. Soc.*, 39, 1170–1177, 2019.

5

Superconductors for Energy Storage

Navneet Kaur*, **Mona, Ranjeet Kaur, Jaiveer Singh and Shweta Rana**†

Department of Chemistry, Panjab University, Chandigarh, India

Abstract

The advent of superconductivity has seen brilliant success in the research efforts made for the use of superconductors for energy storage applications. Energy storage is constantly a substantial issue in various sectors involving resources, technology, and environmental conservation. This book chapter comprises a thorough coverage of properties, synthetic protocols, and energy storage applications of superconducting materials. Further discussion has been made on structural aspects along with the superconducting properties of various superconducting materials. The categorization of the material has been done based on the temperature required for the transition between superconducting and normal state (low-temperature superconductors [LTS] and high-temperature superconductors [HTS]). It has been established that various superconducting materials are usually used as wires because of many added advantages like improved efficiency and high value of electric current density by controlling structural attributes. The major applications of these superconducting materials are in superconducting magnetic energy storage (SMES) devices, accelerator systems, and fusion technology. Starting from the design of SMES devices to their use in the power grid and as a fault, current limiters have been discussed thoroughly. This chapter analyzes superconducting materials for magnetic energy storage technology and is expected to give directions and achieve further progress in the future.

Keywords: Low-temperature superconductors, high-temperature superconductors, energy storage applications, SMES

**Corresponding author*: neet_chem@yahoo.co.in

†*Corresponding author*: shweta0402@gmail.com

Inamuddin, Tariq Altalhi and Sayed Mohammed Adnan (eds.) Electroceramics for High Performance Supercapacitors, (95–134) © 2024 Scrivener Publishing LLC

5.1 Introduction

5.1.1 Background

The development of energy storage devices for renewable energy (solar and wind energy) has been a significant research interest considering the shortcomings of conventional energy sources like natural gas, coal, and petroleum and increased environmental awareness [1]. However, these renewable energy sources do not provide security of supply on demand and hence are inefficient towards energy storage applications. Hence, suitable energy storage systems (ESS), e.g., fuel cells, flywheel, supercapacitor, battery, the superconductor is always in demand and can offer on-demand energy supply along with renewability [2–4]. Among all types of ESSs, intensive use of superconductors for energy storage applications is the landmark of successful research efforts made after the advent of superconductivity as they offer fast response time (milliseconds), high energy efficiency (95%), long life, and good charging/discharging capability [4–6].

Superconducting materials allow the flow of electricity below a temperature known as transition temperature (Tc) [7]. Depending upon the critical magnetic field, superconducting materials are of two types; type-I superconductors [2] exhibit a single critical magnetic field and undergo an abrupt change [51] from superconducting to a normal state. These are often called soft superconductors and include pure metals [8, 9]. In contrast, type-II superconductors possess normal superconducting regions that co-occur with two critical magnetic fields. This is attributable to the greater value of the magnetic penetration depth than the coherence length [96] defined as the average electron pair size [10]. Due to possession of the superconducting condensation energy as well as beneficial magnetic field penetration, type-II superconductors have an upper edge over type-I superconductors. Usually, high-temperature superconductors belong to this class. The choice of superconducting material has been limited to compounds having Tc lower than 110 K due to difficulty arising because of synthetic procedures [8, 9].

5.1.2 Superconducting Properties

Superconducting materials epitomize the trailblazing prospect for the advancements in electric power generation and energy storage applications such as magnetic energy storage and power transmission lines [7]. Usually, various superconducting materials are fashioned into wires because of the added advantages of improved efficiency and higher electric current density with negligible resistance attributed to the decreased weight and size [11, 12]. These wires are characterized by some fundamental properties [13, 14].

(a) Superconducting transition temperature (Tc), which is the temperature till the material manifests the superconducting behavior
(b) Critical field (Bc_2), that is the maximal magnetic field ousted by the superconductor during the pinning phenomenon
(c) Critical current density (Jc), which defines the maximum value of current to be carried by the superconductor

In addition to the above characteristics, superconducting materials must possess some other basic requirements like better uniformity, mechanical strength and stability, long length, and low ac losses [29]. The correlation of three characteristics of the superconducting state in a wire is shown in Figure 5.1.

The capacity of an industrial superconductor to transport high currents in the superconducting state in the prevalence of strong magnetic fields is the most critical need. The Bc_2 and Tc values depend on the types of material used while Jc is determined by the microstructure of the materials. The Bc_2, Tc, and Jc must be high in value for efficient energy storage applications. By selecting materials of high Hc_2 and Tc, one can model the Jc values by controlling growth techniques [15, 16]. The maximum possible Jc value depends on the extrinsic defects of the material, which may also be created into the material artificially by various growth techniques. Thus, new effective pinning mechanisms are being implemented to improve the performance of superconductors.

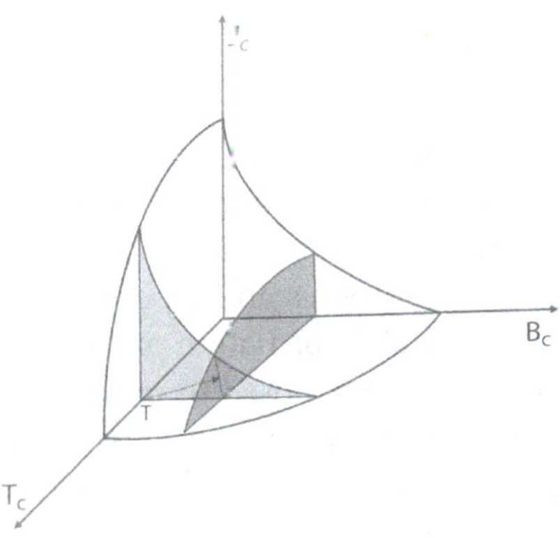

Figure 5.1 Corraletion between Tc, Jc and Bc_2 [15].

To explore the use of superconductors in energy storage, efforts are being done to the development of new technologies for producing complicated wires or tapes of kilometer lengths. The wire must be capable of regaining equilibrium despite a disruption that causes temperature zones to surpass Tc locally. The Stekly criteria is now employed to determine the magnet's stability and it leads to the following general principles [15]:

- The difference (Tc vs. T_b) should be as significant as feasible.
- The wire's radius should be as little as feasible. In general, subdividing the wire to create a multifilamentary structure is thermally more advantageous.
- To achieve a high thermal transmission to the cooling media, the filaments must be surrounded by a high-conductive matrix.

5.1.3 Synthetic Methodology

The superconducting materials can be produced by either solid or solution state reactions [17]. The powder preparation for superconductor materials is achieved by solid-state reactions, which ensure adequate homogeneity and low residual carbon content. However, the method of solid-state reaction for the preparation of the superconductor powder suffers from time constraints and severe chemical inhomogeneity on an atomic level. So, this is replaced by other solution-based procedures such as pyrolysis and oxalate co-precipitation [35]. For some of the superconducting materials, even the melt-cast process has been employed for synthesis. Ivanovskii *et al.* [18] discussed an improved solid-state method for the synthesis of iron-based superconducting materials that offered simpler routes for the fabrication of superconductor material. Apart from that, these materials are also explored as superconductor films. Different techniques such as pulsed laser deposition (PLD) [19] electron beam evaporation [20], molecular beam epitaxy (MBE) [21], metal-organic chemical vapor deposition (MOCVD), magnetron sputtering [22], hybrid physical-chemical vapor deposition (HPCVD) [23] and metal-organic deposition (MOD) [24] have been used to deposit high-Tc superconductor films.

These materials are cast into wires and tapes for energy storage applications. Conventional mechanical deformation procedures like extrusion, wire drawing, rolling, etc. have long been used to make LTS wires, together with suitable heat treatments for annealing and microstructure control. The term "thermomechanical processing" is used to describe these types of industrial processes. These processes were immediately extended to HTS wire and tape processing. HTS wire manufacture began using mixed oxide powders rather than solid metal precursor components and is known as powder-in-tube (PIT) or oxide powder-in-tube (OPIT) [24]. The major obstruction for a given wire or tape is to boost its critical current for the working magnetic field and temperature. It can be dealt with by enhancing pinning strength up to the maximum possible value and the maximal irreversibility field, except for the cubic NbTi and Nb_3Sn, where the Bc_2 value is near B_{irr} [25].

In the present chapter, we have discussed low-temperature (LTS) and high-temperature superconductors (HTS), which are classified based on the transition temperature. The advantages and extensive use of HTS over LTS have also been discussed in this chapter. Further, the appropriate use of LTS and HTS in making wires and tapes for energy storage applications has been discussed.

5.2 Low-Temperature Superconductors

The superconductors showing conversion at a temperature of ~ 20K are known as low-temperature superconductors (LTS). To achieve such a low temperature, a cooling system like liquid helium is used, which makes LTS very costly and limits their applicability. Nb-Ti (alloy) and Nb_3Sn (A15) with Tc up to 9 and 18 K, respectively, are well-known Type-II LTS superconductors for large-scale applications in magnets and energy storage devices. Despite having stability issues because of the requirement of expensive refrigeration, they are comparatively more economic than other conventional conductors. They provide added advantages for large-scale applications, which require high current and high magnetic field. They can be fabricated as round wires upholding distinct filament structures, and high current density, thus making them more reliable. Over 95% of superconducting magnets have been manufactured using Nb-Ti and Nb_3Sn and thus, are often named "technical superconductors."

5.2.1 Nb-Ti-Based LTS

Niobium-titanium (NbTi) alloy has been widely used as a low-temperature superconductor in various types of magnets as its critical temperature is nearly 9.7 K and it can fabricate superconducting magnets possessing magnetic fields reaching up to 10 T [26, 27]. The ability of NbTi to show superconductivity was discovered by Berlincourt and Hake in 1962 with a superconductivity value of 4.2 K [28]. Due to the advantages like good mechanical workability and deformation ability, low processing cost, and more reliability and stability, the niobium-titanium alloy has been extensively fabricated into wires [29]. The Jc value of NbTi wire has been increased to 3470 A/mm^2 in a magnetic field of 5 T at temperature 4.2 K by using its 61 filaments [30]. NbTi superconducting wires must be multi-filamentary to minimize the superconducting losses i.e. eddy current loss and hysteresis loss [31]. For this, Nb–Ti alloy is pierced into various copper tubes and placing them into a single Cu tube eventually to make a composite, which is thurst out to get a thin wire [29]. This obtained wire of Nb–Ti alloy possesses a high critical current density (Jc) value because a cell structure is formed in which several dislocations, which serve as flux pinning centers, get introduced during the extrusion and drawing process. Moreover, the superconductivity of the alloy relies on the composition of Nb and Ti, where the higher the number of α-Ti pinning centers, the lower will be the cost of the alloy along with the high hardness of the NbTi filaments [32, 33]. Accordingly, 46–50 wt.% of Ti in the NbTi alloy makes it appropriate for critical current density [34–36].

5.2.2 Nb_3Sn-Based LTS

Nb_3Sn is an A_3B type intermetallic compound of niobium and tin of simple β-tungsten structure, whose critical temperature is about 18 K at 0 T. Nb_3Sn was found to be a superconductor in 1954 by the Matthias and group [37]. Kunzler *et al.* in 1961 first designed an Nb_3Sn powder containing Nb wire showing superconductivity in fields up to 8.8 T [38]. Nb_3Sn multifilament and twisted wires were discovered in the early 1970s; however, their practicality for magnets was realized in the late 1970s [39]. Nb_3Sn can carry a large current density, by which they can produce strong magnetic fields in comparison to Nb-Ti and could be used to make high-power magnets and electric power [40]. The addition of Hf or Zr to Nb_3Sn could further increase the maximum Jc in a magnetic field, making it a possibility to be used at 16 T [41]. Despite being able to be operative at a high magnetic field, it had limited applicability due to its brittle nature. Thus, due to their stability requirement, they are more expansive than Nb-Ti-based superconductors.

Some magnets have been manufactured by using Nb_3Sn tapes, which were developed by a surface diffusion method. However, the Nb_3Sn wire is practically more important. Nb_3Sn wires (composition of 18-25% at Sn) have been designed to date, with Tc ranging from 6-18K. Various processes used to manufacture Nb_3Sn wires include the bronze process, the internal-tin (IT) process, and the powder in tube (PIT) process [42] (Figure 5.2). In the bronze process, the wire compositing a bronze (Cu-Sn alloy) tube with Nb core is formed by heating up to 600-700°C. Sn of the bronze tube reacts with the Nb core at high temperature, synthesizing Nb_3Sn wires.

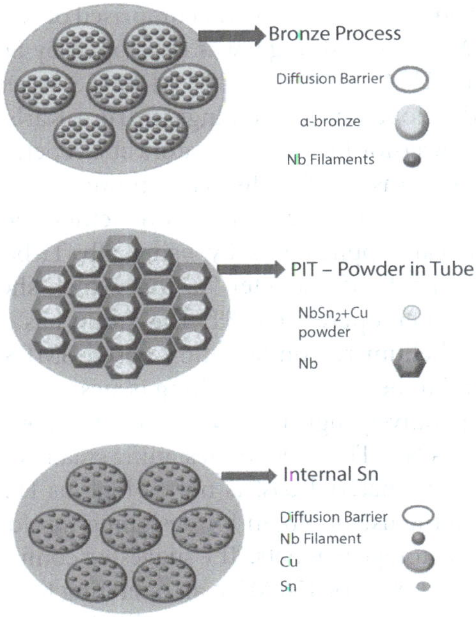

Figure 5.2 Bronze powder in the tube and Internal tin processes for fabricating Nb_3Sn.

In the IT process, the filament regions involve a Sn or Sn-alloy core by Nb or Nb-alloy rods expanding into the Cu environment, surrounded by a diffusion barrier in addition to a pure Cu stabilizer. On the other hand, in the powder-in-tube (PIT) method, the Nb tube packed with Nb and Sn powders is heated, which results in the formation of a Nb_3Sn wire.

The formed Nb_3Sn wires could be used to fabricate superconducting magnets, possessing the ability to generate higher magnetic fields up to 10 T and more. Usually, multifilamentary wires are used to fabricate Nb_3Sn wires embedded into a metal tube that is formed by inserting various single-core wires into a metal tube, drawn, and heated to get a multifilamentary wire in the end. During this fabrication, annealing is also carried out as Cu–Sn alloys undergo work hardening.

With the successful design of superconducting wires of Nb_3Sn and Nb-Ti, it becomes possible to manufacture energy storage systems based on superconductors SMES. The first successful installation of SMES using the NbTi wires for commercial power application was done by the USA situated Los Alamos National Laboratory (LANL). Yuan *et al.* [43] reported the installation of 30 MJ SMES devices based on Nb-Ti that can provide stability support to Bonneville Power Authority's Pacific Intertie installed in 1982 which has demonstrated the successful operation of SMES in power system [18]. Later on, a micro-SMES unit comprised of Nb-Ti alloy with the capacity of 1–10 MJ energy storage, was developed by Superconductivity Inc. situated in the USA. In 1988, a 188 kJ SMES based on a Cu/NbTi mixed wire was developed by Forschungszentrum Karlsruhe (Germany) to deliver pulsed power for linear accelerators at a repetition rate of 10 Hz [18]. These SMES systems had fast discharge power.

Bhunia *et al.* [44] presented the formulation method for designing SMES devices for small-scale applications by using Nb–Ti-based Rutherford-type cable with filaments of diameter 7.5 μm, which showed the critical current of 4000 A when operated @ 5T. The group has designed a 5 MJ/ 0.5 MW/150 MPa helium re-condensation-based SMES unit [53]. They claimed the method to be safe for quenching issues.

Despite of comparatively high Tc of Nb_3Sn but they are costly due to their brittle structure. Thus Nb- Ti is used for designing small-scale SMES systems generally. But still, the material cost is not as high as HTS. Luongo *et al.* [46] have presented the use of Nb_3Sn for designing toroidal superconducting magnetic energy storage magnets. The suggested configuration results in total (usable) energy storage of 450 MJ at an operating temperature of 4.5 K.

Mikkonen *et al.* [47] also presented the Nb3Sn-based SMES applicable to UPS devices. They provided an alternative to reduce the cost of the cryogen system (using liquid He conventionally) by rising the operation temperature to around 10 K and using Nb_3Sn as a coil material. A conduction-cooled Nb_3Sn SMES with an operating temperature of 10 K, resulted in a magnet energy of about 210 kJ.

The use of these superconducting materials for energy storage is completely based on a state of zero resistivity which is achieved at very low temperatures. Some LTS found uses in various energy storage applications which are listed in Table 5.1. Thus, the cooling system is required to realize the superconducting transition. Owing to very low critical temperature up to ~20 K, LTS require liquid He for cooling, which is very costly. Later, in 1986 various other materials i.e., HTS (discussed later) having much improved critical temperature was discovered.

Table 5.1 Various LTS materials used in energy storage applications.

Class	Compounds	Critical parameters	Applications	Ref.
Nb and Ti	Nb-Ti	Tc = 9.5K, Bc = 14T	SMES SFCL	[43, 44 45]
Nb and Sn	Nb_3Sn	Tc = 18.3, Bc = 28T	SMES UPS	[46] [47]

5.3 High-Temperature Superconductors

High-temperature superconductors (HTS) are defined as superconductors with transition temperatures greater than 20 K [48]. HTS often composed of alloys or complicated oxide ceramics which is a focal point in energy storage applications. J. Georg Bednorz of Germany and K. Alex Muller of Switzerland were awarded the Nobel Prize in physics in 1986 for their invention of ceramic cuprate in $LaBaCuO_4$, a superconductor with a transition temperature of around 30 K [49]. HTS is classified as a Type II superconductor due to its partial Meissner effect and incomplete diamagnetism. Which have higher critical magnetic fields and are mechanically tougher than Type I superconductors. They are frequently found in a condition that is a combination of normal and superconducting areas. Abrikosov [50] demonstrated in 1957 that a lattice of quantum vortices with a rapid cutoff to the vortex core led to the generation of the mixed state of a type II superconductor instead of superconducting condensate that gradually fade towards the vortex core. The observation was that the vortices form a regular structure known as a vortex lattice. A process called flux pinning is possible in a vortex state. As magnetic forces cannot permeate type-I superconductors, so this process is not possible in type-I superconductors. The vortex state is named after the fact that conventional material filaments are surrounded by superconducting current vortices

Based on materials used in energy storage applications, HTS is broadly divided into the following categories.

5.3.1 Cuprate-Based HTS

Bednorz and Müller's [49] discovery that superconductivity occurs in the La-Ba-Cu-O system at temperatures above 30 K heralded the start of a new era in energy storage research. The discovery triggered a global hunt for novel cuprate superconductors with greater critical temperatures. Within a year, the first cuprate superconductor with a transition temperature significantly higher than the boiling point of nitrogen, $YBa_2Cu_3O_{7-x}$ with Tc of 93 K, was discovered [57]. The other families in HTS include;

- $(La, M)_2CuO_4$ (M: Sr or Ba)
- $REBa_2Cu_3O_{7-\delta}$ (RE: rare earth element or yttrium)
- $Bi_2Sr_2Ca_{n-1}Cu_nO_{2n+4}$
- $Tl_2Ba_2Ca_{n-1}Cu_nO_{2n+4}$, $TlM_2Ca_{n-1}Cu_nO_{2n+3}$ (M: Sr or Ba), and $HgBa_2Ca_{n-1}Cu_nO_{2n+2}$

The maximum critical temperatures for cuprate superconductors range from 39K for the La-214 family to 135K for the Hg-12 (n-1) n family [58, 59].

Cuprate-based HTS has anatomy which is similar to a distorted and perovskite structure having multiple layers and oxygen deficiencies. All cuprate superconductors have a layered crystal structure that includes conducting CuO_2 layers sandwiched between insulating metal oxide layers. These additional metal oxide layers function as charge carrier reservoirs. The more layers of CuO_2, the higher the value of Tc.

Because electrical currents pass through holes formed in the oxygen sites available in the sheets of CuO_2, the structure exhibits substantial anisotropy in normal conducting and superconducting states. This can be seen from the fact that the electrical conductivity value is much higher when the applied field is parallel to the CuO_2 plane as opposed to perpendicular (Figure 5.3) [54].

The factors that influence the value of critical temperatures and in turn the energy storage parameters include chemical compositions, crystal structure, cation substitutions, and oxygen content. Cuprate high-temperature superconductors are generally nonstoichiometric oxides with variable oxygen contents. The number of charge carriers in the planes of CuO_2 influences their physical characteristics. They generally exhibit orthorhombic or tetragonal crystal structures. There is an insignificant difference between "a" and "b" (lattice parameters) having values close to 0.38 nm which is due to the comparable structural characteristic of the CuO_2 planes. The number of CuO_2 sheets within the CuO_2 blocks may be varied

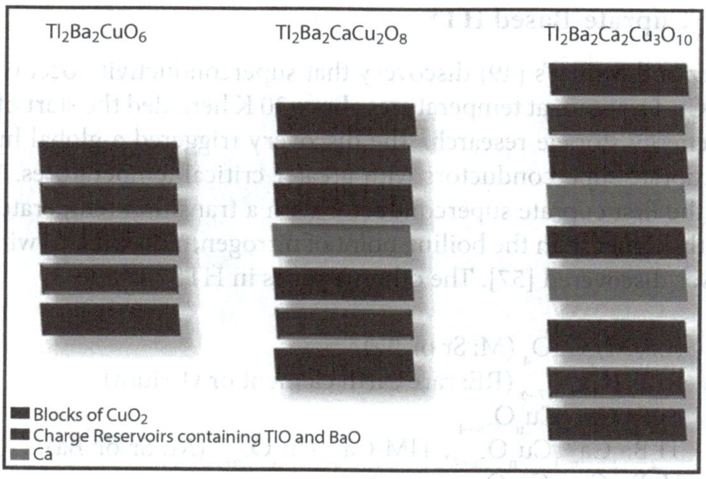

Figure 5.3 The layered structure of cuprate based HTS.

from 1 to n in most cuprate HTS families which leads to the predictable increase of the "c" lattice parameter with increasing "n." The lattice parameters are closely related to the chemical composition of cuprate superconductors and hence can be varied depending on the synthetic conditions [55]. For example, the value of parameter "c" increases in the case of $HgBa_2CaCu_2O_{6+\delta}$ (a=b= 0.3856 and c= 1.2652) when the number of CuO_2 planes in base material increases to $HgBa_2Ca_2Cu_3O_{8+\delta}$ (a=b= 0.3853 and c= 1.5818) [52].

Besides this, the charge carrier density of CuO_2 planes of Cuprate-based HTS can also be increased by the doping process. For example, the number of electrons that can be transferred from the charge carrier reservoir to the CuO_2 planes is reduced in the case of La_2CuO_4 when La^{3+} is largely replaced by Ba^{2+}. To keep the charge neutrality, one Cu^{3+} ion is produced in the CuO_2 planes for every Ba^{2+} ion supplied to the LaO double layers. The Cu^{3+} flaws act as moveable holes under normal conducting conditions [57]. Tokura *et al.* [58] discovered the first electron-doped cuprate superconductor $Pr_{2-x}Ce_xCuO_{4-\delta}$ in 1989. Wherein skeleton Pr had a valency of +3 and Ce had a valency of +4. Electron doping of the CuO_2 planes made by the substituting Ce^{4+} for Pr^{3+} resulted in an enhancement of overall conductivity offered by the compound at a critical temperature of 22.4K. The phase diagram can be used to determine the similarities and differences in the characteristics of both types of cuprates i.e. hole-doped as well as electron-doped (Figure 5.4). Both types exhibit the existence of a pseudogap phase up to the optimum doping level. The presence of a linear trend in their phase diagram indicates that their physics is two-dimensional [56].

Among all families of Cuprate-based HTS, in particular, YBCO (cuprate-based HTS) seems a very attractive candidate for energy storage applications owing to their high mechanical capabilities, large current capacity, and high temperatures at which they operate. Successful testing has been carried out since the early experiments in the 1970s, but their high cost acted as a barrier at the industrial level. For SMES, the YBCO-coated conductor or second-generation (2G) HTS wire carries huge importance. At high magnetic flux densities, their current capacity remains high even as temperature rises, hitting 1000 MA^{-2} at 20 K under 13 T. The value of 2G cables will continue to climb in the future since they are always developing and advancing [59]. In the first decade of this century, the French agency Délégation Générale pour l'Armement (DGA) had begun a program in charge of army research to produce an HTS made up of SMES which was employed as rail electromagnetic launchers/guns in partnership with Néel institute and G2Elab. This DGA endeavor culminated in the creation of an

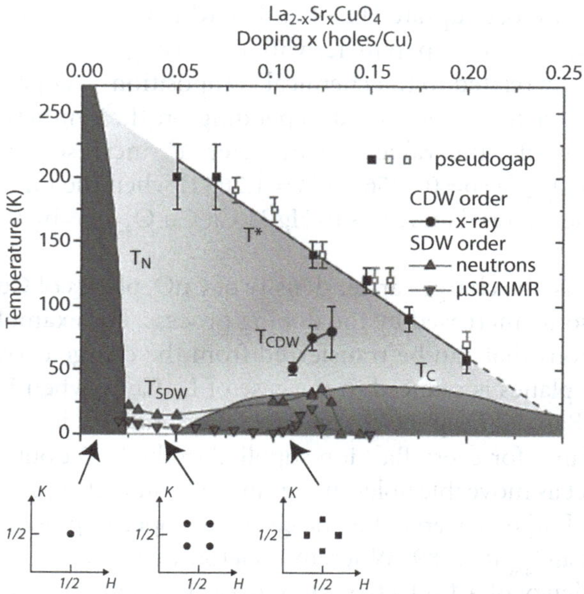

Figure 5.4 Phase Diagram of cuprate-based superconductors [reproduced with permission from Ref. 56].

HTS SMES for 800 kJ (425 kJ realized) that runs at 20 K and needs cooling for conduction purposes [60].

5.3.2 Iron-Based Pnictides (Pn) and Chalcogenides (Ch) as HTS

These are two-dimensional materials that also exhibit superconducting properties and hence can be employed as superconducting magnetic energy storage components in the energy storage device. These materials are made up of repeating units of a square lattice of Fe^{2+} ions, which are coordinated tetrahedrally with Ch ions or Pn (P and/or As). LaFePO was the first iron-based superconductor with Tc = 4 K found [61]. Later, superconductivity was discovered in LaNiAsO with Tc of 2.4 K and LaNiPO with Tc of 3K [62]. The value of Tc for $LaFeAsO_{1-x}F_x$ (x=0.08) was increased to 26 K by using a doping approach in which the substitution of phosphorus with arsenic and fraction of O atoms with that of fluorine [63].

These are generally characterized by their multiband and multiorbital electronic structure in which all the iron 3d orbitals hybridize with 4p orbitals of As and Se [64, 65]. They have a strong coupling and contribute to itinerant conducting electrons as well as localized magnetic moments

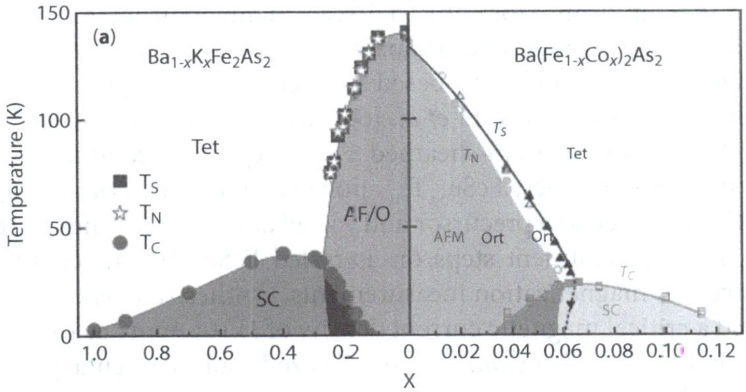

Figure 5.5 Phase diagram of $Ba_{1-x}K_xFe_2As_2$ and Ba $(Fe_{1-x}Co_x)_2As_2$ [reproduced with permission from Ref. 56].

which enhanced their suitability to be used as a superconducting energy store. Based on their Fermi surface topology iron-based HTS can be divided into two systems (a) one including both fermi surfaces of electron and hole and (b) the other containing only electron Fermi surfaces. Iron-based high-temperature superconductors are further categorized into four prototype families which are 1111,122,111 and 11. The surface topology of the fermi level and band structure of iron-based superconductors in the 11,111,122, and 1111 series are quite comparable, with the Fe 3d states dominating the low energy electronic structure [68].

Figure 5.5 shows the phase diagrams for $Ba_{1-x}K_xFe_2As_2$ and Ba $(Fe_{1-x}Co_x)_2As_2$ which indicate that superconductivity and antiferromagnetic order exist simultaneously in both cases [63].

Due to the presence of layered crystal architectures in iron-based HTS, the upper critical fields are anisotropic. The value of anisotropy factor $B_{c2}^{ab}B_{c2}^{c}$ of Sm-1111 at temperatures close to critical temperature is 7.3 and for (Ba, K)-122 this value comes out to 2.9 [66]. The top critical fields of Sm-1111, Nd-1111, Ba-122, Ca-122, Sr-122, and $K_{0.58}Fe_{1.56}Se_2$ reach or surpass 100 T at zero temperature indicating that these HTS materials can be used for energy storage applications even at very high value of the critical magnetic field which in turn diversify their practical applications in various fields [66].

The members of 122-type are the most important for energy applications among all iron-based superconductors due to the very high value of $Hc_2 > 70$T at 20K, low anisotropy (2 for 122), and simplicity in production. The world's first 100 m-class 122-type Fe-based wire was created which revealed the significance for industrial-scale manufacturing [67]. Magnetic levitation, energy storage, and compact magnetic resonance devices all are benefited from large bulk iron-based superconductor magnets with polycrystalline microstructures. Li *et al.* [68] used the ex-situ powder-in-tube approach to synthesize Nb-sheathed $FeSe_{0.5}Te_{0.5}$ superconducting tapes. In the synthesis of tapes, $FeSe_{0.5}Te_{0.5}$ polycrystalline material of superior properties was used as a precursor and varied annealing settings were used as the last heat-treatment steps on as-rolled $FeSe_{0.5}Te_{0.5}$ tapes. By using resistance and magnetization measurements, synthesized $FeSe_{0.5}Te_{0.5}$ tapes delivered a critical magnetic current density of $1x10^4$ Acm^{-2} at 15.7 K operating temperature. Xiao *et al.* [69] synthesized multifilamentary 122-type iron pnictides with excellent mechanical strength and a high value of filling factor, which is crucial for boosting engineering applications. In this work, the authors employed roller-die drawing to construct 19-filamentary $Sr_{0.6}K_{0.4}Fe_2As_2$/Ag/Monel composite wires and tapes. Magnetic characterization revealed the critical current density (Jc) values of $Sr_{0.6}K_{0.4}Fe_2As_2$ wires and tapes to be $2.7x10^3$ and $4.2x10^3$ Acm^{-2} at 4.2 K and 5 T respectively. The large value of mass density and roughness present in grains of the filaments contributed to the high Jc value in tapes, a significant parameter in the energy application.

5.3.3 MgB_2-Based HTS

The discovery of superconductive MgB_2 at Tc = 39 K in 2001 by Akimitsu *et al.* [70] was surprising given that it had been known since the 1950s. The absence of d- & f-shells in such binary metallic compounds plays no role in coulomb correlation in the conduction electron system. The intercalation of B-layers which resembled graphitic sheet, with Mg increases conduction as well as superconductive and normal state anisotropy; however, unlike organic superconductors, this does not limit effective dimensionality due to the stacking of isolated aromatic rings, making it an appropriate component in superconducting energy storage systems. Aside from that, the discovery of two energy gaps (at 1.8 and 6.8 m eV) and significant superconductive anisotropy (~ 6-9) poses a challenge to a more detailed theoretical investigation that can explain these findings in terms of two-band superconductivity based on the large anharmonicity of the involved phonon mode and a modification of its coupling with the different sheets of the electronic conduction band.

MgB_2 has a significant role in future superconducting energy storage components used in making SC wires which finds various applications having working temperatures up to 20 K as it is cheaper and easily available.

A high Tc of 39 K indicates its extreme type-II SC nature owing to coherence lengths of 4.4 nm and transparency of grain boundaries to current. The very low value of normal state resistivity of 0.38 cm for MgB_2 (at 42 K), which was equivalent to the copper wire but greater than polycrystalline Nb_3Sn and especially beneficial for quench avoidance [71]. Suo *et al.* [72] synthesized MgB_2 mono-core wires using iron tubes with inner diameters of 5mm and outer diameters of 8mm by filling MgB_2 powder in iron tubes. The synthesized composite powder was later drawn into a wire with a diameter of 2mm, which was cold-rolled into the tape of a thickness of 0.375mm. MgB_2/Fe tape was given heat treatment in an inert atmosphere for 30 minutes at 1223 K. The heat treatment enhanced the connection of the MgB_2 grains in the tape core, which are the characteristic requirements for achieving high critical current density values. This highlights the role of synthetic methodology in drawing critical parameters.

MgB_2 wires with commercially available critical current densities at magnetic fields of 5 T have potential use in SMES coils. To investigate the suitable twist pitch, Yagai *et al.* [73] synthesized cables with multi-strand having a nominal current value of 600 A for 400 mm inner diameter double-pancake (DP) coils using wind-and-react (W&R) and react-and-wind (R&W) methods. Here Rutherford-type cable consisting of eight (W&R) or ten wires (R&W) was reacted and then used for assembling the DP coils. Five-stacked DP coils with 512 turns were used to construct a 30 kJ SMES coil and demonstrate voltage fluctuation correction on a BUS line of 48 V DC in a microgrid comprised of sustainable energy sources and a liquid hydrogen supply system.

5.3.4 Hydrides-Based HTS

According to the traditional superconductivity theory of Bardeen-Cooper-Schrieffer (BCS) [74], a desirable combination of high-frequency phonons, strong coupling of electron & phonon, and a large density of states were needed to attain high Tc with no theoretical upper bound. Because hydrogen atoms produce the required high-frequency phonon modes along with strong interaction of electron and phonon, making it is suitable for more use of metallic hydrogen and hydrogen-dominated covalent compounds as they may theoretically meet these conditions. Numerous simulations supporting this idea suggest that transition temperatures between 50–235 K can be achieved for various hydrides. Drozdov *et al.* [75] investigate sulfur hydride, which has a Tc of 80 K at 90 GPa pressure. With magnetic field and magnetic susceptibility studies, the authors observed a rapid decrease in resistivity to zero as well as a decrease in transition temperature, confirming the Tc of 203 K for the H_2S-based superconductor. According to them, the phase responsible for high-Tc superconductivity in this system was most likely H_3S which was produced from H_2S via pressure breakdown. These discoveries encourage the pursuit of superconductivity at a standard temperature in additional hydrogenous materials which in turn open the doors for energy storage in superconducting magnets at room temperature. Binary hydrogen-rich compounds have been explored including the binding of the majority of the periodic table elements to hydrogen. According to BCS theory [74], the smaller the relative molecular mass, the greater the possibility of a higher Tc. In this theory, the doping of lighter metals with hydrogen is an interesting concept regarding superconducting properties.

Based on the literature survey [76], some suggestions for rationalizing metal hydrides in the periodic table have been collected which are as follows;

(i) In Mendeleev's periodic table, the lability belt constitutes the vast majority of HTS metal hydrides such as Sc-Y-La-Ac (d^1 belt), Mg-Ca-Sr-Ba-Ra (d^0 belt), and Th that make up the high-Tc hydrides (s^2d^2). These elements are suitable to be used in superconducting energy storage due to their electrical lability which results in significant electron-phonon interaction.

(ii) Higher values of Tc can be obtained by transferring 0.3e per hydrogen atom from metal atoms.

(iii) The superconductivity of hydrides deteriorated drastically with the increased participation of d- and f-electrons. Also, with an increase in the number of f-electrons, the critical temperatures of lanthanoid- and actinoid-based hydrides decrease almost uniformly.

(iv) The pressure required to stabilize hydrides reduces the group in the periodic table. Superconducting polyhydrides such as UH_7 and PaH_8 in actinoids get stabilized with a pressure of only 50 GPa.

The literature shows the applications of these findings. Xie *et al.* [69] have produced extremely compressed hydrides ZrH_3 and Zr_4H_{15} at low pressures (30-50 GPa) in diamond anvil cells. These hydrides were synthesized using two separate reaction pathways at an ambient temperature of 1500 K by laser heating. The electrical resistance measurement and the dependence of Tc on the applied magnetic field of the sample revealed the presence of two superconducting transitions at 6.4 and 4.0 K at 40 GPa, which corresponds to the critical temperature of ZrH_3 and Zr_4H_{15}. Zhong *et al.* [77] have demonstrated superconductivity in four energetically stable and metallic tellurium hydrides of stoichiometric ratios as H_4Te, H_5Te_2, HTe, and HTe_3 at 140 GPa. Two hydrogen-rich hydrides H_4Te and H_5Te_2 had shown intriguing layered structures intercalated by quasi-molecular H_2 and linear H_3 units respectively. They are both superconductors at high temperatures with Tc values ranging from 46 to 104 K. Aside from the high-frequency H_2 and H_3 vibrations, the intermediate-frequency phonons generated by H-Te wagging and H-Te-H bending vibrations are the most important in superconductive nature which further enhance their utility in energy applications.

5.4 Superconductors in Energy Applications

In 1970, Ferrier developed the use of superconducting coils to store magnetic energy [77]. To store energy, an electric current must pass through a superconducting coil. According to Faraday's law of induction, this produces both an electric field and a changing magnetic field over time. This results in the coil being able to store energy in both magnetic and electric forms, which can then be retrieved quickly. The superconducting nature of the coil is a must otherwise Joule effect will waste the energy in a very short time [85].

In DC operation, superconductors have current densities 100 times that of copper and have very low resistance. These properties provide superconducting power applications with several excellent advantages like high efficiency, small size, and low weight in comparison to conventional devices. Furthermore, superconductors possess the unique ability to switch between superconducting and normal states under controlled conditions. This phase shift may lead to a large change in their resistivity value and thus, opens up new applications that are not currently possible with ordinary materials. As a result, the likelihood of real energy applications based on superconductors is increasing continuously [59]. Various HTS materials used in energy storage applications are listed in Table 5.2.

5.4.1 Superconducting Magnetic Energy Storage

Superconducting magnetic energy storage (SMES) is a technique that stores energy directly in form of electrical energy and provides moderate specific energy density at a high rate of power density. The magnets

Table 5.2 Various HTS materials used in energy storage applications.

Class	Compounds	Critical parameters	Applications	Ref.
Hg-HTS $Hg_mBa_2Ca_{n-1}Cu_nO_{2n+m+2}$ m = 1, 2 n = 1, 2, 3 . . .	Hg-1201 Hg-1212 Hg-1223	Tc= 94 Tc=128 Tc=135	Superconducting wires and tapes	[101] [102] [103]
LMCO type or 214-type L= La, Pr, Nd, Sm,Eu, Sr	$La_{2-X}Sr_xCuO_4$ La_2CuO_{4+x} $La_2CuO_4F_x$ Sr_2CuO_{3+x} $Sr_{2-x}Ba_xCuO_{3+y}$	Tc=51 Tc=35 Tc=35 Tc=95 Tc=98	Superconducting wires and tapes	[104] [105] [106] [107] [108]
REBCO type or 123-type RE = Y, La, Pr, Nd, Sm, Eu, Gd, Tb, Dy, Ho, Er, Tm, Yb, Lu	Y-123, YBCO Yb-123 Nd-123, NBCO Gd-123 Er-123 $YSr_2Cu_3O_{7.5}$	Tc=93 Tc=88.2 Tc=96 Tc=94 Tc=92 Tc= 60	SFCL, Fusion technology and FACTS.	[109] [110] [111] [112] [113] [114]
Bi-Cuprates or BSCCO $Bi_mSr_2Ca_{n-1}Cu_nO_{2n+m+2}$ m = 1, 2 n = 1, 2, 3....	Bi-1212 Bi-2212 Bi-2223 Bi-2234	Tc= 102 Tc= 96 Tc= 110 Tc= 110	SMES, Fusion technology and Uninterruptible power source (UPS)	[115] [116] [117] [118]

(*Continued*)

Table 5.2 Various HTS materials used in energy storage applications. (*Continued*)

Class	Compounds	Critical parameters	Applications	Ref.
Tl- Cuprates $Tl_mBa_2Ca_{n-1}Cu_nO_{2n+m+2}$ m = 1, 2 n = 1, 2, 3 . . .	Tl-1223 Tl-1234 Tl-2212 Tl-2223 Tl-2234	Tc= 133.5 Tc= 127 Tc= 110 Tc= 128 Tc= 113	Superconducting wires and tapes	[119] [119] [120] [121] [121]
1111-type Iron oxy pnictides $RFeAsO_{1-x}F_x$ R=La and lanthanoids	$LaO_{0.89}F_{0.11}FeAs$ $CeFeAsO_{0.84}F_{0.16}$ $La_{0.7}Y_{0.3}O_{0.9}F_{0.1}FeAs$	Tc= 26 Tc= 41 Tc= 38.5	Superconducting wires, magnets and tapes	[63] [122] [123]
$RFeAsO_{1-x}F_x$ R=La and lanthanoids	$SmFeAsO_{0.9}F_{0.11}$ $PrFeAsO_{0.89}F_{0.11}$ $NdFeAsO_{0.89}F_{0.11}$	Tc= 43 Tc= 52 Tc= 52		[124] [125] [126]
RFeAsO R = Er, Gd, Sm, Nd, La, Pr	$SmFeAsO_{0.85}$ $GdFeAsO_{1-Y}$ $ErFeAsO_{1-y}$	Tc= 55 Tc= 53.5 Tc= 45		[127] [128] [129]
RFeAsOH R = lanthanoids	$SmFeAsO_{1-x}H_x$ $LaFeAsO_{0.65}H_{0.35}$	Tc= 55 Tc= 52		[130] [131]

(*Continued*)

Table 5.2 Various HTS materials used in energy storage applications. (*Continued*)

Class	Compounds	Critical parameters	Applications	Ref.
122-type Non-oxy iron pnictides Ae, AFe_2As_2 Ae: Ca, Ba, Sr A: alkali metal	$Ba_{0.6}K_{0.4}Fe_2As_2$ $Sr_{0.6}K_{0.4}Fe_2As_2$ $Ca_{0.6}Na_{0.4}Fe_2As_2$ $Sr_{0.6}Na_{0.4}Fe_2As_2$	Tc= 38 Tc= 30 Tc= 18 Tc= 26	Superconducting wires, magnets and tapes.	[132] [133] [133] [134]
111 types Non-oxy iron pnictides AfeAs	Li_xFeAs Na_xFeAs	Tc= 18 Tc= 9	Superconducting wires, magnets and tapes.	[135] [136]
11 types Iron chalcogenides Fe (Se, Te)	$Fe_{1.01}Se$ $FeTe_{0.5}Se_{0.5}$ $Fe_{1.13}Te_{0.85}Se_{0.1}$ $FeTe_{0.75}S_{0.25}$	Tc= 8 Tc= 14 Tc= 2	Superconducting wires, magnets and tapes.	[137] [138] [139, 140]
245 types $A_{0.8}Fe_{1.6}Se_2$ or $(A_2Fe_4Se_5)$ A: K, Cs, Rb, Tl	$K_{0.8}Fe_{1.78}Se_2$ $Cs_{0.8}(FeSe_{0.98})_2$ $Rb_{0.8}Fe_{1.6}Se_2$	Tc= 30 Tc= 27.4 Tc= 32.4	Superconducting wires and tapes	[66] [141] [142]
42622 $Sr_4TM_2O_6Fe_2(As,P)_2$ TM: transition metal	$Sr_4V_2O_6Fe_2As_2$ $Sr_4Sc_2O_6Fe_2P_2$	Tc= 36 Tc= 15.6	Superconducting wires and tapes	[143] [144]

(*Continued*)

Table 5.2 Various HTS materials used in energy storage applications. (*Continued*)

Class	Compounds	Critical parameters	Applications	Ref.
Hydride based	LiH_6 LiH_8 BeH_2 MgH_4 MgH_6 MhH_{12} $AlH_3(H_2)$ KH_6	Tc= 38 Tc= 71 Tc= 97 Tc= 37 Tc= 271 Tc= 60 Tc= 146 Tc= 70	Superconducting wires, magnets and tapes.	[75]
MgB_2 based	MgB_2	Tc = 39	Used in SMES.	[70]

and coils made up of superconducting material are used to store magnetic energy when introduced with direct current at positive voltage under a closed short circuit situation. SMES acts as a current source during discharging because, with the opening of a short circuit, the energy stored in form of current is transferred to load under negative electric potential. The value of load resistance decides the discharging time of a SMES device because discharging time is calculated by the ratio of inductance to the load resistance value [79].

Global advancement had represented various scales of SMES in energy applications. However, the variation in design elements depending on the intended application demonstrates the disparity in the anticipated cost of SMES. In general, the SMES system is made up of four parts which are shown in (Figure 5.6) [80].

(i) Superconducting magnet and supporting structure:
It is equipped with a superconducting coil, a superconducting magnet, and coil protection. A circulating current forms the superconducting coil that stores energy in the magnetic field at the heart of a SMES system. Two factors that influence the amount of stored energy are as;

(a) shape and size of coil: the amount of energy stored in the coil directly depends on the size of the coil.
(b) conductor properties that influence maximum current.

The two most prevalent magnet topologies used here comprise solenoid and toroid. Solenoids are more typically used than toroid configurations

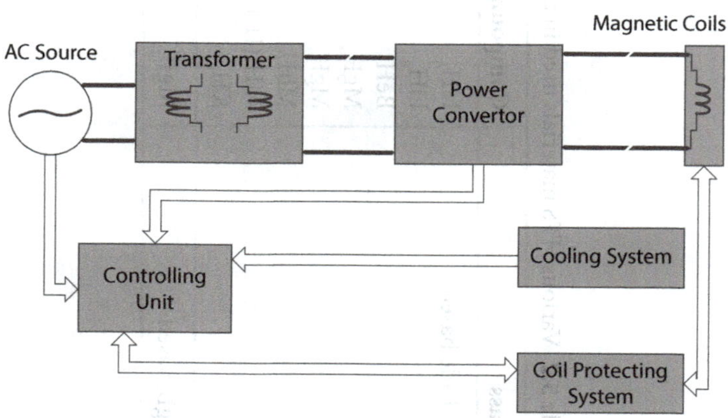

Figure 5.6 Schematic design of a SMES system.

the reason being the reduced conductor number and low cost exhibited by them.

(ii) Cooling system:
A cryogenic refrigerator also known as a cryogenic system, is made up of a cryostat, a compressor, vacuum enclosures, coolant, and other components. Usually, helium is chosen to act as a coolant because it is the only substance that is not present in solid form at desired temperatures (4.2 K) for the superconducting state. For this, one or more gaseous helium compressors are present in which a vacuum enclosure is used to receive the compressed form of helium and converts it to liquid helium which in turn is used by the coil.

(iii) Power conditioning system:
It consists of inverters, rectifiers, and electronic circuits and is commonly known as a power conversion system. Here, the converters that convert DC currents to AC currents and vice versa are commonly utilized because the majority of grids run in alternating current (AC). Based on the use of different converters and other circuits, SMES systems are grouped into three types: thyristor-based SMES, voltage source converter (VSC)-based SMES, and current source converter (CSC)-based SMES.

(iv) Control system:
It is used to create a link between grid power demand and power flow to and from the SMES coil. It also checks the status of the SMES coil and regulates other devices such as the refrigerator to guarantee safety. Control systems are frequently comprised of controlling devices or circuits such as microcontrollers and DSPs.

The superconducting conductor must meet several requirements to be useful in magnetic energy storage, including [59];

i. high engineering current densities (Jc) at high magnetic fields (B_c)
ii. mechanical stress/deformation support to integrate the mechanical function
iii. cheaper as the present SMES system is quite costly
iv. the high possible value of operating temperature (Tc).

In LTS, NbTi conductors presently fulfill almost requirements, but their working temperature is disappointingly low, at or slightly above the liquid helium temperature of 4.2 K. even though 4 K cryogenics has been mastered, it remains highly expensive both in terms of capital as well as the operational expenditures [81]. Another significant advancement was the introduction of HTS "current leads" because HTS materials create a lot of opportunities for SMES such as the ability to operate at higher temperatures which lower cryogenic operating costs and most importantly cryocooler costs. These materials greatly reduce related losses which contribute significantly to overall loss [82].

The temperature at which a refrigeration cycle operates has a significant effect on the energy storage efficiency of a SMES device. For example, at operating temperatures of 4.2 K, 20 K, and 77 K, the input power required to remove a heat load of 1 W is 70.4, 14, and 2.9 W respectively. Refrigeration efficiency calculations illustrated the capability to run superconductive equipment at 77 K rather than 4.2 K resulting in a considerable reduction in cooling costs. Owing to this problem HTS materials are preferred over LTS materials in most superconducting energy storage applications [59].

In this regard, Zimmermann *et al.* [83] synthesized a second-generation (2G) HTS tape for use in grid-scale SMES. A 2G HTS SMES system was designed that used tapes made up of Yttrium-Barium-Copper-oxide (YBCO) at 22 K. The intended storage capacity was set at 1 MJ with a maximum output power of 100 kW. The magnet was constructed from a set of double pancake coils to maximize storage limit while using the lowest tape length possible. The resulting coil design's inductance was calculated analytically and used to evaluate the magnet's total storage capacity. As synthesized YBCO tapes deliver 1 MJ of energy at 22 K operating temperature, a total storage capacity of 1.14 MJ was available. Abhinav *et al.* [84] developed a 2.5MJ SMES solenoidal magnet out of 2G (SuperPower, YBCO with Tc of 90K and magnetic field of 0T) HTS tape. The impact of the operational current (which is passed through a single superconducting tape) was studied. The HTS SMES was designed by keeping in mind a reference magnetic flux of 3.5T. In solenoidal magnets, it has been found that parallel fields are larger than perpendicular fields. This causes enormous Lorentz forces to act on HTS tape, which can lead to structural instability and failure. It has been revealed that greater currents may be employed to minimize the entire length of the superconductor, hence lowering the overall cost of the device.

When comparing various energy storage devices using the Ragon plot, SMES lies in between conventional capacitors and batteries as far as energy density is concerned and is comparable to electrochemical capacitors but with high power density potential. This comparison of various energy storage technologies shows that SMES is more of a power source rather being an energy source like batteries. As a result, SMES is a suitable option for high power generation of up to 100 MW within a few seconds [85].

5.4.1.1 *Use of SMES in the Power Grid: Flexible AC Transmission System (FACTS)*

A FACTS is a static power-electronics device that increases the control and power transmission capabilities of the power grid. SMES with energy ranging from tens to hundreds of megajoules can be used as FACTS. As far as the first superconducting application is concerned then SMES first of all employed as a FACT which was operated in a grid [86]. The SMES unit in a FACTS device can regulate active and reactive power at the common connection point in quadrant operations. The power system can be linked to the SMES coil using either CSC or VSC [87].

(a) Current source converter configuration: In this configuration, a two-series six-pulse step-down coupling transformer links the SC coil with the three-phase network. Since the current flowing through a superconducting inductor is unidirectional, it is possible to regulate both active and reactive power by modifying the sign of the voltage across the inductor terminals, which is then changed by adjusting the firing angles 1 and 2 of the two converter stations. Feedback signals such as generator shaft speed variation or network frequency as well as voltage deviation at the point of common connection are utilized to regulate power transfer, both active and reactive, between the SMES unit and the 3-phase network. The changes in firing angles 1 and 2 are zero during normal operation which leads to the voltage through the SC coil remaining constant. In this case, there will be no power exchange between the SMES unit and the power system.

(b) Voltage source converters:
In this technique, SMES coil and power system are integrated through a voltage source converter that allows for decoupled regulation of actual and reactive power yet VSC enables continuous rated reactive power supply even with extremely low coil current. Figure 5.7 shows a schematic of SMES coil and the ac network integrated through VSC [88].

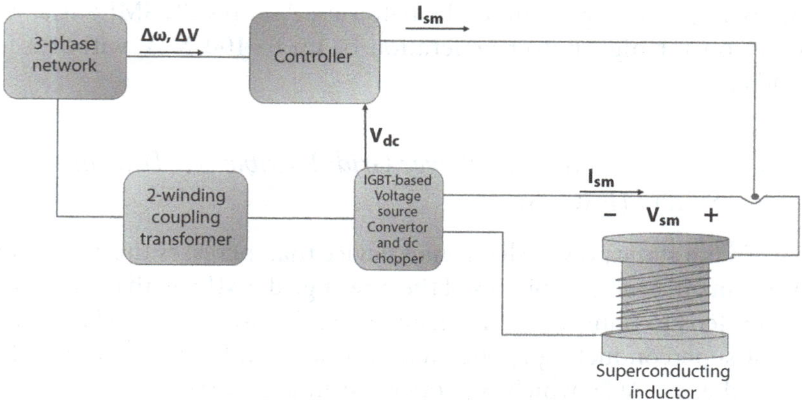

Figure 5.7 Schematic diagram of the SMES unit with VSC and dc chopper.

HTS-based technology is economical when compared to LTS due to the development of ceramic-based HTS which work at comparable high temperatures of 160K with the use of cheaper liquid Nitrogen as a cryogenic component in SMES. The Bonneville Power Authority in the United States used a 30 MJ SMES to attenuate low-frequency power oscillations in the 1980s [87]. For over a year this SME operated in real-world grid situations transmitting around 1200 hours of power. This amounted to almost 10^6 cycles for the magnet.

5.4.1.2 *Use of SMES as Fault Current Limiters*

In the current system, various components of the grid along with interconnections have outgrown electrification. These components of electrification are built in such a way that they can function in various situations like transformer loss in a substation which frequently mandates the functioning of more such transformers in the same or neighboring substations. As a results fault current in practically every transmission and distribution system is growing. Technically the growth is due to two factors: (a) the greater the number of interconnections, the lower the effective system impedance and (b) the total power available at any location grow over time [89].

Faults in the transmission and distribution systems can occur almost everywhere. Because faults are very strong than that of rated current, which can lead to huge loss to a variety of components. When a malfunction lasts long enough, the damage is generally produced by increasing forces in proportion to the square of the current or by overheating.

It is not feasible (or cost-effective) to substitute older network components just to manage larger fault currents. Hence, some technique for minimizing them is required. SFCLs (Superconducting Failure Current Limiters) are used to restrict current in the grid when a fault occurs. In this design when a defect in the gridline is identified, a superconductor is quenched (heated). As the superconductor is quenched, its resistance increases, and the current is redirected to other grid lines. This is done while avoiding interference with the larger grid. When the fault is fixed, the SFCL's temperature drops and it becomes undetectable to the rest of the grid [90]. In laboratories and businesses all across the world, three unique types of SFCLs are being produced named as resistive, shielded core, and saturated (or saturable) core. Later two versions are inductive type FCLs as they employ a ferromagnetic core. Till now, SCFCLs are unable to find practical utility but a first pre-commercial prototype use at the medium voltage level is perceptible in near future. The field experiment of various SCFCL types has already been conducted showing the technical capability at this voltage level [91].

5.4.2 Use of Superconductors in Accelerator System

The first large-scale industrial application of high-temperature superconductor (HTS) materials was as "current leads" for low-temperature superconductor (LTS) magnets in accelerators. Large research infrastructure facilities like Fermilab in the United States, European Council for Nuclear Research (CERN), and the International Thermonuclear Experimental Reactor (ITER) are the industry drivers in important areas like cost reduction and performance reliability for LTS (NbTi and Nb_3Sn) and HTS using current lead technology [92].

Accelerators employ superconductors for two reasons: performance and cost. Normal resistive iron-based magnets have a magnetic field limit of 1.8 T due to iron saturation, however, a superconducting magnet may attain at least 10 times this amount [93]. The dipole magnets are employed to bend the particle beams in circular accelerators. The more powerful the particle bending and concentrating, the smaller the machine and the more defined the interaction zones.

The use of HTS "current leads" to deliver large currents from a room-temperature magnet power source to cryogenic LTS magnets was proposed shortly after the discovery of HTS [94]. HTS "current leads" are now important components that can be acquired commercially from a range of sources and are used in all applications that use an LTS/HTS magnet. Wire/tape and bulk-based solutions are available which may be made from

Bi-2212, Bi-2223, and YBCO [59]. HTS materials have been utilized at the Large Hadron Collider (LHC) at CERN in Geneva, Switzerland/France for "current leads" to power the LTS magnets (Figure 12.1) that transmit up to 13 000 A. [92]. With an order amount of 31 km of Bi–2223 tape, this was the first large-scale industrial application of HTS [92].

Apart from these, HTS is also being investigated for use in a few other areas relevant to the accelerator industry including focusing elements, insertion devices, bending magnets, and high filed ion sources. Various programs are running across the world that seek to develop HTSs for use in the most promising enabling areas such as "current leads," sharply focused components, and dipole magnet inserts. Except for "current leads," prototypes have been constructed and tested but the long-term dependability of HTS technologies in a genuine accelerator or storage ring has not been tested yet and is still a lacuna that needs to be addressed.

5.4.3 Use of Superconductors in Fusion Technologies

Superconductor technology has long been associated with the idea of magnetic confinement producing nuclear fusion. Nuclear fusion is swiftly emerging as a key source of potential energy with the first tokamak reactors intended for full nuclear operation (ITER) nearing completion and a significant new research tokamak (JT60SA) beginning commissioning. The success of magnetic confinement for fusion depends on the application of superconductor technology. The information and experiences gained by introducing this technology to ITER and JT60SA in parallel with newly designed superconducting materials are paving the road for various approaches to commercial fusion reactors. Several fusion devices in the process of being built by utilizing superconducting magnets include JT-60SA, EAST, WEST, ITER, and KSTAR. NbTi or Nb_3Sn CICCs were used to fabricate superconducting magnets to be used in fusion devices [95].

For the fusion device, the key parameter is the magnetic field and as the magnetic field increases, the value of plasma confinement duration decreases. HTSs are presumed to be a good solution for high-current fusion magnet "current leads" also suggested by MIT in SPARC [96]. An aluminum alloy-jacketed Nb_3Sn superconductor with indirect cooling via cooling panels within the coil has been proposed as a suitable magnet system for the LHD-type reactor force-free helical reactors (FFHR) [97]. However, the fundamental technical challenges of HTS technology as well as its high cost make it unsuitable for the winding of fusion magnets. For the hybrid magnet, the greatest alternative is the design scheme that produces high-field magnets. In this regard, hybrid HTS-Sn_3Sn-NbTi coils were designed for the EU DEMO CS coil [97] and Nb_3Sn and NbTi hybrids were produced for the Chinese Fusion Engineering Test Reactor (CFETR) CS modular coil. A hybrid CS coil has two advantages first it reduces the outer radius of the magnet and second, it increases the magnetic flux generated. As a consequence, hybrid magnets are adopted as the industry standard for producing a high magnetic field in pulsed tokamaks [99].

High-field hybrid superconducting magnets are attractive options for future fusion devices. Nonetheless, there are certain worries and roadblocks. Because of its substantial hysteresis loss, Nb_3Sn is unsuitable for CS and PF magnets. When the magnetic field crosses 16 T then the hybrid is typically HTS (Bi2212, REBCO) and LTS (Bi2212, REBCO) (Nb_3Sn, NbTi) (Nb_3Sn, NbTi). A new HTS CICC structure, heat treatment technology, superconducting magnet material properties, new metals or composite structures possessing large values of yield strength, ductility and elastic modulus, and insulation materials having high radiation resistance are just a few examples of the new technologies that must be developed to meet the technical challenges [95].

5.4.4 Challenges Faced During Superconducting Energy Storage

Superconducting magnet or coil is the costliest part of SMES compared with the cooling system and the rest of the mechanical construction which makes this technique very expensive. Apart from this, at present time SMES systems have a low energy content which forces them to use large-scale storage to enhance the energy storage capacity of SMES. The following material outlines the most pressing issues confronting SMEs today [100].

1. Self-Discharging: The most obvious drawback is the short storage duration. SMES can be conducted for smaller cycles having lengths of a few minutes to several hours, which is even less than the storage time. Because of its incredibly quick self-discharge, SMES has a limited energy storage span daily proportion of 10% to 15%.
2. Low Energy Density: SMES has a small value of energy density, ranging between 0.5 and 5 Wh/kg. SME systems with current energy content are extremely small.
3. High Cost: SMES have a considerable capital cost ranging from $1,000 to $10,000 per kWh, which is much more than the cost of most other technologies.

4. Handling Difficulties: More often, difficulties exist within the materials and the design. The earliest generation of HTS, BSCCO (BiSrCaCuO), for example, although using a high critical current in power applications at high magnetic fields proved challenging. The magnetic field causes the critical current of the magnetic tape to rapidly decrease. It might take a lot of time and money to get the system back up and running after a superconducting material quench. In the event of a superconducting material quench in the system, restoring operational status may be time and money-demanding.
5. Concerns about Health and Environment: SMES is not an ecologically advantageous energy storage technology due to large input in form of energy requirements for cooling purposes and emission of carbon. The powerful magnetic field might damage people's health. High magnetic field exposure commonly results in irregular heart rates, alterations in brain activity, immune system damage, the appearance of skin disorders, and other symptoms.
6. Long Precooling Time: Because a SMES system operates at such a low temperature, it takes about four months to cool the superconducting magnet from room temperature to operating temperature. In the event of a coil breakdown or an emergency energy release, the recovery time is the same.

5.5 Conclusion

Energy storage is the pivotal link considering today's increasing demand for energy and superconductors have a cardinal role to play in them. The present chapter accounts for this role of the superconducting materials for applications in energy storage systems along with the compilation of major downsides. Research and development in superconducting wire and tape are progressing at a rapid pace with a focus on the critical parameter Jc, Tc, and Bc which exhibit the potential to increase the practicality of these materials in energy storage applications. SMES in particular has bright prospects in the electric utility sector. Apart from SMES, superconducting materials find their usage in fusion, FACTS, FCL, and UPS. The practicality of SC's in various energy storage systems is currently limited to "current leads" which reduces cryogenic costs. Future applications will benefit even more from superconducting coil materials, which will make future energy storage devices economical by simplifying cryogenic system requirements due to the high value of critical temperature which would enable them to even be used at room temperature.

Acknowledgments

The authors are grateful to CSIR-New Delhi (grant 09/0135(13579)22/EMR-I and 02(0446)/21/EMR-II) for funding.

References

1. Duffy, P., Fitzpatrick, C., Conway, Y., Lynch, R.P., The growing need for storage, in: *Energy Storage Options and Their Environmental*, R.E. Hester, and R.M. Harrison, (Eds.), pp. 1–41, RSC Publishers, Ingram Publisher Services UK, 2018.
2. Owusu, P.A., Sarkodie, S., Dubey, S., A review of renewable energy sources, sustainability issues and climate change mitigation. *Cogent Eng.*, 3, 1167990, 2016.
3. Shaqsi, A.Z., Sopian, K., Al-Hinai, A., Review of energy storage services, applications, limitations, and benefits. *Energy Rep.*, 6, 288, 2020.
4. Ali, M.H., Wu, B., Dougal, R.A., An overview of SMES applications in power and energy systems. *IEEE Trans. Sustain. Energy*, 1, 38, 2010.
5. Oskouei, M.Z., Åžeker, A.A., Tunçel, S., Demirbaş, E., Gözel, T., Hocaoğlu, M.H., Abapour, M., Ivatloo, B., A critical review on the impacts of energy storage systems and demand-side management strategies in the economic operation of renewable based distribution networks. *Sustainability*, 14, 2110, 2022.
6. Yao, C. and Ma, Y., Superconducting materials: Challenges and opportunities for large-scale applications. *iScience*, 24, 102541, 2021.
7. Kaur, H. and Sharma, A., A review of recent advancement in superconductors. *Mater. Today Proc.*, 37, 3612–3614, 2021.
8. Hake, R.R., Thermodynamics of type-I and type-II superconductors. *J. Appl. Phys.*, 40, 5148, 1969.
9. Jha, A.K. and Matsumoto, K., Superconductive REBCO thin films and their nanocomposites: The role of rare-earth oxides in promoting sustainable energy. *Front. Phys.*, 7, 82, 2019.
10. Aftabi, A. and Mozaffari, M., Fluctuation induced conductivity and pseudo gap state studies of $Bi_{1.6}Pb_{0.4}Sr_2Ca_2Cu_3O_{10+\delta}$ superconductor added with ZnO nanoparticles. *Sci. Rep.*, 11, 4341, 2021.
11. Hosono, H., Tanabe, K., Muromachi, E.T., Kageyama, E.H., Yamanaka, S., Kumakura, H., Nohara, M. Hiramatsu, H., Fujitsu, S., Exploration of new superconductors and functional materials and fabrication of superconducting tapes and wires of iron pnictides. *Sci. Technol. Adv. Mater.*, 16, 033503, 2015.

12. Shiohara, Y., Yoshizumi, M., Takagi, Y., Izumi, T., Future prospects of high Tc superconductors-coated conductors and their applications. Ed.: K. Enpuku, T. Izumi. *Phys. C. Supercond. Appl.*, 484, 1, 2013.
13. Jung, S.G., Kang, J.H., Park, E., Lee, S., Lin, J.Y., Chareev, D.A., Vasiliev, A.N., Park, T., Enhanced critical current density in the pressure-induced magnetic state of the high-temperature superconductor FeSe. *Sci. Rep.*, 5, 16385, 2015.
14. Song, D., Ishida, S., Iyo, A., Nakajima, M., Shimoyama, J., Eisterer, M., Eisaki, H., Distinct doping dependence of critical temperature and critical current density in Ba1-xKxFe$_2$As$_2$ superconductor. *Sci. Rep.*, 6, 26671, 2016.
15. Flükiger, R., Overview of superconductivity and challenges in applications. *Rev. Accel. Sci. Technol.*, 5, 1–23, 2012.
16. Larbalestier, D., Gurevich, A., Feldmann, D.M., Polyanskii, A., High-Tc superconducting materials for electric power applications. *Nature*, 414, 368–377, 2001.
17. Takahei, Y., Tomita, K., Itoh, Y., Ashida, K., Lee, J.-H., Nishimoto, N., Kimura, T., Kudo, K., Nohara, M., Kubozono, Y., Kambe, T., A new way to synthesize superconducting metal-intercalated C60 and FeSe. *Sci. Rep.*, 6, 18931, 2016.
18. Ivanovskii, A.L., New ternary ThCr$_2$Si$_2$-type iron–selenide superconducting materials: Synthesis, properties and simulations. *Phys. C. Supercond. Appl.*, 471, 409, 2011.
19. Wu, X.D., Foltyn, S.R., Dye, R.C., Garcia, A.R., Nogar, N.S., Muenchausen, R.E., Pulsed laser deposition of oxide superconducting thin films. *Thin Solid Films*, 218, 310, 1992.
20. Hammond, R.H., Electron beam evaporation synthesis of A15 superconducting compounds: Accomplishments and prospects. *IEEE Trans. Magn.*, 11, 201, 1975.
21. Ueda, K. and Naito, M., As-grown superconducting MgB$_2$ thin films prepared by molecular beam epitaxy. *Appl. Phys. Lett.*, 79, 2046, 2001.
22. Selvamanickam, V., Chen, Y., Xie, J., Zhang, Y., Guevara, A., Kesgin, I., Majkic, G., Martchevsky, M., Influence of Zr and Ce doping on electromagnetic properties of (Gd,Y)-Ba-Cu-O superconducting tapes fabricated by metal organic chemical vapor deposition. *Phys. C: Supercond. Appl.*, 469, 2037, 2009.
23. Cai, X., Guo, Z., Yang, C., Niu, R., Luo, W., Huang, Z., Wang, H., Feng, Q., Gan, Z., HPCVD thin film MgB$_2$ for superconducting magnetic shielding. *IEEE Trans. Appl. Supercond.*, 29, 1200104, 2019.
24. Ma, Y., Gao, Z., Qi, Y., Zhang, X., Wang, L., Zhang, Z., Wang, D., Fabrication and characterization of iron pnictide wires and bulk materials through the powder-in-tube method. *Phys. C. Supercond. Appl.*, 469, 651, 2009.
25. Arumugam, S., Krishnan, M., Ishigaki, K., Gouchi, J., Pervin, R., Selvan, G.K., Shirage, P.M., Uwatoko, Y., Enhancement of superconducting properties and flux pinning mechanism on Cr$_{0.0005}$NbSe$_2$ single crystal under Hydrostatic pressure. *Sci. Rep.*, 9, 347, 2019.

26. Charifoulline, Z., Residual resistivity ratio (RRR) measurements of LHC superconducting NbTi cable strands. *IEEE Trans. Appl. Supercond.*, 16, 1188, 2016.
27. Berlincourt, T.G., Emergence of Nb-Ti as super magnet material. *Cryogenics*, 27, 283, 1987.
28. Wilson, M.N., Stabilization of superconductors for use in magnets. *IEEE Trans. Magn.*, 13, 440, 1977.
29. Kumakura, H., Development and prospects for the future of superconducting wires. *Jpn. J. Appl. Phys.*, 51, C10003, 2012.
30. Zhang, P., Li, J., Guo, Q., Zhu, Y., Yan, K., Wang, R., Zhang, K., Liu, X., Feng, Y., NbTi superconducting wires and applications, in: *Titanium for Consumer Application*, F. Fores, M. Qian, M. Ninomi (Eds.), pp. 279–296, Elsevier Amsterdam, 2019.
31. Lee, P.J., McKinnell, J.C., Larbalestier, D.C., Microstructure control in high Ti Nb-Ti alloys. *IEEE Trans. Magn.*, 25, 1918, 1989.
32. Vedernikov, G.P., Shikov, A.K., Potanina, L.V., Plashkin, E.I., Nikulenkov, E.V., Gubkin, I.N., Salunin, N.I., Korpusov, V.Y., Development of fine filament NbTi superconducting strands for magnet systems of fusion reactors. *Phys. C. Supercond. Appl.*, 354, 420, 2001.
33. Kanithi, H.C., Valaris, P., Zeitlin, B.A., A novel approach to make fine filament superconductors. *Supercollider*, 4, 41, 1992.
34. Parrel, J.A., Lee, P.J., Larbalestier, D.C., Cold work loss during heat treatment and extrusion of Nb-46.5 wt.% Ti composites as measured by microhardness. *IEEE Trans. Appl. Supercond.*, 3, 734, 1993.
35. Cooley, L., Lee, P.J., Larbalestier, D.C., Conductor processing of low-Tc materials: The alloy Nb-Ti, in: *Handbook of Superconducting Materials*, D.A. Cardwell, D.C. Larbalestier, A.I. Barginski (Eds.), IOP Pub, Bristol, England, 2003.
36. Lee, P.J., Fischer, C.M., Larbalestier, D.C., Naus, M.T., Squitieri, A.A., Starch, W.L., Werner, R.J., Limon, P.J., Abbi, G., Zlobin, A., Gregory, A., Development of high performance multifilamentary Nb-Ti-Ta superconductor for LHC insertion quadrupoles. *IEEE Trans. Appl. Supercond.*, 9, 1571, 1999.
37. Devred, A., *Practical low-temperature superconductors for electromagnet*, CERN, Geneva, 2004.
38. Scanlan, R.M., Malozemoff, A.P., Larbalestier, D.C., Superconducting materials for large scale applications. *Proc. IEEE*, 92, 1639, 2004.
39. Rossi, L. and Zlobin, A.V., *Nb_3Sn accelerator magnets: The early days (1960s-1980s)*, D. Scheorling and A.V. Zlobin (Eds.), pp. 1–5, Springer Nature Switzerland AG. Cham, Switzerland, 2019.
40. Keckert, S., Junginger, T., Buck, T., Hall, D., Kolb, P., Kungler, O., Laxdol, R., Liepe, M., Posen, S., Prokscha, T., Critical field of Nb_3Sn prepared for superconducting cavities. *Supercond. Sci. Technol.*, 32, 075004, 2019.
41. Balachandran, S., Tarantini, C., Lee, P.J., Kametani, F., Su, Y.F., B. Walker, B., Starch, W.L., Larbalestier, D.C., Beneficial influence of Hf and Zr additions to Nb_4at%Ta on the vortex pinning of Nb_3Sn with and without an O source. *Supercond. Sci. Technol.*, 32, 044006, 2019.

42. Godeke, A., Ouden, A.D., Nijhuis, A., Kate, H.H.J., State of the art powder-in-tube niobium–tin superconductors. *Cryogenics*, 48, 308, 2008.
43. Yuan, W. and Zhang, M., Superconducting magnetic energy storage (SMES) systems, in: *Handbook of Clean Energy Systems*, J. Yan (Ed.), pp. 1–16, Wiley Online Library, US, 2015.
44. Bhunia, U., Saha, S., Chakrabarti, A., Design optimization of superconducting magnetic energy storage coil. *Phys. C. Supercond. Appl.*, 500, 25, 2014.
45. Zhu, G., Song, M., Wang, Z., Dai, S., Design of LTS coil used for the combined device of SMES- SFCL. *IEEE Trans. Appl. Supercond.*, 16, 674, 2006.
46. Lungo, C.A., Optimization of toroidal superconducting magnetic energy storage magnets. *Phys. C. Supercond. Appl.*, 354, 110–114, 2001.
47. Mikkonen, R., Kalliohaka, T., Korpela, A., Lehtonen, J., Perala, R., A 0.2 MJ cryogen free Nb_3Sn SMES in UPS application. *Supercond. Sci. Technol.*, 16, 946, 2003.
48. Holla, R.V., Energy storage methods - superconducting magnetic energy storage - A review. *J. Undergrad. Res.*, 5, 49–54, 2015.
49. Bednorz, J.G. and Muller, K.A., Possible high Tc superconductivity in the Ba–La–Cu–O system. *Z. Phys. B*, 64, 189, 1986.
50. Abrikosov, A., On the magnetic properties of superconductors of the second groups. *Sov. Phys. JETP*, 5, 1174, 1957.
51. Wu, M.K., Ashburn, J.R., Torng, C.J., Hor, P.H., Meng, R.L., Gao, L., Huang, Z.J., Wang, Y.Q., Chu, C.W., Superconductivity at 93K in a new mixed-phase, Y–Ba–Cu–O compound system at ambient pressure. *Phys. Rev. Lett.*, 58, 908, 1987.
52. Antipov, E.V., Loureiro, S.M., Chaillout, C., Capponi, J.J., Bordet, P., Tholence, J.L., Putilin, S.N., Marezio, M., The synthesis and characterization of the $HgBa_2Ca_2Cu_3O_{8+\delta}$ and $HgBa_2Ca_3Cu_4O_{10+\delta}$. *Phys. C: Supercond. Appl.*, 215, 1, 1993.
53. Wesche, R. (Ed.), *High-temperature superconductors: Materials, properties and applications*, Kluwer Academic Publishers, Norwell, MA, USA, 1998.
54. Wagner, J.L., Chmaissem, O., Jorgensen, J.D., Hinks, D.G., Radaelli, P.G., Hunter, B.A., Jensen, W.R., Multiple defects in overdoped $Tl_2Ba_2CuO_{6+\delta}$: Effects on structure and superconductivity. *Phys. C: Supercond. Appl.*, 277, 170, 1997.
55. Capponi, J.J., Kopnin, E.M., Loureiro, S.M., Antipov, E.V., Gautier, E., Chaillout, C., Souletie, B., Brunner, M., Tholence, J.L., Marezio, M., High-pressure synthesis and heat treatments of the $HgBa_2Ca_4Cu_5O_{12+\delta}$ and $HgBa_2Ca_5Cu_6O_{14+\delta}$ phases. *Phys. C: Supercond. Appl.*, 256, 1, 1996.
56. Song, Y. and Dai, P., High-temperature superconductors, in: *Experimental Methods in the Physical Sciences*, F. Fernandez-Alonso, and D.L. Price, (Eds.), pp. 145–201, Elsevier, Amsterdam, 2015.
57. Wesche, R. (Ed.), *Physical properties of high-temperature superconductors*, John Wiley & Sons, Southern Gate, Chichester, 2015.
58. Takura, Y., Takagi, H., Uchida, S., A superconducting copper oxide compound with electrons as the charge carriers. *Nature*, 337, 345, 1989.

59. Melhem, Z. (Ed.), *High temperature superconductors (HTS) for energy applications*, Woodhead Publishing, New Delhi, 2012.
60. Tixador, P., Bellin, B., Deleglise, M., Vallier, J.C., Bruzek, C.E., Pavard, S., Saugrain, J.M., Design of a 800 kJ HTS SMES. *IEEE Trans. Appl. Supercond.*, 17, 1707, 2007.
61. Kamihara, Y., Hiramatsu, H., Hirano, M., Kawamura, R., Yanagi, H., Kamiya, T., Hosono, H., Iron based layered superconductor: LaOFePo. *J. Am. Chem. Soc.*, 128, 10012, 2006.
62. Watanabe, T., Yanagi, H., Kamiya, T., Kamihara, Y., Hiramatsu, H., Hirano, M., Hosono, H., Nickel-based oxyphosphide superconductor with a layered crystal structure, LaNiOP. *Inorg. Chem.*, 46, 7719, 2007.
63. Kamihara, Y., Watanabe, T., Hirano, M., Hosono, H., Iron-based layered superconductor $La[O_{1-x}F_x]FeAs$ (x= 0.05-0.12) with Tc = 26 K. *J. Am. Chem. Soc.*, 130, 3296, 2008.
64. Ma, F., Lu, Z.-Y., Xiang, T., Arsenic-bridged antiferromagnetic superexchange interactions in LaFeAsO. *Phys. Rev. B*, 78, 224517, 2008.
65. Singh, D.J., Electronic structure of Fe-based superconductors. *Phys. C: Supercond. Appl.*, 469, 418, 2009.
66. Guo, J., Jin, S., Wang, G., Wang, S., Zhu, K., Zhou, T., He, M., Chen, X., Superconductivity in the iron selenide $K_xFe_2Se_{2(0-x-1.0)}$. *Phys. Rev. B*, 82, 180520, 2010.
67. Zhang, X., Yao, C., Lin, H., Cai, Y., Chen, Z., Li, J., Dong, C., Zhang, Q., Wang, D., Ma, Y., Oguro, H., Awaji, S., Watanabe, K., Realization of practical level current densities in $Sr_{0.6}K_{0.4}Fe_2As_2$ tape conductors for high-field applications. *Appl. Phys. Lett.*, 104, 202601, 2014.
68. Li, X., Zhang, Y., Yuan, F., Zhuang, J., Cao, Z., Xing, X., Zhou, W., Shi, Z., Fabrication of Nb-sheathed $FeSe_{0.5}Te_{0.5}$ tape by an ex-situ powder-in tube method. *J. Alloys Compd.*, 664, 218, 2016.
69. Xiao, Y., Jin, H., Pan, X., Luo, W., Lin, H., Zhao, Y., Fabrication and superconducting properties of 19-Filamentary $Sr_{0.6}K_{0.4}Fe_2As_2$/Ag/Monel composite wires and tapes. *J. Supercond. Nov. Magn.*, 35, 697, 2022.
70. Nagamatsu, J., Nakagawa, N., Muranaka, T., Zenitani, Y., Akimitsu, J., Superconductivity at 39 K in magnesium diboride. *Nature*, 410, 63, 2001.
71. Hishinuma, Y., Kikuchi, A., Takeuchi, T., Yamada, S., Ambient temperature dependence on superconducting properties of MgB_2 wires synthesized with low temperature diffusion process. *J. Phys. Conf. Ser.*, 234, 022014, 2010.
72. Suo, H.L., Beneduce, C., Dhalle, M., Musolino, N., Genoud, J.-Y., Flukiger, R., Large transport critical currents in dense Fe- and Ni-clad MgB_2 superconducting tapes. *Appl. Phys. Lett.*, 79, 3116–3118, 2001.
73. Yagai, T., Mizuno, S., Okubo, T., Mizuochi, S., Kamibayashi, M., Jinbo, M., Takao, T., Makida, Y., Shintomi, T., Hirano, N., Komagome, T., Tsukada, K., Onji, T., Arai, Y., Tomita, M., Miyagi, D., Tsuda, M., Hamajima, T., Design

and demonstration of a double-pancake coil for SMES using MgB_2 multi-strand cable. *J. Phys. Conf. Ser.*, 1054, 012080, 2018.
74. Lv, H.-Y., Chen, M., Feng, Y., Li, W.-J., Zhong, G.-H., Yang, C.-L., Superconductivity of light-metal hydrides. *J. Chin. Chem. Soc.*, 66, 1, 2019.
75. Drozdov, A.P., Eremets, M.I., Troyan, I.A., Ksenofontov, V., Shylin, S.I., Conventional superconductivity at 203K at high pressures in the sulfur hydride system. *Nature*, 525, 73, 2015.
76. Semenok, D.V., Kruglov, I.A., Savkin, I.A., Kvashnin, A.G., Organov, A.R., On distribution of superconductivity in metal hydrides. *Curr. Opin. Solid State Mater. Sci.*, 24, 100808, 2020.
77. Zhong, X., Wang, H., Zhang, J., Liu, H., Zhang, S., Song, H.-F., Yang, G., Zhang, L., Ma, Y., Tellurium hydrides at high pressures: High-temperature superconductors. *Phys. Rev. Lett.*, 116, 057002, 2016.
78. Ferrier, M., *Stockage dénergie dans un enroulement supraconducteur', low temperature and electric power*, pp. 425–432, International Institute of Refrigeration, Low Temperatures and Electric Power, London, 1970.
79. Olabi, A.G., Onumaegbu, C., Wilberforce, T., Ramadan, M., Abdelkareem, M.A., Al–Alami, A.H., Critical review of energy storage systems. *Energy*, 214, 118987, 2020.
80. Zaman, A.A., Ahmed, S., Monira, N.J., An overview of superconducting magnetic energy storage (SMES) and its applications. *International Conference on Nanotechnology and Condensed Matter Physics (ICNCMP)*, 2018.
81. Wilson, M.N., Stabilization, protection and current density: Some general observations and speculations. *Cryogenics*, 31, 499, 1991.
82. Dresner, L. (Ed.), *Stability of superconductors*, Springer, New York City, USA, 1995.
83. Zimmermann, A.W. and Sharkh, S.M., Design of a 1 MJ/100 kW high temperature superconducting magnet for energy storage. *Energy Rep.*, 6, 180, 2020.
84. Kumar, A., Jeyan, J.V.M.L., Agarwal, A., Electromagnetic analysis on 2.5 MJ high temperature superconducting magnetic energy storage (SMES) coil to be used in uninterruptible power applications. *Mater. Today: Proc.*, 21, 1755, 2020.
85. Kondoh, J., Ishii, I., Yamaguchi, H., Murata, A., Otani, K., Sakuta, K., Higichi, N., Sekine, S., Kamimoto, H., Electrical energy storage systems for energy networks. *Energy Convers. Manage.*, 41, 1863, 2000.
86. Boenig, H.J. and Hauer, J.F., Commissioning tests of the Bonneville power administration 30 MJ superconducting magnetic energy storage unit. *IEEE Trans. Power Appar. Syst.*, 104, 302, 1985.
87. Siada, A., Review of flexible AC transmission systems; enabling technologies for future smart grids. *International Conference on High Voltage Engineering and Power System*, IEEE, 2017.
88. Siada, A. and Islam, S., Application of SMES unit in improving the performance of an AC/DC power system. *IEEE Trans. Sustain. Energy*, 2, 109, 2011.

89. Noe, M. and Steurer, M., High-temperature superconductor fault current limiters: Concepts, applications and development status. *Sci. Technol.*, 20, R15, 2007.
90. Xiao, L. (Ed.), *A 35 kV, 1.5 kA spider type of FCL is installed at the Puji substation in China*, Chinese Academy of Sciences Private Communication, Elsevier, Amsterdam, 2009.
91. Kreutz, R., Bock, J., Breuer, F., Juengst, K.P., Kleimaier, M., Klein, H.U., Krischel, D., Noe, M., Steingass, R., Weck, K.H., System technology and test of CURL 10, a 10 kV, 10 MVA resistive high- Tc superconducting fault current limiter. *IEEE Trans. Appl. Supercond.*, 15, 1961, 2005.
92. Ballarino, A., Martini, L., Mathot, S., Taylor, T., Brambilla, R., Large scale assembly and characterization of Bi–2223 HTS Conductors. *IEEE Trans. Appl. Supercond.*, 17, 3121, 2007.
93. Devred, A., Baudouy, B., Baynham, D.E., Boucboul, T., Canfer, S., Overview and status of the next European dipole joint research activity *Supercond. Sci. Technol.*, 19, S67, 2006.
94. Matrone, A., Rosatelli, G., Vaccarone, R., Current leads with high Tc superconducting bus bars. *IEEE Trans. Magn.*, 25, 1742, 1989.
95. Mitchell, N., Zheng, J., Vorpahl, C., Corato, V., Snabria, C., Segal, M., Sorbom, B., Slade, R., Brittles, G., Bateman, R., Miyoshi, Y., Banno, N., Saito, K., Kario, A., Kate, H.T., Bruzzone, P., Wesche, R., Schild, T., Bykovskiy, N., Dudarev, A., Mentink, M., Mangiorotti, F.J., Sedlak, K., Evans, D., Laan, V.D., Weiss, J.D., Liao, M., Liu, G., Superconductors for fusion: A roadmap. *Supercond. Sci. Technol.*, 34, 103001, 2021.
96. Creely, A.J., Greenwald, M.J., Ballinger, S., Brunner, D., Canik, J., Doody, J., Overview of the SPARC tokamak. *J. Plasma Phys.*, 86, 865860502, 2020.
97. Tamura, H., Takahata, K., Mito, T., Imagawa, S., Sagara, A., Mechanical behaviour analysis of superconducting magnet in LHD-type reactor FFHR. *J. Phys. Conf. Ser.*, 97, 012139, 2008.
98. Sarasola, X., Wesche, R., Ivashov, I., Sedlak, K., Uglietti, D., Bruzzone, P., Progress in the design of a hybrid HTS-Nb_3Sn-NbTi central solenoid for the EU DEMO. *IEEE Trans. Appl. Supercond.*, 30, 4200705, 2020.
99. Bykovsky, W.N., Sarasola, X., Sedlak, K., Stepanov, B., Uglietti, D., Bruzzone, P., Central solenoid winding pack design for DEMOR. *Fusion Eng. Des.*, 124, 82, 2017.
100. Yao, L., Yang, B., Cui, H., Zhuhang, J., Ye, J., Xue, J., Challenges and progresses of energy storage technology and its application in power systems. *J. Mod. Power Syst. Clean Energy*, 4, 519, 2016.
101. Putilin, S.N., Antipov, E.V., Chmaissemt, O., Marezio, M., Superconductivity at 94 K in $HgBa_2Cu0_{4+1}$. *Nature*, 362, 226, 1993.
102. Putilin, S.N., Antipov, E.V., Marezio, M., Superconductivity above 120 K in $HgBa_2CaCu_2O_{6+1}$. *Physica C: Supercond. Appl.*, 212, 266, 1993.
103. Schilling, A., Cantoni, M., Guo, J.D., Ott, H.R., Superconductivity above 130K in the Hg-Ba-Ca-Cu-O system. *Nature*, 363, 56, 1993.

104. Bozovic, I., Logvenov, G., Belca, I., Narimbetov, B., Sveklo, I., Epitaxial strain and superconductivity in $La_{2-x}Sr_xCuO_4$ thin films. *Phys. Rev. Lett.*, 89, 107001, 2002.
106. Schirber, J.E., Morosin, B., Merrill, R.M., Hlava, P.F., Venturini, E.L., Kwak, J.F., Nigrey, P.J., Baughman, R.J., Ginley, D.S., Stoichiometry of bulk superconducting $La_2Cuo_{4+Î´}$: A superconducting superoxide. *Physica C: Supercond. Appl.*, 152, 121, 1988.
106. Tissue, B.M., Cirillo, K.M., Wright, J.C., Daeumling, M., Larbalestier, D.C., Conversion of $La_2CuO_{4-Î´}$ to a superconductor by treatment in fluorine gas. *Solid State Commun.*, 65, 51, 1988.
107. Geballe, T.H. and Marezio, M., Enhanced superconductivity in Sr_2CuO_{4-v}. *Physica C: Supercond. Appl.*, 469, 680, 2009.
108. Gao, W.B., Liu, Q.Q., Yang, L.X., Yu, Y., Li, F.Y., Jin, C.Q., Uchida, S., Out-of-plane effect on the superconductivity of $Sr_{2-x}Ba_xCuO_{3+y}$ with Tc up to 98 K. *Phys. Rev. B*, 80, 094523, 2009.
119. Zhang, Y. and Xu, X., Yttrium barium copper oxide superconducting transition temperature modeling through gaussian process regression. *Comput. Mater. Sci.*, 179, 109583, 2020.
110. Lin, J.G., Huang, C.Y., Xue, Y.Y., Chu, C.W., Cao, X.W., Ho, J.C., Origin of the R-ion effect on T_c, in $RBa_2Cu_30_7$. *Phys. Rev. B*, 51, 12900(R), 1995.
111. Williams, G.V.M. and Tallon, J.L., Ion size effects on T_C and interplanar coupling in $RBa_2Cu_30_{7-Î´}$. *Physica C: Supercond. Appl.*, 258, 41, 1996.
112. Stangl, E., Proyer, S., Borz, M., Hellebrand, B., BÃ¤uerle, D., Pulsed-laser deposited $GdBaSrCu_30_{7-Î´}$ and $GdBa_2Cu_30_{7-Î´}$ films. *Physica C: Supercond. Appl.*, 256, 245, 1996.
113. Muralidhar, M., Sakai, N., Machi, T., Miyajiri, T., Hirabayashi, I., Tanaka, S., New method of synthesis and physical properties of thick superconducting Er-123 films. *Physica C: Supercond. Appl.*, 468, 1345, 2008.
114. Cao, Y., Hudson, T.L., Wang, S., Xu, S.H., Xue, Y.Y., Chu, C.W., High-temperature superconducting $YSr_2Cu_3O_{7.5}$ under pressure. *Phys. Rev. B*, 58, 11201, 1998.
115. Eisaki, H., Kaneko, N., Feng, D.L., Damascelli, A., Mang, P.K., Shen, K.M., Shen, Z.-X., Greven, M., Effect of chemical inhomogeneity in bismuth-based copper oxide superconductors. *Phys. Rev. B*, 69, 064512, 2004.
116. Ehmann, A., Sack, S., Lösch, S., Schlichenmaier, M., Wischert, W., Zoller, P., Nissel, T., Huebener, R.P., New family of superconducting copper oxides: Bi cuprates of type 1212. *Physica C: Supercond. Appl.*, 198, l, 1992.
117. Lejay, P., de Rango, P., Sulpice, A., Giordanengo, B., Tournier, R., Retoux, R., Deslandes, S., Michel, C., Hervieu, M., Raveau, B., Superconductivity up to 110 K in $Bi_2Sr_2Ca_2Cu_3O_{10}$ compounds. *Rev. Phys. Appl. (Paris)*, 24, 485, 1989.
118. Lösch, S., Budin, H., Eibl, O., Hartmann, M., Rentschler, T., Rygula, M., Sack, S.K., Huebener, R.P., Structural analysis and superconducting properties of Pb-free $Bi_2Sr_2Ca_3Cu_4O_y$ (n = 4, nominal composition). *Physica C: Supercond. Appl.*, 177, 271, 1991.

119. Iyo, A., Tanaka, Y., Tokumoto, M., Tokiwa, K., Watanaba, T., Ihara, H., High-pressure synthesis of $TlBa_2Ca_{n-1}Cu_nO_y$(n = 3 and 4) with Tc = 133.5 K(n = 3) and 127 K (n =4). *Physica C: Supercond. Appl.*, 357, 324, 2001.
120. Molchanov, V.N. and Simonov, V.I., Superconducting single crystals of $Tl_2Ba_2CaCu_2O_8$ and $YBa_2Cu_4O_8$: Crystal structures in the vicinity of Tc. *Acta Crystallogr.*, 54, 905, 1998.
121. Parkin, S.S.P., Lee, V.Y., Engler, E.M., Nazzal, A.I., Huang, T.C., Gorman, G., Savoy, R., Beyers, R., Bulk superconductivity at 125K in $Tl_2Ca_2Ba_2Cu_3O_x$. *Phys. Rev. Lett.*, 60, 2539, 1988.
122. Chen, G.F., Li, Z., Wu, D., Li, G., Hu, W.Z., Dong, J., Zheng, P., Luo, J.L., Wang, N.L., Superconductivity at 41 K and its competition with spin-density-wave instability in layered $CeO_{1-x}F_xFeAs$. *Phys. Rev. Lett.*, 100, 247002, 2008.
123. Singh, S.J., Prakash, J., Maurya, V.K., Ganguli, A.K., Patnaik, S., Study of upper critical field in 1111-ferropnictide superconductors. *AIP Conf. Proc.*, 1447, 905, 2012.
124. Chen, X.H., Wu, T., Wu, G., Liu, R.H., Chen, H., Fang, D.F., Superconductivity at 43 K in $SmFeAsO_{1-x}F_x$. *Nature*, 453, 761, 2008.
125. Ren, Z.A., Yang, J., Lu, W., Yi, W., Che, G.C., Dong, X.L., Sun, L.L., Zhao, Z.X., Superconductivity at 52 K in iron-based F doped layered quaternary compound $Pr[O_{1-x}F_x]FeAs$. *Mater. Res. Innov.*, 12, 105, 2018.
126. Ren, Z.-A., Yang, J., Lu, W., Yi, W., Shen, X.-L., Li, Z.-C., Che, G.-C., Dong, X.-L., Sun, L.-L., Zhou, F., Zhao, Z.-X., Superconductivity in the iron-based F-doped layered quaternary compound $Nd[O_{11-x}F_x]$ FeAs. *Europhys. Lett.*, 82, 57002, 2008.
127. Ren, Z.-A., Che, G.-C., Dong, X.-L., Yang, J., Lu, W., Yi, W., Shen, X.-L., Li, Z.-C., Sun, L.-L., Zhou, F., Zhao, Z.X., Superconductivity and phase diagram in iron-based arsenic-oxides $ReFeAsO_{1-\delta}$ (Re = rare-earth metal) without fluorine doping. *Europhys. Lett.*, 83, 17002, 2008.
128. Yang, J., Li, Z.-C., Lu, W., Yi, W., Shen, X.-L., Ren, Z.-A., Che, G.-C., Dong, X.-L., Sun, L.L., Zhou, F., Zhao, Z.X., Superconductivity at 53.5 K in $GdFeAsO_{1-\delta}$. *Supercond. Sci. Technol.*, 21, 082001, 2008.
129. Shirage, P.M., Miyazawa, K., Kihou, K., Lee, C.-H., Kito, H., Tokiwa, K., Tanaka, Y., Eisaki, H., Iyo, A., Synthesis of ErFeAsO-based superconductors by the hydrogen doping method. *Europhys. Lett.*, 92, 57001, 2010.
130. Hanna, T., Muraba, Y., Matsuishi, S., Igawa, N., Kodama, K., Shamoto, S., Hosono, H., Hydrogen in layered iron arsenides: Indirect electron doping to induce superconductivity. *Phys. Rev. B*, 84, 024521, 2011.
131. Takahashi, H., Soeda, H., Nukii, M., Kawashima, C., Nakanishi, T., Iimura, S., Muraba, Y., Matsuishi, S., Hosono, H., Superconductivity at 52 K in hydrogen-substituted $LaFeAsO_{1-x}H_x$ under high pressure. *Sci. Rep.*, 5, 7829, 2015.
132. Rotter, M., Tegel, M., Johrendt, D., Superconductivity at 38 K in the iron arsenide $(Ba_{1-x}K_x)$ Fe_2As_2. *Phys. Rev. Lett.*, 101, 107006, 2008.

133. Gil, R. and Clarke, S.J., Structure, magnetism and superconductivity of the layered iron arsenides $Sr_{1-x}NaxFe_2As_2$. *Chem. Mater.*, 23,1009, 2011.
134. Alireza, P.L., Ko, Y.T., Gillett, J., Petrone, C.M., Cole, J.M., Lonzarich, G.G., Sebastian, S.E., Superconductivity up to 29 K in $SrFe_2As_2$ and $BaFe_2As_2$ at high pressures. *J. Phys.: Condens. Matter.*, 21, 012208, 2009.
135. Tapp, J.H., Tang, Z., Lv, B., Sasmal, K., Lorenz, B., Chu, C.W., Guloy, A.M., LiFeAs: An intrinsic FeAs-based superconductor with Tc= 18 K. *Phys. Rev. B*, 78, 060505(R), 2008.
136. Parker, D.R., Pitcher, M.J., Baker, P.J., Franke, I., Lancaster, T., Blundell, S.J., Clarke, S.J., Structure, antiferromagnetism and superconductivity of the layered iron arsenide NaFeAs. *Chem. Commun.*, 16, 2189–2191, 2009.
137. Hsu, F.C., Luo, J.Y., Yeh, K.W., Chen, T.K., Huang, T.W., Wu, P.M., Lee, Y.C., Huang, Y.L., Chu, Y.Y., Yan, D.C., Wu, M.K., Superconductivity in the PbO-type structure Î±-FeSe. *Proc. Natl. Acad. Sci. U.S.A.*, 105, 14262, 2008.
138. Yeh, K.-W., Huang, T.-W., Huang, Y.-L., Chen, T.-K., Hsu, F.-C., Wu, P.M., Lee, Y.-C., Chu, Y.-Y., Chen, C.-L., Luo, J.-Y., Yan, D.-C., Wu, M.-K., Tellurium substitution effect on superconductivity of the Î±-phase iron selenide. *Europhys. Lett.*, 84, 37002, 2008.
139. Xia, Y., Qian, D., Wray, L., Hsieh, D., Chen, G.F., Luo, J.L., Wang, N.L., Hasan, M.Z., Fermi surface topology and low-lying quasiparticle dynamics of parent $Fe_{1+x}Te/Se$ superconductor. *Phys. Rev. Lett.*, 103, 037002, 2009.
140. Awana, V.P.S., Pal, A., Vajpayee, A., Gahtori, B., Kishan, H., Superconductivity and thermal properties of sulphur doped FeTe with effect of oxygen post annealing. *Physica C: Supercond. Appl.*, 471, 77, 2011.
141. Maziopa, A.K., Shermadini, Z., Pomjakushina, E., Pomjakushin, V., Bendele, M., Amato, A., Khasanov, R., Luetkens, H., Conder, K., Synthesis and crystal growth of $Cs_{0.8}(FeSe_{0.98})_2$: A new iron-based superconductor with Tc = 27 K. *J. Phys.:Condens. Matter.*, 23, 052203, 2011.
142. Ksenofontov, V., Medvedev, S.A., Schoop, L.M., Wortmann, G., Palasyuk, T., Tsurkan, V., Deisenhofer, J., Loidl, A., Felser, C., Superconductivity and magnetism in $Rb_{0.8}Fe_{1.6}Se_2$ under pressure. *Phys. Rev. B*, 85, 214519, 2012.
143. Zhu, X., Han, F., Mu, G., Cheng, P., Shen, B., Zeng, B., Wen, H.-H., Transition of stoichiometric Sr_2VO_3FeAs to a superconducting state at 37.2 K. *Phys. Rev. B*, 79, 220512, 2009.
144. Ogino, H., Matsumura, Y., Katsura, Y., Ushiyama, K., Horii, S., Kishio, K., Shimoyama, J.I., Superconductivity at 17 K in (Fe_2P_2) $(Sr_4Sc_2O_6)$: A new superconducting layered pnictide oxide with a thick perovskite oxide layer. *Supercond. Sci. Technol.*, 22, 075008, 2009.

6

Key Factors for Optimizing Energy Density in High-Performance Supercapacitors

M. Rizwan[1]*, Ambreen[2], A. Ayub[2] and F. Aleena[2]

[1]*School of Physical Sciences, University of Punjab, Lahore, Pakistan*
[2]*Department of Physics, University of Punjab, Lahore, Pakistan*

Abstract
Electroceramics with high energy density are very crucial to meet the increasing demands of energy storage devices. Storage devices with high electrochemical performance are the need of the hour. Superior electrochemical performance has a direct tie with parameters, such as high storage density and power density. High-performance supercapacitors can be achieved by simply enhancing energy density. Many factors greatly influence the energy storage density of a supercapacitor. The energy density can easily be tailored by controlling two factors such as capacitance and voltage. The energy density is affected by parameters such as spore size, grain size, surface area, functional group, and band gap. The voltage can be increased by introducing asymmetric supercapacitors or hybrid supercapacitors. The future perspective of new methods to improve energy density is deliberated briefly.

Keywords: Energy density, grain size, double layer supercapacitor, hybrid supercapacitor, pseudo capacitor, surface area, pore size, electrolyte

6.1 Supercapacitor

Electrochemical capacitors are referred to as supercapacitors. The major components for the fabrication of superconductors are the electrodes and electrolytes. The electrodes employed for charging and discharging are made from porous materials of high surface area such as metal oxides [1] and porous carbon. A solid or liquid separator/electrolyte is used to make

**Corresponding author*: rizwan.spr@pu.edu.pk

Inamuddin, Tariq Altalhi and Sayed Mohammed Adnan (eds.) Electroceramics for High Performance Supercapacitors, (135–158) © 2024 Scrivener Publishing LLC

an interface between the electrode and electrolyte. A porous non-reactive sheet of the separator is mandatory to transport ions, for the liquid electrolyte. Solid electrolytes not only separate positive and negative electrodes but also conduct ions.

Due to this unique composition called the electrical double layer, supercapacitors possess high capacitance and low internal resistance therefore, are also termed ultracapacitors. Electrical double layer and pseudo capacitance both are incorporated in supercapacitors to achieve much high capacitance and tremendous increase in energy. Its capacitance is of the order of tens to thousands of farads as compared with conventional capacitors with capacitance ranges in micro-farads and milli-farads. For storing and supplying charge, the electrochemical supercapacitor functions like a rechargeable battery. Yet its charge-storing mechanism is much different than a conventional battery. Therefore, it is regarded as a corresponding charge storage device rather than a battery replacement. In comparison to the batteries, these capacitors offer high efficiency and lifetime because of the lesser chemical phase changes. These characteristics make it useful for civil as well as military devices. They provide a rapidly charged power source (~ 90s) to portable wireless screwdrivers [2]. This characteristic made it useful for grid stabilization [3] and in electronic systems of backup memory [4]. The black box of helicopters and armed vehicles use supercapacitors as an alternating power source [5]. It also finds applications in solar arrays, [6] wind turbines [7], and automotive industries.

Electrochemical supercapacitors also provide fast charging and discharging with a minute of specific energy. These capacitors provide high power density and high energy density than typical fuel cells and batteries respectively. Keeping these characteristics intact, supercapacitors are surely the ideal candidate for an instant and continuous power supply. On the other hand, batteries are expensive and have wild temperature intensification. It is also a valuable resource in electric power trains, trolleybuses as well as electric vehicles.

Supercapacitors are mainly categorized as electric double-layer capacitors, pseudo-capacitor, and hybrid supercapacitors [8].

6.2 Electric Double-Layer Capacitor

An electrical double-layer capacitor (EDLC) is a typical type of supercapacitor. It consists of two electrodes having current collectors made up of metal oxides such as aluminum foil, graphite sheet, and nickel foam. These are then coated with porous carbon materials such as graphene, carbon nanotubes (CNTs), activated carbons (ACs), carbon foams, carbon aerogels, etc. Active carbon powders are commercially used for electrode fabrication with surface area ranges from 1000 to 3000 m^2 g^{-1}. When voltage is supplied, the coulomb's force is responsible for the attraction of the negative charges in the electrolyte towards the positive electrode due to the positive charges accumulated on it. There is scattered distribution of charges on the ions of the electrolyte due to thermal fluctuations. It gives rise to the crowd of negative charges around the electrode. Similarly, positive charges cluster around the positive electrode keeping the system electrically neutral. In this way, two electric double layers are formed in the system, one at each electrode-electrolyte interface with Helmholtz and diffusion layers. Both of these layers are key features for the performance of the capacitor. These layers utilize the fact that the capacitance of the capacitor increases with the increment in the effective surface area of the plates and with the decrease in the distance between them. The working of EDLC is based on the non-faradaic process which sets a disadvantage in energy density. Its energy density is lower than other types of supercapacitors. No chemical reaction occurs in the mechanism of energy storage; therefore, it is reversible in its operation. It can withstand several rounds of charging and discharging because it only depends on the motion of ions here. This fact makes it much faster than batteries.

6.3 Pseudo-Capacitor

Although EDLC provides towering capacitance and enhanced power so far it restrains energy density. However, commercial demands require giant power density with increased energy storage capacity. Keeping this trend in view, pseudo capacitors are fabricated from the material that undergoes rapid reversible redox reaction at the surface. Pseudo capacitors are based on the faradaic process in which the charge transferred is proportional to the voltage applied. This process results in high energy density. With the voltage application, electrons and holes are generated and charged ions travel toward the opposite terminals. Oxidation and reduction reaction takes place at the anode and cathode respectively. As a result, the faradaic current is generated at the double layer which enhances the energy density. Pseudo-capacitors occupy the gap between batteries and EDLCs. Its galvanostatic charge-discharge (GCD) and cyclic voltammogram (CV) resemble EDLC due to rapid reaction kinematics. It resembles a battery due to redox reactions. There are three different mechanisms for pseudo capacitance listed; intercalation pseudo capacitance, under-potential deposition, and redox pseudo capacitance.

In underpotential deposition, the ions are adsorbed on the monolayer formed by H^+ or metallic ions such as Pd and Cu on the surface of different metals such as gold or platinum. This mechanism provides better reversibility along with rapid charging and discharging. It also results in a fascination with power density [9, 10]. The most customary mechanism is the redox pseudo capacitance, in which charge is exchanged between the electrodes and the electrolyte. This results in the adsorption of ions. Conducting polymers and metal oxides are utilized for redox pseudo capacitance [11, 12].

When a dissolved redox couple is utilized i.e., both oxidant and reductant are dissolved in the electrolyte then their diffusion to or from the electrode surface is the key feature that controls high-power applications. Transition metals are being utilized for undissolved redox couple which results in much higher conductivity and reversibility. It also increases the capacitance and widens the potential range up to 1.4V. Nickel oxide is cheap and found to be suitable for this purpose. In the faradaic process, there is a risk of phase change of the material with time which minimizes the lifetime Dissolution of the redox couple and also affects the reversibility rate. In an undissolved state, 3D morphology is under control.

The intercalation pseudo-capacitance mechanism does not involve a redox reaction. Excess energy density and larger power density are achieved using bulk electrode materials for the intercalation of the ions. This intercalation is different than the intercalation mechanism of batteries which results in the reduction of power density. A typical example of intercalation is lithium intercalation. It transits technology between electrochemical supercapacitors and acid batteries. In the battery, lithium is propelled thermally on graphite anode which upon discharging impinges upon the cathode with better thermal stability. In this case, the cathode is a transition metal oxide or sulfide such as V_6O_{13}, MoS_2, and TiS_2. When this intercalation mechanism is utilized in pseudo capacitance, it requires a double-layer electrode, lithium source electrode as well as intercalation electrode. In the cathode crystal structure, layer lattice sites are utilized for intercalation. It is not useful for high power application as lithium diffusion rates limits charge rates [13, 14]. Although a pseudo capacitor made up for the flaws of EDLC, it has certain limitations as well. It cannot match the power density and cyclic stability of EDLC.

6.4 Hybrid Supercapacitor

To overcome the limitations and retain the goodness of both the supercapacitors, another supercapacitor was proposed called a hybrid supercapacitor. Hybrid supercapacitors are subjected to a faradaic as well as a non-faradaic process. Resultantly, the hybrid supercapacitor is half EDLC and half pseudo-capacitor. Hybrid supercapacitors typically have three types; battery-type hybrid, asymmetric hybrid, and composite hybrid. The electrode arrangement of the first two types is similar but different materials are used for composition. Out of two electrodes of the battery-type hybrid, one electrode is fabricated with the materials used in electrodes in a typical battery. This part contributes to the elevation of the energy density, whereas its other electrode resembles the electrode of the supercapacitor which results in higher power density.

In the asymmetric hybrid type, the EDLC part contains a negative electrode which is made up of carbon material. The other part is pseudocapacitive and comprises a positive electrode. In some cases, both electrodes are made up of carbon but with different functional groups. However, the former combination is preferred because it results in a longer life cycle, more stable charging-discharging cycles, and enhanced working potential. For the composite hybrid type, the pseudocapacitive material is incorporated with the carbon material to fabricate the electrodes. The pseudocapacitive material can be conducting polymer or metal oxide. However, greater structural stability is observed in the case of carbon incorporation in conducting polymer. It not only increases the potential and corrosion stability but also results in enhanced capacitance [15].

Although the hybrid supercapacitor is the better alternative to EDLC and Pseudoscalar, it has the potential risk of having higher equivalence resistance. It results in decreased efficiency of the device. When the electrode material follows the simple abscrption mechanism, the ions from electrodes disseminate towards the electrolyte responding to the differences in the concentration. This leads to the self-discharging of the supercapacitor. The incorporation of zinc anode can suppress this behavior. It is noteworthy that hybrid supercapacitors do not readily show self-discharging [16, 17].

6.4.1 Electrochemical Performance

The electrochemical efficiency of the supercapacitors is greatly influenced by modifying electrodes and electrolytes. The following fundamental concepts help us to understand the correlating factors affecting the efficiency and performance of supercapacitors.

6.4.2 Capacitance

The capacitance of a capacitor is its ability to store the charge. The correspondence of charge stored between the plates and the differences between their potentials gives the interpretation of capacitance. It depends on the following factors as well.

$$C = \frac{A\varepsilon_o\varepsilon_r}{d} \tag{6.1}$$

Here A = area of the plate,
ε_o = permittivity of the free space,
ε_r = relative permittivity
and
d = thickness of the double layer at the electrode [18–20].

6.4.3 Specific Capacitance

The quantity of energy delivered per unit mass or per unit volume of the active substance is termed specific capacitance. The gathered charge is responsible for the charging and discharging of the capacitor. The specific capacitance is enumerated by the following relation.

$$C_s = \frac{I.\Delta t}{\Delta V.m} \tag{6.2}$$

Here V is the potential difference between the electrodes, t is the discharge time, I is the charging/discharging current, and m is the mass of active material.

6.4.4 Energy Density

The total energy stored per unit volume between the parallel plates of the capacitor is termed the energy density of the capacitor. It can be estimated as follows.

$$E_d = \frac{CV^2}{2m} \tag{6.3}$$

Here, m is the mass of the active material, C is the capacitance of the capacitor and V is the potential difference, and.

6.4.5 Power Density

Power density is the amount of energy transferred per unit volume per unit of time. It is calculated as:

$$P_d = \frac{V^2}{R.m} \text{ or } \frac{E}{t} \tag{6.4}$$

Here He is the energy density, m is the mass of the active material, R is the resistance, t is the discharge time, and V is the potential difference between the plates of the capacitor [21, 22].

6.4.6 Cyclic Stability

The number of charging/discharging cycles of the capacitor before it reaches a certain reduced capacity is termed cyclic stability. To check the stability of the material potential-time graph is plotted [23]. In the above formulas, it is perceived that for increasing the energy density, capacitance, and potential difference can be increased. Increased area of the plates and decreased distance between them will result in elevated capacitance. Another factor affecting the capacitance is the dielectric medium. The presence of capacitance decreases the surface charge density and the electric field between the plates which in turn increases the capacitance. Modification of the electrode material also aids the enhancement of the capacitor. Double layer formation and dielectric constant is material dependent. Therefore, the material of the electrode is the key factor in controlling the electrochemical performance and accuracy of the supercapacitor. The electrode material is modified either by varying the pore size or by adding a heteroatom or functional group. Studies showed that pore size modification does not guarantee the rise of capacitance [24]. However, the agreement of pore size with the ion size increases the capacitance to a considerable extent [25–27]. If pores with a diameter less than 0.4 nm are associated with the specific surface area then capacitance shows no considerable increase [28]. The stability of electrolyte and electroactive materials greatly influences power and energy density [29].

6.5 The Energy Density of Supercapacitor

As described in the previous section, energy density depends upon the capacitance of the capacitor and the potential difference between the plates. Energy density varies directly with the capacitance and double power of the potential difference. Therefore, the greater the capacitance, the greater will be the energy density. For potential difference, its fluctuation greatly influences the energy density. The factors that can influence these two parameters will be the controlling factors for the energy density of the supercapacitors.

6.5.1 Optimization of High Energy Density

The energy density is a key parameter that decides the electrical performance of a capacitor and plays a pivotal role in the breakdown strength of a storage device. The energy density of a basic supercapacitor is restricted to 10 Wh $kg^{-1.}$ This small value has limited the application of supercapacitors to airplane cabin switches. Electro ceramics with superior storage density can support a higher value of electric field close to breakdown strength. On the other hand, ceramics that have a poor energy density tend to have pores that lead to short circuits even at a moderate electric field. The energy density of a supercapacitor is given as

$$E= (1/2)\ CV^2 \tag{6.5}$$

where V is the voltage [30].

There are many methods to obtain high energy density electro-ceramics including optimization of sintering parameters such as temperature, time, and heating rate. The addition of certain foreign constituents can also help with the energy density of ceramics, as this will help in the optimization of sintering conditions. Many parameters can increase energy density some are shown in Figure 6.1 [31].

6.5.1.1 Pore Size

The pore size of the electrode material used for the supercapacitor greatly affects the capacitance and thus the energy density. Variations of pore size

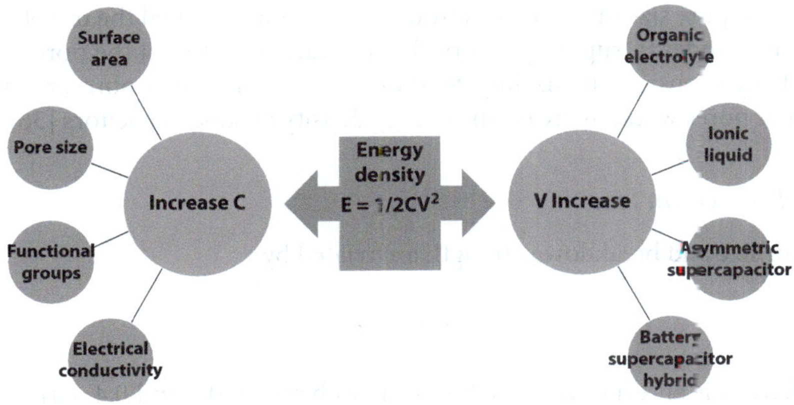

Figure 6.1 Factors affecting storage density of supercapacitor [31].

play a vital role in the charging and discharging process of the capacitors [32]. There are three different sizes of pores

- Macropores (>50 nm)
- Micropores (< 2 nm)
- Mesopores (2-50 nm)

Micropores in certain electrode materials tend to have a double electrical layer that produces large pores and ultimately diminishes the conductivity of electrode material. Mesopores are the most suitable option for double-layer capacitance without causing any damage. It is possible to control the pore size by tailoring the pre-carbonization temperature and quantity of the activator [33].

6.5.1.2 *Surface Area*

Usually, the greater surface area is attributed to high capacitance and thus a greater storage density but there is not a linear relationship between the two parameters. The surface area where the charge is deposited and absorbed is related to pore size and is termed a specific surface area. Surface area and pore size are related as micropores and mesopores give higher specific surface area. The specific surface area with pore size <0.4 nm does not contribute to storage density [34]. Pore size and capacitance are related. There is a relation between the size of electrolyte ions and pore size, capacitance is greater when the pore size and ions of electrolyte are of the same size [35]. Greater capacitance has been achieved by tailoring the surface area and pore size of carbon electrodes. This has accelerated the use of carbon electrodes in supercapacitors. The interaction between the pores and electrolyte ions is still puzzling. Studies suggest that smaller pore sizes and proper pores would increase the energy density of supercapacitors [36].

6.5.1.3 Grain Size

Grain size and breakdown strength are related by

$$\mathrm{BDS} \propto G^{-a} \tag{6.6}$$

Here, a is an exponent which has values between 0.2 and 0.4. Grin size greatly affects the energy storage properties of ceramics. It was suggested that ceramics with finer grain size have a low value of leakage current in comparison to ceramics with coarse grain. Energy storage properties can be optimized with high density and fine grain size. Forming a solid solution and the inclusion of foreign constituents can also help in tailoring the grain size to a fine value. Ultrathin coating before Sintering can also help reduce the grain size. The relationship between energy storage properties and grain size for different energy storage ceramics is shown in Figure 6.2 [37].

6.5.1.4 Functional Groups

Apart from pore size and surface area, the surface functional group also greatly affects the capacitance and hence the storage density. Functional groups can increase the wettability which results in greater capacitance due to redox reactions. It was reported that N(8.2%-11.9%)-doped mesoporous

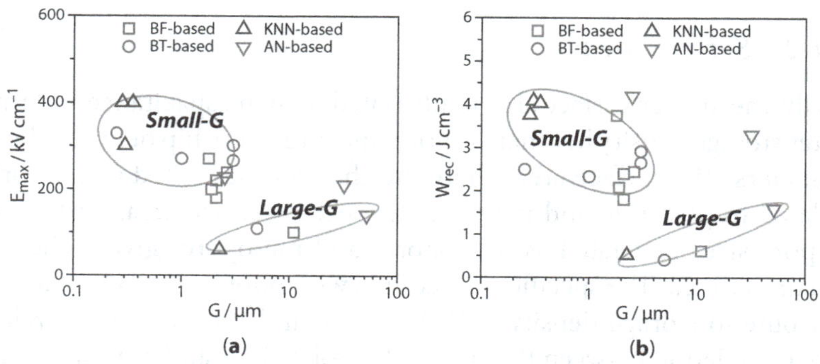

Figure 6.2 Relationship between Energy storage properties and grain size (a) Grain size vs. E_{max} (b) Grain size vs. W_{rec} [37].

C-layer had an energy density of 41 Wh kg^{-1} [38]. The introduction of surface functional groups has the prospect to increase the capacitance. Nitrogen-doped Carbon materials for storage devices can be synthesized in two ways. Many functional carbon materials are derived directly from natural resources which are economical and eco-friendly. The amount of nitrogen introduced is very important as high content can in turn reduce capacitance. There has been many studies devoted to understanding the relationship between functional group and their effect on capacitance, but more focus needs to be on establishing the correlation between these parameters [39].

6.5.1.5 *Band Gap*

The band gap is usually referred to as the space between the valence and conduction bands. Band gap greater than 4 eV is for insulators, 0–4 eV for semiconductors, and 0 eV for metals. The breakdown strength is given as

$$BDS=1.36x10^7\ (E_g/4)^3\ (V/cm) \tag{6.7}$$

Semiconductors that have large band gap tends to have larger BDS. The band gap of semiconductors can be analyzed via theoretical and experimental techniques. Activation energy is half of the band gap and can be enhanced via doping and thus increasing the BDS. A higher value of BDS suggests superior energy density. The highest band gap is exhibited by $NaNbO_3$; thus, it can be introduced in other ceramics to increase the capacitance.

6.5.2 Effect of Voltage

The role of voltage apart from capacitance is essential for determining energy density as its square is proportional to the E, where ($E = ½\ CV^2$). An increase in operating voltage of threefold leads to a rise in energy of about one order of magnitude for the same capacitance. The common potential difference for electrolyte solution systems is less than 1.0 V which clarifies why the power density of a typical supercapacitor device is relatively low. [40].

Li-ion BSHs served as the bridge between Li-ion batteries (LIBs) and supercapacitors and attracted international consideration due to the large specific capacity of Li-ion-type electrodes, In IL electrolyte systems the maximum voltage devices were often accomplished where the voltage that can reach more than 3 V and is comparable to that of standard Li-ion batteries. ILs are desirable options for next-generation electrolytes due to their large potential windows (>3 V) and strong chemical as well as physical capabilities. Due to its wide electrochemical stability window which spans 2.0 to 6.0 V particularly around 4.5 V. Employing ILs to raise the working potential is a promising technique to obtain large energy concreteness. Furthermore, the lack of a solvent in ILs without solvation shells can offer well-identified ion sizes, allowing for the optimization of the pore diameters of electrodes. Recently created porous carbon with optimum pore sizes, which is consistent with earlier studies showing that 0.7 nm size openings produce superior capacitance. The upper limits of the $EMIMBF_4$ ion solution electrolytes are 0.48 and 0.76 nm, respectively [41].

Stock highly porous flakes revealed a high capacitance (246 Fg^{-1}) and when combined with an $EMIMBF_4$ IL solution of a high voltage e.g. 3.5 V, the calculated energy density was 103W h kg^{-1} that is based on the weight of the electrode layer. The capacitance is reduced by the fact that ILs usually have poor electronic conductivity and high viscosity. Compositions of ILs and organic solutions have gained popularity as a solution to this problem [42].

The superior-energy-density supercapacitors construed on an $EMIMBF_4$/A mixed electrolyte can attain an operating voltage of up to 3.5 V and have a density of up to 35 W h kg^{-1}. It is predicted that increases in working voltage will make it possible to have a high energy density. Developing more acceptable electrolytes with higher operational potentials, high conductivities of ions, ideal ionic radius, appropriate viscosity values throughout a wide temperature range, and suitable porous structures to adjust to IL sizes will be the most pressing task ahead. The study is broken into various sections for clarity even though many elements affect energy density and work together to make it better. If the aforementioned contributing elements and difficulties are not further studied and treated concurrently, the maximum energy density cannot be achieved by handling any single issue [43].

6.5.3 Asymmetric Supercapacitors

Asymmetric supercapacitors (ASCs) are constructed from 2 electrode supplies that are different from one another and have the particular advantage of having a broad working voltage range, which greatly improves their energy density. Normally metal oxides are used as supercapacitor electrodes, the most popular materials are using are RuO2, MnO2, and $Ni(OH)_2$. To create ASCs, alternative materials including porous carbon can be employed as the other electrode by Moore J, *et al.* [1]. ASCs using aqueous electrolytes for instance possess potential windows bigger than 2.0 V. ASCs have an energy concreteness of about 100 W h kg^{-1} [44].

Based on these characteristics and using chemical or ionic-liquid electrolytes which have greater operating voltages will cause a higher ASC energy density. Contrarily, Misra *et al.* described a tandem ASC with a power density that was 61% greater than that of individual ASCs and a high operational potential of 4.5 V to provide a broader voltage gap. However, the structure of pseudo-capacitor materials is altered by repeated electrochemical processes which greatly reduce their stability. In addition compared to EDLC devices, devices made from these material types are more challenging to prepare [45, 46].

6.5.4 Negative Electrode Materials

Carbon-based elements are the finest possible options for negative electrocatalysts due to their inexpensive cost, wide availability, lack of toxicity, and superior electronic conductivity, electrocatalysts are used in ASCs. Midst the numerous carbonaceous materials graphene, carbon nanotubes and AC have drawn a significant amount of attention. ASC was created by Kim *et al.* using MnO2/SiC nanoneedle composites as the optimistic electrode and functionalized AC as the negative electrode. The improved ASC displayed a maximum energy density of 30.06 Whkg^{-1} and could work in a voltage space of 0-1.9 V. A three-dimensional electrode association with vertical alignment carbon nanotubes that were grown up effectively on carbon nanofibers was recently created by Qiu *et al.* [47] enabling a large specific energy of 70.7 Wh kg^{-1} (established on the electrode material mass) and 97% accumulation even after 20,000 charging and discharging phases. In comparison to AC and CNTs graphene has demonstrated a strong mix of appropriate performance characteristics (mechanical stability, surface energy, and conductance) leading to improved electrochemical performances. The energy density level is raised to 90 Wh kg^{-1} presented by Liu *et al.* [48] that prohibits the again stacking of graphene nanoplatelets and allows the creation of a porous structure that is exposed to ionic solutions [46].

6.5.5 Positive Electrode Materials

Metal oxides are an excellent candidate as materials for positive electrodes. RuO_2, MnO_2, and Ni $(OH)_2$ are interesting choices for positive electrocatalysts in ASCs due to their high specific permeability and broad potential window. Interdigitated supercapacitors constructed of 3D porous RuO_2

nanoparticles attached to graphene sheets were reported recently by Kaner *et al.* [58]. These electrodes showed a phenomenal rate capability and a very high capacitance of 1,139 F*g*$^{-1}$. In addition, ASCs used graphene sheets/RuO_2 as the positively charged electrode and an AC negative electrode showed a very high energy density of 55 Wh*kg*$^{-1}$ at a power density of 12 kW*kg*$^{-1}$. Limited surface area and poor electrical properties are the two significant issues that prevent the practical usage of MnO_2. To solve these problems it has been widely researched to combine a large surface area and electrical conductivity materials with nanostructured MnO_2 [49].

In a study by Wu *et al.* to study the properties of ASCs graphene was used as a negatively charged electrode and a MnO_2 graphene composites as a positive electrode in Na_2So_4 solutions. The graphene/MnO2 ASC device functioned in a large potential window of 0-2.0 V and had a high energy density of 30.4 W h *kg*$^{-1}$ according to the weight of the active material. The 3D UGF network in the Ni$(OH)_2$-and-ultrathin-graphite (UGF) composite has great electrical conductivity and permeability. ASCs using Ni$(OH)_2$/UGF as the positive electrodes and graphite oxides as the negative anode displayed a very significant power density of 44 kW*kg*$^{-1}$ in comparison to many conventional commonly produced supercapacitors [50].

The new supercapacitors should have an energy density close to 100 Wh *kg*$^{-1}$. In addition to the wide operating potential window in ASCs, the development of new cathodes with logical designs is necessary to provide higher surface areas, improved electrical properties, and efficient ion-diffusion networks to achieve maximum power density. Further research is needed to determine how to combine different capacitive materials to create composites that have larger surface areas, lots of porosity, great electronic conductivity, and large voltage windows. In the future, a thorough comprehension of these synergistic effects will be necessary. With these developments, it is possible to maximize factors like component selection and electrode mass loaded to achieve a high power concentration and true capacitive characteristics [51].

6.5.6 Battery-Supercapacitor Hybrid (Bsh) Device

The creation of new materials and enhanced energy storage device designs is necessary to achieve both high energy densities and high power densities [52]. An auspicious power storage device configuration is a battery-supercapacitor hybrid (BSH) device which consists of one battery charge electrode and a high-rate capacitive electrode. This has gathered a lot of attention due to the device's capability to simultaneously have a significant amount of energy (wider operating voltage and greater capacity) at a high power density [53]. BSH devices are divided into the following categories: Li-ion BSH, Na-ion BSH, acidic BSH, and alkaline BSH are based on the various category of electrodes and electrolytes.

6.5.6.1 *Lithium-Ion BSH*

Li-ion BSHs gained international interest since they filled the gap between LIBs and supercapacitors owing to their high specific capacitance of Li-ion-type electrodes. The creation of hybrid battery-type electrodes with nanostructures is a viable method for raising system performance. Nb_2O_5 carbon central Nano crystal electrodes and BSHs with power density as high as 63 Wkg^{-1} were reported by Lim *et al.* [54]. Because of the high voltage range of the cathode, Li-ion BSHs are manufactured by using a battery-type lithium-intercalation electrode and capacitive carbon electrode which is also beneficial and typically has high operational potentials. A thorough contrast of aqueous Li-ion BSHs made from AC and $LiCoO_2$, $LiMn_2O_4$ and $LiNi_{1/3}Co_{1/3}Mn_{1/3}O_2$ was presented by Xia *et al.* [55] The described devices however showed sluggish energy storage dynamics due to the electrolyte cathodes' pristine condition. The power and the energy concentrations were therefore limited to 900 and 40 W kg^{-1} correspondingly. The introduction of nanostructures could encourage an improvement in overall performance. Li-ion BSHs with carbon nanowires were fabricated that resembled peapods that were doped with Li_3VO_4 and showed an energy density of 136.4 Wkg^{-1}at 532 Wkg^{-1} based on the number of active materials. Yu *et al.* [56].

6.5.6.2 *Na-Ion BSH*

In Na-ion BSHs, carbon/carbon pairing has been studied extensively. Intercalation carbon was employed as the anode while capacitive carbon was employed as the electrode. However, the device's electrochemical characteristics were poor because of the relatively limited hard carbon capacity in Na ion electrolytes. For the device's characteristics to be improved the electrode's smaller scale design is important. A carbon/carbon Na-ion BSH was recently described by Ding *et al.* and the resultant carbon materials were extremely brittle, thin, and permeable. Based on the weight of the active material this Na-ion BSH demonstrated high energy and power densities (201, 76, and 50 W kg–1 at 285, 6,500, and 16,500 W kg^{-1} correspondingly). As battery-type electrolytes for Na-ion BSHs, several alternative Na-ion battery substrates have been employed; for example, Xia *et al.*

demonstrated Na-ion BSHs with Na0.5MnO_2/Fe_3O_4 which produced an energy density of 81W kg^{-1} at 647 W kg^{-1} [57].

K-ion BSH devices can be created which resemble Li-ion BSH and Na-ion BSH in design. Although different capacitive electrodes made from Li-ion and Na-ion BSHs may be employed, using electrodes made from K-ion electrolyte batteries still presents considerable difficulties. This is because the parent materials are limited and the ionic radius of K^+ is considerably larger than that of Li^+ or Na^+ [58].

6.5.6.3 *Acidic BSH*

Even though lead-acid batteries were created more than half a century ago, they are still among the greatest economic rechargeable batteries. Acidic BSHs are produced when lead-acid batteries are hybridized with SC. Lead-carbon capacitors are the best BSHs due to their high voltage of around 2.0 V. Additionally, the method for recycling PbO_2 and sulfuric acid has been optimized and is now self-sustaining. Lead-carbon capacitors have a low electrochemically active surface of PbO_2, which slows down quick redox processes it has a low energy capacity and a poor specific energy density (15–30 W kg^{-1}).

6.5.6.4 *Alkaline BSH*

Nickel-cadmium (Ni-Cd) batteries represent the most established alkaline battery technology since they have been in use for about 100 years. Alkaline BSHs are hybrid systems that use carbon materials as the capacitive electrodes and alkaline solutions as the electrolytes. The other electrode uses transition metal oxides or hydroxides which behave like batteries. $NiMoO_4$ nanowires array conductors were created by Lou *et al.* on various substrates. The resulting $NiMoO_4$/AC alkaline BSH produced densities of power and energy that were reasonably high (60.9 W kg^{-1}at 850 W kg^{-1} and 41.1 W kg^{-1}at 17,002 W kg^{-1}) [59].

For regenerative alkaline batteries like Ni-Fe batteries, iron oxides are among the few anode alternatives due to their affordability, environmentally friendly nature, and abundance. Iron oxide used in alkaline BSHs is not often been researched. The limitations of Fe-oxide electrodes include their comparatively poor conductivity and destruction during cycling or at a high-density concentration of current. Li *et al.* developed a Fe_3O_4-carbon binder-free nanowires array anode and provided a “carbon shell shielding” solution. The electrode’s integration was maintained with the use of a simple carbon coating that efficiently limited volume expansions and potential structural deformation the carbon shell also increased the electrode's electrical properties [60].

As several BSH categories are still in their early stages of development and still need significant improvements, their properties particularly their energy and energy density cannot yet match those of high-tech batteries and supercapacitors. Based on the so far made advances certain issues and potential, future improvements for next-generation BSHs are mentioned below.

1. The slow oxidation processes that characterized battery-type electrodes limit their power capabilities. At the present, the most common methods for solving this issue, involve designing different nanostructures to reduce the ion transport route and using nanoscale coatings with conductive species to improve conductivity and stability. Future research efforts could focus on developing nanoscale doping methods to achieve high-power attributes in addition to the aforementioned strategies.
2. Research into cutting-edge electrode and electrolyte materials is still greatly desired, especially for green Na-ion BSHs. Making high power density and high energy density Na-ion BSH devices is extremely difficult. Theory, modeling, and simulators, as well as experimental and different computational techniques, are needed to address this. Here we've covered recent developments in the design of high-performance energy storage devices, including BSHs and both symmetric and asymmetric superconductors. To overcome the current shortage of lower power densities, these conversations highlighted several strategies to raise the capacitance/working voltages of supercapacitors.

6.6 Future Outlook

Below is a list of potential future trends. First, irrespective of the type of supercapacitor, a thorough investigation of new electrode and electrolyte materials is still necessary. Theory, modeling and simulations among other computational and experimental studies are necessary to do this. The design choices for electrodes and electrolyte materials can be influenced by such computational research. The development of high-energy-density symmetric supercapacitors (EDLCs) is still a challenging task [61].

Future research should concentrate on increasing the specific capacitance by improving the appropriate specific surface area, pore diameter, and volume optimization and provision of surfaces with functional groups to enhance the supercapacitor contribution. This will increase the capacitance and working voltage. Additionally, using different ILs with voltages up to 3.0 V can considerably boost energy density. Additionally, a potential breakthrough trend is the synergistic influence of various elements. To fully comprehend how the pores and electrolyte ions interact, though is still quite difficult. Taking into account the state of development *in situ* measurement experiments in conjunction with modeling and simulation will assist in identifying the underlying tool which may allow for the expectation of the best potential energy density requires the right electrolytes, pore diameter, and surface energy [62].

The wide working voltage window of ASCs which significantly boosts energy density is their clear advantage. To achieve better energy densities, it is also important to continue researching the incorporation of different capacitive materials into composites. To truly understand how the pores and electrolytes ions interact, though is still quite difficult. Taking into account the state of development *in situ* measurement experiments in conjunction with modeling and simulation will assist in identifying the underlying apparatus, which may allow for the estimation of the ideal surface area, pore diameter, and electrolyte for the highest possible energy density. The deal with large voltage windows of ASCs, which significantly improves energy density, is their massive advantage. To achieve better energy densities, it is also important to continue researching the incorporation of different capacitive materials into composites.

Future research must put in a lot of effort to gain a thorough understanding of this synergistic action to integrate the various capacitive composite materials. Given these developments, it is possible to attain large energy densities and true capacitive qualities by optimizing factors like the composition and mass loads of capacitive synthetic structures. Using high-capacity battery-type electrodes, BSH systems demonstrate prospective energy-storing device architecture to attain a [41] great energy density. These cannot though be included any further in high-power applications due to slow redox processes. New approaches of diverse structures that can reduce the ion conduction pathway and Nanoscale coating with conducting species that can improve conductivity and stability are the main strategies to deal with this. Future studies should also concentrate on developing Nano scale-doped materials to give BSHs their high-power characteristics. The movement of electric vehicles (EVs) can be significantly improved by increasing the energy concreteness depending on device mass such as the energy density of the forthcoming supercapacitor which is close to 100 W kg^{-1}. Because of their benefits of long cycle life, enhanced security, better security, and notably quick charging times, supercapacitors have significant potential to compete with or perhaps substitute Li-ion batteries in uses such as EVs.

6.7 Conclusion

In this chapter, the most important factors that control the electrochemical performance of a supercapacitor are deliberated. One of the important parameters that decide the electrochemical performance is storage density which is directly proportional to capacitance and voltage. Increasing these parameters can result in a superior storage device. The parameters such as grain size, pore size, band gap, surface area, and a functional group that directly controls capacitance are discussed. Voltage can be tailored by employing different asymmetric supercapacitors and hybrid supercapacitors such as lithium-ion, sodium, acid, and alkaline battery supercapacitor hybrid. The future outlook of potential trends in the field of supercapacitors is also deliberated.

References

1. Merrill, M., Montalvo, E., Campbell, P., Wang, Y., Stadermann, M., Baumann, T., Biener, J., Worsley, M., Optimizing supercapacitor electrode density: Achieving the energy of organic electrolytes with the power of aqueous electrolytes. *RSC Adv.*, 4, 42942–42946, 2014.
2. Miller, J.R. and Burke, A., Electrochemical capacitors: Challenges and opportunities for real-world applications. *Electrochem. Soc. Interface*, 17, 53, 2008.
3. Luta, D.N. and Raji, A.K., Optimal sizing of hybrid fuel cell-supercapacitor storage system for off-grid renewable applications. *Energy*, 166, 530–540, 2019.
4. Wang, D.-G., Liang, Z., Gao, S., Qu, C., Zou, R., Metal-organic framework-based materials for hybrid supercapacitor application. *Coord. Chem. Rev.*, 404, 213093, 2020.
5. Yu, A., Chabot, V., Zhang, J., *Electrochemical supercapacitors for energy storage and delivery: Fundamentals and applications*, pp. 370–375, Taylor & Francis, Oxfordshire, 2013.
6. Yun, J., Song, C., Lee, H., Park, H., Jeong, Y.R., Kim, J.W., Jin, S.W., Oh, S.Y., Sun, L., Zi, G., Stretchable array of high-performance micro-supercapacitors

charged with solar cells for wireless powering of an integrated strain sensor. *Nano Energy*, 49, 644–654, 2018.

7. de Carvalho, W.C., Bataglioli, R.P., Fernandes, R.A., Coury, D.V., Fuzzy-based approach for power smoothing of a full-converter wind turbine generator using a supercapacitor energy storage. *Electr. Power Syst. Res.*, 184, 106287, 2020.
8. Kim, B.K., Sy, S., Yu, A. *et al.*, Electrochemical supercapacitors for energy storage and conversion, in: *Handbook of Clean Energy Systems*, J. Yan (Ed.), pp. 1–25, Wiley, Chichetser, 2015.
9. Yue, L., Wang, X., Sun, T., Liu, H., Li, Q., Wu, N., Guo, H., Yang, W., Ni-MOF coating MoS2 structures by hydrothermal intercalation as high-performance electrodes for asymmetric supercapacitors. *Chem. Eng. J.*, 375, 375121959, 2019.
10. Vickers, N.J., Animal communication: When i'm calling you, will you answer too? *Curr. Biol.*, 27, R713–R715, 2017.
11. Yang, K., Fan, L.-Z., Guo, J., Qu, X., Significant improvement of electrochemical properties of AlF3-coated $LiNi_{0.5}Co_{0.2}Mn_{0.3}O_2$ cathode materials. *Electrochim. Acta*, 63, 363–368, 2012.
12. Cheng, C. and Ngan, A.H., Reversible electrochemical actuation of metallic nanohoneycombs induced by pseudocapacitive redox processes. *ACS Nano*, 9, 3984–3995, 2015.
13. Ling, T., Da, P., Zheng, X., Ge, B., Hu, Z., Wu, M., Du, X.-W., Hu, W.-B., Jaroniec, M., Qiao, S.-Z., Atomic-level structure engineering of metal oxides for high-rate oxygen intercalation pseudocapacitance. *Sci. Adv.*, 4, 6261, 2018.
14. Jin, T., Li, H., Li, Y., Jiao, L., Chen, J., Intercalation pseudocapacitance in flexible and self-standing V_2O_3 porous nanofibers for high-rate and ultra-stable K ion storage. *Nano Energy*, 50, 462–467, 2018.
15. Muzaffar, A., Ahamed, M.B., Deshmukh, K., Thirumalai, J., A review on recent advances in hybrid supercapacitors: Design, fabrication and applications. *Renew. Sustain. Energy Rev.*, 101, 123–145, 2019.
16. Huang, Z., Chen, A., Mo, F., Liang, G., Li, X., Yang, Q., Guo, Y., Chen, Z., Li, Q., Dong, B., Phosphorene as cathode material for high-voltage, anti-self-discharge zinc ion hybrid capacitors. *Adv. Energy Mater.*, 10, 2001024, 2020.
17. Huang, Z., Wang, T., Song, H., Li, X., Liang, G., Wang, D., Yang, Q., Chen, Z., Ma, L., Liu, Z., Effects of anion carriers on capacitance and self-discharge behaviors of zinc ion capacitors. *Angew. Chem.*, 133, 1024–1034, 2021.
18. Sun, J., Li, Z., Wang, J., Hong, W., Gong, P., Wen, P., Wang, Z., Yang, S., Ni/Bi battery based on $Ni(OH)_2$ nanoparticles/graphene sheets and Bi_2O_3 rods/graphene sheets with high performance. *JALCOM*, 643, 231–238, 2015.
19. Xia, X., Tu, J., Zhang, Y., Chen, J., Wang, X., Gu, C., Guan, C., Luo, J., Fan, H.J., Porous hydroxide nanosheets on preformed nanowires by electrodeposition: Branched nanoarrays for electrochemical energy storage. *Chem. Mater.*, 24, 3793–3799, 2012.

20. Wu, Z.S., Parvez, K., Li, S., Yang, S., Liu, Z., Liu, S., Feng, X., Müllen, K., Alternating stacked graphene-conducting polymer compact films with ultra-high areal and volumetric capacitances for high-energy micro-supercapacitors. *Adv. Mater.*, 27, 4054–4061, 2015.
21. Cheng, Y., Zhang, H., Lu, S., Varanasi, C.V., Liu, J., Flexible asymmetric supercapacitors with high energy and high power density in aqueous electrolytes. *Nanoscale*, 5, 1067–1073, 2013.
22. Chen, H., Hu, L., Chen, M., Yan, Y., Wu, L., Nickel–cobalt layered double hydroxide nanosheets for high-performance supercapacitor electrode materials. *Adv. Funct. Mater.*, 24, 934–942, 2014.
23. Pershaanaa, M., Bashir, S., Ramesh, S., Ramesh, K., Every bite of Supercap: A brief review on construction and enhancement of supercapacitor. *J. Energy Storage*, 50, 104599, 2022.
24. Wu, Y. and Cao, C., The way to improve the energy density of supercapacitors: Progress and perspective. *Sci. China Mater.*, 61, 1517–1526, 2018.
25. Simon, P. and Gogotsi, Y., Materials for electrochemical capacitors in nanoscience and technology. *Nat. Mater.*, 7, 320–329, 2010.
26. Miao, L., Duan, H., Wang, Z., Lv, Y., Xiong, W., Zhu, D., Gan, L., Li, L., Liu, M., Improving the pore-ion size compatibility between poly (ionic liquid)-derived carbons and high-voltage electrolytes for high energy-power supercapacitors. *Chem. Eng. J.*, 382, 122945, 2020.
27. Heimböckel, R., Hoffmann, F., Fröba, M., Insights into the influence of the pore size and surface area of activated carbons on the energy storage of electric double layer capacitors with a new potentially universally applicable capacitor model. *Phys. Chem. Chem. Phys.*, 21, 3122–3133, 2019.
28. Wu, S. and Zhu, Y., Highly densified carbon electrode materials towards practical supercapacitor devices. *Sci. China Mater.*, 60, 25–38, 2017.
29. Yaqoob, L., Noor, T., Iqbal, N., An overview of supercapacitors electrode materials based on metal organic frameworks and future perspectives. *Int. J. Energy Res.*, 46, 3939–3982, 2022.
30. Cheng, Y., Zhang, H., Lu, S., Varanasi, C.V., Liu, J., Flexible asymmetric supercapacitors with high energy and high power density in aqueous electrolytes. *Nanoscale*, 5, 1067–1073, 2013.
31. Wu, Y. and Cao, C., The way to improve the energy density of supercapacitors. *Prog. Perspect.*, 61, 1517–1526, 2018.
32. Gong, Y., Li, D., Luo, C., Fu, Q., Pan, C., Highly porous graphitic biomass carbon as advanced electrode materials for supercapacitors. *Green Chem.*, 19, 4132–4140, 2017.
33. Vijayan, B.L., Misnon, I.I., Anilkumar, G.M., Yang, C.-C., Jose, R.J., Void-size-matched hierarchical 3D titania flowers in porous carbon as an electrode for high-density supercapacitive charge storage. *JALCOM*, 858, 157649, 2021.
34. Wu, S. and Zhu, Y., Highly densified carbon electrode materials towards practical supercapacitor devices. *Sci. China Mater.*, 60, 25–38, 2017.

35. Zhu, Y., Murali, S., Stoller, M.D., Ganesh, K.J., Cai, W., Ferreira, P.J., Pirkle, A., Wallace, R.M., Cychosz, K.A., Thommes, M.J., Carbon-based supercapacitors produced by activation of graphene. *Sci.*, 332, 1537–1541, 2011.
36. Xu, Y., Lin, Z., Zhong, X., Huang, X., Weiss, N.O., Huang, Y., Duan, X., Holey graphene frameworks for highly efficient capacitive energy storage. *Nature*, 5, 1–8, 2014.
37. Qi, H., Xie, A., Tian, A., Zuo, R., Superior energy-storage capacitors with simultaneously giant energy density and efficiency using nanodomain engineered $BiFeO_3$-$BaTiO_3$-$NaNbO_3$ lead-free bulk ferroelectrics. *Adv. Energy Mater.*, 10, 1903338, 2020.
38. Chen, L.-F., Zhang, X.-D., Liang, H.-W., Kong, M., Guan, Q.-F., Chen, P., Wu, Z.-Y., Yu, S.-H., Synthesis of nitrogen-doped porous carbon nanofibers as an efficient electrode material for supercapacitors. *ACS Nano*, 6, 7092–7102, 2012.
39. Lin, T., Chen, I.-W., Liu, F., Yang, C., Bi, H., Xu, F., Huang, F., Nitrogen-doped mesoporous carbon of extraordinary capacitance for electrochemical energy storage. *Sci.*, 350, 1508–1513, 2015.
40. Hou, J., Jiang, K., Wei, R., Tahir, M., Wu, X., Shen, M., Wang, X., Cao, C., Popcorn-derived porous carbon flakes with an ultrahigh specific surface area for superior performance supercapacitors. *ACS Appl. Mater. Interfaces*, 9, 30626–30634, 2017.
41. Hou, J., Jiang, K., Tahir, M., Wu, X., Idrees, F., Shen, M., Cao, C., Tunable porous structure of carbon nanosheets derived from puffed rice for high energy density supercapacitors. *J. Power Sources*, 371, 148–155, 2017.
42. Xu, Y., Lin, Z., Zhong, X., Huang, X., Weiss, N.O., Huang, Y., Duan, X., Holey graphene frameworks for highly efficient capacitive energy storage. *Nat. Commun.*, 5, 1–8, 2014.
43. Largeot, C., Portet, C., Chmiola, J., Taberna, P.-L., Gogotsi, Y., Simon, P., Relation between the ion size and pore size for an electric double-layer capacitor. *J. Am. Chem. Soc.*, 130, 2730–2731, 2008.
44. Ali, Z., Tahir, M., Cao, C., Mahmood, A., Mahmood, N., Butt, F.K., Tanveer, M., Shakir, I., Rizwan, M., Idrees, F., Solid waste for energy storage material as electrode of supercapacitors. *Mater. Lett.*, 181, 191–195, 2016.
45. Khalid, S., Cao, C., Wang, L., Zhu, Y., Microwave assisted synthesis of porous $NiCo_2O_4$ microspheres: Application as high performance asymmetric and symmetric supercapacitors with large areal capacitance. *Sci. Rep.*, 6, 1–13, 2016.
46. Kim, M. and Kim, J., Development of high power and energy density microsphere silicon carbide–MnO_2 nanoneedles and thermally oxidized activated carbon asymmetric electrochemical supercapacitors. *Phys. Chem. Chem. Phys.*, 16, 11323–11336, 2014.
47. Qiu, Y., Li, G., Hou, Y., Pan, Z., Li, H., Li, W., Liu, M., Ye, F., Yang, X., Zhang, Y., Vertically aligned carbon nanotubes on carbon nanofibers: A hierarchical three-dimensional carbon nanostructure for high-energy flexible supercapacitors. *Chem. Mater.*, 27, 1194–1200, 2015.

48. Liu, C., Yu, Z., Neff, D., Zhamu, A., Jang, B.Z., Graphene-based supercapacitor with an ultrahigh energy density. *Nano Lett.*, 10, 4863–4868, 2010.
49. Hwang, J.Y., El-Kady, M.F., Wang, Y., Wang, L., Shao, Y., Marsh, K., Ko, J.M., Kaner, R.B., Direct preparation and processing of graphene/RuO_2 nanocomposite electrodes for high-performance capacitive energy storage. *Nano Energy*, 18, 57–70, 2015.
50. Wu, Z.-S., Ren, W., Wang, D.-W., Li, F., Liu, B., Cheng, H.-M., High-energy MnO_2 nanowire/graphene and graphene asymmetric electrochemical capacitors. *ACS Nano*, 4, 5835–5842, 2010.
51. Ji, J., Zhang, L.L., Ji, H., Li, Y., Zhao, X., Bai, X., Fan, X., Zhang, F., Ruoff, R.S., Nanoporous $Ni(OH)_2$ thin film on 3D ultrathin-graphite foam for asymmetric supercapacitor. *ACS Nano*, 7, 6237–6243, 2013.
52. Armand, M. and Tarascon, J.-M., Building better batteries. *Nature*, 451, 652–657, 2008.
53. Li, B., Dai, F., Xiao, Q., Yang, L., Shen, J., Zhang, C., Cai, M., Nitrogen-doped activated carbon for a high energy hybrid supercapacitor. *Energy Environ. Sci.*, 9, 102–106, 2016.
54. Lim, E., Jo, C., Kim, H., Kim, M.-H., Mun, Y., Chun, J., Ye, Y., Hwang, J., Ha, K.-S., Roh, K.C., Facile synthesis of Nb2O5@ carbon core–shell nanocrystals with controlled crystalline structure for high-power anodes in hybrid supercapacitors. *ACS Nano*, 9, 7497–7505, 2015.
55. Wang, Y.-G., Luo, J.-Y., Wang, C.-X., Xia, Y.-Y., Hybrid aqueous energy storage cells using activated carbon and lithium-ion intercalated compounds: II. Comparison of $LiMn_20_4$, $LiCo_{1/3}Ni_{1/3}Mn_{1/3}0_{2\ and}$ $LiCoO_2$ positive electrodes. *J. Electrochem. Soc.*, 153, A1425, 2006.
56. Shen, L., Lv, H., Chen, S., Kopold, P., van Aken, P.A., Wu, X., Maier, J., Yu, Y., Peapod-like Li_3VO_4/N-doped carbon nanowires with pseudocapacitive properties as advanced materials for high-energy lithium-ion capacitors. *Adv. Mater.*, 29, 1700142, 2017.
57. Ding, Y., Yang, B., Chen, J., Zhang, L., Li, J., Li, Y., Yan, X., Nanotube-like hard carbon as high-performance anode material for sodium ion hybrid capacitors. *Sci. China Mater.*, 61, 285–295, 2018.
58. Jabeen, N., Hussain, A., Xia, Q., Sun, S., Zhu, J., Xia, H., High-performance 2.6 V aqueous asymmetric supercapacitors based on *in situ* formed $Na_{0.5}$ MnO_2 nanosheet assembled nanowall arrays. *Adv. Mater.*, 29, 1700804, 2017.
59. Peng, S., Li, L., Wu, H.B., Madhavi, S., Lou, X.W., Controlled growth of $NiMoO_4$ nanosheet and nanorod arrays on various conductive substrates as advanced electrodes for asymmetric supercapacitors. *Adv. Energy Mater.*, 5, 1401172, 2015.
60. Li, R., Wang, Y., Zhou, C., Wang, C., Ba, X., Li, Y., Huang, X., Liu, J., Carbon-stabilized high-capacity ferroferric oxide nanorod array for flexible solid-state alkaline battery–supercapacitor hybrid device with high environmental suitability. *Adv. Funct. Mater.*, 25, 5384–5394, 2015.

61. Qin, J., Zhou, F., Xiao, H., Ren, R., Wu, Z.-S., Mesoporous polypyrrole-based graphene nanosheets anchoring redox polyoxometalate for all-solid-state micro-supercapacitors with enhanced volumetric capacitance. *Sci. China Mater.*, 61, 233–242, 2018.
62. Zhang, J. and Zhao, X., On the configuration of supercapacitors for maximizing electrochemical performance. *ChemSusChem*, 5, 818–841, 2012.

7

Optimization of Anti-Ferroelectrics

M. Rizwan[1*], M.A. Salam[1], K. Aslam[1] and A. Ayub[2]

[1]*School of Physical Sciences, University of the Punjab, Lahore, Pakistan*
[2]*Department of Physics, University of the Punjab, Lahore, Pakistan*

Abstract
The quest for extraordinary energy storage materials has always been a keen interest of researchers in industry and academia. In past decades huge efforts have been made to make excellent antiferroelectric ceramics that store more energy than the usual materials, and this research have proven to be quite fruitful. This chapter will cover different properties, techniques, materials, challenges, and future perspectives on optimizing antiferroelectric ceramic systems for energy storage purposes. Some of the challenges that are faced during the synthesis of antiferroelectrics are energy conversion efficiency and working of capacitors at high power as well as the problem of thermal energy. Practical applications of phase transition of antiferroelectric in the real world are also addressed. Different ways of optimization of energy storage materials, such as domain size engineering and doping are deliberated. In the end, the whole conversation is concluded with the point that these energy storage devices have a bright future ahead and that intense research work is required to make this perfect for common use.

Keywords: Antiferroelectric materials, energy storage devices, phase transition, lead zirconate, energy conversion efficiency

7.1 Introduction

Currently, there are two energy storage devices in the industry capacitors and batteries. Batteries typically convert electrical energy to chemical energy but due to the slow flow rate of charge carriers' batteries give less output. On the other hand, capacitors must release energy after a short

**Corresponding author*: rizwan.spr@pu.edu.pk

Inamuddin, Tariq Altalhi and Sayed Mohammed Adnan (eds.) Electroceramics for High Performance Supercapacitors, (159–174) © 2024 Scrivener Publishing LLC

interval of storing charge [1]. After Comparing them both capacitors have an edge on batteries due to high power output and because some dielectric materials have unique applications that make it a promising aspect for the future. Pulsed power innovations and the fast-growing need for a power supply with a pulse have made it more desirable to make capacitors that have a high energy density, better efficiency, and good discharge current.

In capacitors between the conducting electrodes of metal, there is a dielectric material sandwiched which is an insulator. If someone wants to have a dielectric capacitor that is organic and has high output energy density then one shall try to study benzo cyclobutene, $PbTiO_3$, or TiO_3. The reason to name these organic materials is that they can bear electric field strength of high magnitude and still give high energy density. One bad thing about these materials is that they possess low melting points which makes them thermally unstable. On the other hand, looking at inorganic dielectric material gives us not only high energy densities but also high melting points which means they are more thermally stable than the organic materials used in capacitors. Another feature is that the inorganic dielectric material responds more quickly to charging and discharging making it so much better than the organic materials of the dielectric [2].

In Figure 7.1 most of the research done to date is lead-based and very little work is done on lead-free materials [3].

The focus of research on AFE is to increase the energy density and enhance discharge speed to get a high-power energy density.

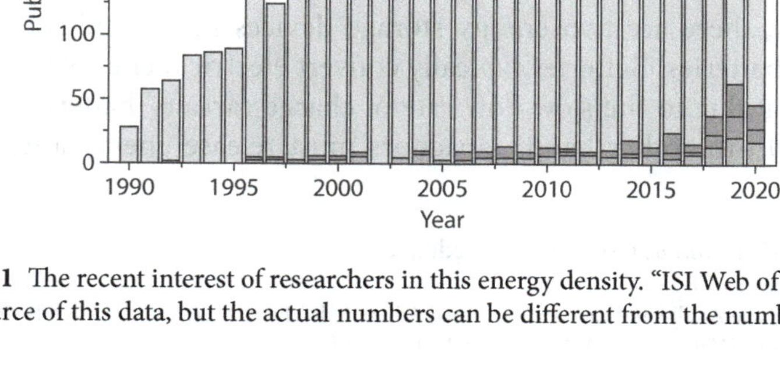

Figure 7.1 The recent interest of researchers in this energy density. "ISI Web of Science" is the source of this data, but the actual numbers can be different from the numbers seen here [3].

7.2 Energy Storage Properties

In the great race of making devices more advanced, lighter, and smaller the demand for energy storage devices and energy conversion devices has also risen which eventually leads to intense research in this area. If we look at the properties of dielectric materials, they possess high charging and discharging rate and high stability of temperature for different supercapacitors and batteries. The two most important properties of antiferroelectric are good breakdown strength and a small hysteresis loop [4]. The AFE materials are most discussed because of the transition between AFE and FE. These are nonpolar materials that possess high polarization and can store high energy which is mainly field-induced transition. The dipoles are in the opposite direction aligned and by applying a sufficient dc field we can change the direction of dipoles in the direction dc field. Meaning changing it to ferroelectric from antiferroelectric because of the small difference in free energy [5].

To calculate stored energy density or the recoverable energy density we should integrate the electric field with polarization.

$$W_{st} = \int_0^{Pmax} EdP \text{ (upon charging)} \tag{7.1}$$

$$W_e = -\int_{Pmax}^{Pr} EdP \text{ (upon discharging)} \tag{7.2}$$

$$\eta = \frac{Wre}{Wst} \tag{7.3}$$

The relationship between applied electric field and polarization is known as linear dielectrics. Due to low polarization and small dielectric constants the energy density is about 1 Jcm^{-3} in linear dielectrics.

Due to the absence of a hysteresis loop their energy density is quite high. When we apply an electric field the oppositely aligned dipoles of AFE are aligned in the direction of the field but once we remove the field it goes back to the initial state. This phenomenon generates the famous double P-E hysteresis loop which is shown in Figure 7.2 in the graph between polarization and Electric field [3].

In this figure, we see the process explained above about how a double hysteresis loop is formed and FE is again reversed to become AFE.

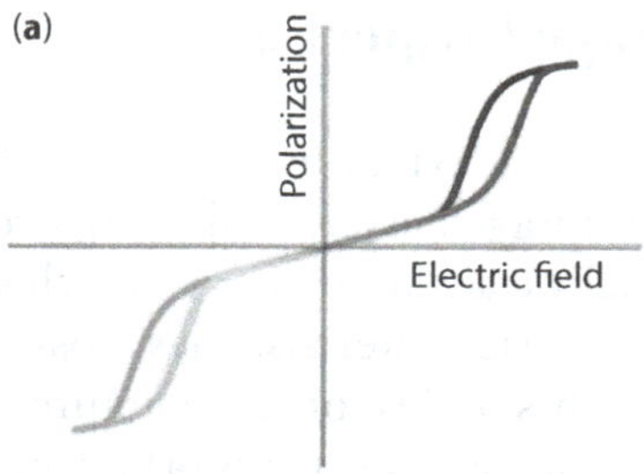

Figure 7.2 A typical loop between electric field and polarization [3].

7.3 Antiferroelectric for Energy Storage

Ferroelectric materials have vast applications including Random access memory, ultrasonic motors, and the topic of our interest energy storing capacitors. Materials that exhibit double hysteresis loop polarization without having the remanent polarization are known as ferroelectric materials, as stated by little [6].

If we dig deep into dielectric materials, they offer high permittivity and can operate at high temperatures which leads the way to making capacitors that have high energy density. The first perovskite ferroelectric material was $PbZrO_3$ because it had dielectric properties. Because the induced transformation in $PbZrO_3$ from AFE to FE due to electricity was only achievable at high temperatures. Another feature impacting phase transition and energy density is pressure. It has been seen that under increased pressure less electric field is required to do the phase shift from antiferroelectric to ferroelectric.

Dielectric materials have the following types

a) Linear Dielectric (LD)
These are the kind of materials in which the polarization induced is dependent upon the applied Electric Field. Examples of these kinds of materials are Mica and Paper [7].

b) Ferroelectric (FE)
In Ferroelectric materials even if we stop applying an electric field the materials remain permanently magnetic. Lead Zirconate and Lead titanate are examples of ferroelectric materials.

c) Antiferroelectric (AFE)
These materials possess orderly arranged dipoles that can have alternate arrangements. These materials possess the

property of phase transition at certain temperatures. Lead Zirconate is an example of antiferroelectric material.

Different materials could be used to form antiferroelectric materials that could store energy some are based on lead and others are lead-free. Every material has a unique way of developing techniques and properties. Here we will the difference between them.

7.3.1 Lead-Based Antiferroelectric

The first perovskite ferroelectric material was $PbZrO_3$ because it had dielectric properties. Because the induced transformation in $PbZrO_3$ from AFE to FE due to electricity was only achievable at high temperatures and the reason for that was the breakdown electric field being higher than the critical field of transformation [8].

Many efforts and research have been made to reduce the transformation field lower than the breakdown by using different substitutions of different impurities such as La^{+3}, Sr^{+2}, and Ti^{+4}. Lead Zirconate the material that is discussed above melts at 1200°C and has a curie temperature of about 230°C. Near the curie temperature, the ferroelectric phase of rhombohedral free energy is equal to the orthorhombic phase of antiferroelectric [9].

At the start it was about $PbZrO_3$ since then numerous calculations have been done for energy storage as well as for other scientific reasons. $PbZrO_3$ has high stability so making a phase transition by using an electric field is difficult at room temperature. There have been reports that if we add 0–1 mol% $PbMnWO_3$ in $PbZrO_3$ it makes it softer which makes it use a less electric field to do the transition and give much more max polarization. Most of the applications of PZ in ceramics are limited by the high critical switching required at room temperature.

7.3.2 Lead-Free Antiferroelectric

Results from different research prove that $NaNbO_3$ and AgNbO3-based AFE should be excellent replacements for lead-based AFE materials. The main purpose of research is to form perovskite that is lead-free and change or tune their salient features including transition due to field [10].

Despite all those efforts it is still not possible to replace the lead-based AFE because its properties and features are still better than the lead-free AFE. Still, a lot of effort is required to discover such materials that are lead-free as well as have high energy storage capability and conversion performance.

Due to a lot of elements in perovskite group and its Due to a lot of elements in perovskite group and its compounds, it is better to do some theoretical investigation to find a suitable solution that could replace lead-based AFE and solve the problem of low-energy-density transition at high temperatures. AFE $Bi_{1-x}Nd_xFeO_3$ is the first system predicted by Xu *et al.* that could give an energy density of about 100J/Cm^3 and efficiency of about 80% which is lead-free AFE [11]. Another approach that could be used to find a replacement for lead-based AFE is to do a replacement of ions in the perovskite structure with a suitable match. If we replace Pb ions with aliovalent then perovskites will have new formulas such as AB(V) X_6. This should also be remembered that ferroelectricity is also present in other compounds that have been reported such as $BiNbO_4$. there should be more choices for antipolar phonons to get mixed with other modes and give more AFE. If the compound is thought through, then we might get a family of perovskite or their derivative that have polymorphs of polar and anti-polar that could be future antiferroelectric material [12]. Trying to prove or discuss the performance or phase stability on of direct substitution basis would be difficult. So usually theory-experiment integration method is used. The tolerance factor (t) is one way to calculate the phase stability of different perovskite materials. In simple words, if $t < 1$ then the phase of AFE is stable. By decreasing the tolerance factor, we can increase the antiferroelectricity.

By using calculations from density function theory (DFT) different AFE materials can be confirmed. Then by synthesizing them experimentally we can study their phase stability. After getting results from these experimental procedures, we can check which candidate is most suitable for application in AFE or modify the element according to our needs. A complete setup that could do all the computational work is quite expensive. But if we could use the data already known then by using machine learning we could get a suitable candidate for AFE.

We could use different factors like ionic radius and electronegativity to predict the desired AFE. The phase transition of $PbZrO_3$ susceptibilities was examined by using First Principle Molecular Dynamics (FPMD). Examining phase transition by using the kinetics model will be another area of interest for researchers in the coming future.

7.3.3 Challenges

AFE Materials display a great abeyant for high power production, solid-state cooling appliances, pyroelectric energy transformation, electrical energy transmitter in form of digital displacement, and some very high energy density condensers. Research for Lead-Free AFE materials has received consistent stress and should lead to productive insight in the future. For AFE materials we shall discuss the present challenges and a few strategies to reform complete energy storage performance.

7.4 Explosive Energy Conversion

By using this equation

$$W = \frac{pr2}{2(\varepsilon 0 * \varepsilon r * \rho)} \tag{7.4}$$

P_r, ε_0, ε_r, and ρ are reminder partitions of the stimulating FE stage. From the above equation we can calculate energy storage density per unit load in the FE stage, and density of bulk respectively. In polycrystalline AFEs the P_r is generally less than 40μC/cm². The most challenge in reaching higher explosive energy showing in AFEs is the low P_r. At the time of the transition between AFE to FE stage, it is easy to notice that it can achieve induced metastable FE stage in AFE media. To improve the P_r of the induced FE stage we put forward three strategies Morph tropic, phase boundary, domain engineering, and crystallographic composition of polycrystalline AFE.

A means of attaining important development of P_r of the field-induced FE segment is offered by texturing of crystallography of AFE potteries. Phase conversion of stress-induced AFE-FE can be made by high pulse voltage such as greater than 100kV, high current such as greater than 100A, and high power such as 10MW respectively. A good approach to improve AFEs media as energy transformation performance by crystallographic schemes.

7.5 Energy Storage and High-Power Capacitors

To increase the energy storage products such as (efficiency and energy density) of the dielectric condensers, the consumption of AFE media is successfully approached. The most challenge of increasing one parameter at the cost of other is faced by the state of art AFE media. Particularly, the energy efficiency of the free lead AFEs is commonly very low approximately (less than 80 % of the entire energy) which gives us high energy excess of approximately (more than 20% of the entire energy). Not long ago 90% efficiency having an energy density of 6.3 J/cm^3 has been described in $AgNbO_3$-0.55$AgTaO_3$ AFE potteries by establishing the form of heterogeneity. Instead of making a ferroelectric media that shows high electrostriction, we should be considered pottery fabrication methods. The fabrication of AFE pottery will be donated to the chemical accesses such as the atmosphere for impurity.

7.6 Thermal-Electric Energy Interconversion

In the previous 2 sections, the thin films exhibit enormous ECE because they can stand with high electric fields. The thin films of electro-caloric AFE can be used to pump a little amount of heat. A very large number of fields without electric power crash cannot be supported by Electro caloric effects. Over the last few years, the basic reason is that the ECE in AFEs has been accessed. The transformation of heat energy between the layers of electrocaloric in a well-designed cooling instrument and the rest of the caloric path can be used by the electrodes of metals. Now timely it can be seen that electro-caloric effects are displayed by the furthermore study of AFE MLCCs and ECE remains an open effect by research prospects. Within the last 5-10 years, particularly AFE materials have been developed and in smaller markets some AFE materials like PLZT potteries are obtainable. Understanding the scientific development of AFEs materials for different energy storage devices and applications is provided by the following strategies

a) Focus on the chemical configuration, Crystallographic projects, and MLCCs manufacturers.
b) The evolutions between AFE and FE positions of the field-dependent stage are being explored by nature.
c) Entire energy presentations, general consistency, and physical properties have been recognized.

7.7 Optimization

7.7.1 Phase Structure Engineering

The underlying architect for the most part acts in support of the practical fashioner, who regularly gives the administration in completing a design task. In the structural designing field, he helps the transportation engineer, water-powered engineer, or clean architect by giving the designs expected to execute their ventures. In building development, he is one of the planner's key partners. Likewise, the primary specialist helps mechanical, synthetic, or electrical architects in planning the large equipment or offices expected for their tasks. He might move his whole mastery and action into maritime engineering or aeronautical designing and become an expert in the plan of boat or plane designs. Thus, a primary designer should have a different encounter to use his maximum capacity. Periods of a primary designing task are depicted underneath exhaustively.

A structural engineering project can be divided into three phases:

- Planning
  This is the first step in which we plan how will we engineer the project in a certain way that may be most efficient.
- Design
  In this step, we design the project either theoretically on computer simulation or paper. Here we just try to predict certain things that might happen with the structure during synthesizing.
- Construction
  The previous two steps lead us to our final step where we construct or synthesize the structure of the material and then do the calculations.

7.7.1.1 *Planning Phase in a Structural Engineering Project*

The arranging stage includes a thought of the different necessities and variables that influence the overall design and aspects of the construction. This prompts the decision of one or maybe a few elective kinds of designs that offer the best broad arrangement. The essential thought is the capability of the design, whether it is to encase or house, to convey, or to help in space. Numerous auxiliary contemplations are likewise involved, including as stylish, humanistic, legitimate, monetary, financial, ecological, or asset protection factors. What's more, there are underlying and constructional prerequisites and restrictions that likewise may influence the primary kind chosen.

7.7.1.2 *Design Phase*

The planning stage includes point-by-point contemplations of the elective arrangements, developed in the arranging stage. It prompts the assurance of the most reasonable extents, aspects, and subtleties of the relative multitude of choices being considered for the development of underlying components and associations. As a rule, before the last plan stage is reached, the best arrangement has been distinguished and the last development plans are ready for this determination. Sporadically, the decision is reliant upon monetary and constructional highlights that cannot be precisely assessed besides by aggressive offering, so last bid plans must be ready for the serious other options.

7.7.1.3 Construction Phase

The development stage includes the acquisition of materials, hardware, workforce, shop creation of individuals, and sub-congregations. It likewise incorporates their transportation to the site, genuine field development, and erection exercises nearby. During this stage, some upgrades might be required. Purposes behind this upgrade can be unexpected establishment hardships or then again if predetermined materials can't be secured, or for some other explanation.

The underlying model is the plan innovation that targets deciding the proper sizes and materials of primary individuals that structure a design, the decided sizes and materials ought to figure out protected and workable construction at the satisfactory expense (least expense).

This makes sense of various stages followed for the achievement of foundational layout work of various designs either entire or individual from the construction.

The following phases are involved.

a) Preliminary structural design
   In this stage, the sizes (aspects) of various underlying individuals shaping design are proposed in estimated by alluding to experience and code necessity. The proposed elements of the individuals are the ones utilized in the next phase of the plan which is load assessment.
b) Estimation of loads
   This elaborates the assessment of the measure of loadings that the design should continue its lifetime; this incorporates wind loads, live loads, and self-weight.
c) Structural analysis
   In primary examination we should decide the impacts of loadings on the construction; this includes the assurance of

inner powers or inner opposition of the underlying individuals and diversion at various places of design.

d) Safety and serviceability check

In this stage, the sizes and materials of primary individuals are checked, if they can endure the impacts of loadings which are inward powers and redirections found in the examination stage. The security and usefulness checking of primary individuals on loadings are done per standard plan code prerequisites of a specific country. On the off chance that the prerequisites are fulfilled, the plan drawings and development determination are ready, and the development stage begins.

f) Revised structural design

If the necessity was not met in the security and usefulness check stage, this stage comes whereby primary part aspects and materials are changed.

So, we will have underlying individuals from various properties, this makes us rehash stages from primary investigation to realize the stacking impacts on adjusted individuals.

The reiteration continues up to somewhere safe and secure and usefulness check until the prerequisites are fulfilled, with the goal that the design to be developed can be protected and functional.

7.7.2 Grain Size Engineering

As a viral portion of micro-electro-mechanical system devices, the high energy storage thicknesses of thin film dielectric capacitors have stimulated increased consideration of industrial and scientific facts. Due to the lack of non-renewable energy sources, the efficiency of thin film capacitors' energy storage has increased gradually. To achieve high energy-storage capacity and an increased ECE through the right management of grain size, the impact of grain size upon electrical characteristics, energy-storage performance, and ECE of the thick films were carefully examined [13].

At the same applied electric field compared $Bi_{0.5}Na_{0.5}TiO_3$ (BNT) based having higher soaked polarization and $K_{0.5}Na_{0.5}NbO_3$ (KNN) based materials to achieve Maximum Polarization P_{max}. Due to higher remnant polarization. We can synthesize the grain at a low temperature of approximately (473K) and control the size and shape of grains by using the endothermal Method. So, by using Hydrothermal methods, it is authoritative to make a lead-free ferroelectric tinny film [14].

7.7.3 Domain Engineering

Domain engineering is the complete course of reusing area information in the development of new programming frameworks. it is a basic idea in conscious programming reuse and product offering design. A critical thought in methodical programming reuse is the spaces. Most associations work in a couple of spaces. They over and over form similar frameworks inside a given space with varieties to meet different client needs. As opposed to building each new structure variation without any preparation, huge reserve funds might be achieved by reusing fragments of past structures in to fabricate new ones. The most common way of recognizing regions, bouncing them, and finding shared characteristics and changes among the structure in the space is called space examination [15]. Space designing spotlights on catching information assembled during the computer programming process. By creating reusable curios, the parts can be reused in new programming structures for minimal price and high quality. this produces not just a bunch of programming execution parts pertinent to the spaces yet in addition reusable and configurable necessities and design.

7.7.3.1 Phase

Area designing when contrasted with application designing. The results of each period of area designing feed into both ensuing periods of space designing as well as comparing ease in application designing. Studies on lead zirconate thin films that depended on the film's thickness revealed that the released and induced charges were regulated by size effects related to extrinsic and intrinsic mechanisms through the intrinsic switching of time [16].

7.7.3.2 Domain Analysis

Space examination is utilized to characterize the area, gather data about the area, and produce a space model. Using highlight models (at first, considered as a component of the element situated spaces examination technique), space examination plans to distinguish the normal focuses in an area and the differing focuses in the domain. using space examination, the improvement of configurable necessities by a conventional application designing methodology is conceivable.

7.7.3.3 *Domain Design*

Space configuration takes the area model delivered during the space examination stage and expects to create conventional engineering to which all structures inside the area can confirm. Similarly, that application designing purposes the useful and non-utilitarian requirements to deliver a plan, the area design period of spaces designing takes the configurable necessities created during the space investigation stage and creates a configurable, normalized answer for the group of structures. The advanced generation of better-performance antiferroelectric materials can be chosen concerning the incommensurate phase [17]. Space configuration expects to create structural examples which tackle an issue normal across the structure inside the space, despite varying prerequisite configurations. For the improvement of examples during space configuration, engineers should likewise accept care to distinguish the extent of the example and the level to which the setting is relevant to the example. Restriction of setting is urgent: an excess of setting brings about the example not being relevant to numerous structures, and too little setting brings about the example being inadequately strong to be useful. A valuable example should be both regularly repeating and of superior grade.

7.7.4 Doping

Undoubtedly, the biggest roadblock to semiconductor development that takes this class of materials into account is the failure to dope such materials. Overcoming this obstruction may involve an entirely new development. Due to their higher energy storage density compared to ferroelectric, antiferroelectric materials that exhibit double ferroelectric hysteresis loops are drawing more interest. This could be done by doping different materials like Zr, Nb, and Ti [18].

There are three key methods for failing to use drugs:

a) Due to its low dissolvability, the optimal corruption molecule cannot be introduced into the host valuable stone. Models suggest enormous contaminating particles for small hosts expensive stones or deceptively inactive toxins.
b) The optimum doping dissolves in the host, but it does so at a deep level as opposed to a shallow one, leaving the deterioration unionized at normal temperatures. Such "localized centers" do occur, and they integrate.

c) The poison molecule is both flammable and dissolvable, but when it moves free carriers, a sudden delivery of an oppositely charged neighborhood distortion structures reviews and prevents the conscious doping from being expelled.

For most electrical and optoelectronic applications, doped semiconductors are useless. The primary obstacle to semiconductor development when using a class of materials is unquestionably the inability to dope those materials. Overcoming this obstruction may result in whole new development.

7.8 Conclusion

Antiferroelectric devices are the future of energy-storing devices. All that is needed is to find suitable and proper materials that have high energy density and good thermal ability. The reported materials like $PbZrO_3$ and some lead-free materials have shown huge applications and have revolutionized energy storage in capacitors. Within the next five years, the search for new AFEs materials with high-energy presentations is predictable by an increasing effort. For the development of energy efficiency of AFEs materials, we may recommend a road map that may underwrite it. It is also seen that there are many techniques available in the current era to find, think about, design, and then implement the idea in the industry so the day is not far when we see a successful lead-free antiferroelectric material replacing lead-based energy storage devices.

References

1. Winter, M. and Brodd, R., What are batteries, fuel cells, and supercapacitors? *Chem. Rev.*, 104, 4245–4270, 2004.
2. Feng, Q.-K., Zhong, S.-L., Pei, J.-Y., Zhao, Y., Zhang, D.-L., Liu, D.-F., Zhang, Y.-X., Dang, Z.-M., Recent progress and future prospects on all-organic polymer dielectrics for energy storage capacitors. *Chem. Rev.*, 122, 3820–3878, 2021.
3. Zhuo, F., Qiao, H., Zhu, J., Wang, S., Bai, Y., Mao, X., Wu, H.-H., Perspective on antiferroelectrics for energy storage and conversion applications. *Chin. Chem. Lett.*, 32, 2097–2107, 2021.
4. Billah, S.M.R., Dielectric polymers, in: *Functional Polymers*, M.A.J. Mazumder, H. Sheardown, A. Al-Ahmed (Eds.), pp. 241–288, Springer, Switzerland, 2019.

5. Liu, Z., Lu, T., Ye, J., Wang, G., Dong, X., Withers, R., Liu, Y., Antiferroelectrics for energy storage applications: A review. *Adv. Mater. Technol.*, 3, 1800111, 2018.
6. Haertling, G.H., Ferroelectric ceramics: History and technology. *J. Am. Ceram. Soc.*, 82, 797–818, 1999.
7. Tahalyani, J., Akhtar, M.J., Cherusseri, J., Kar, K.K., Characteristics of capacitor: Fundamental aspects, in: *Handbook of Nanocomposite Supercapacitor Materials I*, K.K. Kamal (Ed.), pp. 1–51, Springer, Switzerland, 2020.
8. Singh, K.J.F., Antiferroelectric lead zirconate, a material for energy storage. *Ferroelectrics*, 94, 433–433, 1989.
9. Chao, W., Gao, J., Yang, T., Li, Y., Excellent energy storage performance in La and Ta co-doped $AgNbO_3$ antiferroelectric ceramics. *J. Eur. Chem. Ceram. Soc.*, 41, 7670–7677, 2021.
10. Yang, D., Gao, J., Shu, L., Liu, Y.-X., Yu, J., Zhang, Y., Wang, X., Zhang, B.-P., Li, J.-F., Lead-free antiferroelectric niobates $AgNbO_3$ and $NaNbO_3$ for energy storage applications. *J. Mater. Chem. A*, 8, 23724–23737, 2020.
11. Liu, C., Li, W., Fan, J., Mai, Y., A brief review on the lead element substitution in perovskite solar cells. *J. Energy Chem.*, 27, 1054–1066, 2018.
12. Tan, X., Ma, C., Frederick, J., Beckman, S., Webber, K.G., The antiferroelectric↔ ferroelectric phase transition in lead-containing and lead-free perovskite ceramics. *J. Am. Ceram. Soc.*, 94, 4091–4107, 2011.
13. Gao, H., Hao, X., Zhang, Q., An, S., Kong, L.B., Electrocaloric effect and energy-storage performance in grain-size-engineered PBLZT antiferroelectric thick films. *J. Mater. Sci. Mater. Electron.*, 27, 10309–10319, 2016.
14. Chao, W., Tian, L., Yang, T., Li, Y., Liu, Z., Excellent energy storage performance achieved in novel $PbHfO_3$-based antiferroelectric ceramics via grain size engineering. *Chem. Eng. J.*, 433, 133814, 2022.
15. Jiang, J., Meng, X., Li, L., Guo, S., Huang, M., Zhang, J., Wang, J., Hao, X., Zhu, H., Zhang, S.-T., Ultrahigh energy storage density in lead-free relaxor antiferroelectric ceramics via domain engineering. *Energy Storage Mater.*, 43, 383–390, 2021.
16. Bharadwaja, S. and Krupanidhi, S., Backward switching phenomenon from field forced ferroelectric to antiferroelectric phases in antiferroelectric $PbZrO_3$ thin films. *J. Appl. Phys.*, 89, 4541–4547, 2001.
17. Ge, G., Shi, C., Chen, C., Shi, Y., Yan, F., Bai, H., Yang, J., Lin, J., Shen, B., Zhai, J., Tunable domain switching features of incommensurate antiferroelectric ceramics realizing excellent energy storage properties. *Adv. Mater.*, 34, 2201333, 2022.
18. Zhao, L., Liu, Q., Gao, J., Zhang, S., Li, J.F., Lead-free antiferroelectric silver niobate tantalate with high energy storage performance. *Adv. Mater.*, 29, 1701824, 2017.

8

Super Capacitive Performance Assessment of Mixed Ferromagnetic Iron and Cobalt Oxides and Their Polymer Composites

Mohammad Faraz Ahmer[1]*, Qasim Ullah[2] and Mohammad Kashif Uddin[3]

[1]*Department of Electrical and Electronics Engineering, Mewat Engineering College, Nuh, Gurugram University Haryana, India*
[2]*Physical Sciences Section, School of Sciences, Maulana Azad National Urdu University, Hyderabad India*
[3]*Department of Chemistry, College of Science, Majmaah University, Al Majmaah, Riyadh, Kingdom of Saudi Arabia*

Abstract

There is growing quest for search of novel electrode materials for fabricating supercapacitors in the interest of fulfilling requirement of the escalating eco – friendly energy storing / conversion systems. In case of supercapacitors, the main focus has been on developing nanocomposite materials that are capable to allow fast charging / discharging rates, long cyclic stability, enlarged surface area and high specific capacitance. To meet such requirements, magnetic transition metallic oxides (MTMOs), conductive polymers (CPs) and MTMO / CP nanocomposites have been extensively examined as supercapacitor electrode materials. This book chapter highlights the research progress regarding developments of mixed ternary iron / cobalt ferromagnetic oxides and their polymer nanocomposites as promising electrode fabricating materials for high performance capacitor usage.

TMOs possessing multiple oxidation states are capable to undergo multiple redox reactions and hence capable to demonstrate excellent pseudo-capacitively. On the other hand, CPs exhibited remarkable electrical conductivity and high charge storing capacity. Thus, TMO / CP nanocomposites are promising electrode materials with multifold untapped future opportunities for use in energy storing/ conversion devices.

Corresponding author: farazahmer007@gmail.com

Inamuddin, Tariq Altalhi and Sayed Mohammed Adnan (eds.) Electroceramics for High Performance Supercapacitors, (175–202) © 2024 Scrivener Publishing LLC

Keywords: Supercapacitor, polymer composites, ferromagnetic material, conducting polymers, electrode, cobalt oxide, iron oxide

8.1 Introduction

Concerning to fulfill the escalating global energy need accompanied with the reduction of consumption of fossil fuels, new technologies have to be developed for generating stable electrochemical system (ECSs) for energy storage via transformation of chemical energy into electric power. Among current ECSs (fuel cells, batteries and capacitors), supercapacitors (SCs) have been in extensive demand as energy storing and conversion systems because of superior power density, fast charging / discharging capability, wider operating temperature range, eco – friendliness, affordable cost and long life – span [1, 2]. As a result, SCs have emerged as an attractive option for multiple potential uses covering the spectrum range from portable electronic devices to hybrid commercial electric devices / vehicles [3–6]. SCs are electrical devices, developed to store energy and bridging the void space between traditional capacitors and batteries. The main components constituting a supercapacitor (Figure 8.1) are (a) an electrolyte, (b) couple of electrodes with opposite charges (+ve and –ve)

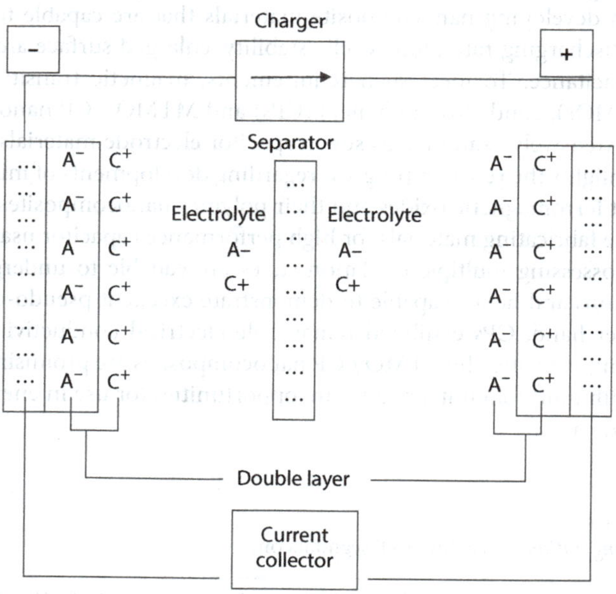

Figure 8.1 Working principle of supercapacitor cations (C^+) and anions (A^-) in solution.

and (c) a separator. In addition, a current collector can be considered as fourth component.

8.1.1 Electrolyte

An electrolyte in most cases is liquid which is electronically non - conductor but behaves as ionic conductor. Aqueous salt solutions, ionic liquids and molten salts covering the following requirements can be used as safer electrolytes in SCs.

- (i) Adequate ionic conductivity
- (ii) High thermal and chemical resistance
- (iii) Non - toxicity
- (iv) Cost effectiveness and
- (v) Non - corrosivity and inertness towards components of supercapacitor assembly.

Besides influencing cyclic life, capacitivity and power / energy density of SCs, electrolyte maintains the charge balance between the coupled electrodes. Though, the aqueous electrolytes are cheaper, eco - friendly and demonstrate high conductivity but their operating voltage range is small due to low water electrolysis potential difference (1.23 V). On the other hand, organic electrolytes having higher potential window (> 2.8V) suffer from lower ionic conductivity and high flammability [7]. In fact, tetraethylammonium tetrafluoroborate solubilized in acetonitrile / propylene has been popular organic electrolyte for use in SCs as it provides temperature operational range of 50 to 70°C and high potential window (3.5 V) [8, 9]. Ionic liquids (ILs) with huge reserve of latent electrochemical performance (potential window 4-6 V) and low flammability have ample opportunities for their extensive usage in supercapacitors applications [10–12]. However, high viscosity of ILs has been their drawback.

8.1.2 Separator

In SCs, the function of separator is to ensure transfer of ionic charge through unhindered migration of ions without undergoing any chemical transformation. Though several materials (glass, paper, ceramics etc.) can be used as separator but polymer - based separators have received popularity due to their inherent flexibility as well as porosity [13].

8.1.3 Current Collector

The main contribution of current collector in capacitors is to allow free conduction of electrons from electrode surface to the external circuit. In addition to metallic alloys, carbon cloth, metal foams and Ni - mesh have been commonly used as current collectors. A detailed overview of current collectors has been provided by M. Arvani *et al.* [14].

8.1.4 Supercapacitor Electrode Materials

Electrode is the most fundamental element of SCs and the electrochemical performance of SCs mainly based upon the composition of electrode material, the voltage range and the nature of electrolyte. Depending upon the use of active electrode materials and charge - storage mechanisms, three types of SCs namely, EDLCs (electric double layer capacitors), PSCs (pseudocapacitors) and HSCs (hybrid supercapacitors) have been identified [15, 16]. EDLCs are generally made of carbonaceous materials like activated carbon (AC), graphene (G), carbon nanotubes (CNTs), reduced graphene oxide / graphene oxide (rGO / GO), carbon dots (C - dots), carbon nanofibres (CNFs), carbon cloths (CC) etc. store charge electrostatically as a result of creation of electrical bilayer of opposing charges at the junction of electrode surface and electrolyte solution. In this case, no electron transfer reaction takes place and the capacitance arised due to accumulation of charges based on the degree of surface area of electrode. Therefore, carbon materials with appreciable surface area have been popular choice to EDLCs [17–20]. Contrary to EDLCs, PSCs accumulate energy through reversible redox reactions of electroactive species occurring at the surface of electrode and hence conducting polymers and various transition metallic oxides have been preferred to fabricate PSCs [21–25]. Based on the type of used electrode material, SCs can store and / or release energy via single process (non - Faradaic or Faradaic) or through both the processes (Faradaic plus non - Faradaic). Furthermore, a third group of SCs known as "hybrid supercapacitors" has been created by coupling PSCs and EDLCs.

Hybrid SCs combine the favorable supercapacitive features of EDLC (high electrical conductivity and good cyclability) and PSC (high energy density and superior capacitance) as these are constructed from composite of either two - or three - components (conductive polymers, metallic oxides and / or carbon - based matter) in different compositional ratio.

In the past, lot of redox metallic oxides (MnO_2, Fe_2O_3, MoO_2, NiO, RuO_2, V_2O_5, $NiCo_2O_4$, $CoMoO_4$, $NiMoO_4$, $MnMoO_4$, $NiMn_2O_4$, $CoFe_2O_4$, $MnFe_2O_4$, $CoMn_2O_4$, $NiCo_2O_4$ and $MnCo_2O_4$ etc.) have been admirably utilized as electrode fabrication materials to achieve improved supercapacitive performance. Additionally, mixed multicomponent transition metal oxides, especially ternary metal oxide nanostructured materials in the form of single metallic phase have been found superior electrode material for wide range applications in energy - related systems. Mixed multi component metal oxides have demonstrated better supercapacitive performance compared to their single metal oxide component through providing additional oxidation states to facilitate multiple pseudocapacitive redox reactions [25, 26]. Notwithstanding this, transition mixed metal oxides (TMMOs) integrated with conductive polymers have emerged as novel pseudocapacitive materials for usage in multiple green energy related research areas [27–29].

8.2 Ferromagnetic Electrode Materials

The materials that can be easily magnetized when exposed to an external magnetic field and remain magnetized even after the withdrawal of the applied external field are considered ferromagnetic. Most of the ferromagnetic materials are metals (Ni, Fe, Co etc), metallic alloys containing Ni, Fe or Co and some compounds of rare earth metals. The maximum temperature at which a ferromagnetic metal exhibits ferromagnetism is called Curie temperature. The Curie temperature (Tc) values of different magnetic materials are presented in Table 8.1.

Due to their large piezoelectric - coupling constant, ferroelectric materials have received considerable attention for use in microphones, capacitors, tapes and transducers. Among magnetic materials, inorganic perovskite oxides and spinel ferrites have demonstrated superior electrochemical performance in supercapacitors. The ferromagnetic oxides of Fe, Co, Ni and Mn have been widely applied in fabrication of novel high-performance supercapacitors. In addition to outers s-electrons in bond formation, the multiple oxidation states due to involvement of variable number of inner d-electrons have facilitated the utility of ferromagnetics in combination of conducting polymers for supercapacitor applications. In fact, several combinations of ferromagnetic transition metal oxides and conjugated conducting polymer systems including polyaniline (PANI), polypyrrol (PPy) or poly (3, 4-ethylenedioxythiophene) (PEDOT) with/without carbon

Table 8.1 Curie temperature of some ferro (-)/ferrimagnetic materials [30].

Ferromagnetic material	Curie temperature (K)
Co	1388
Ni	627
Fe	1043
CrO_2	386
Fe_2O_3	948
Fe_2O_3.FeO	858
Fe_2O_3.CuO	728
Fe_2O_3.MgO	713
NiO. Fe_2O_3	858

Note: Except CrO_2, all other oxides behave as ferrimagnetic substances.

have been successfully synthesized and utilized in energy accumulating appliances.

The aim of present chapter is to assess the supercapacitive performance of mixed ferromagnetic iron and cobalt oxides and their polymer composites as electrode materials through compilation of scattered literature in concise form. The electrochemical performance of mixed (iron oxides, cobalt oxides and iron - cobalt oxides) and their composites with commonly used conducting polymers (PANI, PPy, PEDOT) has been reviewed covering the period of last decade.

8.3 Mixed Ferromagnetic Iron and Cobalt Oxides

The spinel structured MFe_2O_4 and MCo_2O_4 [M is divalent transition metal cation] materials have been prominent contender for utilization in supercapacitor fabrication as a result of their better supercapacitive accomplishment compared to single component metal oxides. The mixed oxides generated by partial substitution of Fe in Fe_3O_4 and Co in Co_3O_4 by other metallic cations with ionic radius in the range of 0.6 to 1.0 A° have shown better capacitive performance. For example, recently developed manganese zinc ferrites nanoneedles have shown much impressive supercapacitive performance associated with remarkable columbic efficacy [31].

Thus, the charge stockpiling capability of Fe_3O_4 for supercapacitors can be considerably enhanced through converting into ternary metal oxide nanoparticles. Generally, co – precipitation, microemulsion, thermal decomposition, electrodeposition/electrospinning and hydrothermal synthetic methods have been used to produce magnetic ferrite nanoparticles [32–36]. In general, hydrothermal method has been most popular to synthesize ternary metal oxides in different controllable structural morphologies at moderate temperature using water soluble metallic precursors. This environmentally benign procedure is simple and useful to produce electrode materials in high purity.

Originating from the arrangement of involved cations, ferrites can be normal ferrites like $ZnFe_2O_4$ and $CdFe_2O_4$, intermediate ferrites (e.g., $MnFe_2O_4$) and inverse ferrites (Co/Ni Fe_2O_4). Like spinel ferrites, cobalt oxide (Co_3O_4) has been an important electrode material to develop mixed transition metal spinels. As a result, numerous spinel cobaltites have been formulated via partial substitution of Co by Ni, Zn, Mn, Cu etc. in Co_3O_4. The developed ternary metal cobaltites have shown excellent electrical conductivity, exceptional stability, promising eco – friendliness and affordable cost effectiveness. In fact, mixed ternary metal oxide electrode materials in various dimensional (1, 2 and 3 – D) nanostructures have been synthesized to utilize their broad – ranged supercapacitive capabilities. In order to maximize the supercapacitive execution in terms of charge storage capacity, ease of ion – transfer during charging/discharging process, cycling stability and energy/power density, mixed metal oxides have been produced in different morphological architectures as listed in Table 8.2.

The supercapacitive performance characteristics of mixed ferromagnetic ternary iron and cobalt oxides have been summarized in Tables 8.3–8.6.

Table 8.2 Electrochemical performance of ternary metal oxide electrode materials in different architectural morphologies.

Morphological structure	Ternary metal oxide	(Capacitance, F/g) / current density	Symbol	Reference
Nanorods	$ZnCo_2O_4$ @ Ni foam	(1400 / 1 A/g) with capacity retention of 97% over 1000 cycles at 6 A/g	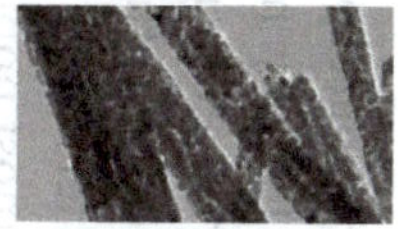	[37]
Nanotubes	$NiCo_2O_4$	(1647 / 1 A/g), cyclic stability (93.6%) capacity retention for 3000 cycles	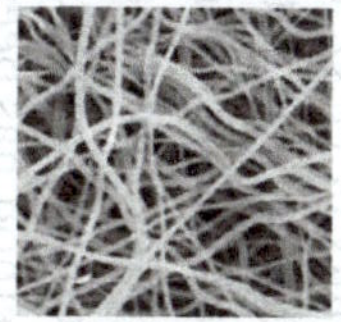	[38]
Nanosheets	$NiCo_2O_4$	(999 / 20 A/g), capacity retention of 84.4% @ current density (10 A/g) for 3000 cycles	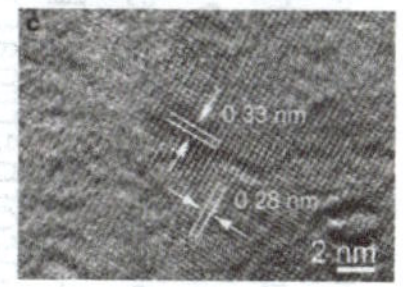	[39]
	$NiCo_2O_4$, Porous nanosheets	(2658 / 2 A/g) with superior cyclic life due to the formation of $NiCo_2O_4$ nano multilayers on the flexible carbon fabric surface		[40]
	$NiCo_2O_4$ @ $NiCo_2O_4$ and $NiCo_2O_4$ @ NiO	(1925 / 0.5 Ag^{-1}) and (2210 / 0.5 A/g) respectively exhibiting good cyclic stability as well as rate capability		[41]

(*Continued*)

Table 8.2 Electrochemical performance of ternary metal oxide electrode materials in different architectural morphologies. (*Continued*)

Morphological structure	Ternary metal oxide	(Capacitance, F/g) / current density	Symbol	Reference
Nanowire arrays	$NiCo_2O_4$	Cell areal capacitance (161 mF / cm^2) at mA / cm^2 with cyclic stability over 3000 cycles under bent state	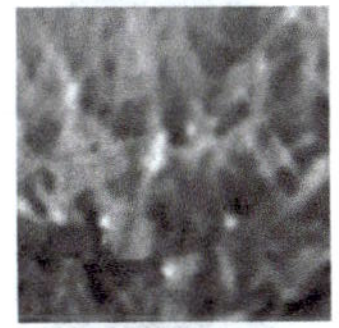	[42]
Core - shell nanowire structures	$NiCo_2O_4$ @ MnO_2 on Ni foam	Specific capacitance (112 / 1 mA / cm^2) with maximum energy density (35 Wh / kg)	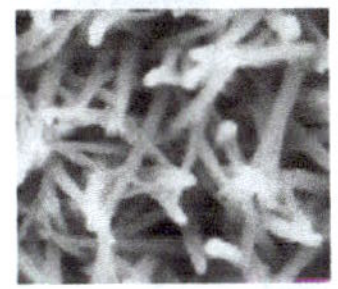	[43]
	$NiCo_2O_4$ @ Ni	Specific capacitance (1792 / 5 mA / cm^2) with capacity retention (87.5%) for 5000 cycles		[44]
	$CuCo_2O_4$ @ MnO_2	(327, 1.25 A/g) with 90% retention of original capacitance of current density (6.25 A/g) in aqueous electrolyte		[45]
	$NiCo_2O_4$ @ $Co_xNi_{(1-x)}$ double hydroxide sheet	(1.64 F / cm^2), 2 mA / cm^2. Excellent energy (33 Wh / kg) and power (41.25 Kw / kg) densities		[46]

(*Continued*)

Table 8.2 Electrochemical performance of ternary metal oxide electrode materials in different architectural morphologies. (*Continued*)

Morphological structure	Ternary metal oxide	(Capacitance, F/g) / current density	Symbol	Reference
Core / shell nanoflake arrays	$NiCo_2O_4$ @ $NiCo_2O_4$	(1.55 F / cm^2) 2 mA / cm^2. capacity retention (98.6%) after 4000 cycles	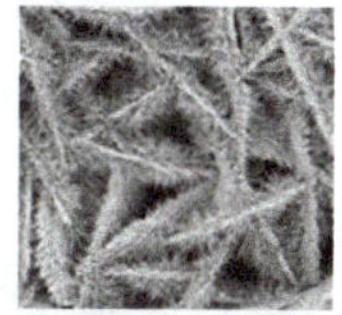	[47]
Thin film	$NiCo_2O_4$	(580, 1 Ag^{-1}) along with power (32 Wh / kg) and energy (4 kw / kg) densities associated with good cyclic stability	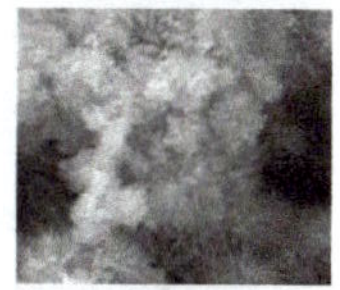	[48]
Sea – urchins	$NiCo_2O_4$	(1650, 1A/g) with retention capacitance (91%) over 2000 cycles at 8 A/g	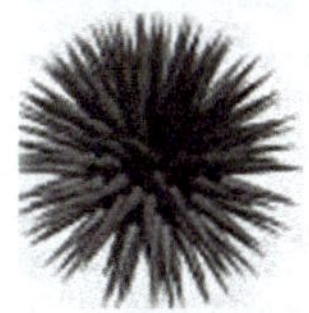	[49]
Nano flower	$NiCo_2O_4$ with uniform diameter (500 nm)	(1191, 1 A/g), good cyclic performance and excellent capacity retention	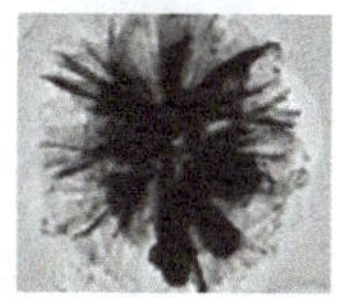	[50]

(*Continued*)

Table 8.2 Electrochemical performance of ternary metal oxide electrode materials in different architectural morphologies. (*Continued*)

Morphological structure	Ternary metal oxide	(Capacitance, F/g) / current density	Symbol	Reference
Nano spheres	$CuFe_2O_4$	(334, 1 A/g) with original capacitance retention (88%) for 600 cycles	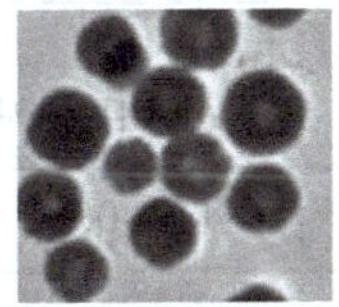	[51]
Sub – micro hollow spheres	$NiCo_2O_4$	(678, 1 A/g), cyclic stability (87%) after 3500 cycles at current density of 10 A/g	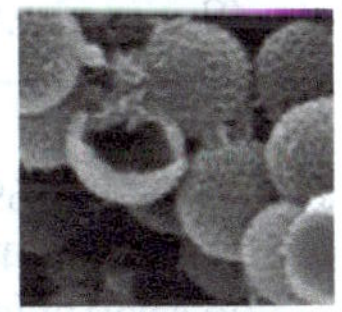	[52]
Network	$NiCo_2O_4$	(587, 2 A/g) along with 6% loss in original capacitance after 3500 charging / discharging continues cycles	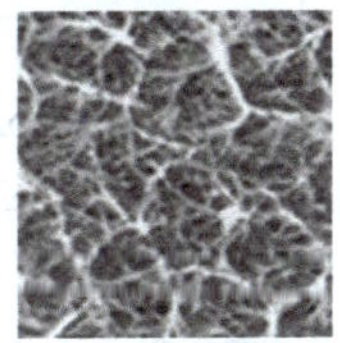	[53]

Table 8.3 Supercapacitive performance characteristics of mixed ternary ferromagnetic iron oxide electrode materials.

Electrode material	Remark	Reference
PEDOT / $NiFe_2O_4$	The PEDOT - $NiFe_2O_4$ composite with excellent capacitance (251 F/g) exhibited excellent stability against charging / discharging cycles (i.e. over 500 cycles)	[54]
PANI / $CoFe_2O4$ / graphene	The ternary composite obtained by dispersion of $CoFe_2O_4$ nanoparticles on graphene sheet with consequent coating of PANI demonstrated excelent capacitance (1133.3 F/g) at scan rate of $1 mVs^{-1}$ along with 96% capacity retention over 5000 cycles.	[55]
$ZnFe_2O_4$	Cyclic stability (83% capacity retention after 8000 cycles) alongwith energy (42 Wh / kg^{-1}) and and power (5 Kw kg^{-1}) densities.	[56]
$MnFe_2O_4$	Specific capacitance (282.4 F/g) with cyclic stability (85.8%) for 2000 cycles	[57]
$MnFe_2O_4$	Specific capacitance (88.4 F/g) and 69.2% original capacitance retention over 2000 cycles	[58]
$MnFe_2O_4$	Capacitance of 25.2 F/g along with energy (12.6 Wh / kg) and power (0.74 W / kg) densities.	[59]
$CoMnFeO_4$	12% loss of original capacitance (770 F/g) over 8000 cycles	[60]

(Continued)

Table 8.3 Supercapacitive performance characteristics of mixed ternary ferromagnetic iron oxide electrode materials. (*Continued*)

Electrode material	Remark	Reference
$Ni_{1-x}Mg_x Fe_2O_4$	Specific capacitance (≈ 260 F/g) with cycling stability of 88.79% over 1000 cycles associated with power (143.9 kW / kg) and energy (11.96 Wh / kg) densities respectively	[61]
$NiAl_{0.1} Fe_{1.9}O_4$	98.7% retention of original specific capacitance (250.9 F/g) after 1000 cycles	[62]
$Co_{0.5}Ni_{0.5} Fe_2O_4$	Original capacitance (630.0 F/g) with 82% retention for 1500 cycles associated with energy density of 7.43 Wh / kg and power density (60.45 W kg^{-1}) demonstrates excellent performance.	[63]
$Mg_{1-x}Zn_xFe_2O_4$	Specific capacitance (484.6 F/g), energy density (108 Wh / kg) and power density (0.5 KW / kg)	[64]

Table 8.4 Supercapacitive performance characteristics of mixed ternary ferromagnetic iron oxide – polymer composites with / without carbon material.

Electrode material	**Remark**	**Reference**
$CoFe_2O_4$ / PANI / graphene	Capacitance (1133 F/g) at 1m Vs^{-1} scane rate for three – electrode system along with excellent cyclability (96% original capacitance retention) for charging / discharging 5000 cycles	[65]
Mn ferrite / PANI / graphene	Capacitance (454.8 F/g) at 0.2 A/g current density	[66]
M – type hexaferrite / PANI / graphene	Specific capacitance (342 F/g) at scane frequency (10 m Vs^{-1}).	[67]
$MnFe_2O_4$ / PANI / graphene	This ternary composed used to fabricate negative electrode in hybrid supercapacitors showed capacitance (241 F / g) at 0.5 mA / cm^2 which was 7.5 times more compared to the capacitance displayed by $MnFe_2O_4$	[68]
$MnFe_2O_4$ / PANI / carbon black	Capacitance (206 F/g) with energy density (16 Wh / kg) and cyclic stability of 75% for 10^5 cycles	[69]
$CoFe_2O_4$ / PANI / rGO	Length capacitance (1.41 F m^{-1}) and energy density (270 x 10^{-8} Wh / cm). Useful sandwiched covalently grafted nanocomposite to fabricate flexible fibre supercapacitor.	[70]

(*Continued*)

Table 8.4 Supercapacitive performance characteristics of mixed ternary ferromagnetic iron oxide – polymer composites with / without carbon material. (*Continued*)

Electrode material	Remark	Reference
$NiFe_2O_4$ / PEDOT: PSS / rGO	Capacitance (1090 F/g) along with energy density (660 Wh / kg) at current density of 0.5 A/g. PEDOT : PSS acted as support layer for $NiFe_2O_4$ nanoparticles	[71]
$CoFe_2O_4$ / PANI / graphene	Excellent supercapacitive parameters, energy density (240 Wh kg^{-1}), power density (2680 W kg^{-1}) and capacitance (1123 F/g) with 98.2% cyclic stability for 2000 cycles	[72]
$MnFe_2O_4$ / PANI	86.7% original capacitance (371 F/g) retention over 1000 cycles	[73]
$CuFe_2O_4$ / PANI / acetylene black	Specific capacitance (732.35 F/g), energy (26.757 Wh kg^{-1}) and power (3165.25 W kg^{-1}) densities with 78% capacity retention for 5000 cycles	[74]
Fe_2O_3 / MnO_2 / PEDOT / rGO	Specific capacitance (287 F/g), power density (1900 W / kg) and energy density (11 Wh kg^{-1}) for 4 A/g current density. The composite is made of mixed metal oxides (MnO_2 plus Fe_2O_3) in the form of fine coating on PEDOT / rGO sheet	[75]

Table 8.5 Supercapacitive performance characteristics of ferromagnetic mixed ternary cobalt oxide electrode materials.

Electrode material	Remark	Reference
$NiCo_2O_4$ @ MnO_2	Retention of original specific capacitance (112 F/g in 1M NaOH) without loss for 8000 cycles	[76]
$NiCo_2O_4$ / CoO	Specific capacitance (908 F/g) and 75% retention of capacity for 3000 cycles	[77]
Co_3O_4 / $CoMoO_4$	Specific capacitance (1062.5 F/g) with energy (31.64 Wh / kg) as well as power (7270 W kg^{-1}) densities and cyclability (90.38%) for 2000 cycles	[78]
$FeCo_2O_4$	Capacitance (407 F/g) with energy density (3 Wh / kg), power density (3780 W kg^{-1}) and appreciable charge / discharge cycling stability for 2000 cycles without any loss in original capacitance	[79]
$ZnCo_2O_4$	Specific capacitance (812 F/g) with 88% cycling stability for 5100 cycles.	[80]

(Continued)

Table 8.5 Supercapacitive performance characteristics of ferromagnetic mixed ternary cobalt oxide electrode materials. (*Continued*)

Electrode material	Remark	Reference
$MnCo_2O_4$ @ $NiMoO_4$	Capacitance (1244 F/g) with original capacitance retention upto 93% after 8000 cycles and excellent energy density (42 Wh / kg)	[81]
$MnCo_2O_4$ @ graphene	Remarkable electrochemical performance parameters such as specific capacitance (406.5 F/g) with energy (20.32 Wh / kg) and power (300 kW / kg) densities and 95% capacity retention for 5000 cycles	[82]
$FeCo_2O_4$	Capacitance (960 F/g) with energy (34.5 Wh / kg) and power (6391.7 W / kg) densities in association of 94% capacitance retention after 10000 cycles	[83]
$ZnCo_2O_4$ @ $NiMoO_4 \cdot H_2O$	Specific capacitance (3.53 F cm^{-2}) with retention of 88% after 5000 charging/discharging cycles	[84]
Zn – Ni – Co oxide @ $NiMoO_4$	Specific capacitance (87.5 mA h/g), energy (70 Wh / kg) and power (5115 W kg^{-1}) densities with 91% retention of original capacitance for 10000 cycles	[85]

Table 8.6 Supercapacitive performance of mixed ternary ferromagnetic cobalt oxide – polymer composites with / without carbon material.

Electrode material	Remark	Reference
Co_3O_4 / MnO_2 / PPy	Capacitance (782 F/g) in 1.0 KOH at 0.5 A/g current density with retention of about 98% original capacitance value at 5.0 A/g	[86]
$ZnCo_2O_4$ / PPy	Capacitance (1559 F/g) at current density (2.0 mA / $cm^{2)}$ with 10% loss in original capacitance for 5000 cycles at 10.0 mA / cm^2	[87]
$NiCo_2O_4$ / PANI	Capacitance (901 F/g) at 1 A/g current density with successful original capacitance retention of 91% over 3000 cycles	[88]
$NiCo_2O_4$ / PPy / Carbon fibre	Areal capacitance (1.44 F / cm^2) at 2 m A / cm^2 and good cycling stability (80.5%) for 5000 charging/discharging cycles at 10 mA / cm^2 current density	[89]
$CuCo_2O_4$ / PANI	Energy density (76 Wh / kg) and power density (599 W kg^{-1}) with only 6% loss in original capacitance (403 F/g) for 3000 cycles	[90]
$MgCo_2O_4$ / PPy / Ni foam	Specific capacitance (1079.6 F/g) at 1.0 A g^{-1} with capacity retention of 97.4% for 1000 cycles	[91]

(Continued)

Table 8.6 Supercapacitive performance of mixed ternary ferromagnetic cobalt oxide – polymer composites with / without carbon material. (*Continued*)

Electrode material	Remark	Reference
$MnCo_2O_4$ / PPy	Specific capacitance (2364.0 F/g) in 6.0 M KOH at current density of 5.0 m Vs^{-1} with cyclic stability (85.5%) for 10^4 cycles	[92]
$NiCo_2O_4$ @ PEDOT	Excellent capacitance (1775 F/g) with energy and power densities of 898 Wh / kg and 1.25 Kw kg^{-1} respectively along with 95% conserved original capacitance for 5000 cycles	[93]
$ZnCo_2O_4$ / PANI / N – dopted graphene	Capacitance (720 F/g) was retained to the level of 96% over 10^4 cycles	[94]
Co_3O_4 / Ag / PPy	Specific capacitance (355.64 F/g) at 1.4 A/g current density with excellent conservation of original capacitance upto 3000 charge / discharge cycles	[95]

8.4 Conclusion

This chapter intends to summarize the available current literature on electrochemical supercapacitive performance of mixed ferromagnetic ternary oxides of iron and cobalt alongwith their composites with conducting polymers. In order to remove the drawbacks (poor conductivity, inferior cyclic stability, volume change during charging / discharging processes) of metal oxides, conducting polymers have been added to magnetic oxides to improve cyclability and electronic conductivity. However, the performance of electrode materials effectively depend upon the polymerization techniques used for generating polymers and the architectural morphologies of the resulted individual pseudocapacitor materials (CP or MTMO) and their composites. The composite materials remove the drawbacks of individual components and further ameliorate the supercapacitive accomplishment of energy accumulating systems.

Though, noticable advancements regarding the development of magnetic ternary metal oxides nanostructures and their polymeric composites for supercapacitor usage have been made in current years, some issues have still to be solved through:

(a) adequate control upon dimensions and architectural morphology of electrode materials
(b) prevention of agglomeration formation of electrode material particles and their protection from mechanical degradation
(c) facilitating unhindered ion mobility between active electrode surface and the liquid electrolyte
(d) developing new more flexible current collector systems to provide effective transfer of both ion as well as electron to external circuit through the entire electrode.

References

1. Raza, W., Ali, F., Raza, N., Luo, Y., Kim, K.H., Yang, J., Kumar, S., Mahmood, A., Kwon, E.E., Recent advancements in supercapacitor technology. *Nano Energy*, 52, 441, 2018.
2. Yu, G., Xie, X., Pan, L., Bao, Z., Cui, Y., Hybrid nanostructured materials for high-performance electrochemical capacitors. *Nano Energy*, 2, 213, 2013.
3. Wang, G., Zhang, L., Zhang, J., A review of materials for electrochemical supercapacitors. *Chem. Soc. Rev.*, 41, 797, 2012.

4. Mohd Abdah, M.A.A., Azman, N.H.N., Kulandaivalu, S., Sulaiman, Y., Review of the use of transition-metal-oxide and conducting polymer-based fibres for high-performance supercapacitors. *Mater. Des.*, 186, 108199, 2020, https://doi.org/10.1016/j.matdes.2019.108199.
5. Palchoudhury, S., Ramasamy, K., Gupta, R.K., Gupta, A., Flexible supercapacitors: A materials perspective. *Front. Mater.*, 5, 83, 2019.
6. Shown, I., Ganguly, A., Chen, L.-C., Chen, K.-H., Conducting polymer-based flexible supercapacitor. *Energy Sci. Eng.*, 3, 2, 2015.
7. Xia, L., Hu, D., Yu, Chen, G.Z., Electrolytes for electrochemical energy storage. *Mater. Chem. Front.*, 1, 584, 2017.
8. Huang, B., Sun, X.–Z., Zhang, X., Zhang, D.-C., Ma, Y.-W., Organic electrolytes for activated carbon-based supercapacitors with flexible package. *Acta Phys. Chim. Sin.*, 29, 1998, 2013.
9. Jäckel, N., Weingarth, D., Zeiger, M., Aslan, M., Grobelsek, I., Presser, V., Comparison of carbon onions and carbon blacks as conductive additives for carbon supercapacitors in organic electrolytes. *J. Power Sources*, 272, 1122, 2014.
10. Buzzco, M.C., Evans, R.G., Compton, R.G., Non-haloaluminate room-temperature ionic liquids in Electrochemistry - A review. *Chem. Phys. Chem.*, 5, 1106, 2004.
11. Zhao, D., Huang, Q., Jin, X.B., Wei, X.-J., Capacitance at the electrode/ionic liquid interface. *Acta Phys. Chim. Sin.*, 26, 1239, 2010.
12. Chen, G.Z., Supercapacitor and supercapattery as emerging electrochemical energy stores. *Int. Mater. Rev.*, 62, 173, 2017, http://dx.doi.org/10.1080/09506608.2016.1240914.
13. Szubzda, B., Szmaja, A., Ozimek, M., Mazurkiewicz, S., Polymer membranes as separators for supercapacitors. *Appl. Phys. A*, 117, 1801, 2014.
14. Arvani, M., Keskinen, J., Lupo, D., Honkanen, M., Current collectors for low resistance aqueous flexible printed supercapacitors. *J. Energy Storage*, 29, 10184, 2020.
15. Miller, E.E., Hua, Y., Tezel, F.H., Materials for energy storage: Review of electrode materials and methods of increasing capacitance for supercapacitors. *J. Energy Storage*, 20, 30, 2018.
16. Muzaffar, A., Ahmed, M.B., Deshmukh, R., Thirumalai, J., A review on recent advances in hybrid supercapacitors: Design, fabrication and applications. *Sustain. Energy Rev.*, 101, 123, 2019.
17. Wang, F., Wang, H., Mao, J., Aligned-graphene composites: A review. *J. Mater. Sci.*, 54, 36, 2018.
18. Chen, X., Paul, R., Dai, L., Carbon – based supercapacitors for efficient energy storage. *Natl. Sci. Rev.* 4, 453, 2017.
19. Chen, T. and Dai, L., Carbon nanomaterials for high-performance supercapacitors. *Mater. Today*, 16, 272, 2013.

20. Ke, O. and Wang, J., Graphene-based materials for supercapacitor electrodes: A review. *J. Mater.*, 2, 37, 2016.
21. Liu, J., Jiang, J., Cheng, C., Li, H., Zhang, J., Gong, H., Fan, H.J., Co_3O_4 nanowire@MnO_2 ultrathin nanosheet core/shell arrays: A new class of high - performance pseudocapacitive materials. *Adv. Mater.*, 23, 2076, 2011.
22. Yuan, C., Wu, H.B., Xie, Y., Lou, X.W., Mixed transition metal oxides: Design, synthesis and energy-related applications. *Angew. Chem. Int. Ed.*, 53, 1488, 2014.
23. Naresh, V., Elias, L., Martha, S.K., Poly(3,4-ethylenedioxythiophene) coated lead negative plates for hybrid energy storage systems. *Electrochim. Acta*, 301, 183, 2019.
24. Wang, H., Lin, J., Shen, Z.X., Polyaniline (PANi) based electrode materials for energy storage and conversion. *J. Sci. Adv. Mater. Devices*, 1, 225, 2016.
25. Chen, D., Wang, Q., Wang, R., Shen, G., Ternary oxide nanostructured materials for supercapacitors: A review. *J. Mater. Chem. A*, 3, 10158, 2015.
26. Sahoo, S., Zhang, S., Shim, J.J., Porous ternary high performance supercapacitor electrode based on reduced graphene oxide, $NiMn_2O_4$ and polyaniline. *Electrochim. Acta*, 216, 386, 2016.
27. Mondal, M., Ghosh, D., Giri, S., Shakir, I., Das, C.K., Polyaniline-wrapped nanorods as electrode materials for supercapacitor energy storage applications. *RSC Adv.*, 4, 58, 3083, 2014.
28. Banerjee, J., Datta, K., Kader, M.A., Nayak, S.K., An overview on the recent developments in polyaniline based supercapacitors. *Polym. Adv. Technol.*, 30, 1902, 2019, https://doi.org/10.1002/pat4624.
29. Ramya, R., Sivasubramanian, R., Sangaranarayanan, M.V., Condunting polymers-based electrochemical supercapacitors – progress and prospects. *Electrochim. Acta*, 101, 109, 2013.
30. Spaldin, A.M., *Magnetic materials: Fundamentals and applications*, 2nd Ed., Cambridge University, Press, Cambridge, England, 2010.
31. Ismail, F.M., Ramadan, M., Abdellah, A.M., Ismail, I., Allam, N.K., Mesoporous spinel manganese zinc ferrite for high-performance supercapacitors. *J. Electroanal. Chem.*, 817, 111, 2018.
32. Lu, A.H., Salabas, E.L., Schuth, F., Magnetic nanoparticles: Synthesis, protection, functionalization and application. *Angew. Chem. Int. Ed.*, 46, 1222, 2007.
33. Boutonnet, M., Logdberg, S., Svensson, E.E., Recent developments in the application of nanoparticles prepared from w/o microemulsion in heterogeneous catalysis. *Curr. Opin. Colloid Interface Sci.*, 13, 286, 2008, https://doi.org/10.1016/j.cocis.2007.10.001.
34. Dominguez, M.S., Boutonnet, M., Solans, C., A novel approach to metal and metal oxide nanoparticle synthesis: The oil-in-water microemulsion reaction method. *J. Nanopart. Res.*, 11, 1823, 2009, https://doi.org/10.1007/s11051-009-9660-8.

35. Jana, N.R., Chen, Y., Peng, X., Size and shape controlled magnetic (Cr, Mn, Fe, Co, Ni) oxide nanocrystals via a simple and general approach. *Chem. Mater.*, 16, 3931, 2004, https://doi.org/10.1021/cm049221k.
36. Faraji, M., Yamini, Y., Rezaee, M., Magnetic nanoparticles: Synthesis, stabilization, functionalization, characterization and applications. *J Iran. Chem. Soc.*, 7, 1, 2010, https://doi.org/10.1007/BF03245856.
37. Liu, B., Liu, B., Wang, Q., Wang, Q., Xiang, Q., Chen, D., Shen, D., New energy storage option: Toward $ZnCo_2O_4$ nanorods/nickel foam architectures for high-performance supercapacitors. *ACS Appl. Mater. Interfaces*, 20, 10011, 2013.
38. Li, L., Peng, S., Cheah, Y., The, P., Wang, J., Wee, G., Ko, Y., Wong, C., Srinivasan, M., Electrospun porous $NiCo_2O_4$ Nanotubes as advanced electrodes for electrochemical capacitors. *Chem. Eur. J.*, 19, 5892, 2013.
39. Deng, F., Yu, L., Cheng, G., Lin, T., Sun, M., Ye, F., Li, Y., Synthesis of ultrathin mesoporous $NiCo_2O_4$ nanosheets on carbon fiber paper as integrated high-performance electrodes for supercapacitors. *J. Power Sources*, 251, 202, 2014.
40. Du, J., Zhou, G., Zhang, H., Cheng, C., Ma, J., Wei, W., Chen, L.B., Wang, T., Ultrathin porous $NiCo_2O_4$ nanosheet arrays on flexible carbon fabric for high-performance supercapacitors. *ACS Appl. Mater. Interfaces*, 5, 15, 7405, 2013.
41. Zhou, W., Kong, D., Jia, X., Ding, C., Cheng, C., Wen, G., $NiCo_2O_4$ nanosheet supported hierarchical core–shell arrays for high-performance supercapacitors. *J. Mater. Chem. A*, 22, 6310, 2014.
42. Wang, Q., Wang, X., Liu, B., Yu, G., Hou, X., Chen, D., Shen, G., $NiCo_2O_4$nanowire arrays supported on Ni foam for high-performance flexible all-solid-state supercapacitors. *J. Mater. Chem. A*, 1, 2468, 2013.
43. Xu, K., Li, W., Liu, Q., Li, B., Liu, X., An, L., Chen, Z., Zou, R., Hu, J., Hierarchical mesoporous $NiCo_2O_4$@MnO_2 core–shell nanowire arrays on nickel foam for aqueous asymmetric supercapacitors. *J. Mater. Chem.*, 2, 4795, 2014.
44. Yang, W., Gao, Z., Ma, J., Zhang, X., Wang, J., Liu, J.Y., Hierarchical $NiCo_2O_4$@NiO core–shell hetero-structured nanowire arrays on carbon cloth for a high-performance flexible all-solid-state electrochemical capacitor. *J. Mater. Chem. A*, 2, 1448, 2014.
45. Wang, Q., Xu, J., Wang, X., Liu, B., Hou, X., Yu, G., Wang, P., Chen, D., Shen, G., Core–shell $CuCo_2O_4$@ MnO_2 nanowires on carbon fabrics as high-performance materials for flexible, all-solid-state, electrochemical capacitors. *ChemElectroChem*, 1, 559, 2014.
46. Huang, L., Chen, D., Ding, Y., Feng, S., Wang, Z.L., Liu, M., Nickel–cobalt hydroxide nanosheets coated on $NiCo_2O_4$ nanowires grown on carbon fiber paper for high-performance pseudocapacitors. *Nano Lett.*, 13, 3135, 2013.
47. Liu, X., Shi, S., Xiong, Q., Li, L., Zhang, Tang, H., Gu, C., Wang, X., Tu, J., Hierarchical $NiCo_2O_4$@$NiCo_2O_4$ core/shell nanoflake arrays as

high-performance supercapacitor materials. *ACS Appl. Mater. Interfaces*, 25, 8790, 2013.

48. Gupta, V., Gupta, S., Miura, N., Electrochemically synthesized nanocrystalline spinel thin film for high performance supercapacitor. *J. Power Sources*, 195, 3757, 2010.
49. Wang, Q., Liu, B., Wang, X., Ran, S., Wang, L., Chen, D., Shen, G., Morphology evolution of urchin-like $NiCo_2O_4$ and their applications as psuedocapacitors and photoelectrochemical cells. *J. Mater. Chem.*, 22, 21647, 2012.
50. An, C., Wang, Y., Huang, Y., Xu, Y., Xu, C., Jiao, L., Yuan, H., Novel three-dimensional $NiCo_2O_4$ hierarchitectures: Solvothermal synthesis and electrochemical properties. *CrystEngComm*, 16, 385, 2014.
51. Zhu, M., Meng, D., Wang, C., Diao, G., Facile fabrication of hierarchically porous $CuFe_2O_4$ nanospheres with enhanced capacitance property. *ACS Appl. Mater. Interfaces*, 5, 13, 6030, 2013.
52. Yuan, C., Li, J., Hou, L., Lin, J., Pang, G., Zhang, L., Lian, L., Zhang, X., Template-engaged synthesis of uniform mesoporous hollow $NiCo_2O_4$ sub-microspheres towards high-performance electrochemical capacitors. *RSC Adv.*, 3, 18573, 2013.
53. Yuan, C., Li, J., Hou, L., Lin, J., Zhang, X., Xiong, S., Polymer-assisted synthesis of a 3D hierarchical porous network-like spinel $NiCo_2O_4$ framework towards high-performance electrochemical capacitors. *J. Mater. Chem. A*, 1, 11145, 2013.
54. Sen, P. and De, A., Electrochemical performances of poly(3,4-ethylenedioxythiophene)–NiFe. *Electrochim. Acta*, 55, 4677, 2010.
55. Xiong, P., Huang, H.J., Wang, X., Design and synthesis of ternary cobalt ferrite/graphene/polyaniline hierarchical nanocomposites for high-performance supercapacitors. *J. Power Sources*, 425, 937, 2014.
56. Vadiyar, M.M., Bhise, S.C., Kolekar, S.S., Chang, J.Y., Ghule, K.S., Ghule, A.V., Low-cost flexible 3-D aligned and cross linked efficient $ZnFe_2O_4$ nano – flakes electrode on stainless steel mesh for asymmetric supercapacitors. *J. Mater. Chem. A*, 4, 3504, 2016.
57. Kwon, J.M., Kim, J.H., Kang, S.H., Choi, C.J., Rajesh, J.A., Ahn, K.S., Facile hydrothermal synthesis of cubic spinel AB_2O_4 type $MnFe_2O_4$ nanocrystallites and their electrochemical performance. *Appl. Surf. Sci.*, 413, 83, 2017.
58. Guo, P., Zhen, L., Shuibo, L., Jing, X., Guanglei, W., Hongliang, L., Zhao, X.S., Electrochemical properties of colloidal nanocrystal assemblies of manganese ferrite as the electrode materials for supercapacitors. *J. Mater. Sci.*, 52, 5359, 2017.
59. Singh, G. and Chandra, S., Electrochemical performance of $MnFe_2O_4$ nano-ferrites synthesized using thermal decomposition method. *Int. J. Hydrog. Energy*, 43, 4058, 2018.
60. Ghadimi, L.S., Arsalani, N., Ahadzadeh, I., Hajalilou, A., Lotf, E.A., Effect of synthesis route on the electrochemical performance of $CoMnFeO_4$

nanoparticles as a novel supercapacitor electrode material. *Appl. Surf. Sci.*, 494, 440, 2019.

61. Wongpratat, U., Tipsawat, P., Khajonrit, J., Swatsitang, E., Maensiri, S., Effects of nickel and magnesium on electrochemical performances of partial substitution in spinel ferrite. *J. Alloys Compd.*, 831, 154718, 2020.
62. Ramadevi, P., Sangeetha, A., Kousi, F., Shanmugavadivu, R., Structural and electrochemical investigation on pure and aluminium doped nickel ferrite nanoparticles for supercapacitor application. *Mater. Today Proc.*, 02, 888, 2020.
63. Sharifi, S., Yazdani, A., Rahimi, K., Effect of Co^{2+} content on supercapacitance properties of hydrothermally synthesized Ni_{1-x} $CoxFe_2O_4$ nanoparticles. *Mater. Sci. Semicond Process.*, 108, 104902, 2020.
64. Uke, S.J., Mardikar, S.P., Bambole, D.R., Kumar, Y., Chaudhari, G.N., Sol-gel citrate synthesized Zn doped $MgFe_2O_4$ nanocrystals: A promising supercapacitor electrode material. *Mater. Sci. Energy Technol.*, 3, 446, 2020.
65. Xiong, P., Huang, H.J., Wang, X., Design and synthesis of ternary cobalt ferrite/graphene/polyaniline hierarchical nanocomposites for high-performance supercapacitors. *J. Power Sources*, 245, 937, 2014.
66. Xiong, P., Hu, C., Fan, Y., Zhang, W., Zhu, J., Wang, X., Ternary manganese ferrite/graphene/polyaniline nanostructure with enhanced electrochemical capacitance performance. *J. Power Sources*, 266, 384, 2014.
67. Bhattacharya, P., Dhibar, S., Hatui, G., Mandal, A., Das, T., Das, C.K., Graphene decorated with hexagonal shaped M-type ferrite and polyaniline wrapper: A potential candidate for electromagnetic wave absorbing and energy storage device applications. *RSC Adv.*, 4, 17039, 2014.
68. Sankar, K.V. and Selvan, R.K., The ternary $MnFe_2O_4$/graphene/polyaniline hybrid composite as negative electrode for supercapacitors. *J. Power Sources*, 275, 399, 2015.
69. Zha, D., Xiong, P., Wang, X., Strongly coupled manganese ferrite/carbon black/polyaniline hybrid for low-cost supercapacitors with high rate capability. *Electrochim. Acta*, 185, 218, 2015.
70. Sankar, K.V. and Selvan, R.K., Fabrication of flexible fiber supercapacitor using covalently grafted $CoFe_2O_4$/grapheme oxide/polyaniline and its electrochemical performances. *Electrochim. Acta*, 213, 469, 2016.
71. Hareesh, K., Shateesh, B., Joshi, R.P., Dahiwale, S.S., Bhoraskar, V.N., Haran, S.K., Dhole, S.D., PEDOT:PSS wrapped $NiFe_2O_4$/rGO tertiary nanocomposite for the supercapacitor application. *Electrochim. Acta*, 20 106, 2016.
72. Mousa, M.A., Khairy, M., Shehab, M., Nanostructured ferrite/graphene/polyaniline using for supercapacitor to enhance the capacitive behavior. *J. Solid State Electrochem.*, 21, 995, 2017.
73. Arsalani, N., Tabrizi, A.G., Ghadimi, L.S., Novel PANI/$MnFe_2O_4$ nanocomposite for low-cost supercapacitors with high rate capability. *J. Mater. Sci. Mater. Electron.*, 29, 6077, 2018.

74. Das, T. and Verma, B., Synthesis of polymer composite based on polyaniline-acetylene black-copper ferrite for supercapacitor electrodes. *Polymer*, 168, 61, 2019.
75. Azman, N.H.N., Sulaiman, Y., S. Mamat, Md., Nazir, M., Lim, H.N., Novel poly(3,4-ethylenedioxythiophene)/reduced graphene oxide incorporated with manganese oxide/iron oxide for supercapacitor device. *J. Mater. Sci.: Mater. Electronics.*, 30, 1458, 2019.
76. Xu, K., Li, W., Liu, Q., Li, B., Liu, X., An, L., Chen, Z., Zou, R., Hu, J., Hierarchical mesoporous $NiCo_2O_4$@MnO_2 core–shell nanowire arrays on nickel foam for aqueous asymmetric supercapacitors. *J. Mater. Chem.*, 2, 4795, 2014.
77. Tang, Q., Chen, M., Wang, L., Wang, G., A novel asymmetric supercapacitors based on binder-free carbon fiber paper@nickel cobaltite nanowires and graphene foam electrodes. *J. Power Sources*, 273, 654, 2015.
78. Zhou, M., Lu, F., Shen, X., Xia, W., He, H., Zeng, X., One-pot construction of three dimensional $CoMoO_4/Co_3O_4$ hybrid nanostructures and their application in supercapacitors. *J. Mater. Chem. A*, 3, 21201, 2015.
79. Pendashteh, A., Palma, J., Anderson, M., Marcilla, R., Nanostructured porous wires of iron cobaltite: Novel positive electrode for high-performance hybrid energy storage devices. *J. Mater. Chem. A*, 3, 16849, 2015.
80. Ramachandran, T. and Hamed, F., Electrochemical performance of plate-like zinc cobaltite electrode material for supercapacitor applications. *J. Phys. Chem. Solids*, 121, 93, 2015.
81. Mehrez, J.A.A., Owusu, K.A., Chen, Q., Li, L., Hamwi, K., Luo, W., Mai, L., Hierarchical $MnCo_2O_4$@$NiMoO_4$ as free-standing core–shell nanowire arrays with synergistic effect for enhanced supercapacitor performance. *Inorg. Chem. Front.*, 6, 857, 2019.
82. Saren, P., Adhikari, A.D., Khan, S., Nayak, G.C., Self-assembled GNS wrapped flower-like $MnCo_2O_4$ nanostructures for supercapacitor application. *J. Solid State Chem.*, 271, 282, 2019.
83. Lalwani, S., Munjal, M., Singh, G., Sharma, R.K., Layered nanoblades of iron cobaltite for high performance asymmetric supercapacitors. *Appl. Surf. Sci.*, 476, 1025, 2019.
84. Chen, C., Wang, S., Luo, X., Gao, W., Huang, G., Zeng, Y., Zhu, Z., Reduced $ZnCo_2O_4$@$NiMoO_4{\cdot}H_2O$ heterostructure electrodes with modulating oxygen vacancies for enhanced aqueous asymmetric supercapacitors. *J. Power Sources*, 409, 112, 2019.
85. Bandyopadhyay, P., Saeed, G., Kim, N.H., Lee, J.H., Zinc-nickel-cobalt oxide @$NiMoO_4$ core-shell nanowire/nanosheet arrays for solid state asymmetric supercapacitors. *Chem. Eng. J.*, 384, 123357, 2020.
86. Wang, B., He, X., Li, H., Liu, Q., Wang, J., Yu, L., Yan, H., Li, Z., Wang, P., Optimizing the charge transfer process by designing Co_3O_4@PPy@MnO_2 ternary core–shell composite. *J. Mater. Chem. A*, 2, 12968, 2014.

87. Chen, T., Fan, Y., Wang, G., Yang, Q., Yang, R., Rationally designed hierarchical $ZnCo_2O_4$ polypyrrole nanostructures for high-performance supercapacitor electrodes. *RSC Adv.*, 5, 74523, 2015.
88. Jabeen, N., Xia, Q., Yang, M., Xia, H., Unique core–shell nanorod arrays with polyaniline deposited into mesoporous $NiCo_2O_4$ support for high-performance supercapacitor electrodes. *ACS Appl. Mater. Interfaces*, 8, 6093, 2016.
89. Chen, T., Fan, Y., Wang, G., Zhang, J., Chuo, H., Yang, R., Rationally designed carbon fibre @ $NiCo_2O_4$ @ polypyrrol core–shell nanowire array for high-performance supercapacitor electrodes. *Nano*, 11, 1650015, 2016.
90. Omar, F.S., Numan, A., Duraisamy, N., Ramly, M.M., Ramesh, K., Ramesh, S., Binary composite of polyaniline/copper cobaltite for high performance asymmetric supercapacitor application. *Electrochim. Acta*, 227, 41, 2017.
91. Gao, H., Wang, X., Wang, G., Hao, C., Zhou, S., Huang, C., An urchin-like $MgCo_2O_4$@PPy core–shell composite grown on Ni foam for a high-performance all-solid-state asymmetric supercapacitor. *Nanoscale*, 10, 10190, 2018.
92. Wang, F., Lv, X., Zhang, L., Zhang, H., Zhu, Y., Hu, Z., Zhang, Y., Ji, J., Jiang, W., Construction of vertically aligned PPy nanosheets networks anchored on $MnCo_2O_4$ nanobelts for high-performance asymmetric supercapacitor. *J. Power Sources*, 393, 169, 2018.
93. Deshagani, S., Liu, X., Wu, B., Deepa, M., Nickel cobaltite@poly(3,4-ethylenedioxypyrrole) and carbon nanofiber interlayer based flexible supercapacitors. *Nanoscale*, 11, 2742, 2019.
94. Kathalingam, A., Ramesh, S., Yadav, H.M., Choi, J.H., Kim, H.S., Kim, H.S., Nanosheet-like $ZnCo_2O_4$@nitrogen doped graphene oxide/polyaniline composite for supercapacitor application: Effect of polyaniline incorporation. *J. Alloys Compd.*, 830, 154734, 2020.
95. Iqbal, J., Numan, A., Ansari, M.O., Jagadish, P.R., Jafer, R., Bashir, S., Mohamad, S., Ramesh, K., Ramesh, S., Facile synthesis of ternary nanocomposite of polypyrrole incorporated with cobalt oxide and silver nanoparticles for high performance supercapattery. *Electrochim. Acta*, 348, 136313, 2020.

9

Transition Metal Oxides with Broaden Potential Window for High-Performance Supercapacitors

Nawishta Jabeen[1]*, Ahmad Hussain[2] and Jazib Ali[3]

[1]*Department of Physics, Fatima Jinnah Women University, Rawalpindi, Pakistan*
[2]*Department of Physics, The University of Lahore, Sargodha Campus, Sargodha, Pakistan*
[3]*Center for Hybrid and Organic Solar Energy (CHOSE), University of Rome Tor Vergata, Rome, Italy*

Abstract

The utilization of transition metal oxides (TMOs) as electrodes of supercapacitors (SCs) and energy storage devices has attained significant consideration. Various authors around the globe have reported the improvement in energy density of SCs by broadening the potential window (V), and here in this chapter, TMOs electrodes for SCs are debated to operate in expanded potential windows (~2.6 V) in aqueous electrolytes for asymmetric supercapacitors (ASCs). Initially, the grouping of nanoscale polyaniline (PANI) as an electrochemically active component and $NiCo_2O_4$ as a conductive scaffold to form $NiCo_2O_4$@PANI nanorod arrays (NRAs) structure is discussed as an electrode for SCs. The fabricated electrode has operated in a broadened potential window (−0.2 to 0.8 V) and in 1 M H_2SO_4 electrolyte has reported the better specific capacitance (901 F g^{-1}) measured at 1 A g^{-1}. Moreover, the capacitance retention of ~91% after 3000 cycles at 10 A g^{-1} is also the highlight of the material. Afterward, a modified charge storage mechanism of potassium (K) ions intercalated α-MnO_2 has been debated for the first time, and it is reported that as the potential window for the material is expanded from 0 to 1.2 V for cyclic voltammetry (CV) measurements, development in specific capacitance occurs due to emergence of redox peaks. In the next section, the influence of high Na content in the *Birnessite* ($Na_{0.5}MnO_2$) nanosheet assembled nanowall arrays (NWAs) is observed with an extended operating potential window

Corresponding author: saba_sahar_2010@yahoo.com

Inamuddin, Tariq Altalhi and Sayed Mohammed Adnan (eds.) Electroceramics for High Performance Supercapacitors, (203–232) © 2024 Scrivener Publishing LLC

(0-1.3 V) against Ag/AgCl electrode. $Na_{0.5}MnO_2$ NWAs cathode has shown the specific capacitance 366 F g^{-1}. Notably, $Na_{0.5}MnO_2//Fe_3O_4$@C ASC is designed with a 2.6-V aqueous operating potential window reporting the improved energy density (81.7 Wh kg^{-1}) and brilliant rate capability. Furthermore, Bi_2O_3-based electrode materials possessing broaden potential window (−1.2 to 0) are discussed as anode materials for SCs. This chapter will open new horizons for researchers and scientists to visualize the importance of broadening the operating potential window phenomenon to boost the energy density of the SCs.

Keywords: Supercapacitor, anode, cathode, potential window, transition metal oxides

9.1 Introduction of Transition Metal Oxides (TMOs)

With the advancement in energy storage application technology, the pollution in the environment and the depletion of traditional fossil resources have become vital issues in the human society of developing countries. Herein, the detailed analysis of the supercapacitors (SCs) has been presented as a better alternative approach for the energy consumption areas like portable electronics and electric-based vehicles. SCs lie among the energy storage devices possessing the ability to display long cycle life, fast charge and discharge, high power density, and most importantly SCs are environmental protection and show safety [1, 2]. Though, for the utilization of SCs as high-performance devices, a few fundamental issues are necessary to be addressed, including the low energy density and poor cycling ability [3]. Recently, scientists have brought uniqueness to this field by introducing the pseudo-capacitors and asymmetric supercapacitors (ASCs) by designing the composites for anode and cathode materials with the presence of transition metal oxide electrodes to achieve the extended potential window, higher energy density, and higher specific capacitance in comparison with traditional electric double layer capacitors (EDLCs) [4]. It is reported that commercial carbon-based SCs show less energy density (10 Wh kg^{-1}), which is not acceptable as compared to batteries, and hence such devices are not capable to meet the requirements of market demands [5]. To overcome such kind of problems, researchers have focused their interest on the TMOs as capable electrodes for pseudo-supercapacitors. Various transition metals oxides, MnO_2, FeO_x, RuO_2, and Bi_2O_3 have achieved considerable attention as electrode materials for SCs which demonstrate a broad potential window to enhance the energy density [6]. Moreover, these TMOs are preferred due to low cost, easy availability, and high theoretical specific capacitance [7]. But still, the low ion transport properties have deprived their electrical conductivity and restricted their actual electrochemical properties for energy storage devices.

Keeping given above discussion, herein this chapter, we aim to describe the feature studies, up-to-date achievements, and novelty presented by researchers for transition-metal-oxide-based materials (MnO_2, FeO_x, and Bi_2O_3, etc) with enhanced electrochemical performance as electrode materials. Moreover, the ion transmission performance via high power density and energy density depending on the broader potential window and stable cycling ability will be addressed. Another important aspect of the study is to focus on the structure-dependent intrinsic capacitive behavior of α-MnO_2 and δ-MnO_2 nanostructures as SCs electrodes by comparing them in three different potential windows. Their charge storage mechanism in the enlarged potential windows through understanding the alkali cations intercalation/deintercalation in the tunnel and layered structures of MnO_2 will be focused. Carbon-coated layer Fe_3O_4@C composite materials as negative electrode material for SCs have shown better-quality electrochemical performance with broad negative potential window for ASCs. Finally, an expanded potential window of 2.6 V aqueous ASC is designed in terms of integrated $Na_{0.5}MnO_2$ NWAs as cathode and Fe_3O_4@C nanorods arrays (NRAs) as the anode, with excellent cycling stability, improved energy density, and power density, and high rate performance [8]. The achievements in the field of TMOs as electrode materials in SCs are described in this chapter, which may provide simple and effective approaches to understand the concept of broad potential window effects in the performance of SCs electrodes. To achieve high performance and high energy density for SCs, the selection of electrode materials is the most important step regarding the fabrication of SCs for determining the electrochemical performance of SCs. Important selection criteria for the choice of electrode materials are their microstructure, electrochemical properties, and morphology.

9.2 Redox-Based Materials

The widely used materials for SC electrodes are carbon nanotubes (CNTs), activated carbon (AC), graphene, template carbons, and carbon-based hybrids [9]. Such materials not only possess the ability to present high surface density and better conductance but also show some major drawbacks which restrict their specific capacitance (10–50 $\mu F\ cm^{-2}$) for such electrode surfaces [10]. However, pseudo-capacitance can be varied 10 to 100 times larger as compared to EDLC capacitance. SCs with materials showing redox reactions show pseudo-capacitance which is vastly required in the future developed advanced energy storage devices [11]. SCs of this type have shown the character to store electric charges in the double layer, as well as perform rapid and reversible surface redox reactions [12]. Generally, such materials are further categorized into two categories: conducting polymers and electroactive metal oxides [13].

9.3 Conducting Polymers

The conjugated bond system is the backbone of the polymer materials and is the main reason for describing them as conducting polymers. Conducting polymers are commonly fabricated by the electrochemical oxidation method of the monomer and the chemical oxidation method of the monomer [14]. Polythiophene, polyaniline, and polypyrrole are frequently considered polymers in the field of SCs. The charge storage mechanism for conducting polymer includes the gathering of charges via proton doping interactions all over the backbone of polymer materials [15]. These conducting polymers during the reduction process can behave like n-doped with (counter) cations while during the oxidation process they behave like p-doped with (counter) anions. These two charge/discharge processes can easily be described by equations as follow [16]:

$$Cp + ne^{-} \Leftrightarrow (C^{+})_n Cp^{n-} \quad \text{(N-type)} \tag{9.1}$$

$$Cp \Leftrightarrow Cp^{n+}(A^{-})_n + ne^{-} \quad \text{(P-type)} \tag{9.2}$$

Controlled nanoscale conducting polymer electrodes have drawn the considerable focus of research to be utilized in SCs owing to their low band gaps, suitable morphology, better charge-discharge rate, and less cost. Controlled morphology and dimensions of conducting polymers offer noticeable advantages [17]. (a) High surface area can escalate the possibility of providing the maximum interaction area of electrolyte solution and causing the improvement of charge and discharge rates by improved charge uptake into the conducting polymer. (b) Small path lengths ease the rapid ions transportation throughout the backbone of conducting polymer. (c) Less material and large space can decrease strain and improve cycle life.

The electrochemical activity of conducting polymers in a developed state is generally a serious problem because of the volumetric shrinking and swelling during the ejection of counter ions (doped ions) [18]. Conductance issues can be improved by fabricating composite electrodes like conductive polymer and carbon materials or metal oxide compounds. Composite materials can bear the stress generated by volume changes, so the cycle stability can be improved. Jabeen *et al.*, have reported rationally designed novel core-shell $NiCo_2O_4$@PANI nanorod arrays (NRAs). The morphology was characterized and compositional analysis was performed finally, heterostructure was utilized as an electrode for SCs with a -0.2-0.8 V broaden potential window (Figure 9.1a) [19]. This potential window is twice the time larger compared to only $NiCo_2O_4$ materials which can hardly operate between 0 and 0.5 V [20]. $NiCo_2O_4$ conductive core offers a highly porous morphology, while electrochemically active component nanoscale PANI layer. Through implementing the refined and evenly coated PANI around the $NiCo_2O_4$ conductive core, the synthesized electrode material has displayed a much better specific capacitance of ~901 F g^{-1} at 1 A g^{-1} and outstanding retention capacitance coefficient of ~91% even after performing 3000 cycles at the current density of 10 A g^{-1} (Figure 9.1c), these electrochemical performance is much improved than the earlier reported PANI-based pseudo-capacitors [19].

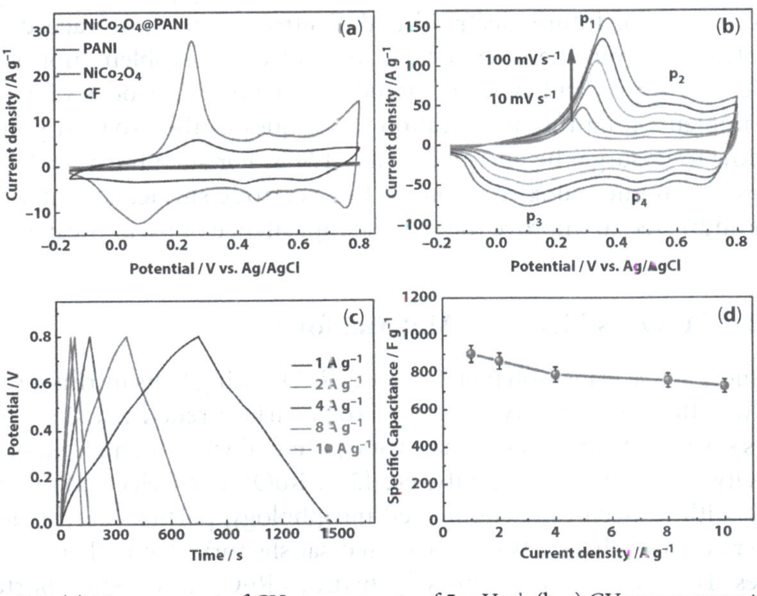

Figure 9.1 (a) Measurement of CV at a scan rate of 5 mV s^{-1}. (b-c) CV measurements and charging-discharging of $NiCo_2O_4$@PANI NRAs at variable scan rates and current densities. (d) The plot of average specific capacitances of $NiCo_2O_4$@PANI NRAs [19].

9.4 Electroactive Metal Oxides or Transition Metal Oxides (TMOs) as Electrodes for SCs

TMOs are an alternative significant class of redox-based electrode materials for pseudo-capacitors, which can provide excellent electrochemical properties, good energy density, and stability [21]. TMOs possess the ability to electrostatically store energy like carbon-based electrode materials and with suitable potential windows TMOs perform the electrochemical faradaic reactions among ions and electrode materials. Common requirements for the utilization of TMOs in SCs are [22]: (a) TMOs must be electronically conductive; (b) two or more oxidation states of the TMOs can exist simultaneously for the continuous range without any phase change (c) ions can spontaneously intercalate/de-intercalate into the lattice sites of oxides during the process of reduction and during the process of oxidation is extracted from the lattice sites, letting the simplistic inter-conversion among O^{2-} and OH^- [23].

V_2O_5, RuO_2, Co_3O_4, MnO_2, Fe_3O_4, and NiO are the common TMOs that are investigated with significant interest as electrode materials to be utilized in SCs [24]. But they show the low energy densities for the existing practical SCs and fail to overcome the ever-rising power consumption requirements of future electrical and electronic energy storage devices. Scientists have put their best efforts to resolve this problem, not only by fabricating the hybrid types of pseudo-capacitive electrodes of SCs but also implementing the modification techniques to the broaden potential window to upsurge the energy density of SCs. For such purpose, fast and reversible faradic redox reactions at the electrode surface are vital issues to be addressed to improve the specific capacitance of pseudo-capacitors.

9.4.1 MnO_2 as Electrode Material for SCs

The most active transition metal oxide is RuO_2 owing to its intrinsic reversibility, better conductivity, and numerous surface redox reactions. RuO_2 offers several advantages such as a wide potential window, high theoretical capacity, good thermal stability, etc [25]. RuO_2 as an electrode material along with a specifically engineered morphology, particle size, structure, and crystalline phase has demonstrated satisfactory electrochemical outcomes. The specific capacitances for hydrous RuO_2 have been reported to lie between 200-1300 F g^{-1} [26]. As SCs electrode, the major drawback of RuO_2 is its expensiveness, rareness, and environmental pollution effects. Nevertheless, there is a continuous search for alternative materials which should be abundant and low cost, such alternative TMO must have the abilities where its metal ions can reversibly transform to multiple valence states and possess the competence to substitute not only RuO_2. Manganese oxide (MnO_x) is reported as a renowned multi-valence (Mn^{2+}, Mn^{3+}, and Mn^{4+}) material, along with the existence of various polymorphs [27]. Nowadays, MnO_x has become a widely studied material owing to its environment-friendly nature, abundantly found, low toxicity, broad potential window, and excellent theoretical capacity (1370 F g^{-1}) [28]. Hence herein, MnO_2 has been selected as electrode material in our discussion of this chapter. In 1999, Goodenough and Lee were the first who fabricated the amorphous $MnO_2 \cdot xH_2O$ by a co-precipitation method in KCl aqueous electrolyte and utilized the material in SCs as an electrode with a specific capacitance of ~200 F g^{-1} [29]. But, during the co-precipitation fabrication process, the redox reaction occurred so rapidly, that it became difficult to control the morphology of the material as well as the structure.

Manganese oxide can reside in various crystalline structures, which include α, β, γ, δ and λ of MnO_2 [30]. The description and presence of these various structures of MnO_2 can be explained depending on the size of the tunnel resolute by the number of octahedral subunits ($n \times m$). α-MnO_2 comprises the MnO_6 octahedra connected at the corners to achieve the tetragonal unit cell with 1-dimensional, 1D (2 × 2), and (1 × 1) tunnels. (2 × 2) tunnel size is about 4.6 Å, larger enough to insert/extract the alkali cations within the tunnel [31]. Similarly, β-MnO_2 involves a single string of edge-shared MnO_6 octahedrons to achieve a 1D (1 × 1) tunnel. For β-MnO_2 tunnel size is 1.89 Å, which is narrow as compared to α-MnO_2, hence it becomes difficult to adjust alkali cations within the tunnel [32]. Moreover, the structure of γ-MnO_2 is a bit complex, as it contains the random intergrowths of pyrolusite (1 × 1) and ramsdellite (1 × 2) domains [31]. Furthermore, δ-MnO_2 is a 2D layered structure containing the inter-layer spacing of ~7 Å. The much larger size of inter-layer spacing for δ-MnO_2 allows for adjustment of significant cations quantity, Ca^{2+}, Na^+, Li^+, or K^+, and water molecules amid the sheets of MnO_6 octahedra. Besides, 3D spinel structure has been reported for λ-MnO_2 [33].

The morphology and crystal structure of the fabricated electrodes are the defining parameters of the electrochemical properties of the SCs. Several research groups reports have focused on the engineering and alteration of the MnO_2 morphologies and achieving effective capacitive properties outcomes [34]. Wu *et al.* compared the morphology-dependent specific capacitances of MnO_2 nanorods and nanowires (243 F g^{-1} and 350 F g^{-1}) measurements were employed with similar parameters. They concluded that the smaller diameter of nanowires provides a thin track for ion diffusion with better active sites for the transfer of charge. On the other hand, MnO_2 nanotubes can settle high changes in volume during the charge-discharge cycle, and show improvement in the cycle life of the electrode [35]. The urchin structured or hollow sphere MnO_2 materials possess highly mesoporous specific surface area, which can establish improved cycling stability and capacitive properties [36]. Park *et al.*, have successfully synthesized the MnO_2 thin film by following the gel-mediated electrodeposition technique and demonstrated a better areal loading capacity of ~52.55 mF cm^{-2} [37]. Among several polymorphs of MnO_2, a δ-MnO_2 nanosheet array is a famous polymorph, which offers nearly 4.5 times larger surface area than another planar form. δ-MnO_2 nanosheet arrays offer a stable structure for the intercalation/deintercalation of cations, which results in improved charge/discharge ability, specific capacitance, and cycling ability [38]. Fabrication of nanostructured MnO_2 electrodes by rational manipulation/modification in morphologies can result in a porous structure which also improves the capacitive performances of electrodes.

Along with the improvement of the structure and morphologies of MnO_2, the charge storage mechanism is another important parameter for understanding. Meanwhile, the storage mechanism of MnO_2 depends upon the intercalation/deintercalation of alkali cations and protons of MnO_2. The type of MnO_2-based polymorph offering the suitable lattice to settle alkaline cations can play a dynamic role to establish the electrochemical properties of SCs. Brousse and his co-workers were the pioneer to illustrate the comparison study for the five polymorphs of MnO_2 and confirmed that electrochemical analysis of the material is governed by tunnel sizes of MnO_2 [39]. Moreover, they found that large tunnel sizes of α-MnO_2 are suitable to rapidly accommodate the alkaline cations, causing the creation of excellent capacitive properties. Munichandraiah *et al.* reported a similar kind of conclusion, where the electrochemical performance of various types of MnO_2 polymorphs was measured and it was concluded that electrochemical performance declines with the following pattern: $\alpha \approx \delta > \gamma > \lambda > \beta$ [40]. Charge storage mechanisms proposed earlier were incapable of fully understanding the electrochemical behavior of MnO_2. Commonly, there exist two mechanisms to describe charge storage behavior. First is reliant on the electrolyte's cations absorption by the surface of MnO_2 as follows [41]:

$$(MnO_2)_{surface} + M^+ + e^- \ (MnOOM)_{surface} \ (\mathrm{M^+= K^+, Na^+, and\ Li^+\ etc.}) \tag{9.3}$$

The second step is expressed by the cations of electrolyte intercalation/deintercalation in MnO_2 [41].

$$MnO_2 + M^+ + e\ MnOOM \tag{9.4}$$

Depending upon Mn^{4+}/Mn^{3+} redox reactions, the theoretical capacitance of MnO_2 is related to cation adsorption or intercalation.

9.4.2 Pseudo-Capacitive Behavior of α-MnO_2 by Cation Insertion

In recent years, several research groups have proposed the improvement in the electrochemical performances of SCs by the intercalation/deintercalation of cations into the MnO_2-based electrodes and perceived that such insertion of cations in the MnO_2 counterpart can assist ion diffusion. Among various polymorphs of MnO_2, α-MnO_2 contains body-centered tetragonal possessing (2 × 2) and (1 × 1) tunnels, which are capable to allow the insertion of alkaline cations [31]. Recently, Jabeen *et al.* have successfully reported the capacitive properties of K^+ introduced α-MnO_2 (K_xMnO_2) NRAs for the broaden potential windows (Figure 9.2) [42].

As the K_xMnO_2 structure contains a (2 × 2) tunnel with a tunnel size of 4.6 Å, where the insertion of K^+ into the tunnel is ideal. During the fabrication, firstly during charging the K^+ ions might be deintercalation from the tunnel, causing the intercalation of the H_2O molecule alongside. Then during the discharge process, K^+-ions from electrolytes start to intercalate and accommodate into the tunnel making the structure stabilize. As the Na^+ cation possesses a smaller radius than K^+-ions, hence during faradic activity the diffusion of Na^+ is easier resulting in the establishment of improved pseudo-capacitance [43]. Hence it can be stated that K_xMnO_2 NRAs as electrode material display better electrochemical properties owing to rapid reversible intercalation/deintercalation of Na^+-ions at the solid phase lattice sites. Figure 9.2b is representing the CV of the K^+ inserted MnO_2 electrode for varying potential windows (0-0.8, 0-1.0 and 0-1.2 V) at a 5 mV s^{-1} scan rate. CV curves demonstrate distinctive behaviors in different potential windows. For the 0-0.8 V potential windows, the CV curve demonstrated an ideally rectangular curve, for the double-layer capacitive electrodes, such CV shape is regarded as a characteristic CV curve. Moreover, a noticeable current leap arises at 1.0 V during the charging process, supposed to be water decay alongside oxygen evaporation. Previously it was reported that for MnO_2-based electrodes, the upper cut-off potential was always adjusted under 1.0 V during electrochemical measurement to

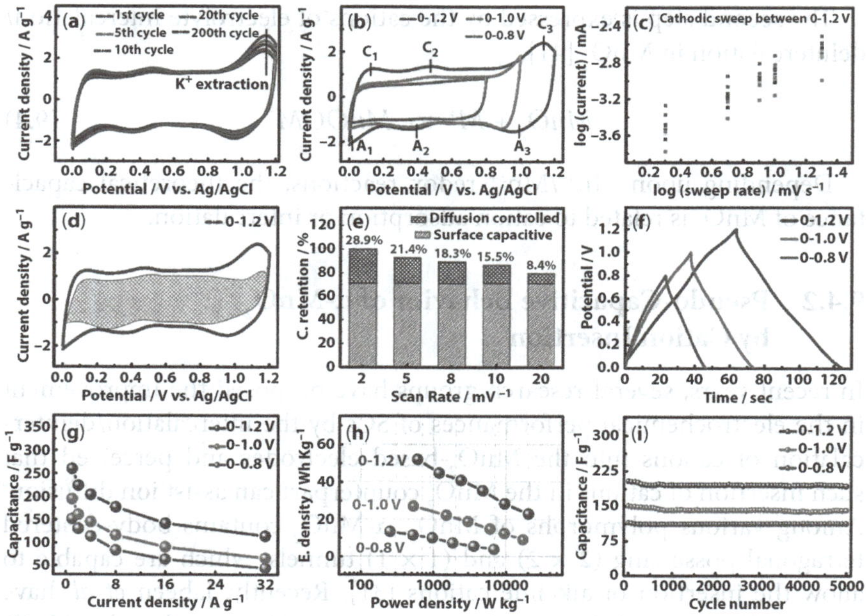

Figure 9.2 (a-e) CV of K^+ introduced α-MnO_2 cathode and capacitance separation analysis of K_xMnO_2. (f-i) Charge and discharge curves, rate capabilities, Ragone plots, and cycle performances of K^+ introduced α-MnO_2 cathode at varying potential windows [42].

evade the water decomposition process [44]. In this work, the upper cut-off potential is varied to 1.2 V, and between 1.0 and 1.2 V additional couple of redox peaks appeared, current leap at this stage cannot be associated with water decomposition but can be related to reversible redox reactions. The capacitive contribution was evaluated by applying Dunn's method on the K_xMnO_2 NRAs electrode. At a fixed potential for CV measurements overall current contributions are supposed to come from surface-controlled and diffusion-controlled processes for pseudo-capacitive materials which are calculated as follows [45]:

$$i(V) = K_1 v + K_2 v^{1/2} \tag{9.5}$$

Usually, both sides of Equation 9.5 are divided by the square root of the scan rate for analytical purposes, hence achieved Equation 9.6 becomes as follows;

$$i(V)/v^{1/2} = K_1 v^{1/2} + k_2 \tag{9.6}$$

In Equation 9.5, $i(V)$ represents the current at some specific voltage, k_1 and k_2 are the constants of scan rate, while scan rate is represented by v, the current contribution from surface capacitive effects is represented by k_1v and current contribution from the diffusion-controlled intercalation is presented by $k_2v^{1/2}$. Linear behavior was determined from slow scan rate CVs between 1 to 5 m Vs^{-1} and the current permits to calculate of k_1 (b-values) and k_2 for anodic/cathodic scans by the slopey-axis intercepts of a straight line for every provided voltage (Figure 9.2c). Herein, it becomes easier to quantitatively distinguish the currents ascending during capacitive processes and arising from Na^+ insertion, which is differentiated from the CV curve by the area under the shade (Figure 9.2d). For the total charge storage phenomenon of the K_xMnO_2 NRAs electrode, the surface capacitive contributions are dependent on varying scan rates presented in Figure 9.2e. Surface capacitive contribution at 2 mV s^{-1} lower scan rate is 71% of total charge storage, the surface capacitive contribution portion of total charge storage is much greater than diffusion-controlled contribution. At 4 A g^{-1} current density, charging/discharging curves for K_xMnO_2 NRAs electrode is presented in Figure 9.2f for different potential windows. At the broaden potential window 0-1.2 V, a couple of voltage plateaus are observable in charging/discharging curves, wherein the extension of the potential window has enhanced charge storage performance. Under the influence of different potential windows, the comparison among the varying current densities dependent on specific capacitance is presented (Figure 9.2g). The reported specific capacitance of the K_xMnO_2 NRAs electrode tends to 260 F g^{-1} at 1 A g^{-1} for the potential window of 0-1.2 V and this same potential window with a current density of 32 A g^{-1}, electrode still displays much capacitance of 115 F g^{-1}. For the upper cut-off potential (1.2 V), the K_xMnO_2 NRAs electrode displays the enhancement in energy density as well (Figure 9.2h). K_xMnO_2 NRAs electrode delivers the energy density of 52 Wh kg^{-1} at 1 A g^{-1} for potential window 0 to 1.2 V. To highlight the working stability of the K_xMnO_2 NRAs electrode under 5000 cycles, a comparison study under different varying potential windows and at 4 A g^{-1} current density is presented in Figure 9.2i. For 0-0.8, 0-1.0, and 0-1.2 V potential windows and even after 5000 cycles K_xMnO_2 NRAs electrode has displayed capacitance retentions of 96%, 96%, and 95%, respectively [42]. Results confirm that with the extension of the potential window, the K_xMnO_2 NRAs electrode is a strong candidate for future SCs with better energy density.

The study has also been expanded to the comparison of electrochemical performances of pre-inserted K^+ ions α-MnO_2 nanorod arrays (K^+-free α-MnO_2 NRAs) as electrode material and K_xMnO_2 NRAs electrode [42]. In CV analysis for K^+-free α-MnO_2 NRAs, the current density has increased with the extension of the potential window but there exists no redox peak. In the article, the capacitive performance of potassium-free α-MnO_2 NRAs is also investigated under varying from scan rates 5 to 800 mV s^{-1} and varying current densities (1 to 32 A g^{-1}). GCD measurements were taken at 0-1.2 V potential window. The rectangular-shaped CV response was obtained for each potential window, indicating the capacitive behavior with the surface adsorption/desorption of alkali cations inside the tunnels of the K^+-free α-MnO_2 electrode crystal. For a detailed comparative study of electrochemical performance under different potential windows specific capacitances and energy densities of both K_xMnO_2 NRAs and K^+-free α-MnO_2 NRAs electrodes are illustrated in Table 9.1. It can be observed from Table 9.1 that by varying the upper cut-off potential for K_xMnO_2 NRAs and K^+-free α-MnO_2 NRAs electrodes the columbic efficiencies were decreased to 96.3% and 89%, respectively. Moreover, for 4 A g^{-1} current density and after 5000 charging/discharging cycles, the K^+-free α-MnO_2 NRAs electrode under the 0-1.2 V potential window has shown the 88% of capacitance retention, whereas the K_xMnO_2 NRAs electrode has shown the 95% under same conditions [42].

Depending on the prescribed study the previously reported redox reaction for MnO_2 was revised as follows [42]:

$$M_xMnO_2\ MnO_2 + xM^+ + xe^- \quad (M^+ = H^+, Na^+, K^+) \tag{9.7}$$

Usually, MnO_2 or M_xMnO_2 are considered to be utilized as cathode material in SCs, where the low valence Mn^{3+} is required for the charging process initially. For stoichiometric MnO_2 theoretically, the only charge storage phenomenon is double-layer capacitance as it is hard to oxidize Mn^{4+} further. During the fabrication of MnO_2-based materials specific content of alkaline cations, all the time persists in MnO_2 and further some amount of alkaline cations can be intercalated in MnO_2 through the process of discharge, presence of such cations in the form of M_xMnO_2 are important to increase the pseudo-capacitive performance. Hence the theoretical capacitive value (1370 F g^{-1}) of MnO_2 is achievable in the form of M_xMnO_2 [46]. Hence, better specific capacitance can be presented by K_xMnO_2 NRAs electrode for SCs as compared to K^+-free α-MnO_2 NRAs electrode.

9.4.3 $Na_{0.5}MnO_2$ Nanosheet Assembled Nanowall Arrays for ASCs

In literature about MnO_2-base materials applications in SCs, it is reported that the content of alkaline cations insertion in MnO_2 is kept low, while the cation/Mn ratio must be kept below 0.3, it can restrict the pseudo-capacitive

Table 9.1 Electrochemical performance under varying potential windows comparison between K+-free α-MnO_2 NRAs and K_xMnO_2 NRAs electrodes [42].

Electrodes	Potential window (V vs. Ag/AgCl)	At 1 A g^{-1}, Specific capacitance (F g^{-1})	After 5000 cycles, capacitance retention (%)	At 1 A g^{-1}, energy density (Wh Kg^{-1})	At 4 A g^{-1}, coulombic efficiency (%)
K_xMnO_2	0-0.8 V	152	96	13.47	99
MnO_2		110	95	9.7	100
K_xMnO_2	0-1.0 V	195	96	27	97
MnO_2		145	92	20.1	94
K_xMnO_2	0-1.2 V	260.5	95	52	96.3
MnO_2		184	88	36.8	89

influence of MnO_2 [47]. However, it is still a big challenge to insert the high cations content in MnO_2 along with keeping the stable nanostructure of the material. In this report, Jabeen *et al.*, have utilized the high Na content in MnO_2 in the form of Birnessite $Na_{0.5}MnO_2$ nanosheet assembled nanowall arrays (NWAs) fabricated on the carbon cloth substrate. Herein the unique hierarchical architecture (nanosheets/nanowalls) has shown the enhanced surface area electrode, while the high Na-ion insertion allows the electrode to deliver improved specific capacitance. Notably, in the study authors have reported the prolonged potential window (0-1.3 V) versus Ag/AgCl for $Na_{0.5}MnO_2$ NWAs electrode for the first time [8].

It is reported that to electrochemically oxidize Mn_3O_4 NWAs into *Birnessite* $Na_{0.5}MnO_2$ hierarchical NWAs after 500 typical CV cycles have been performed with a specific scan rate (10 mV s^{-1}) in 0 to 1.3 V potential windows. At the first cycle, a large irreversible anodic peak was observed towards the potential limit, indicating the electrochemical oxidation process. With further continuous potential cycling, the irreversible anodic peak decreases rapidly and almost disappears at the 50th cycle, indicating that the electrochemical oxidation proceeds quickly with cycling. Subsequently, for both anodic and cathodic scans, the current has increased significantly with the cycling process for the whole potential range, showing improved capacitive performance of the electrode. After 100 cycles the CVs shape appear to be more symmetric accompanied by a couple of redox peaks and the current keeps on increasing slightly further up to 500 cycles, suggesting a complete phase transformation of Mn_3O_4 NWAs into *Birnessite* $Na_{0.5}MnO_2$ hierarchical NWAs. Along with the increased CV area, specific capacitance has also stabilized and increased significantly (Figure 9.3b).

For the evaluation of the electrochemical performance of *Birnessite* $Na_{0.5}MnO_2$ hierarchical NWAs, at 10 mV s^{-1} scan rate and under varying 0-1.0, 0-1.2, and 0-1.3 V potential windows, CV curves were measured (Figure 9.3c). There appeared a couple of redox peaks at 0.58 V for the anodic scan and 0.69 V for the cathodic scan, when the CV curve of *Birnessite* $Na_{0.5}MnO_2$ hierarchical NWAs electrode was measured for 0-1.0 V potential window, which correspond to the Mn^{3+}/Mn^{4+} reversible redox reaction along with the intercalation/deintercalation of Na^+ ions [48]. With the further extension of potential window 0-1.3 V, not only those redox peaks were pronounced but also a couple of new redox peaks appeared at 0.79 V and 0.96 V. Appearance of new redox peaks and increment of the current density for the potential window 0-1.3 V show that redox reaction for Mn^{3+}/Mn^{4+} is not fully done yet and also the sodium (Na^+) ions are not completely extracted from $Na_{0.5}MnO_2$ counterpart under adjusting the upper cutoff potential less than 1 V. Herein this study, Jabeen *et al.*, have

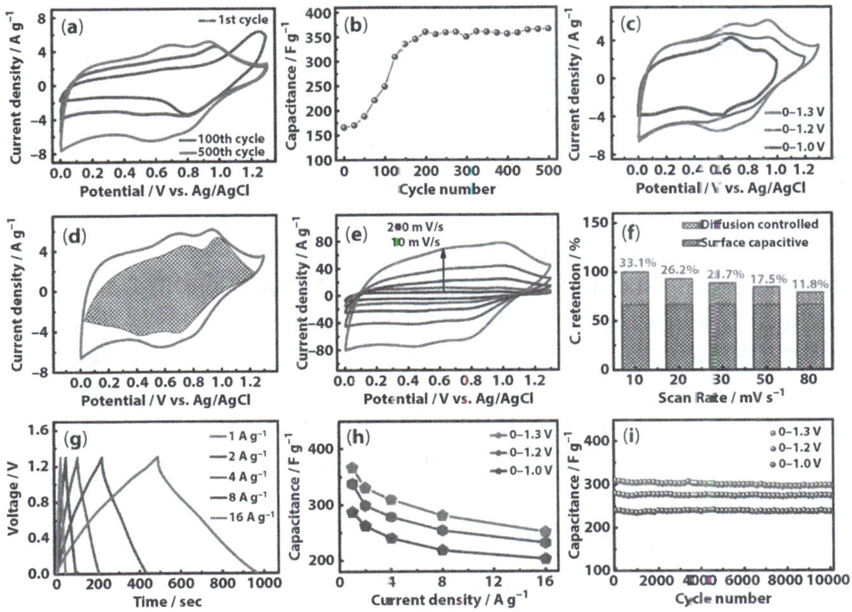

Figure 9.3 (a, b) CV curves and specific capacitance of Mn_3O_4 at varying cycling stages. (c-e) CV curves for $Na_{0.5}MnO_2$ NWAs electrode under varying potential windows. (g-i) GCD curves, rate capabilities, and cycle performance of $Na_{0.5}MnO_2$ NWAs electrode under varying potential windows [8].

introduced the concept of utilizing high Na^+-ions for *Birnessite* $Na_{0.5}MnO_2$ NWAs electrode to function at the enlarged potential window (0-1.3 V). For understanding the phenomenon of storing charge in $Na_{0.55}MnO_2$ NWAs electrode Dunn's method is utilized to separate the current distribution among the diffusion control method and surface control method [45]. The shaded portion in the CV curve of Figure 9.3d is representing the surface-controlled capacitance contribution of the electrode prepared by material $Na_{0.55}MnO_2$ NWAs. CV curves of the $Na_{0.55}MnO_2$ NWAs electrode under variable scan rates are presented in Figure 9.3e. It is obvious from the CV curves that even at the high scan rate (200 mV s^{-1}), CV curves have demonstrated the ideal rectangular shape. From Figure 9.3f, it can be concluded that there is 67% of total charge storage from surface capacitive contribution at the scan rate of 10 mV s^{-1}. GCD curves measured at varying current densities 1-16 A g^{-1} under the extended potential window 0-1.3 V for $Na_{0.55}MnO_2$ NWAs electrode are presented in Figure 9.3g. From Figure 9.3h, a comparison study of the specific capacitance of $Na_{0.55}MnO_2$ NWAs electrode is demonstrated at a current density of 1 A g^{-1} and under different potential windows, for 0.0-1.0 V, 0.0-1.20 V and 0.0-1.30 V the measured specific capacitances are 287 F g^{-1}, 366 F g^{-1}, and 338 F g^{-1}, respectively. The measured specific capacitance for potential windows 0-1.3 V is larger than previously reported literature [49, 50]. Cycling performance under the effect of extended potential window 0-1.3 V of $Na_{0.55}MnO_2$ NWAs electrode at 4 A g^{-1} for 10,000 continuous charging/discharging cycles is investigated (Figure 9.3i). For the potential window 0-1.3 V, the capacitance retentions remained at 96%, signifying that the broad potential window has not damaged the cycling stability of the $Na_{0.55}MnO_2$ NWAs electrode. Moreover, for the potential window 0-1.0 V, the capacitance retention is 98%, while for 0-1.2 V the capacitance retention is 97%. The reported energy density is 86 Wh kg^{-1} for the potential window of 0-1.3 V at 1 A g^{-1} [8]. Hence the achieved results dictate the potential of $Na_{0.55}MnO_2$ NWAs electrode for practical implementation in energy storage applications.

9.4.4 FeO_x/FeOOH Material as Negative Electrode

Iron oxides (FeOx) are another important TMO, which has drawn attention as negative electrode material due to their good electrochemical performance, source abundance, and environmental friendliness. It is reported that the Fe element can possess varying oxidation states including Fe_3O_4, $Fe(OH)_2$, FeOOH, FeO, and Fe_2O_3, among these states Fe_3O_4, Fe_2O_3, and FeOOH are regarded as showing the most stable phases for energy storage devices as electrodes of SCs [51]. Iron oxides/hydroxides perform the faradaic reactions in aqueous electrolytes as follows [52];

$$FeO_x + yM^+ + ye^- \leftrightarrow M_yFeO_x\ (M= Na^+ , K^+, Li^+) \quad (9.8)$$

Usually, iron oxides/hydroxides show similar kinds of CV curves irrespective of their non-similar crystal compositions. Recently in various reports the CV performance of iron oxides/hydroxides is vastly reliant on the operating potential windows and iron oxides/hydroxides for the varying potential windows (0-0.8 V and 0-1.0 V, versus Ag/AgCl) have demonstrated the rectangular CV curves with no clear indication of redox peaks. Usually, it is described that the pseudo-capacitive performance of iron oxides/hydroxides-based electrodes is largely dependent on the redox reaction between Fe^{3+} and Fe^{2+} [53]. For the development of a highly efficient FeO_x electrode, it will be a very unique approach to introduce the anion faradic reaction, with the novelty of employing cations and anions simultaneously in a single electrode. No doubt researchers and scientists have put their best efforts to explore the diversity in the electrode materials to fabricate reliable daily life energy storage devices in the form of SCs. However, there is still a need to bring a lot of effort to modify the fabrication techniques, and chemical and physical properties of the materials to achieve the best merits of the materials as electrodes of SCs.

9.4.5 Carbon-Stabilized Fe_3O_4@C Nanorod Arrays as an Efficient Anode for SCs

Fe_3O_4 contains the inverse spinel-type cubic structure with Fe^{2+} ions occupying the octahedral sites while Fe^{3+} ions occupy both tetrahedral as well as octahedral sites [54]. Fe_3O_4 is usually explored as a negative electrode for ASCs owing to their abundant nature and low cost. Although pure Fe_3O_4 possesses the highest conductivity among all the iron-based structures, the low specific capacitance (60–80 F g^{-1}) is a big issue that limits its applications [55]. To solve this problem, many researchers tried to fabricate hybrid nanocomposites. Lately, Fe_3O_4-multiwalled carbon nanotubes (MWCNTs) and Fe_3O_4-carbon nanofibers (CNFs) were synthesized successfully with an improved specific capacitance of 135 F g^{-1} and 120 F g^{-1}, respectively [56]. Despite all efforts, the specific capacitances and capacitance retention are still very low and the potential ranges are only between -0.8-0 and -1.0-0 V. Jabeen *et al.*, have successfully synthesized core-shell structured Fe_3O_4@C nanorods arrays (NRAs) and operated it in -1.3-0 V negative operating potential window. As a negative electrode material, Fe_3O_4@C NRAs can be utilized for highly-efficient ASCs [8].

Variable oxidation states along with the high conductivity ($\sigma = 2\times10$ 4 S m^{-1}) as compared to other TMOs, Fe_3O_4 has achieved considerable attention. Moreover, there exist the possibility of discrepancy in the Fe-ions valence states ($Fe^{3+} \leftrightarrow Fe^{0}$), which compels the Fe_3O_4 to display a strong theoretical capacity character in an alkaline aqueous solution [57]. Under these circumstances and due to the multi-phased nature Fe_3O_4 can create structural deformation/dissolution and huge volumetric expansion. For Fe_3O_4, serious electrolytic hydrogen evolution eventually causes drastic capacity decay which occurs after a few hundred cycles [58]. To overcome this issue, the selection of narrow operating can evade the possibility of several unnecessary phase transformation processes, and create the balance between capacities and cycling performance.

Recently, much attention has been dedicated to escalating/diffusing the nanoscaled Fe_3O_4 into several carbon-based materials like carbon nanosheets/nanorods/nanotubes/nanowires and graphene, etc. Furthermore, their electrochemical properties are mostly evaluated between 0.8 and 1.0 V potential ranges. Expectedly, the existence of strong covalent bonding with conductive carbon has resulted in up to 1000 times improvement in the capacitive properties of such electrode material [59]. Iron oxide/hydroxide can show high values of specific capacitance in the broader negative operating potential window up to -1.3-0 V. But it must be noticed that for such large potential window cycling performance of Fe_3O_4-based electrodes is damaged as Fe starts to dissolute into the electrolyte [60]. To overcome this issue and support the Fe_3O_4-based material in the ASCs, an ultrathin carbon layer is coated on Fe_3O_4 nanorod arrays (NRAs) to achieve the stable electrochemical performance of the material as an electrode [8]. Core-shell structured Fe_3O_4@C NRAs with a diameter of 80-100 nm and a shell's thickness of 5-10 nm has been successfully synthesized. Broaden negative operating potential window of -1.3-0 V has been implemented to analyze the electrochemical performance of Fe_3O_4@C NRAs as an electrode for ASCs.

9.4.6 Electrochemical Performance of Fe_3O_4 and Fe_3O_4@C NRAs as Anode

Typical CV analysis at variable potential windows (-1.3-0, -1.2-0, and -1.0-0 V) for Fe_3O_4@C NRAs electrode measured at 10 mV s^{-1} scan rate are demonstrated in Figure 9.4a [8]. For the potential windows -1.0-0 V and −1.2 to 0 V, CV curves have exhibited alike rectangular shapes confirming the ideal pseudo-capacitive performance, while a pair of redox peaks start to appear at -0.8 V for anodic scan and at -0.9 V for a cathodic scan when the cutoff potential is varied to -1.3 V, these couple of redox peaks are corresponding to Fe^0/Fe^{3+} redox coupling [60]. At variable scan rates 10-200 mV s^{-1}, CV curves of Fe_3O_4@C NRAs anode are illustrated in Figure 9.4b. Well-maintained ideal rectangular shape CV curves are visible even at a high scan rate (200 mV s^{-1}). For variable current densities 1-16 A g^{-1}, GCD curves of Fe_3O_4@C NRAs electrode are presented between -1.3-0 V. GCD curves are symmetric and substantially prolonged. Specific capacitance versus current density for varying potential windows of Fe_3O_4@C NRAs anode has been presented in Figure 9.4d, and specific capacitance of 344 F g^{-1} has been reported at 1 A g^{-1} between -1.3-0 V potential window [8].

It is evident from Figure 9.4d that Fe_3O_4@C NRAs anode has delivered the specific capacitance of 199 F g^{-1} at 16 A g^{-1} and between 1.3-0 V negative operating potential window. The comparison between the electrochemical performances of carbon-free Fe_3O_4 NRAs electrode and Fe_3O_4@C NRAs electrode is performed. Variable current densities 1-16 A g^{-1} dependent

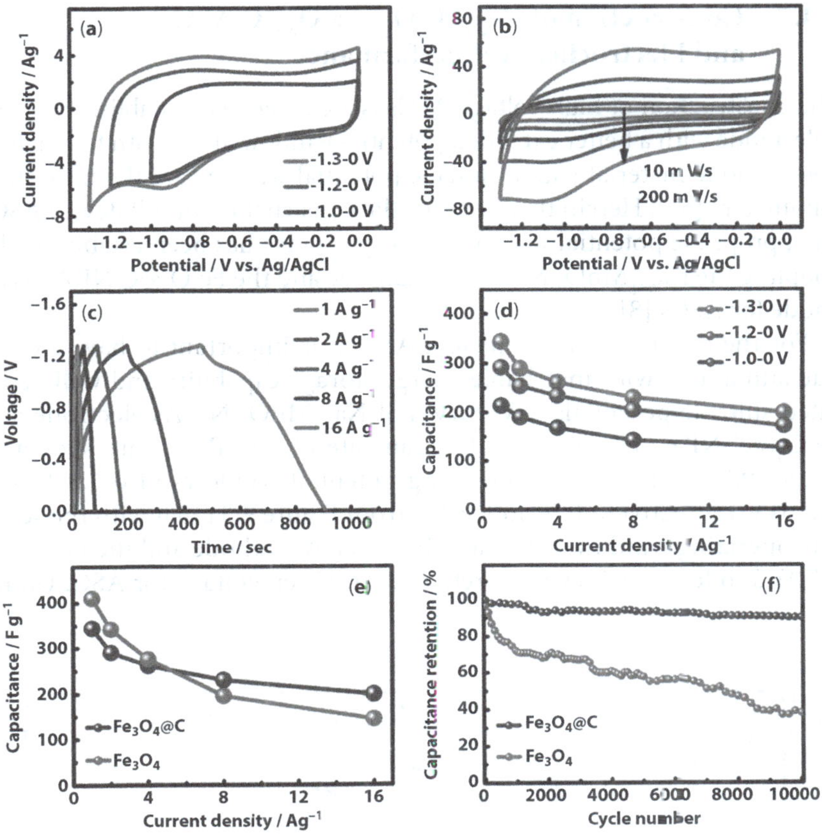

Figure 9.4 (a-b) At varying scan rates typical CV curves of Fe_3O_4@C, (c-d) Charging/discharging curves, and rate capabilities of the Fe_3O_4@C NRAs anode at different current densities and different potential windows. Comparison of (e) Rate capabilities Fe_3O_4 and Fe_3O_4@C NRAs electrodes (f) Cycle performance of Fe_3O_4 and Fe_3O_4@C NRAs electrodes [8].

specific capacitance for carbon-free Fe_3O_4 NRAs and Fe_3O_4@C NRAs electrodes is illustrated in Figure 9.4e, where it is clear that Fe_3O_4@C NRAs anode has shown the better specific capacitance as compared to Fe_3O_4 NRAs even for the higher current densities and extended negative potential windows of 0 to 1.3 V. Figure 9.4f shows that even after 10,000 GCD cycles, Fe_3O_4@C NRAs electrode has shown the capacitance retention of 95%, confirming the better cycling stability, while Fe_3O_4 NRAs have only retained 38% of its initial capacitance [8]. Such outcomes confirm the potential of Fe_3O_4@C NRAs as excellent electrode material to be utilized in ASCs.

9.4.7 Construction of $Na_{0.5}MnO_2$//Fe_3O_4@C ASC and Electrochemical Performance

The construction of high voltage ASCs is a challenge to establish the suitable anode with a better extended potential window along with the matchable cathode material with a suitable potential window are the important parameters [61]. Herein this work for the construction of full device ASCs an appropriate potential window and capacitance has been established by coupling the $Na_{0.55}MnO_2$ NWAs as a cathode and the Fe_3O_4@C NRAs as an anode for ASCs [8].

For the construction of efficient ASC, it is important to have a cathode and anode with matchable charge storage capability and well-separated suitable potentials. CV curves of $Na_{0.5}MnO_2$ NWAs electrode and Fe_3O_4@C NRAs electrode at the scan rate of 10 mV s^{-1}, are shown in Figure 9.5a with separate operating potential windows of 0-1.3 V and -1.3-0 V, respectively. It is noticeable from Figure 9.5a that with the separate operating windows, the $Na_{0.5}MnO_2$ NWAs cathode and the Fe_3O_4@C NRAs anode can achieve theoretically 2.6 V cell voltage for ASC. Under

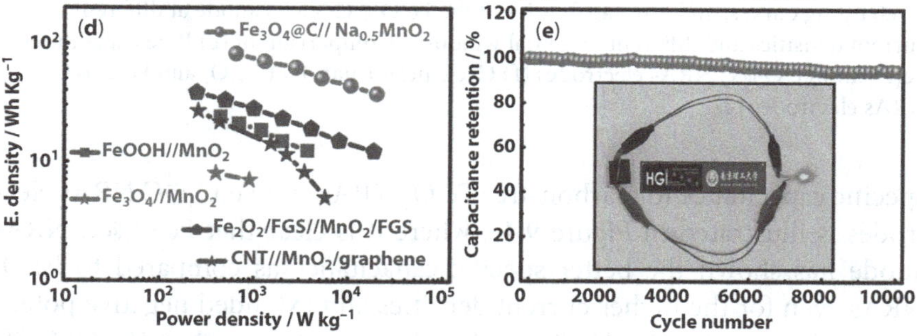

Figure 9.5 (a) Separate potential windows CV curves of $Na_{0.5}MnO_2$ NWAs electrode and Fe_3O_4@C NRAs electrode. (b) For different potential windows, CV curves of $Na_{0.5}MnO_2$//Fe_3O_4@C ASC. (c) GCD plots of $Na_{0.5}MnO_2$//Fe_3O_4@C ASC, (d) Ragone plots of $Na_{0.5}MnO_2$//Fe_3O_4@C ASC and previously reported ASCs. (e) Cycling stability performance of $Na_{0.5}MnO_2$//Fe_3O_4@C ASC for 0-2.6 V (Inset: the optical image of the $Na_{0.5}MnO_2$//Fe_3O_4@C ASC device illuminating a 2.2 V LED) [8].

50 mV s^{-1} scan rate, CV curves of full device $Na_{0.5}MnO_2$//Fe_3O_4@C ASC have been demonstrated in Figure 9.5b with the upper cutoff voltages from 0 to 2.6 V. Here the CV curves of the full cell are also of ideal rectangular shape which was also the feature for individual CV curves for $Na_{0.55}MnO_2$ NWAs electrode and Fe_3O_4@C NRAs electrode for the high cell voltage (2.6 V) [8]. Figure 9.5c is presenting the GCD curves under various current densities for the potential window 0-2.6 V of $Na_{0.5}MnO_2$//Fe_3O_4@C ASC. $Na_{0.5}MnO_2$//Fe_3O_4@C ASC has demonstrated the significant specific capacitance of 88 F g^{-1} at 0.5 A g^{-1} between 0-2.6 V, much improved than earlier reports [62].

A state-of-the-art comparison for energy density versus power density depending on GCD curves for varying current densities of $Na_{0.5}MnO_2$//Fe_3O_4@C ASC is shown in Figure 9.5d with previously reported ASCs [63–65]. The present $Na_{0.5}MnO_2$//Fe_3O_4@C ASC has shown the ability to perform 81.7 Wh kg^{-1} energy density at 647.5 W kg^{-1} power density. $Na_{0.5}MnO_2$//Fe_3O_4@C ASC has not only demonstrated excellent power capability, but it also shows stable cycling performance even at 0-2.6 V extended operating potential window in Figure 9.5e. 93% capacitance retention as compared to initial capacitance at 2 A g^{-1} for $Na0_{.5}MnO_2$//Fe_3O_4@C ASC has been observed even after the 10,000 charging/discharging cycles. From Figure 9.5e, the inset optimizes the practical implementation of the $Na_{0.5}MnO_2$//Fe_3O_4@C ASC. Prototype fabricated $Na_{0.5}MnO_2$//Fe_3O_4@C ASC has been connected to the circuit with the red light emitting diode (LED) of 2.2 V. Further it is reported that the full cell device was kept continuously powered on with the different bending states to observe the stability performances of the device and resulted in the excellent flexibility. Moreover, it is reported that the $Na_{0.5}MnO_2$//Fe_3O_4@C ASC device has maintained its ideal rectangular shape CV curves without severe deterioration under the scan rate range 10-1600 mV s^{-1} for an operating potential window of 0 to 2.6 V.

Schematic elaboration of $Na_{0.5}MnO_2$//Fe_3O_4@C ASC with the explanation of capacitive performance at 2.6 V is presented in Figure 9.6. The electrochemical oxidation process for the fabrication of $Na_{0.5}MnO_2$ NWAs offers a high overpotential to evaluate the oxygen, which becomes the reason to extend the potential window of the $Na_{0.5}MnO_2$ NWAs electrode. Moreover, *Birnessite* $Na_{0.5}MnO_2$ contains a layered structure with an interlayer spacing of 7 Å, which is supporting to facilitate the alkaline-based cations intercalation and deintercalation easily [8].

Herein, a unique approach is followed to allow high Na content insertion in MnO_2 and established the hierarchical nanosheets assembled nanowall morphology to achieve $Na_{0.5}MnO_2$ NWAs electrode and ultrathin carbon

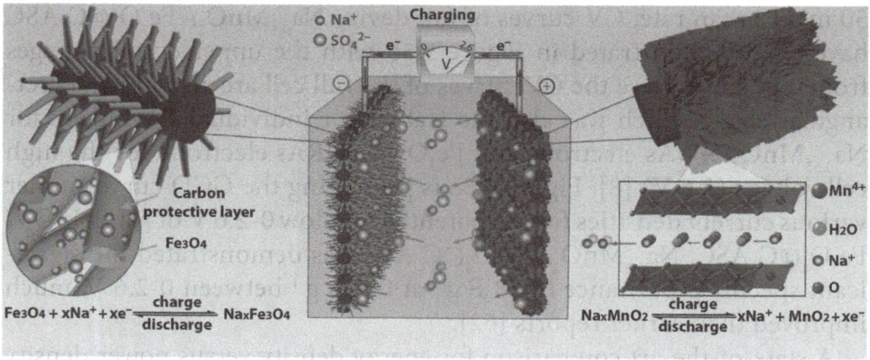

Figure 9.6 Schematic illustration of $Na_{0.5}MnO_2//Fe_3O_4$@C ASC, describing unique electrode structure and charge-storage mechanism between $Na_{0.5}MnO_2$ NWAs cathode and Fe_3O_4@C anode [8].

layer is coated around Fe_3O_4 NRAs as the anode. The above outcomes clearly demonstrate that by coupling the Fe_3O_4@C NRAs and $Na_{0.5}MnO_2$ NWAs, a high voltage stable 2.6 V, ASC device can successfully be engineered, with improved power capability, better energy density, and stable cycling performance [8].

9.4.8 Highly Efficient $NiCo_2S_4$@Fe_2O_3//MnO_2 ASC

Due to the establishment of matchable and a suitable combination of anode and cathode material, it is still challenging to fabricate the ASCs consisting of better energy and power densities. Moreover, usually, anode materials (carbon materials, 100–200 F g^{-1}) display less specific capacitance and low operating voltage window (< 2 V), which restricts their utilization in the applications. Jia *et al.* reported the synthesis of a hybrid $NiCo_2S_4$@Fe_2O_3 nanoneedle array to operate as an electrode (anode) for SCs. Fabricated hybrid $NiCo_2S_4$@Fe_2O_3 nanoneedle array at a scan rate of 5 mV s^{-1}, demonstrated excellent specific capacitance (342 F g^{-1}). MnO_2 nanosheet arrays are utilized as cathode material in ASCs, which have performed under 0 to 1.3 V, the extended operating potential window. Besides, as MnO_2 cathode offers the extended operating potential window, which efficiently varies the ASC voltage up to 2.3 V. It is reported that at a power density of 196 mW cm^{-3}, reported ASC full cell has shown the ability to deliver 2.29 mWh cm^{-3} volumetric energy density, confirming it as a device for the future electronic and energy storage devices [66].

9.4.9 Bi_2O_3 as Negative Electrode with Broaden Potential Window

Bismuth oxide (Bi_2O_3) is among the various TMOs which has attained the significant attention of researchers because of its abundance, less cost, efficiency, environmentally friendly, and high theoretical specific capacitance. But it is observed that due to the poor electrical conductivity of Bi_2O_3 as a negative electrode, its electrochemical properties are restricted [67]. Gujar *et al.* have reported the successful electrochemical deposition of Bi_2O_3 thin film, which was further implemented for SCs. The Bi_2O_3 thin film has demonstrated 98 F g^{-1} specific capacitance [68]. Later on, Tong's research group made the successful fabrication of hierarchical rippled Bi_2O_3 nanobelts, which has shown a specific capacitance of 250 F g^{-1} [69]. Quite a lot of methods are monitored to solve the conductivity relevant issues of Bi_2O_3-based materials, to make them capable and further employ it as the electrode in SCs. Wang *et al.* reported the fabrication of a composite of activated carbon Bi_2O_3 to work as the negative electrode in SCs, material at the current density of 1 A g^{-1} has demonstrated the specific capacitance 332.6 F g^{-1} [70]. Scientists and researchers have made considerable progress in the electrochemical properties of the Bi_2O_3 to work as the negative electrode in energy storage devices and they have achieved significant success.

9.5 Conclusion

SCs have attained considerable attention due to their efficient charge storage phenomenon and better electrochemical performance among energy storage devices. Exclusive core-shell $NiCo_2O_4$@PANI NRAs were discussed to elaborate on the importance in broaden potential window and utilization of conducting polymers for energy storage devices, where core-shell $NiCo_2O_4$@PANI NRAs have displayed the tremendous specific capacitance of 901 F g^{-1} at 1 A g^{-1}. Then K_xMnO_2 NRAs electrode was investigated in detail, where the K_xMnO_2 NRAs electrode has shown 52 Wh kg^{-1} energy density at 1 A g^{-1} current density. K_xMnO_2 NRAs electrode has displayed 96% capacitance retentions after 5000 cycles for the 0 to 1.2V potential window. The extended operating window has been reported for $Na_{0.5}MnO_2$ NWAs electrode (0–1.3 V), along with 366 F g^{-1} specific capacitance. High Na^+ content addition is the main reason for such better specific capacitance and excellent rate performance of $Na_{0.5}MnO_2$ NWAs cathode. Moreover, ASC has been constructed by coupling the $Na_{0.5}MnO_2$ NWAs (cathode), and

Fe_3O_4@C NRAs (anode). Fe_3O_4@C NRAs anode has also performed stable electrochemical properties for the extended negative potential window (−1.3 to 0 V). Hence, $Na_{0.5}MnO_2$//Fe_3O_4@C ASC has shown the pseudo-capacitive properties for a high voltage of 2.6 V. $Na_{0.5}MnO_2$//Fe_3O_4@C ASC has illustrated the 81.7 Wh kg^{-1} energy density. Such significant performance and better efficient ASCs are capable to be utilized in the forthcoming generation energy storage applications. Finally, the implementation of Bi_2O_3-based material as a highly negative electrode (−1.2 to 0 V) material for SCs is discussed. This study is helpful to optimize the electrochemical performance outcomes of the transition metal oxide-based electrodes to operate at the broad potential window and also to utilize them in energy storage applications of future generations.

References

1. Li, H., Han, C., Huang, Y., Huang, Y., Zhu, M., Pei, Z., Xue, Q., Wang, Z., Liu, Z., Tang, Z., Wang, Y., An extremely safe and wearable solid-state zinc ion battery based on a hierarchical structured polymer electrolyte. *Energy Environ. Sci.*, 11, 941–951, 2018.
2. Ajdari, F.B., Kowsari, E., Shahrak, M.N., Ehsani, A., Kiaei, Z., Torkzaban, H., Ershadi, M., Eshkalak, S.K., Haddadi-Asl, V., Chinnappan, A., Ramakrishna, S., A review on the field patents and recent developments over the application of metal organic frameworks (MOFs) in supercapacitors. *Coord. Chem. Rev.*, 422, 213441, 2020.
3. Yan, J., Li, S., Lan, B., Wu, Y., Lee, P.S., Rational design of nanostructured electrode materials toward multifunctional supercapacitors. *Adv. Funct. Mater.*, 30, 1902564, 2020.
4. Hong, J., Lee, Y.W., Ahn, D., Pak, S., Lee, J., Jang, A.R., Lee, S., Hou, B., Cho, Y., Morris, S.M., Shin, H.S., Highly stable 3D porous heterostructures with hierarchically-coordinated octahedral transition metals for enhanced performance supercapacitors. *Nano Energy*, 39, 337–345, 2017.
5. Wong, S.I., Sunarso, J., Wong, B.T., Lin, H., Yu, A., Jia, B., Towards enhanced energy density of graphene-based supercapacitors: Current status, approaches, and future directions. *J. Power Sources*, 396, 182–206, 2018.
6. Dai, M., Zhao, D., Wu, X., Research progress on transition metal oxide based electrode materials for asymmetric hybrid capacitors. *Chin. Chem. Lett.*, 31, 2177–2188, 2020.
7. Weng, W., Lin, J., Du, Y., Ge, X., Zhou, X., Bao, J., Template-free synthesis of metal oxide hollow micro-/nanospheres via Ostwald ripening for lithium-ion batteries. *J. Mater. Chem. A*, 6, 10168–10175, 2018.

8. Jabeen, N., Hussain, A., Xia, Q., Sun, S., Zhu, J., Xia, H., High-performance 2.6 V aqueous asymmetric supercapacitors based on *in situ* formed $Na_{0.5}MnO_2$ nanosheet assembled nanowall arrays. *Adv. Mater.*, 29, 1700804, 2017.
9. Jian, X., Liu, S., Gao, Y., Tian, W., Jiang, Z., Xiao, X., Tang, H., Yin, L., Carbon-based electrode materials for supercapacitor: Progress, challenges and prospective solutions. *J. Electr. Eng.*, 4, 75–87, 2016.
10. Cai, M., Outlaw, R.A., Butler, S.M., Miller, J.R., A high density of vertically-oriented graphenes for use in electric double layer capacitors. *Carbon*, 50, 5481–5488, 2012.
11. Raza, W., Ali, F., Raza, N., Luo, Y., Kim, K.H., Yang, J., Kumar, S., Mehmood, A., Kwon, E.E., Recent advancements in supercapacitor technology. *Nano Energy*, 52, 441–473, 2018.
12. Akinwolemiwa, B., Peng, C., Chen, G.Z., Redox electrolytes in supercapacitors. *J. Electrochem. Soc.*, 162, A5054, 2015.
13. Snook, G.A., Kao, P., Best, A.S., Conducting-polymer-based supercapacitor devices and electrodes. *J. Power Sources*, 196, 1–12, 2011.
14. Namsheer, K. and Rout, C.S., Conducting polymers: A comprehensive review on recent advances in synthesis, properties and applications. *RSC Adv.*, 11, 5659–5697, 2021.
15. Zhao, Z., Xia, K., Hou, Y., Zhang, Q., Ye, Z., Lu, J., Designing flexible, smart and self-sustainable supercapacitors for portable/wearable electronics: From conductive polymers. *Chem. Soc. Rev.*, 50, 12702–12743, 2021.
16. Snook, G.A., Kao, P., Best, A.S., Conducting-polymer-based supercapacitor devices and electrodes. *J. Power Sources*, 196, 1–12, 2011.
17. Xue, Y., Chen, S., Yu, J., Bunes, B.R., Xue, Z., Xu, J., Lu, B., Zang, L., Nanostructured conducting polymers and their composites: Synthesis methodologies, morphologies and applications. *J. Mater. Chem. C*, 8, 10136–10159, 2020.
18. Ibanez, J.G., Rincón, M.E., Granados, S.G., Chahma, M.H., Quintero, O.A.J., Uribe, B.A.F., Conducting polymers in the fields of energy, environmental remediation, and chemical–chiral sensors. *Chem. Rev.*, 118, 4731–4816, 2018.
19. Jabeen, N., Xia, Q., Yang, M., Xia, H., Unique core–shell nanorod arrays with polyaniline deposited into mesoporous $NiCo_2O_4$ support for high-performance supercapacitor electrodes. *ACS Appl. Mater. Interfaces*, 8, 6093–6100, 2016.
20. Pu, J., Wang, J., Jin, X., Cui, F., Sheng, E., Wang, Z., Porous hexagonal $NiCo_2O_4$ nanoplates as electrode materials for supercapacitors. *Electrochim. Acta*, 106, 226–234, 2013.
21. Samantara, A.K. and Ratha, S., *Materials development for active/passive components of a supercapacitor: Background, present status and future perspective*, Springer, Singapore, 2017.

22. Yi, T.F., Wei, T.T., Mei, J., Zhang, W., Zhu, Y., Liu, Y.G., Luo, S., Liu, H., Lu, Y., Guo, Z., Approaching high-performance supercapacitors via enhancing pseudocapacitive nickel oxide-based materials. *Adv. Sustain. Syst.*, 4, 1900137, 2020.
23. Yuan, C., Wu, H.B., Xie, Y., Lou, X.W.D., Mixed transition-metal oxides: Design, synthesis, and energy-related applications. *Angew. Chem., Int. Ed. Engl.*, 53, 1488–1504, 2014.
24. Jabeen, N., Hussain, A., Elsaeedy, H.I., Rahman, A.U., Tarique, M., Unique hierarchical architecture of SnO_2 hexagonal interconnected nanolayered arrays as negative electrode for high performance asymmetric supercapacitors. *Mater. Chem. Phys.*, 303, 127796, 2023.
25. Majumdar, D., Maiyalagan, T., Jiang, Z., Recent progress in ruthenium oxide-based composites for supercapacitor applications. *ChemElectroChem*, 6, 4343–4372, 2019.
26. Grace, A.N. and Ramachandran, R., Advanced materials for supercapacitors, in: *Eco-Friendly Nano-Hybrid Materials for Advanced Engineering Applications*, S.A. Kumar (Ed.), pp. 99–128, Apple Academic Press, CRC Press, Taylor & Francis Group, United States, 2017.
27. Hussain, A., Nawaz, S., Jabeen, N., Zafar, R., Qaiser, M.A., Abbas, Z., Ahmed, F., Khan, M.U., Waseem, M., Aslam, S., Enhanced ferroelectric and piezoelectric response by MnO_2 added $Bi_{0.5}(K_{0.2}Na_{0.8})_{0.5}TiO_3$ ceramics. *J. Solid State Chem.*, 306, 122716, 2022.
28. Tian, S., Zhao, C., Nie, P., Wang, H., Xue, X., Lin, L., Chang, L., Electrochemical deposition enables freestanding CoNi layered double hydroxide/MnO_X electrode with enhanced electrochemical properties for asymmetric supercapacitors. *Energy Technol.*, 7, 1900680, 2019.
29. Lee, H.Y. and Goodenough, J.B., Supercapacitor behavior with KCl electrolyte. *J. Solid State Chem.*, 144, 220–223, 1999.
30. Zhang, H., Wu, A., Fu, H., Zhang, L., Liu, H., Zheng, S., Wan, H., Xu, Z., Efficient removal of Pb (II) ions using manganese oxides: The role of crystal structure. *RSC Adv.*, 7, 41228–41240, 2017.
31. Rodriguez-Romero, J., Ruiz de Larramendi, I., Goikolea, E., Nanostructured manganese dioxide for hybrid supercapacitor electrodes. *Batteries*, 8, 263, 2022.
32. Thackeray, M.M., Manganese oxides for lithium batteries. *Prog. Solid State Ch.*, 25, 1–71, 1997.
33. Jiang, Y., Ba, D., Li, Y., Liu, J., Noninterference revealing of "layered to layered" zinc storage mechanism of δ-MnO_2 toward neutral Zn–Mn batteries with superior performance. *Adv. Sci.*, 7, 1902795, 2020.
34. Kim, M., Hwang, Y., Kim, J., Process dependent graphene/MnO_2 composites for supercapacitors. *Chem. Eng. J.*, 230, 482–490, 2013.
35. Wu, M.S., Electrochemical capacitance from manganese oxide nanowire structure synthesized by cyclic voltammetric electrodeposition. *Appl. Phys. Lett.*, 87, 153102, 2005.

36. Huang, M., Zhang, Y., Li, F., Zhang, L., Ruoff, R.S., Wen, Z., Liu, Q., Self-assembly of mesoporous nanotubes assembled from interwoven ultrathin birnessite-type MnO_2 nanosheets for asymmetric supercapacitors. *Sci. Rep.*, 4, 3878, 2014.
37. Park, S., Nam, I., Kim, G.P., Han, J.W., Yi, J., Hybrid MnO_2 film with agarose gel for enhancing the structural integrity of thin film supercapacitor electrodes. *ACS Appl. Mater. Interfaces*, 5, 9908–9912, 2013.
38. Ghodbane, O., Pascal, J.L., Favier, F., Microstructural effects on charge-storage properties in MnO_2-based electrochemical supercapacitors. *ACS Appl. Mater. Interfaces*, 1, 1130–1139, 2009.
39. Brousse, T., Toupin, M., Dugas, R., Athouel, L., Crosnier, O., Belanger, D., Crystalline MnO_2 as possible alternatives to amorphous compounds in electrochemical supercapacitors. *J. Electrochem. Soc.*, 153, A2171, 2006.
40. Devaraj, S. and Munichandraiah, N., Effect of crystallographic structure of MnO_2 on its electrochemical capacitance properties. *J. Phys. Chem. C*, 112, 4406–4417, 2008.
41. Pang, S.C., Anderson, M.A., Chapman, T.W., Novel electrode materials for thin-film ultracapacitors: Comparison of electrochemical properties of sol-gel-derived and electrodeposited manganese dioxide. *J. Electrochem. Soc.*, 147, 444, 2000.
42. Jabeen, N., Xia, Q., Savilov, S.V., Aldoshin, S.M., Yu, Y., Xia, H., Enhanced pseudocapacitive performance of α-MnO_2 by cation preinsertion. *ACS Appl. Mater. Interfaces*, 8, 33732–33740, 2016.
43. Zhu, M., Meng, W., Huang, Y., Huang, Y., Zhi, C., Proton insertion enhanced pseudocapacitance based on the assembly structure of tungsten oxide. *ACS Appl. Mater. Interfaces*, 6, 18901–18910, 2014.
44. Wei, C., Xu, C., Li, B., Du, H., Nan, D., Kang, F., Anomalous effect of K ions on electrochemical capacitance of amorphous MnO_2. *J. Power Sources*, 234, 1–7, 2013.
45. Wang, J., Polleux, J., Lim, J., Dunn, B., Pseudocapacitive contributions to electrochemical energy storage in TiO_2 (anatase) nanoparticles. *J. Phys. Chem. C*, 111, 14925–14931, 2007.
46. Ou, T.M., Hsu, C.T., Hu, C.C., Synthesis and characterization of sodium-doped MnO_2 for the aqueous asymmetric supercapacitor application. *J. Electrochem. Soc.*, 162, 5124–5132, 2015.
47. Xia, H., Zhu, X., Liu, J., Liu, Q., Lan, S., Zhang, Q., Liu, X., Seo, J.K., Chen, T., Gu, L., Meng, Y.S., A monoclinic polymorph of sodium birnessite for ultrafast and ultrastable sodium ion storage. *Nat. Commun.*, 9, 1–10, 2018.
48. Athouel, L., Moser, F., Dugas, R., Crosnier, O., Belanger, D., Brousse, T., Variation of the MnO_2 birnessite structure upon charge/discharge in an electrochemical supercapacitor electrode in aqueous Na_2SO_4 electrolyte. *J. Phys. Chem. C*, 112, 7270–7277, 2008.

49. Xiao, W., Xia, H., Lu, L., Electrochemical synthesis and supercapacitive properties of ε-MnO_2 with porous/nano flaky hierarchical architectures. *J. Electrochem. Soc.*, 156, 627–633, 2009.
50. Dubal, D.P., Dhawale, D.S., Salunkhe, R.R., Lokhande, C.D., Conversion of chemically prepared interlocked cube like Mn_3O_4 to birnessite MnO_2 using electrochemical cycling. *J. Electrochem. Soc.*, 157, 812–817, 2010.
51. Zeng, Y., Yu, M., Meng, Y., Fang, P., Lu, X., Tong, Y., Iron-based supercapacitor electrodes: Advances and challenges. *Adv. Energy Mater.*, 6, 1601053, 2016.
52. Singh, A.N., Mondal, R., Rath, C., Singh, P., Electrochemical performance of delafossite, $AgFeO_2$: A pseudo-capacitive electrode in neutral aqueous Na_2SO_4 electrolyte. *J. Electrochem. Soc.*, 168, 120512, 2021.
53. Guan, C., Liu, J., Wang, Y., Mao, L., Fan, Z., Shen, Z., Zhang, H., Wang, J., Iron oxide-decorated carbon for supercapacitor anodes with ultrahigh energy density and outstanding cycling stability. *ACS Nano*, 9, 5198–5207, 2015.
54. Rowan, A.D., Patterson, C.H., Gasparov, L.V., Hybrid density functional theory applied to magnetite: Crystal structure, charge order, and phonons. *Phys. Rev. B*, 79, 205103, 2009.
55. Du, X., Wang, C., Chen, M., Jiao, Y., Wang, J., Electrochemical performances of nanoparticle Fe_3O_4/activated carbon supercapacitor using KOH electrolyte solution. *J. Phys. Chem. C*, 113, 2643–2646, 2009.
56. Zhou, G., Wang, D.W., Li, F., Zhang, L., Li, N., Wu, Z.S., Wen, L., Lu, G.Q., Cheng, H.M., Graphene-wrapped Fe_3O_4 anode material with improved reversible capacity and cyclic stability for lithium ion batteries. *Chem. Mater.*, 22, 5306–5313, 2010.
57. Sasidharan, M., Gunawardhana, N., Yoshio, M., Nakashima, K., α-Fe_2O_3 and Fe_3O_4 hollow nanospheres as high-capacity anode materials for rechargeable Li-ion batteries. *Ionics*, 19, 25–31, 2013.
58. Lin, T.W., Dai, C.S., Hung, K.C., High energy density asymmetric supercapacitor based on NiOOH/Ni_3S_2/3D graphene and Fe_3O_4/graphene composite electrodes. *Sci. Rep.*, 4, 7274, 2014.
59. Zhu, X., Zhu, Y., Murali, S., Stoller, M.D., Ruoff, R.S., Nanostructured reduced graphene oxide/Fe_2O_3 composite as a high-performance anode material for lithium ion batteries. *ACS Nano*, 5, 3333–3338, 2011.
60. Liu, J., Zheng, M., Shi, X., Zeng, H., Xia, H., Amorphous FeOOH quantum dots assembled mesoporous film anchored on graphene nanosheets with superior electrochemical performance for supercapacitors. *Adv. Funct. Mater.*, 26, 919–930, 2016.
61. Cheng, Y., Zhang, H., Lu, S., Varanasi, C.V., Liu, J., Flexible asymmetric supercapacitors with high energy and high power density in aqueous electrolytes. *Nanoscale*, 5, 1067–1073, 2013.
62. Yang, J., Li, G., Pan, Z., Liu, M., Hou, Y., Xu, Y., Dong, H., Sheng, L., Zhao, X., Qiu, Y., Zhang, Y., All-solid-state high-energy asymmetric supercapacitors

enabled by three-dimensional mixed-valent MnO_x nanospike and graphene electrodes. *ACS Appl. Mater. Interfaces*, 7, 22172–22180, 2005.

63. Khomenko, V., Pinero, E.R., Frackowiak, E., Beguin, F., High-voltage asymmetric supercapacitors operating in aqueous electrolyte. *Appl. Phys. A*, 82, 567–573, 2006.
64. Jin, W.H., Cao, G.T., Sun, J.Y., Hybrid supercapacitor based on MnO_2 and columned FeOOH using Li_2SO_4 electrolyte solution. *J. Power Sources*, 175, 686–691, 2008.
65. Cottineau, T., Toupin, M., Delahaye, T., Brousse, T., Belanger, D., Nanostructured transition metal oxides for aqueous hybrid electrochemical supercapacitors. *Appl. Phys. A*, 82, 599–606, 2006.
66. Jia, R., Zhu, F., Sun, S., Zhai, T., Xia, H., Dual support ensuring high-energy supercapacitors via high-performance $NiCo_2S_4@Fe_2O_3$ anode and working potential enlarged MnO_2 cathode. *J. Power Sources*, 341, 427–434, 2017.
67. Sinha, P., Banerjee, S. *et al.*, Transition metal oxide/activated carbon-based composites as electrode materials for supercapacitors, in: *Handbook of Nanocomposite Supercapacitor Materials*, K.K. Kar (Ed.), pp. 145–178, Springer Nature, Switzerland AG, 2020.
68. Gujar, T.P., Shinde, V.R., Lokhande, C.D., Han, S.H., Electrosynthesis of Bi_2O_3 thin films and their use in electrochemical supercapacitors. *J. Power Sources*, 161, 1479–1485, 2006.
69. Zheng, F.L., Li, G.R., Ou, Y.N., Wang, Z.L., Su, C.Y., Tong, Y.X., Synthesis of hierarchical rippled Bi_2O_3 nanobelts for supercapacitor applications. *ChemComm*, 46, 5021–5023, 2010.
70. Wang, S.X., Jin, C.C., Qian, W.J., Bi_2O_3 with activated carbon composite as a supercapacitor electrode. *J. Alloys Compd.*, 615, 12–17, 2014.

10

Aqueous Redox-Active Electrolytes

Ranganatha S.

Dept. of Chemistry, Presidency University, Rajanakunte, Bengaluru, India

Abstract

It is necessary to improve the supercapacitors' energy particulars due to low energy storage capacity and charge/discharge tolerance. Electrolytes are considered to be an important part of the output delivery of electrochemical supercapacitors. Organic electrolytes are being used in the majority of commercially marketed electrochemical supercapacitors, which has some advantages, such as a high operating voltage. Organic alternatives, on the other hand, are more expensive than aqueous ones. Electrolytes are costly, combustible, and hazardous in a few instances. It is a safe bet to say that. Even though aqueous electrolytes are subjected to a low workable voltage, they exhibit far quicker charge carrier rates than non-aqueous electrolytes and do improve the efficiency of supercapacitors. As a result, research works are being done concentrating voltage and energy density in supercapacitor devices by expanding the workable potential range of aqua-based electrolytes. This book chapter summarizes the most recent developments related to the concerned interest and gives an overview of aqua-based electrolytes.

Keywords: Supercapacitors, electrolytes, aqueous electrolytes, non-aqueous electrolytes, polymer electrolytes, gel electrolytes

10.1 Introduction

Global warming is accelerating, and the world's access to fossil fuels is diminishing. Society must adapt to sustainable resources which are reusable. Because of this, advancement in sustainable energy technologies has been seen as a significant concern around the world. Most of these reusable energy resources are reliant on weather conditions around the country.

Email: kamath.ranganath@gmail.com

Inamuddin, Tariq Altalhi and Sayed Mohammed Adnan (eds.) Electroceramics for High Performance Supercapacitors, (233–254) © 2024 Scrivener Publishing LLC

Electrochemical supercapacitors/ultracapacitors, fuel cells, and batteries are the most competent and widely employed among various energy storage technologies [1]. The greatest common feature of these systems is the phenomenon taking place at electrode/electrolyte interfaces in these devices.

Supercapacitors have gained much interest in academia and industry because of the appreciable rate of energy delivery along with high cyclability to par with fuel cells and batteries [2]. Electrochemical supercapacitors are grouped into three kinds concerning their charge storage process: (i) EDLC or electric double layer, (ii) pseudo, and (iii) hybrid [3]. Activated carbon which behaves as EDLC is used in practically all commercially available supercapacitors because of their technical maturity. Compared with rechargeable fuel cells and battery systems, supercapacitors face the most critical obstacle of low values for storage capacity (10 Watt hour per kg) [4]. As a result, massive investigations made to improve the energy density of these systems [5].

The charge storage of supercapacitors is directly proportional to capacitance and the square of operating voltage. As a result, increasing capacitance and working potential are seen as possible strategies for improving high-charge storage supercapacitors. By selecting high-capacity materials as electrodes and an electrolyte possessing a high working voltage, a high energy density can be achieved. As voltage (square of) and energy stored are directly proportional enhancing the workable voltage range rather than improving the specific capacitance seems to be a successful approach to obtaining higher charge storage. Therefore, establishing a novel electrolyte with a wide voltage range is the primary parameter to consider when searching for novel negative and positive electrodes.

10.2 Electrolyte Requirements for High-Performance Supercapacitors

10.2.1 Conductivity

Electrolytes play a key role in imparting supercapacitor device characteristics such as power and energy density, cycle life, and safety. The performance of electrolytes is strongly ruled by the factors of conductivity and ionic mobility. Aqueous electrolytes stand superior compared to the non-aqueous and solid ones as they possess low dynamic viscosity. The conductivity of the electrolyte is dependent on the properties of species like ionic mobility, the concentration of charge carriers' elementary charge, and the magnitude of charges carried. All the properties are sensitive to the solvation effect, migration of solvated ions, and lattice energy of the salt [6]. Hence, solvents, additives, and salts will significantly influence the overall conductivity of the electrolytes.

10.2.2 Salt Effect

Each type of salt is typical in producing conductivity as ionic species interact differently with the solvent with varied ionic sizes. In addition, the concentration of the salt determines the conductivity. The optimum concentration of salt is significant as the number of free ions is ascendant at lower concentrations which results in higher conductivity. This is also true in the case where there is a balance between viscosity and free ions. In the situation at a very high concentration of salt, there can association of neutral ions with that of cations and anions which decreases the conductivity by minimizing the available free ions. Also, in the case of highly viscous ionic liquid electrolytes, with the increase in solution concentration, conductivity falls [7–14].

10.2.3 Solvent Effect

In the case of liquid and gel electrolytes, the composition becomes very vital in managing the conductivity. The properties of an electrolyte like viscosity and dielectric constant greatly control the conductivity as viscosity is associated with the mobility of the ions in salt and dielectric constant is associated with the dissociation of salts. As per the literature solvents exhibiting appreciable viscosity also possess high values for dielectric constants [15]. So, while designing supercapacitor devices it is recommended to consider a mixture of solvents with low viscosity (e.g., dimethyl carbonate) and high dielectric constant (e.g., ethylene carbonate). Research reports show that solvent systems of single component exhibit relatively lower conductivity than that of binary solvent-based electrolytes. This advocates the superior conductivity of solvent systems with high dielectric constant and low viscosity. Kamath *et al.* [16] investigated the kinetic and thermodynamic factors to formulate the solvent systems for high-power sodium-ion batteries and they found ethylene carbonate–dimethyl carbonate and ethylene carbonate–ethyl methyl carbonate was superior.

10.2.4 Electrochemical Stability

The two important supercapacitor characteristics, namely safety and cycle life are mainly linked to electrochemical stability. The electrochemical stability window can be equated to the lower and upper limits of electrolytic redox reactions. This stability is not only limited to the composition of the electrolyte but also to the compatibility of the electrode with that of the electrolytic solution. Electrochemical study at varying temperatures with the help of analytical techniques, such as cyclic voltammetry and linear sweep voltammetry, is very important [6].

10.2.5 Thermal Stability

During the testing cycle supercapacitor, devices encounter safety concerns due to heat release and operating temperature, which may lead to electrolytic decomposition. This makes thermal stability a major issue to address during the study. Device thermal stability is sensitive to two parameters: electrode/electrolyte interaction and thermal stability of electrolyte. Constituents in the electrolyte, including additive if any, decides the thermal stability of the electrolyte which can be studied with the help of thermal techniques like DSA/DSC [17–24].

10.3 Effect of the Electrolyte on Supercapacitor Performance

Concerning supercapacitors, liquid or solid electrolytic materials are one of the most important parts, since they possess current carrying capacity, allowing for charge balancing during the electrochemical process [25, 26]. Electrolyte's ionic conductivity which can affect the electrochemical series resistance of the supercapacitors, and stability range (electrochemical), which determines the operating voltage of the supercapacitors, are the two key features of electrolytes for supercapacitors. Therefore, as mentioned in the previous sections, both energy storage and the rate of energy delivery will rise. As a result, for improved capacitive performance in supercapacitors, electrolytes with a broader workable and stable voltage range and higher ionic conductance will be preferred. The quality of the electrolyte which constitutes, the radius and nature of the ion, strength, and ion-solvent behavior, all have a substantial impact on supercapacitor performance. Also, the action of electrolyte ions and electrodes has a substantial impact on supercapacitor capacitive performance. The mismatch in electrolytic ion size and the carbonaceous electrode's porosity, for example, imparts a significant impact on charge storage ability in the case of supercapacitors.

Electrolytic solutions in supercapacitors aid in the stabilization of other critical supercapacitor properties. Voltage drop, rate capability, temperature stability, number of charge/discharges, discharge when no load and environmental benignity are all factors to consider when using supercapacitors in practice. Figure 10.1 depicts the influence of electrolytes on different supercapacitor characteristics, which affect the device's strength.

In the representation, the first circle contains supercapacitors with electrolytes; the second circle contains electrolytes and electrochemical supercapacitors, and circle 3 contains electrolytes and electrochemical supercapacitors. The parameters that strongly influence the functioning of the supercapacitor are found in the second circular region. Electrolyte factors influencing the parameters in the third circular are shown (circle 2). Share carriage and movement of electrolyte ions and the resistance they have for mobility, for example, impact directly influence supercapacitor electrochemical series resistance (ESR) (see Figure 10.1). The parameters within each circle, on the other hand, affect each other. As depicted in the second circle, the more the series resistance lower will be the rate of energy delivery. It demonstrates that the qualities of electrolytic solutions specified in the third circular region are critical in determining supercapacitor performance in one way or another. Different electrolytes are designed and

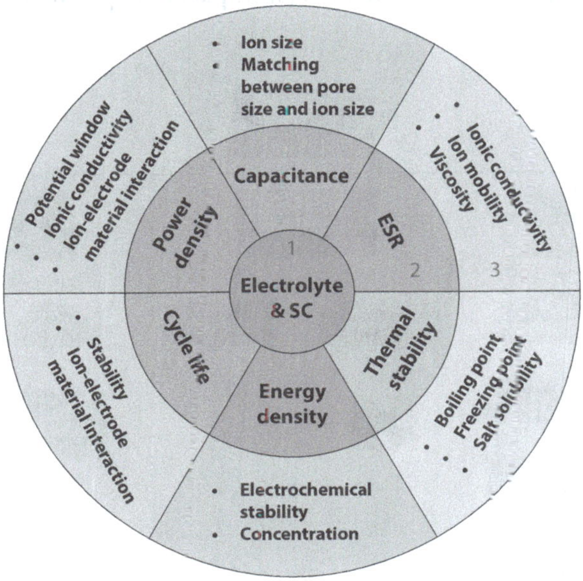

Figure 10.1 Influence of electrolyte nature on various supercapacitor characteristics (reused with permission [27]).

published by scientists for Supercapacitors. Based on its physical state it is primarily liquid and solid state. Based on aqua, organic or ionic nature, liquid electrolytes can be classified. Electrolytes based on polymers, gel polymers, and inorganic-based solids are three types of solid or quasi-solid electrolytes [27, 28]. The schematic in Figure 10.2 depicts the general classification of electrolytes. So far, no single electrolyte has just been found to meet all of the requirements for supercapacitors. Between the two crucial electrolyte properties of conductance and stability range, there is always a trade-off. Supercapacitors with aqueous electrolytes, for example, have significant conductance and charge storage in comparison. However, its stability range is restricted by the electrolyte's small breakdown (One-volt limit), ending up with the supercapacitors with a small value for energy storage. Supercapacitors with electrolytes sourced from organic or ionic sources, on the other hand, can be operated at greater voltages and have significant energy storage than those aqua based. Furthermore, the solid-state has the benefit of not having the outflow problems associated with liquid electrolytes, although they often have lesser ionic conductivity. As a result, each electrolyte possesses its inherent benefits and limitations.

Therefore, many methodologies are used to formulate novel and effective electrolytes with a broader working voltage range, and better conductance with a wider temperature range of operation. This will allow researchers to take advantage of the beneficial impacts of specific electrolytes on

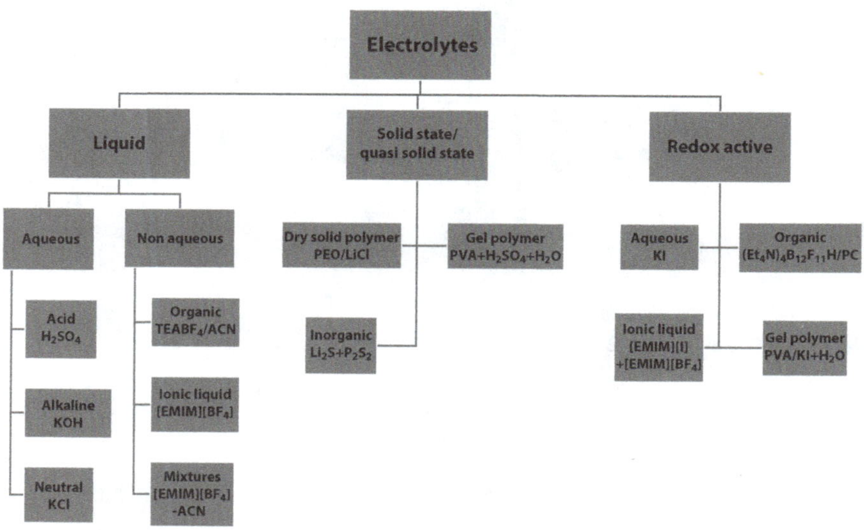

Figure 10.2 Classification of electrolytes for supercapacitors (reused with permission [27]).

supercapacitor performance metrics like energy storage, rate of energy delivery, etc. Detailed outlook on typical electrolytic forms for supercapacitors, like aqua and non-aqua-based electrolytes, will be presented in the following subsections.

10.3.1 Aqueous Electrolytes

Because of their narrow voltage window, aqueous electrolytes are usually not a great choice for practical supercapacitor devices when it comes to energy density studies. This could explain why most practical supercapacitors employ nonaqueous (organic) electrolytes rather than the inorganic electrolyte. Electrolytes in an aqueous solution are less effective than electrolytes in an aqueous solution. Even though aqueous electrolytes have insufficient cell voltage, they have been extensively used in the literature since 1997 as they appear to be less expensive and may be easily managed in the laboratory.

To keep moisture out of ionic liquids and organic electrolytes, extensive purification processes in a highly restricted environment are required. These characteristics of aqua-based electrolytes help to understand the design and function of supercapacitors. Aqueous electrolytes, in general, have a very high conductivity of higher magnitude than organic or ionic liquid electrolytes. The aqueous electrolyte's greater conductivity makes it ideal for lowering solution resistance leading to supercapacitors with much higher power density.

Some typical factors should be considered when evaluating the comprehensive performance of aqua-based electrolytes, like the original size of the ions and hydrated counterparts, ionic movement modifying the electrolytic conductance, and charge storage. Acidic, basic, and neutral are the three types of aqueous electrolytes. KOH, H_2SO_4, and sodium sulfate are commonly used aqueous electrolytes, respectively.

10.3.2 Acidic Electrolytes

Because of extraordinarily significant conductance (0.8 cm^{-1} at room temperature for 1 molar sulphuric acid), sulphuric acid is a very commonly utilized aqueous acid electrolyte in supercapacitors [29]. Because of the direct relation between concentration and the ionic conductance of the electrolytic solution, appropriate molar concentrations for achieving appreciable conductance at a given temperature have already been researched. When the concentration of the electrolyte is high or low, conductance drops quickly. As a result, the majority of research investigations, particularly for carbon-based supercapacitors, use a 1 M H_2SO_4 solution.

10.3.2.1 Sulfuric Acid Electrolyte-Based EDLC and Pseudocapacitors

Many researchers recently observed the specific capacitance found with the electrolyte sulphuric acid is substantially greater compared to that of specific capacitance obtained in a neutral for carbon-based capacitors (EDLCs). Furthermore, the equivalent series resistance is substantially lesser compared to the neutral one because of the high ionic conductivity of H_2SO_4. A group investigated electric double-layer capacitor behavior w.r.t. activated carbon in the electrolyte of sulphuric acid and discovered higher electrolyte conductivity improving the specific capacitance [30]. Many publications over the last few years have claimed that carbon-based materials can give capacity in the scale of 100-300 Farads per gram. When compared to commercial electrolytes, certain reported values are frequently greater. Changes in specific capacitance could mimic the unique interactions between electrode materials and ions of electrolyte generated by different electrolytes. As previously stated, charge storage of EDLCs is severely decreased due to the limited voltage range of aqua electrolyte. So, massive exercises are considered to improve the electrochemical supercapacitor storage capacity by studying alternative approaches, such as exploiting pseudocapacitive behavior in electrodes.

The sulphuric acid, when employed as the electrolyte, contributes to the pseudocapacitance owing to redox-active reactions associated with the carbon surface's functionalities, adding to the usual double-layer capacitance. Adding various heteroatoms to the carbon materials surface, such as nitrogen, oxygen, and boron, could improve the pseudocapacitance contributions [31]. Heteroatom doping not only boosts charge storage capacity with improving cyclability in aqueous electrolytes but at higher potentials too. In an aqua electrolyte, redox-type electrodes, such as oxides and sulfides of metal, and polymers that electrically conduct have substantially greater expected capacity values than carbonaceous materials [32]. Because metallic compounds are extremely responsive to the environment and acidity/basicity, they are often unstable in electrolytes with lower pH values below 7, limiting their usage in commercial goods. Ruthenium oxide (RuO_2), as is widely known, is one of the superior electrodes that has been thoroughly investigated for its pseudocapacitance wherein sulphuric acid is the electrolyte. Because of the ease with which the proton can be inserted into the amorphous structure, non-crystalline Ruthenium oxide produces a significant capacitance of 10^3 Farads/gram in the electrolytes of low pH. Regrettably, because of higher prices and less availability of Ru sources, their practical application has been limited.

10.3.2.2 H_2SO_4 Electrolyte-Based Hybrid Supercapacitors

Constructing a hybrid supercapacitor is a very efficient and reliable technique to boost energy storage in the electrolytes of the water base. The highest symmetric supercapacitor EMF employing the same electrodes in a water-based electrolyte is limited due to the gas evolution reactions. Asymmetric supercapacitors combine two alternate electrodes in distinct working potentials, resulting in a broader functional voltage range in an aqueous electrolyte. There have been many studies on the performances of symmetric supercapacitors in electrolytes of the type strongly acidic nature, as like combination of carbonaceous material along with metal oxides of lead and ruthenium, and carbon with varied weight and characteristics in the electrodes. In the acidic electrolyte, the carbon/PbO_2 asymmetric supercapacitor supplied an energy density of 25–30 Watt hour per kilo gram, showing a significantly higher value compared to symmetric carbonaceous capacitors (3–6 Wh/kg). Polymers that are electrically conducting in nature and carbonaceous asymmetric supercapacitors, like metal oxide, have provided enough energy density for commercial use. In the case of polyaniline employed as a +ve, carbonaceous material as –ve one at a wider voltage window (negative 1 to positive 1 V), storage capacity may reach up to 11.46 Wh/kg [33]. Polyaniline has found restricted application in the real world because of weak stability, despite having a larger energy density than symmetric carbon capacitors. The utilization of sulphuric acid in the case of polymer systems can increase stability. In contrast to polymer in the solid state, liquid H_2SO_4 has great thermal stability. So, the stability and energy density of supercapacitors in liquid-based electrolytes may be increased. The utilization of sulphuric acid as the electrolyte in the case of polymer-based electrodes can increase stability. Considering all these characteristics, there is a scope to enhance the charge storage of supercapacitors when liquid-based electrolytes are employed. In the case of ruthenium oxide and carbon-based symmetric electrochemical supercapacitors, sulphuric acid gives a storage capacity of roughly 20 Watt-hour per kilogram, which is double compared to the electrolyte related to polymer gel low pH [34].

10.3.3 Alkaline Electrolytes

Electrolytes of alkaline nature have been used widely by the research community because acidic electrolytes are typically not suited for various economical metallic and metal compounds (Ni, Co, Eu, etc.). Due to the much higher conductance of about 0.6 Siemen per centimeter, potassium hydroxide (KOH) is the much often utilized aqueous alkaline electrolyte.

10.3.3.1 Alkaline Electrolyte-Based EDLC and Pseudocapacitors

In aqueous KOH, the charge storage capacity of carbonaceous material-based devices is comparable with sulphuric acid electrolytes. As a result, significant effort has been made to improve EDLC material energy density in the basic electrolyte by raising capacity and increasing working potential. Few of the approaches include:

1. doping some pseudocapacitance functional groups into carbon materials to increase specific capacitance,
2. finding out highly capacitive electrode materials of pseudocapacitive in nature,
3. developing novel hybrid materials which can contribute both EDLC and pseudocapacitance, and
4. designing high-performance asymmetric supercapacitors possessing a wide voltage range.

As stated earlier, redox reactions associated with functionalized carbon materials take place as a result of electrolyte ions interacting with the grafted reactive groups. According to reports, potassium hydroxide was found to be helpful for the doping or functioning of carbon-based electrodes to improvise pseudocapacitance. Possession of reactive moiety with oxygen w.r.t. carbonaceous materials can improve the overall capacitance of the electrode by increasing the pseudocapacitance contribution in potassium hydroxide electrolyte [35]. It is widely understood that the interaction of ions of electrolyte and electrode plays an important part in pseudocapacitance contribution as a result of this. Some oxides of metal, sulfides, and hydroxides, like Co_3O_4, MnO_2, NiO, $NiCo_2O_4$, CoS, nickel hydroxide, etc., have extraordinarily high predicted energy storage and are studied for supercapacitor usage in potassium hydroxide, e.g., in the electrolyte of 2 M potassium hydroxide, charge storage of Co_3O_4 nanosized films attained extraordinarily greater values of about one thousand and four hundred Farads per gram [36]. In the same way, while metal sulfides related to cobalt, manganese, nickel, etc. possess lesser value for faradaic capacitance in potassium hydroxide, electrochemical conversion of sulfides into various electroactive products like nickel hydroxide, cobalt hydroxide may increase the capacitance of electrodes. The operating temperature and supercapacitor working possibly be influenced by parameters related to electrolytes including the type of ion, ionic size, and concentrations. Because the pH of potassium hydroxide electrolyte will be high, corrosion of the surface of the electrode may happen during the usage of high electrolyte concentration is utilized. As a result, optimizing the strength of electrolyte in order in minimising current collector corrosion. The overall performance of an electrochemical supercapacitor is sensitive to the ionic nature and concentration in the electrolyte. Insertion and disinsertion of the electrolytic ion can determine the extent to which the material's pseudocapacitance. Because of Li^+ ions' small ionic radius, Misnon *et al.* [37] were able to produce greater energy characteristics of manganese oxide in lithium hydroxide compared to potassium hydroxide as the electrolyte The smaller the ion, easy is the intercalation and de-intercalation which leads to result in good faradaic processes. Moreover, the influence of different electrolytes of water base on $NiCo_2O_4$ nanomaterials in a wider temperature range was examined, with potassium hydroxide electrolyte obtaining the maximum energy density when compared to sodium hydroxide and lithium hydroxide. The ion mobility in KOH increased dramatically due to the reduced size of Potassium ions, facilitating quick redox reactions of electrode and electrolyte [39, 40]. In addition to cations, anions pose a crucial role in electrochemical supercapacitor function. A research group investigated the effect of negative ions on the charge storage behavior of potassium-based alkaline (potassium hydroxide) and inert (potassium chloride) in depth [41]. They observed less bulky hydroxide ions could improve the faradaic processes of sulfide of cobalt and graphene composites with potassium hydroxide. There are fewer reports accessible for comparative investigations of a variety of alkaline electrolytic phenomena and therefore mechanisms stay unclear

Pseudocapacitive materials have low cyclic stability in alkaline electrolytes in contrast with EDLC materials, which could be due to the electrolyte's recurrent faradaic reactions. A previous study looked into using carbon materials to extend the cycle life in redox-type electrodes (composites). Composites expanded the operating potential range of alkaline electrolytes while also improving electrode stability. Fe_2O_3 nanodots/N-doped graphene hybrid, for example, exhibited significantly high cycle life stable up to 75.3 percent over 1 lakh charge/discharges in potassium hydroxide [42], which could be owing to the pyrrolic Nitrogen atoms in graphene promoting the composite's transfer of electron processes.

10.3.3.2 Alkaline Electrolyte-Based Hybrid Supercapacitors

For hybrid supercapacitors, a series of alkaline solutions have been researched to boost charge storage over a long voltage window. When asymmetric electrodes are utilized, the applied potential of potassium hydroxide can be increased by 1.7 V. In the KOH, asymmetric carbon/metal hydroxides (carbon/nickel hydroxide 1.7 V and carbon/Cobalt hydroxide) 1.6 Volts) and C/Ruthenium oxide (1.4 Volts) capacitors are seen to provide remarkable capacity storage. Most hybrid systems could produce greater capacity storage in the range of 20 and 40 Watt-hour per kilogram as a result of their long voltage range and strong redox reactions, which were close to the values related to that of lithium-ion systems. The performance and operating voltage of an asymmetric device were improved by *in situ* synthesis of electroactive colloids of vanadium with high cation utilization [43]. As a result, building an asymmetric hybrid supercapacitor is an economical solution to enhance the working potential, and it might be utilized in KOH electrolyte applications.

10.3.4 Neutral Electrolyte

Neutral electrolytes have also been thoroughly studied as compared to alkaline and acid electrolytes because of the wider working potential range and lower corrosive properties. A variety of inert electrolytic solutions like lithium chloride, lithium sulfite, sodium sulfate, sodium chloride, potassium chloride, potassium sulfate, and others, have been employed in supercapacitor research to date. Na_2SO_4 neutral electrolyte, in particular, has demonstrated favorable electrochemical responses for electrodes, particularly pseudocapacitance materials.

10.3.4.1 Neutral Electrolyte-Based EDLC and Pseudocapacitors

Compared to the alkaline electrolyte, smaller H^+ and OH^- concentrations in neutral ones allow the voltage of water-splitting reactions to get pushed to a different voltage range, enabling the working voltage range to get extended. At higher cell EMF of 1.6 V in 0.5 Molar sodium sulfate, Demarconnay *et al.* showed outstanding cyclic stability w.r.t. symmetric carbonaceous device even after 10,000 charged-discharge cycles [44]. Because of the smaller ionic size in the Li_2SO_4 electrolyte, the EMF of the device should be able to increase to 2.2 V for the carbonaceous system (Table 10.1).

Because Li^+ ions are smaller, they can speed up the charge storage process in the interface of carbon electrodes/electrolytes and prevent gases like oxygen and hydrogen from escaping at higher potentials. In comparison to H_2SO_4 and KOH electrolytes, the reported working potential of inert electrolytes concerning carbon-based electrode systems is high with less harsh chemically. In a neutral electrolyte, symmetric carbon supercapacitors have been found as a possible contender for devices with increased charge storage and fewer environmental consequence. There have been some similar investigations on the systems with inert electrolytes of different metals, including lithium, potassium, and sodium, to see how ions affect capacitive performance. Several researchers [45, 46] investigated the carbon-based

Table 10.1 Ionic sizes and their conductance values.

Ion type size	Bare ion	Hydrated ion size	Gibbs energy (kcal/mol)	Ionic conductance
	(Å)	(Å)		(S cm^2 mol^{-1})
H^+	1.15	2.80		350.1
Li^+	0.60	3.82	138.4	38.69
Na^+	0.95	3.58	162.3	50.11
K^+	1.33	3.31	179.9	73.5
NH_4	1.48	3.31	–	73.7
Mg^{2+}	0.72	4.28	–	106.12
Ca^{2+}	1.00	4.12	–	119
Ba^{2+}	1.35	4.04	–	127.8
Cl–	1.81	3.32	–	75.31
NO_3–	2.64	3.35	–	71.42
$SO_4{}^2$–	2.90	3.79	–	160.0
OH^-	1.76	3.00	–	198
ClO_4–	2.92	3.38	–	67.3
PO_4–	2.23	3.39	–	207
CO_3–	2.66	3.94	–	138.6

compounds in inert electrolytes and their performance is in the following sequence lithium sulfate > sodium sulfate > potassium sulfate.

Electrochemical supercapacitors' function is influenced not only by the nature of the electrolyte used but also by the preparation of the electrode and conditions at which analysis is carried out, such as rate of scanning, temperature, and potential range. Accordingly, more investigation is necessary to analyze the effect of electrolytes on electrochemical supercapacitor functioning.

In neutral electrolytes, faradaic materials like RuO_2, MnO_2, and vanadium oxide demonstrated good electrochemical supercapacitor performance. The most prevalent pseudocapacitive compound is MnO_2, which has been extensively researched in the inert electrolytic solution. In neutral electrolytes, Li *et al.* [47] emphasized the sequence of charge storage and capacitance of

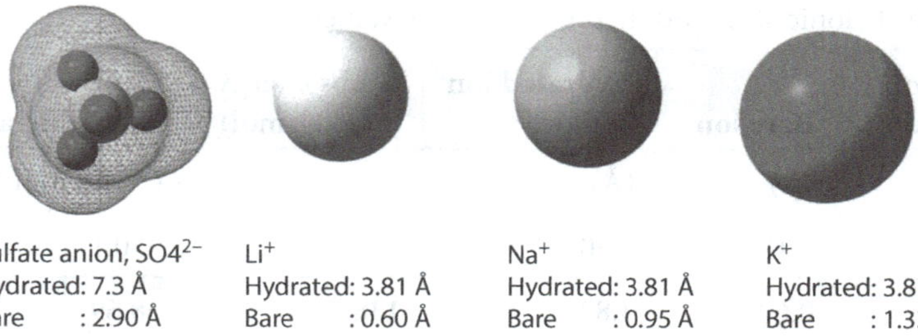

Figure 10.3 Ionic dimension and size in water-based electrolytes as obtained by modeling (reused with permission [48]).

porous manganese oxide electrodes as follows: $Li_2SO_4 > Na_2SO_4 > K_2SO_4$ is the order of importance. This behavior seems to be linked to the sizes of alkali metals both in normal and hydrated conditions, Lithium Sodium and Potassium ions, implying smaller the ionic size better it is functioning. Fic *et al.* demonstrated the same behavior in the case of ruthenium oxide in various inert electrolytes. It is found that ionic motion increases in the sequence of Li^+ Na^+ K^+. Higher movement of ionic Lithium is advantageous to improvise altogether functioning of the faradaic electrodes, according to the shape and size of the ion (sourced from modeling) [45], as illustrated in Figure 10.3.

10.3.4.2 Neutral Electrolyte-Based Hybrid Supercapacitors

Neutral electrolytes were used in devices of different positive and negative electrodes to provide a larger variety of possible windows for achieving enhanced charge storage. Devices with Manganese oxide electrodes electrochemical supercapacitors provided sufficient specific capacitance, their working potential, and total charge storage are limited. In many situations, a device potential of around 1 Volt was used. The MnO_2 cell potential can be greatly improved by using carbon materials (activated carbon and CNT) as the negative electrode [49]. Symmetric devices with manganese phosphate electrodes, on the other hand, may be operated at an extraordinarily high voltage (1.8 V) in the Na_2SO_4 electrolyte, resulting in a high charge storage of about 19 Watt-hour per kilogram [50]. Devices with the same and different types of positive and negative electrodes have generated significant charge storage in an inert electrolytic solution and not in the alkaline. In neutral electrolytes, the rationale in the case of $Mn_3\,(PO_4)_2$'s improved performance and great cycle stability is still unknown. Asymmetric capacitors in inert electrolytic solutions were studied using a variety of cathodes and anodes, some of which are included in Table 10.2. In the 1.5–2.0 V range,

Table 10.2 Few significant water-based electrolytic supercapacitor devices and their output.

Water-based electrolyte/ concentration	Electrode	Cs (F/g)	E ($W\,h\,kg^{-1}$)	Voltage range (V)	Ref
Sulfuric acid/1 M Sulfuric acid/0.5 Molar	RuO_2-carbon nano-onion RuO_2-graphene	570 479	10.62 20.28	1 1.2	[41] [51]
H_2SO_4/1 M	Graphene-mesoporous PANI	510	133	1	[52]
Potassium hydroxide/6 M	Graphene	303	6.5	1	[53]
Potassium hydroxide/2 M	$NiCo_2O_4$	1647.6	38	0.41	[54]
Potassium hydroxide/1 M	$Ni(OH)_2$/graphene	160	48	1.5	[55]
Potassium hydroxide/6 M	Iron nanosheets/graphene	720	140	1.2	[56]
KCl/3 M	Ni $(OH)_2$	718	–	0.5	[57]
NaOH/1 M	Fe_2O_3	178	–	0.5	[58]
Na_2SO_4/1 M	CNT/V_2O_5 nanocomposite//MnO_2/C		16	1.6	[59]
Na_2SO_4/1 M	Hydrous RuO_2	56.66	18.77	1.6	[60]

the voltage range of this set of asymmetric supercapacitors is wider than that of electrolytes of non-neutral pH. The benefit of inert water-based electrolytes is that they not only solve supercapacitor device corrosion concerns but also provide a cheap and benign option for improving the output of supercapacitors with higher working potential and charge storage. The charge/discharge stability of supercapacitors w.r.t. inert aqua electrolytic solutions is currently a developing field.

10.4 Conclusion and Future Research Directions

To summarize, this contribution provides a thorough examination of the evolution and current practices in water-based electrolytic solutions for electrochemical supercapacitors. The impact of these electrolytic solutions parameters, such as conductance, size of ion, workable voltage range, and other factors on supercapacitor output specifications, such as cyclic stability, energy density, specific capacitance, and temperature stability is thoroughly examined. The effect of the interplay between electrodes and electrolytes has been examined in particular. The current discussion demonstrates electrochemical supercapacitors, depending on neutral aqueous electrolytes give various advantages over other electrolyte systems, including low cost, environmental friendliness, and safety. Despite significant progress in this field, numerous challenges remain, like the lesser charge storage and working potential associated with water-based electrolytes.

To address the above issues, future exploration should be in the following path:

1. Extending electrolyte stable potential window values (ESPW): The ESPW values of aqueous electrolytes are determined by the ions which it is composed with. As a result, discovering novel water-based conducting electrolytic salt along with optimization could help to improve the electrolyte stable potential window values.
2. Increasing the effective area of the surface of the faradaic electrode materials: Because energy density is mostly determined by capacitance, the performance of supercapacitors might be improved by increasing the electrode material's charge capacity. The symmetric and asymmetric pseudocapacitive material-based supercapacitors bring better energy density in aqueous electrolytes than EDLC.

3. Building water-based electrolytic solution purity: In a few situations, impurity associated with electrolytes has a detrimental impact on the working voltage range which results in automatic discharging. As a result, developing the purest form of electrolytic solution to increase supercapacitor output is highly considered.

References

1. Ramachandran, R., Saranya, M., Grace, A.N., Wang, F., MnS nanocomposites based on doped graphene: Simple synthesis by a wet chemical route and improved electrochemical properties as an electrode material for supercapacitors. *RSC Adv.*, 7, 2249, 2017.
2. Yu, G., Xie, X., Pan, L., Bao, Z., Cui, Y., Hybrid nanostructured materials for high-performance electrochemical capacitors. *Nano Energy*, 2, 213, 2013.
3. Ramachandran, R., Saranya, M., Kollu, P., Ragupathy, B.P.C., Jeong, S.K., Grace, A.N., Solvothermal synthesis of zinc sulfide decorated graphene (ZnS/G) nanocomposites for novel supercapacitor electrodes. *Electrochim. Acta*, 178, 647, 2005.
4. Conway, B.E., *Electrochemical supercapacitors: Scientific fundamentals and technological applications*, Kluwer Academic/Plenum, New York, 1999.
5. Xia, L., Yu, L., Chen, G.Z., Electrolytes for electrochemical energy storage. *Mater. Chem. Front.*, 1, 584, 2017.
6. Xu, K., Nonaqueous liquid electrolytes for lithium-based rechargeable batteries. *Chem. Rev.*, 104, 4303, 2004.
7. Ponrouch, A., Marchante, E., Courty, M., Tarascon, J.M., Palacín, M.R., In search of an optimized electrolyte for Na-ion batteries. *Energy Environ. Sci.*, 5, 8572, 2012.
8. Bhide, A., Hofmann, J., Katharina, D.A., Janek, J., Adelhelm, P., Electrochemical stability of non-aqueous electrolytes for sodium-ion batteries and their compatibility with $Na_{0.7}CoO_2$. *Phys. Chem. Chem. Phys.*, 16, 1987, 2014.
9. Wang, C.H., Yeh, Y.W., Wongittharom, N., Wang, Y.C., Tseng, C.J., Lee, S.W., Chang, W.S., Chang, J.K., Rechargeable Na/$Na_{0.44}MnO_2$ cells with ionic liquid electrolytes containing various sodium solutes. *J. Power Sources*, 274, 1016, 2015.
10. Feng, J., Zhang, Z., Li, L., Yang, J., Xiong, S., Qian, Y., Ether-based non flammable electrolyte for room temperature sodium battery. *J. Power Sources*, 284, 222, 2015.
11. Wu, F., Zhu, N., Bai, Y., Liu, L., Zhou, H., Wu, C., Highly safe ionic liquid electrolytes for sodium-ion battery: Wide electrochemical window and good thermal stability. *ACS Appl. Mater. Interfaces*, 8, 21381, 2016.

12. Pope, C.R., Kar, M., MacFarlane, D.R., Armand, M., Forsyth, M., O'Dell, L.A., Ion dynamics in a mixed-cation alkoxy-ammonium ionic liquid electrolyte for sodium device applications. *ChemPhysChem*, 17, 3187, 2016.
13. Moreno, S.J., Maresca, G., Panero, S., Scrosati, B., Appetecchi, G.B., Sodium-conducting ionic liquid-based electrolytes. *Electrochem. Commun.*, 43, 1, 2014.
14. Wongittharom, N., Lee, T.-C., Wang, C.-H., Wang, Y.-C., Chang, J.-K., Electrochemical performance of Na/$NaFePO_4$ sodium-ion batteries with ionic liquid electrolytes. *J. Mater. Chem. A*, 2, 5655, 2014.
15. Che, H., Chen, S., Xie, Y., Wang, H., Amine, K., Liao, X.-Z., Ma., Z.-F., Electrolyte design strategies and research progress for room-temperature sodium-ion batteries. *Energy Environ. Sci.*, 10, 1075, 2017.
16. Kamath, G., Cutler, R.W., Deshmukh, S.A., Fard, M.S., Parrish, R., Huether, J., Butt, D.P., Xiong, H., Sankaranarayanan, S.K.R.S., In silico based rank-order determination and experiments on nonaqueous electrolytes for sodium ion battery applications. *J. Phys. Chem. C*, 118, 13406, 2014.
17. Chancelier, L., Diallo, A.O., Santini, C.C., Marlair, G., Gutel, T., Mailley, S., Len, C., Targeting adequate thermal stability and fire safety in selecting ionic liquid-based electrolytes for energy storage. *Phys. Chem. Chem. Phys.*, 16, 1967, 2014.
18. Feng, J., An, Y., Ci, L., Xiong, S., Nonflammable electrolyte for safer non-aqueous sodium batteries. *J. Mater. Chem. A*, 3, 14539, 2015.
19. Gnanaraj, J.S., Zinigrad, E., Asraf, L., Gottlieb, H.E., Sprecher, M., Schmidt, M., Geissler, W., Aurbach, D., A detailed investigation of the thermal reactions of $LiPF_6$ solution in organic carbonates using ARC and DSC. *J. Electrochem. Soc.*, 150, A1533, 2003.
20. Wang, Y., Jiang, J., Dahn, J.R., The reactivity of delithiated $Li(Ni_{1/3}Co_{1/3}Mn_{1/3})O_2$, $Li(Ni_{0.8}Co_{0.15}Al_{0.05})O_2$ or $LiCoO_2$ with non-aqueous electrolyte. *Electrochem. Commun.*, 9, 2534, 2007.
21. Jiang, J. and Dahn, J.R., Effects of solvents and salts on the thermal stability of LiC_6. *Electrochim. Acta*, 49, 4599, 2004.
22. Xia, L., Xia, Y., Liu, Z., A novel fluoro cyclophosphazene as bifunctional additive for safer lithium-ion batteries. *J. Power Sources*, 278, 190, 2015.
23. Zinigrad, E., Asraf, L.L., Salitra, G., Sprecher, M., Aurbach, D., On the thermal behavior of Li bis(oxalato)borate LiBOB. *Thermochim. Acta*, 457, 64, 2007.
24. Kim, G.-Y. and Dahn, J.R., ARC studies of the effects of electrolyte additives on the reactivity of delithiated $Li_{1-x}[Ni_{1/3}Mn_{1/3}Co_{1/3}]O_2$ and $Li_{1-x}[Ni_{0.8}Co_{0.15}Al_{0.05}]O_2$ positive electrode materials with electrolyte. *J. Electrochem. Soc.*, 161, A1394, 2014.
25. Matthes, F.C., Hermann, H., Zimmer, W., The vision scenario for the european union 2011 update for the EU-27, Berlin, 2011.
26. Moseley, P.T. and Garche, J., *Electrochemical energy storage for renewable sources and grid balancing*, Elsevier, Amsterdam, 2014.

27. Zhong, C., Deng, Y., Hu, W., Qiao, J., Zhang, L., Zhang, J., A review of electrolyte materials and compositions for electrochemical supercapacitors. *Chem. Soc. Rev.*, 44, 7484–7539, 2015.
28. Shaplov, A.S., Marcilla, R., Mecerreyes, D., Recent advances in innovative polymer electrolytes based on poly(ionic liquid)s. *Electrochim. Acta*, 175, 18, 2015.
29. Galinski, M., Lewandowski, A., Pniak, I.S., Ionic liquids as electrolytes. *Electrochim. Acta*, 51, 5567, 2006.
30. Torchala, K., Kierzek, K., Machnikowski, J., Capacitance behavior of KOH activated mesocarbon microbeads in different aqueous electrolytes. *Electrochim. Acta*, 86, 260, 2012.
31. Pognon, G., Brousse, T., Demarconnay, L., Belanger, D., Performance and stability of electrochemical capacitor based on anthraquinone modified activated carbon. *J. Power Sources*, 196, 4117, 2011.
32. Augustyn, V., Simon, P., Dunn, B., Pseudocapacitive oxide materials for high-rate electrochemical energy storage. *Energy Environ. Sci.*, 7, 1597, 2014.
33. Khomenko, V., Pinero, E.R., Frackowiak, E., Beguin, F., High-voltage asymmetric supercapacitors operating in aqueous electrolyte. *Appl. Phys. A*, 82, 567, 2006.
34. Muniraj, V.K.A., Kamaja, C.K., Shelke, M.V., RuO_2·nHO nanoparticles anchored on carbon nano-onions: An efficient electrode for solid state flexible electrochemical supercapacitor. *ACS Sustain. Chem. Eng.*, 4, 2528, 2016.
35. Ramachandran, R., Saranya, M., Velmurugan, V., Ragupathy, B.P.C., Jeong, S.K., Grace, A.N., Effect of reducing agent on graphene synthesis and its influence on charge storage towards supercapacitor applications. *Appl. Energy*, 153, 22, 2015.
36. Feng, C., Zhang, J.F., He, Y., Zhong, C., Hu, W.B., Liu, L., Deng, Y.D., Sub-3 nm Co_3O_4 nanofilms with enhanced supercapacitor properties. *ACS Nano*, 9, 1730, 2015.
37. Misnon, I.I., Aziz, R.A., Zain, N.K., Vidhyadharan, B., Krishnan, S.K., Jose, R., High performance MnO_2 nanoflower electrode and the relationship between solvated ion size and specific capacitance in highly conductive electrolytes. *Mater. Res. Bull.*, 57, 221, 2014.
39. Gupta, R.K., Candler, J., Palchoudhury, S., Ramasamy, K., Gupta, B.K., Flexible and high performance supercapacitors based on $NiCo_2O_4$ for wide temperature range applications. *Sci. Rep.*, 5, 15265, 2015.
40. Barzegar, F., Momodu, D.F., Fashedemi, O.O., Bello, A., Dangbegnon, J K., Manyala, N., Investigation of different aqueous electrolytes on the electrochemical performance of activated carbon-based supercapacitors. *RSC Adv.*, 5, 107482, 2015.
41. Ramachandran, R., Grace, A.N., Subramaniam, C.K., Cobalt sulfide-graphene (CoSG) composite based electrochemical double layer capacitors. *MRS Proc.*, 1786, 19, 2015.

42. Liu, L., Lang, J., Zhang, P., Hu, B., Yan, X., Facile synthesis of Fe_2O_3 nano-dots@nitrogen-doped graphene for supercapacitor electrode with ultralong cycle life in KOH electrolyte. *ACS Appl. Mater. Interfaces*, 8, 9335, 2016.
43. Chen, K. and Xue, D., High energy density hybrid supercapacitor: *In-situ* functionalization of vanadium-based colloidal cathode. *ACS Appl. Mater. Interfaces*, 8, 29522–29528, 2016.
44. Demarconnay, L., Pinero, E.R., Beguin, F., A symmetric carbon/carbon supercapacitor operating at 1.6 V by using a neutral aqueous solution. *Electrochem. Commun.*, 12, 1275–1278, 2010.
45. Fic, K., Lota, G., Meller, M., Frackowiak, E., Novel insight into neutral medium as electrolyte for high-voltage supercapacitors. *Energy Environ. Sci.*, 5, 5842, 2012.
46. Chae, J.H. and Chen, G.H., Influences of ions and temperature on performance of carbon nano-particulates in supercapacitors with neutral aqueous electrolytes. *Particuology*, 15, 9–17, 2014.
47. Li, S., Qi, L., Lu, L., Wang, H., Facile preparation and performance of mesoporous manganese oxide for supercapacitors utilizing neutral aqueous electrolytes. *RSC Adv.*, 2, 3298, 2012.
48. Pal, B., Yang, S., Ramesh, S., Thangadurai, V., Jose, R., Electrolyte selection for supercapacitive devices:A critical review. *Nanoscale Adv.*, 1, 3807, 2019.
49. Long, J.W., Belanger, D., Brousse, T., Sugimoto, W., Sassin, M.B., Crosnier, O., Asymmetric electrochemical capacitors—Stretching the limits of aqueous electrolytes. *MRS Bull.*, 36, 513, 2011.
50. Ma, X.J., Zhang, W.B., Kong, L.B., Luo, Y.C., Kang, L., Electrochemical performance in alkaline and neutral electrolytes of a manganese phosphate material possessing a broad potential window. *RSC Adv.*, 6, 40077, 2016.
51. Deng, L.J., Wang, J.F., Zhu, G., Kang, L.P., Hao, Z.P., Lei, Z.B., Yang, Z.P., Liu, Z.H., RuO_2/graphene hybrid material for high performance electrochemical capacitor. *J. Power Sources*, 248, 407, 2014.
52. Wang, Q., Yan, J., Fan, Z.J., Wei, T., Zhang, M.L., Jing, X.Y., Mesoporous polyaniline film on ultra-thin graphene sheets for high performance supercapacitors. *J. Power Sources*, 247, 197, 2014.
53. Wang, H.J., Sun, X.X., Liu, Z.H., Lei, Z.B., Creation of nanopores on graphene planes with MgO template for preparing high-performance supercapacitor electrodes. *Nanoscale*, 6, 6577, 2014.
54. Li, L., Peng, S., Cheah, Y., The, P., Wang, J., Wee, G., Ko, Y., Woung, C., Srinivasan, M., Electrospun porous $NiCo_2O_4$ nanotubes as advanced electrodes for electrochemical capacitors. *Chem. Eur. J.*, 19, 5892, 2013.
55. Wang, H., Liang, Y., Mirfakhrai, T., Chen, Z., Casalomgue, H.S., Dai, H., Advanced asymmetrical supercapacitors based on graphene hybrid materials. *Nano Res.*, 4, 729, 2011.
56. Long, C., Wei, T., Yan, J., Jiang, L., Fan, Z., Supercapacitors based on graphene-supported iron nanosheets as negative electrode materials. *ACS Nano*, 7, 11325, 2013.

57. Lee, J.W., Ahn, T., Kim, J.H., Ko, J.M., Kim, J.D., Nanosheets based mesoporous NiO micro- spherical structures via facile and template-free method for high performance supercapacitors. *Electrochim. Acta*, 56, 4849, 2011.
58. Kulal, P.M., Dubal, D.P., Lokhande, C.D., Fulari, V.J., Chemical synthesis of Fe_2O_3 thin films for supercapacitor application. *J. Alloys Compd.*, 509, 2567, 2011.
59. Qu, Q.T., Shi, Y., Li, L.L., Guo, W.L., Wu, Y.P., Zhang, H.P., Guan, S.Y., Holze, R., $V_2O_5.0.6H_2O$ nanoribbons as cathode material for asymmetric supercapacitor in K_2SO_4 solution. *Electrochem. Commun.*, 11, 1325, 2009.
60. Xia, H., Meng, Y.S., Yuan, G., Cui, C., Lu, L., A symmetric RuO_2/RuO_2 supercapacitor operating at 1.6 V by using a neutral aqueous electrolyte. *Electrochem. Solid-State Lett.*, 15, A60, 2012.

11

Strategies for Improving Energy Storage Properties

A. Geetha Bhavani[1]* and Tanveer Ahmad Wani[2]

[1]*Department of Chemistry, School of Science, Noida International University, Greater Noida, U.P., India*
[2]*Department of Physics, School of Science, Noida International University, Greater Noida, U.P., India*

Abstract
Petro fuels are significant resources to generate energy, which is progressively depleting and moving toward recent advanced technologies fixated on resources like wind and solar, which are renewable. Despite the regular hike in price, demand and supply are rising by economic progress and population. The storage of energy allows flexibility and electricity supply with stability for consumers' demands. This chapter is intended to cater to the comparison of present and advanced technologies and methods, which are beneficial and economic to literature. Advanced materials with technologies on supercapacitors, batteries, pumped hydro storage, flywheel energy storage, and superconducting magnetic energy storage are conferred. Groundbreaking devices of grids (energy) and similar devices and machines are needed for commercialization for scaleup. In this chapter, storage devices were compared with their benefits, challenges, and environmental impacts. Indeed, the outcome of the chapter may provide beneficial information for energy sector-related stakeholders.

Keywords: Energy storage systems, power stations and grid electricity, environmental impacts

11.1 Introduction

Energy sources are active intermediaries due to their complementary and renewable energy sources. These energy resources will be an innovation in

**Corresponding author*: ageethabhavani@gmail.com

Inamuddin, Tariq Altalhi and Sayed Mohammed Adnan (eds.) Electroceramics for High Performance Supercapacitors, (255–268) © 2024 Scrivener Publishing LLC

technology to meet the demand for power supply and costs of the energy storage system, without showing any environmental consequences. The requirements for energy storage are trice by 2030 with the current usage. To meet the high demand the groundbreaking requirement of systems and devices is significant. The environmental effects on fossil fuels and degree of the durability of energy grids are focused on by engineers and everyone to find a significant solution for energy storage. The storage of energy may also provide solutions for avoiding solar and wind power [1]. The solutions may clear the fluctuations between supply and demand by producing the grid in an agreeable and responsive that will also minimize and support the power plants [2]. Figure 11.1 shows the effectiveness of types of equipment (energy storage) that may easily asses by quantifying the spontaneous reactions that lead to the shift in energy and speed loss while the energy storage process. All-inclusive energy storage capacity and most important how fast it can be recharged [3].

Storage of energy is something, not a new process. Since the early 1800s, batteries have been used for energy processes [4]. The new efficient projects of cleaner grids are addressing energy storage solutions [5] in a responsive way. The maximum energy form is fossil fuels, which are the basic due to transportation and storage facilities to help energy generation. The generated energy is feasible due to practical forms of storage, and transportability. Wind and solar energy merely depend on seasons [6]. Renewable

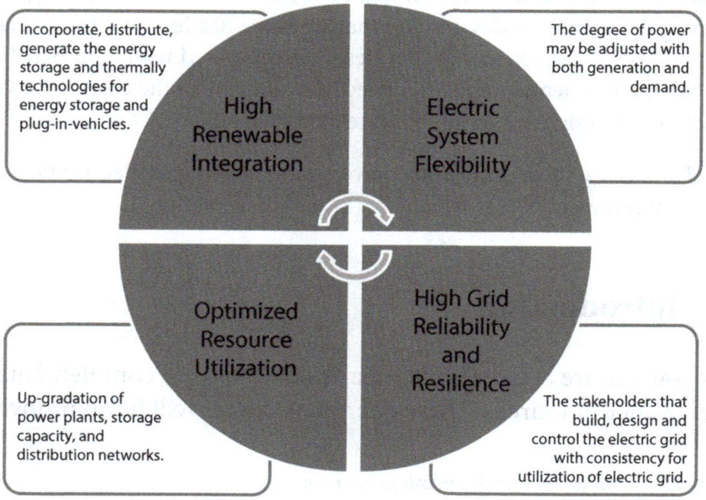

Figure 11.1 The various components of energy storage systems linked with storage applications with dependable electric grid.

energy resources have become eminent on the electrical grid, the interest is growing in a system that can store energy.

The energy storage devices are known as 1) batteries (Li-ion), 2) dielectric 3) electrochemical capacitors, and 4) solid oxide fuel cells (SOFC) [7, 8]. These four classifications are quantified with their energy density and power density. The parameter energy density may alter using perovskite materials having high permittivity. Storage of energy can also help in meeting the electricity demand during peak hours, such as on hot summer days. Electricity becomes more expensive during summertime as the production of electricity is required to increase to meet essential energy demands. The storage of energy allows greater flexibility of the grid as distributors can easily buy electricity during winter or off-peak times when energy is at low cost, it may sell to the grid during peak times, which may use in demand rises [9]. Energy storage is an excellent backup when delay in power plant generation. The flexibility of the grid helps to maximize the storage of energy in Puerto Rico, which aided for the year to all the residents until energy generates. The strength of the grid is increased due to weather conditions that extremely worsen throughout the world, which leads the policy-making and reforms by government officials and infrastructure [10].

11.2 Result and Discussion

Over the years, several methods were derived for energy storage to collect and supply the energy in the grid and used when needed most [11], which represents in Figure 11.2. There are large numbers of technologies used for energy storage, and all these methods have their advantages and disadvantages. Some of the energy storage methods are discussed as follows.

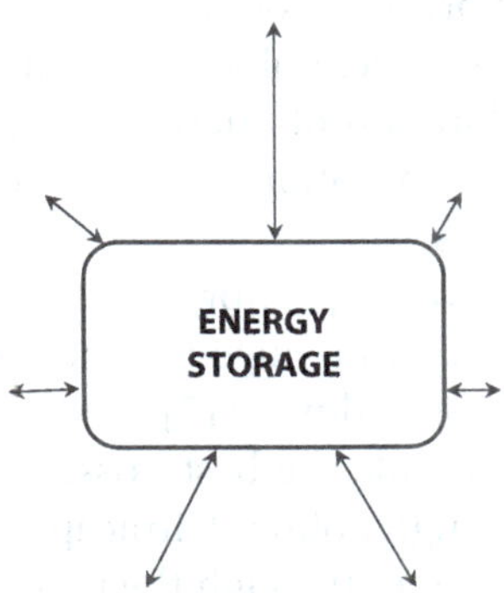

Figure 11.2 Interconnectivity and intraconnectivity of energy storage technologies.

11.2.1 Solid-State Batteries

The most common form used for energy storage is batteries. Solid-state (electrode) batteries like lithium-ion batteries and lead-acid are heavy in energy storage. Advanced lithium-ion is well practiced for more exceptional energy storage capacity with a comparison to other batteries like lead-acid [12]. Advanced lithium-ion is superior for standby provision, and energy for drawn-out periods and can be used at night times by reloading again. This facility may avail in the daytime by charging it. These types of batteries are ideal for a large number of functions, which required energy for long hours of storage capacities. What lacking is the power of the battery. The technology of lead-acid storage battery needs to reach its high for storage in density, as well as power density [13]. However, modifications are done in lithium-ion batteries to increase the power density of the grid. The main task is to increase of battery life cycle in energy storage. The batteries disintegrate or discharge may be possible for every cycle by experiencing or subjection to punitive weather conditions, which also include temperatures. Very frequently maintaining the harsh temperatures may also affect the cost of the whole system.

11.2.2 Ultracapacitor

Supercapacitors are known as ultracapacitors made with electric double-layer capacitors. Ultracapacitors encourage short duration with a huge power density and normally perform thousands of cycles. The ultracapacitors allow low deprivation against the period. The supercapacitors are not having acid or lead, which shows less possibility according to surrounding conditions (temperature) [14]. Ultracapacitors operate as an ideal application in the industrial, and transportation process with purposes of the grid that strive to meet short duration demand of energy supply, and high power demands with present technologies in batteries. Ultracapacitors are not effective for a long duration of energy storage in large numbers and may accompany the large applications which usually met the density and duration of energy demands.

The electrical double-layer capacitors are the best equipment for any system in vehicles that required a huge number of charge cycles or times for the engine to start and shut down [15]. The car batteries are similar to lead storage batteries to provide the best possibility for the car's onboard energy loads, such as heating/cooling. Ultracapacitors are useful in stabilizing renewable energy sources through the upgradation of technologies.

11.2.3 Flywheels

The flywheel spins easily and energy stores without any external pressure. Merry-go-round slows down when people pull energy from it. A flywheel rotates around an axis with maximum speed and energy stores in the form of kinetic energy [16]. The more generators on the grid, the more heavily and faster the flywheel, and the stored energy will be. The capacity with storage of energy is merely dependent on the flywheel spin rate, whereas increasing the spin rate higher the energy stores.

Flywheels are facing tasks very prominently in the form of instability by the commercial industrial sector. While installing the flywheels, we must build retaining walls around them and contain the flywheel so that it will not fall from the axis. The installation may be done over cars and storage of energy will be provided on a megawatt-scale. The flywheels are like supercapacitors, which are feasible by being discharged and charged automatically. The rate optimization is possible through a continuous supply of energy releases whenever required [17]. Flywheels are compared with supercapacitors are shows better energy storage capacity, whereas supercapacitors devices are short-term energy storage devices. These devices are significant for grid energy storage for all commercial applications. Flywheel is mainly known for its mechanical system, eco-friendly and long-lasting technology because of its performance [18].

11.2.4 Pumped Hydroelectric Storage Dams

As per data from the department of energy, 95% of U.S. stored energy is provided by pumped hydroelectric storage dams. This technique usually practices in reservoirs of two, whereas one will be at a low elevation and another high elevation. This method merely depends upon energy demand and energy supply, which hinge on seasons, especially during summer. The consumption of energy indication goes the release of the high elevation (upper reservoir) to low elevation to released water. Through water flow from height, the electricity will generate and also release to the grid [19]. The released excess power will be stored in the grid when the low requirement of electricity, which also sensors indicates the water may go back through the pump to a high reservoir [20]. Pumped hydroelectric storage dams are long backups of energy production technology which enables the highly demanded times required to supply to be very high.

11.2.5 Rail Energy Storage

Rail production is an extension of pumped hydroelectric storage dams. The rocks full of tail cars are loaded arduous when less energy (low grid energy) was required. The rocks are dumbing down from the hill to generate power as well as storage depending on grid requirements. This technology required a huge infrastructure [21]. There are several places in Nevada hills Nevada Public Utilities Commission that is manufacturing energy storage through rail cars and energy is produced and stored in the grid [22].

11.2.6 Compressed Storage of Air

This technique involved using air in compressed form in a deep hole in the side of a hill using motors run by electricity and when high energy demands. The turbine is activated by the air automatically on the rampage to produce demanded power [23]. This method of storing power is used for a year, especially in industries. The advantages of this process are that it does not use any harmful chemical substances.

Many other techniques are commercialized to store energy, which has advantages and disadvantages. The capacity of storage is aimed to improve by practicing novel concepts and methods day by day with prevailing methods [24].

11.2.7 Liquid Air Energy Storage

The grid may also store the excess energy that will be utilized to cool down the surrounding air to convert it into liquid air while proceeding with energy stores. The liquidized air converts gas by the reverse process through the surrounding air. The gas expansion causes the charged turbines [25].

11.2.8 Pumped Heat Electrical Storage

Pumped Heat Electrical Storage technology (PHES) stores energy by using it to power the pump to heat up so that the "cold store" may transfer to the "hot store," this function is similar to the refrigerator. The power pump will be on to energy recuperation by receiving from the hot reservoir and placing it in the cold reservoir. This type of method required huge mechanics to produce a generator for electricity [26]. This method's important advantage is this mechanics reacts within minutes for storage of power in comparison to other methods [27].

11.2.9 Redox Flow Batteries

Redox flow energy reserves excess grid energy through the chemical reduction and oxidation process in liquid electrolyte solutions [28]. Redox batteries have a potential advantage over batteries used with solid-state in the capacity of adaptableness and flexibility. The battery with redox energy flow storage capacity is easily increased by modifying some applications like simply adjusting the size of the tanks that stored the electrolyte [29].

11.2.10 Superconducting Magnetic Energy Storage

A superconducting magnetic energy (SME) device stores power in magnetic pitch. The magnetic pitch generates by flowing electricity through a loop, which is superconducting. The process is lower to critical temperature for cooling [30]. The advantage of this process is very little energy is required in maintaining the electromagnetic field. This electromagnetic field is produced by clearing the coils. Technology is significant output by clearing instant expulsion capacity [31].

11.2.11 Methane

The studies have formulated a technology for the gasification of biomass by using unused or trash products for the stable production of methane. Methane gas is fired in turbines for energy storage and medium. Existing natural gas plants is a technology used in the pipeline for methane energy storage [32].

11.3 Energy Storage Systems Applications

11.3.1 Mills

In the olden days, the streams are also used to run powering machines as water mills for simple daily solicitations. For this purpose currently, dams and reservoirs are used for water storage with energy generation and to release energy [33].

11.3.2 Homes

Growing the usage of the large depletion of energy in buildings required the alternative of producing and storing in the home itself. Household storage saves energy by 40% is achieved by setting up the equipment of the photovoltaic system. Many industries are making batteries with the provision of rechargeability for energy storage. Other generation options are wind and solar residential systems [34]. The battery of lithium-ion ,which is a solid-state battery is well used in the comparison of energy storage in lead-acid batteries. The batteries of lithium-ion are well cast off for small-scale systems due to economic and loftier performance. Using an inverter for electricity generation at home may pass to the grid by selling, where the batteries are not required [35].

11.3.3 Power Stations and Grid Electricity

The tanks made with salt are constructed to produce sufficient hot energy to store. This hot energy is produced after the sun sets and released whenever energy demand rises. For example, the Solana station produces 380 MW with 8 hours of energy storage capacity. Next-generation technology visions around 48% of energy storage capacity [36].

A variable amount of energy is released through many resources of renewable energy like wind, waste, and solar. Better storage capacity of energy easily assists the steadiness of imbalance that occurs in supply and demand. The moment electricity is generated it must be used immediately or transformed into storable forms with the help of methods used for the storage of energy.

11.3.4 Air Conditioning

Energy storage through thermal systems is utilized to condition the air [37]. Energy storage through thermal systems is utilized to cool huge commercial infrastructures. The provision of air conditioning for commercial purposes caused peak electrical demand [38]. Energy storage through thermal systems technology is employed in over 45 countries successfully. At night time this system is running through cooling the filament material and is released on high-temperature days (summers) for cooling [39].

11.3.5 Transportation

The liquid forms of hydrocarbons are commonly used for transport, which are essential energy storage fuels [40]. At present many electric battery vehicles and hybrid types save the depletion of fuels [41]. Hydrogen is another alternative energy to avoid greenhouse gas effects.

Energy storage in the form of power is essential for trolleybuses and trams as the transport facility of the public is in a challenging energy deficit depending on their different usage, it is difficult to obtain a reliable electricity supply through renewable sources [42]. Photovoltaic systems are also an alternative to provide energy public transportation systems during peak hours or hot summer days, which are easily fitted on the building roof.

11.3.6 Electronics

Electrical capacitors are well practiced as an alternative power by flowing directly in electrical circuits [43], which is a significant form of the output of power. They use circuits to resonate radios to certain frequencies. Electrical capacitors effectively control the power flow and voltage in commercial and household transmissions.

11.4 Energy Storage Systems Economics

The economy of any energy capacity depends heavily on required earmarked provision and other effecting aspects to increase the number of advantages. Every technology has its own merits and demerits by addressing economic and technical viabilities of energy storage capacity [44].

Large energy storage systems are associated with much jeopardy:

1. Risks are related to technical and economic feasibilities;
2. The aspects that influence the power quality and quantity supplies are not feasible as per market demands;
3. Risks are in the formulation of regulations and Policies.

By analyzing these risks the conventional methods of investments are counted on discounted cash flow (DCF), which will not sufficient for the evaluation of risks and qualms. The investors will be convent to handle the risks for better commercialization. The most important factors that are related to economic risk are the shortening of power cost, evasion, trading of price, avoidance of grid overflow, large scale of energy output, and carbon-free process for large-scale applications. Energy invested for the storage of energy is periodically collected and segregated with energy quantity is significant [45]. The energy invested for the storage of energy in huge amounts is known for efficiency and is more economic. This method required batteries to assess around lithium-ion 9-10 numbers and lead-acid of 1-2 batteries.

11.5 Impacts on Environment by Electricity Storage

Over a longer period, the energy storage process may have affirmative effects on the environment. Restoring the alternative resource of renewables is highly possible with energy stored. This type of restoration may make electricity generation plants more viable in the long run with high efficiency, and potential, which also affectivity power generates during highly demanded seasons. Another power released by stored energy may get rid of challenging issues like distribution and transmission [46]. The technologies used for storage merely affect the efficiency and nullify potential risk factors of electricity storage systems. The batteries are composed of metal materials like lead and lithium, so disposal and/or recycling may cause an advisee effect on the environment. Indeed energy production, storage, and release also waste electricity.

11.6 Future Prospective

- The drawbacks of batteries need to be diagnosed using software and upgraded with advanced materials and technologies.
- The chemistry of battery materials needs to be tailored to current grid demands [47].
- The atomic and molecular level analysis with using new and powerful tools to characterize and design computationally for the development of efficient, last longer, high charge density and low charge–discharge cycles degradation.
- The usage of composite graphene-based materials to recharge the battery in a faster way.
- The before the commercialization of any novel materials testing partners like industry, academia, and national laboratories' feedback is significant to increase the energy storage capacity [48].
- The membranes like polymer membranes blended with sub-nanometer pores are used as cross membranes instead of battery ions.
- Thermal energy storage needs to integrate with solid oxide fuel cells.

- New technologies like lithium-sulfur materials, high energy anode materials, nanowire battery technology, silicon-based anode materials, silicon nanowire composite materials, regenerable battery electrodes, and electromechanical, zinc-bromide flow batteries are commercialized and known for being highly powerful compared to traditional lithium-ion batteries.
- The new projects need to overlook an electric grid with long storage capacity with specifications like affordability, efficiency, flexibility, reliability, and resiliency [49–52].

11.7 Conclusion

Energy storage systems can be divided into high and small-capacity systems. High-capacity systems are for supporting the electrical grid. The higher capacity system is power configuration and the lower capacity systems are energy configuration. The power configuration systems use in various applications like batteries which provide a large amount of power to the electrical grid in a respectively short time. In the energy configuration, batteries are inserted to provide a fixed steady amount of power into the grid for a longer time.

In general, it is possible to conclude that all energy storage solutions have a lot to offer and provide the highest possible efficiency factors to store energy, reduce overall costs or an economical process and help reduce greenhouse gas CO_2 emissions. This will be the overall goal and target of research and development departments to be a growing and competitive world.

References

1. Sherrill, S.A., Banerjee, P., Rubloff, G.W., Lee, S.B., High to ultra-high power electrical energy storage. *Phys. Chem. Chem. Phys.*, 13, 20714, 2011.
2. Christen, T. and Carlen, M.W., Theory of ragone plots. *J Power Sources*, 91, 210, 2000.
3. Fletcher, N.H., Hilton, A.D., Ricketts, B.W., Optimization of energy storage density in ceramic capacitors. *J. Phys. D. Appl. Phys.*, 29, 253, 1996.
4. Moulson, A.J. and Herbert, J.M., *Electroceramics*, John Wiley & Sons, Ltd., Chichester, UK, 2003.
5. Love, G.R., Energy storage in ceramic dielectrics. *J. Am. Ceram. Soc.*, 73, 323, 1990.

6. Energy storage: Possibilities for expanding electric grid flexibility, National Renewable Energy Laboratory, February 2016, nrel.gov/docs/fy16osti/64764.pdf 2.
7. Li, H., Liu, F., Fan, B., Ai, D., Peng, Z., Wang, Q., Nanostructured ferroelectric-polymer composites for capacitive energy storage. *Small Methods*, 2, 1700399, 2018.
8. Singh, P., Borkar, H., Singh, B.P., Singh, V.N., Kumar, A., Ferroelectric polymer-ceramic composite thick films for energy storage applications. *AIP Adv.*, 4, 087117, 2014.
9. Haertling, G., Ferroelectric ceramics: History and technology. *J. Am. Ceram. Soc.*, 82, 718, 1999.
10. Tilley, R.J.D., Insulating solids, in: *Understanding Solids: The Science of Materials*, R.J.D. Tilley (Ed.), John Wiley & Sons, Ltd., Chichester, UK, 2004.
11. Jena, A.K., Kulkarni, A., Miyasaka, T., Halide perovskite photovoltaics: Background, status, and future prospects. *Chem. Rev.*, 119, 3036, 2019.
12. Batmunkh, M., Zhong, Y.L., Zhao, H., Recent advances in perovskite-based building-integrated photovoltaics. *Adv. Mater.*, 32, 2000631, 2020.
13. Hwang, J., Rao, R.R., Giordano, L., Katayama, Y., Yu, Y., Horn, Y., Perovskites in catalysis and electrocatalysis. *Science*, 358, 751, 2017.
14. Cohen, R.E., Origin of ferroelectricity in perovskite oxides. *Nature*, 358, 136, 1992.
15. Christen, T. and Carlen, M.W., Theory of ragone plots. *J. Power Sources*, 91, 210, 2000.
16. Vorauer, T., Kumar, P., Berhaut, C.L., Chamasemani, F.F., Jouneau, P.H., Aradilla, D., Tardif, S., Pouget, S., Fuchsbichler, B., Helfen, L., Multi-scale quantification and modeling of aged nanostructured silicon-based composite anodes. *Commun. Chem.*, 3, 1, 2020.
17. Elissalde, C. and Ravez, J., Ferroelectric ceramics: Defects and dielectric relaxations. *J. Mater. Chem.*, 11, 1957, 2001.
18. Ravez, J. and Simon, A., Some solid state chemistry aspects of lead-free relaxor ferroelectrics. *J. Solid State Chem.*, 162, 260, 2001.
19. Cohen, R.E., Origin of ferroelectricity in perovskite oxides. *Nature*, 358, 136, 1992.
20. Hao, X., A review on the dielectric materials for high energy-storage application. *J. Adv. Dielectr.*, 3, 1330001, 2013.
21. Moulson, A.Q.J. and Herbert, J.M., *Electroceramics*, John Wiley & Sons, Ltd., Chichester, UK, 2003.
22. Love, G.R., Energy storage in ceramic dielectrics. *J. Am. Ceram. Soc.*, 73, 323, 1990.
23. Jena, A.K., Kulkarni, A., Miyasaka, T., Halide perovskite photovoltaics: Background, status, and future prospects. *Chem. Rev.*, 119, 3036, 2019.
24. Hwang, J., Rao, R.R., Giordano, L., Katayama, Y., Yu, Y., Horn, Y., Perovskites in catalysis and electrocatalysis. *Science*, 358, 751, 2017.

25. Galen, J.S. and Truman, S.S., *Sustainable power technologies and infrastructure*, Acad. Press, Cambridge, 2016.
26. Cowley, R.A., Gvasaliya, S.N., Lushnikov, S.G., Roessli, B., Rotaru, G.M., Relaxing with relaxors: A review of relaxor ferroelectrics. *Adv. Phys.*, 60, 229, 2011.
27. Quadrennial technology review 2015, U.S. Department of Energy, September 2015, energy.gov/quadrennial-technology-review-2015.
28. Whittingham, M.S., History, evolution, and future status of energy storage. *Proc. IEEE*, 100, 1518, 2012.
29. Fletcher, N.H., Hilton, A.D., Ricketts, B.W., Optimization of energy storage density in ceramic capacitors. *J. Phys. D. Appl. Phys.*, 29, 253, 1996.
30. Jena, A.K., Kulkarni, A., Miyasaka, T., Halide perovskite photovoltaics: Background, status, and future prospects. *Chem. Rev.*, 119, 3036, 2019.
31. Bhalla, A.S., Guo, R., Roy, R., The perovskite structure-a review of its role in ceramic science and technology. *Mater. Res. Innov.*, 4, 3, 2000.
32. Fletcher, N.H., Hilton, A.D., Ricketts, B.W., Optimization of energy storage density in ceramic capacitors. *J. Phys. D. Appl. Phys.*, 29, 253, 1996.
33. Burns, G. and Burstein, E., Index of refraction in "dirty" displacive ferroelectrics. *Ferroelectrics*, 7, 297, 1974.
34. Huang, Y., Zhao, C., Wu, B., Wu, J., Multifunctional $BaTiO_3$-based relaxor ferroelectrics toward excellent energy storage performance and electrostrictive strain benefiting from crossover region. *ACS Appl. Mater. Interfaces*, 12, 23885, 2020.
35. Xu, Z., Qiang, H., Chen, Y., Improved energy storage properties of Mn and Y co-doped BS films. *Mater. Lett.*, 259, 126894, 2020.
36. Goodwin, A.L., Opportunities and challenges in understanding complex functional materials. *Nat. Commun.*, 10, 10, 2019.
37. Ioan, S. and Calin, S., A comprehensive review of thermal energy storage. *Sustainability*, 10, 191, 2018.
38. Gabbar, H.A. and Runge, J., *Smart energy grid engineering*, Acad. Press, Cambridge, 2017.
39. Zhifeng, W., *Design of solar thermal power plants*, Acad. Press, Cambridge, 2019.
40. Juan, S. and James, A.D., Catalytic production of liquid hydrocarbon transportation fuels, in: *Catalysis for Alternative Energy Generation*, L. Guczi, and A. Erdohelyi, (Eds.), pp. 29–56, Springer, New York, 2012.
41. Rakesh, A., Navneet, R.S., Fabio, H.R., Delgass, W.N., Sustainable fuel for the transportation sector. *PNAS*, 104, 4828, 2007.
42. George, W.H., Sara, I., Corma, A., Synthesis of transportation fuels from biomass: Chemistry, catalysts, and engineering. *Chem. Rev.*, 106, 4044, 2006.
43. Heddle, T., Capacitors, in: *Calculations in Fundamental Physics: Electricity and Magnetism*, T. Heddle, (Ed.), pp. 1–22, Elsevier, Netherlands, 1971.

44. Ibrahim, H. and Ilinca, A., Techno-economic analysis of different energy storage technologies, in: *Energy Storage*, A.F. Zobaa, (Ed.), pp. 1–40, InTechOpen, London, 2012.
45. Paulo, R.J., Luiz, C.S.R., Sandra, N.M., Ivan, B., Gianfranco, C., Andrea, M., Karel, J., Economic analysis of the investments in battery energy storage systems: Review and current perspectives. *Energies*, 14, 2503, 2021.
46. Bell, A.J. and Deubzer, O., Lead-free piezoelectrics-the environmental and regulatory issues. *MRS Bull.*, 43, 581, 2018.
47. Whittingham, M.S., History, evolution, and future status of energy storage. *Proc. IEEE*, 100, 1518, 2012.
48. Evans, A., Strezov, V., Evans, T.J., Assessment of utility energy storage options for increased renewable energy penetration. *Renew. Sustain. Energy Rev.*, 16, 4141, 2012.
49. López, R. and Agustín, J.L., Techno-economic analysis of grid-connected battery storage. *Energy Convers. Manage.*, 91, 394, 2015.
50. Barcellona, S., Piegari, L., Musolino, V., Ballif, C., Economic viability for residential battery storage systems in grid-connected PV plants. *IET Renew. Power Gener.*, 12, 135, 2018.
51. Foles, A., Fialho, L., Pereira, M., Techno-economic evaluation of the Portuguese PV and energy storage residential applications. *Sustain. Energy Technol. Assess.*, 39, 100686, 2020.
52. Nousdilis, A.I., Kryonidis, G.C., Kontis, E.O., Ntovom, G.A., Panapakidis, I.P., Christoforidis, G.C., Papagiannis, G.K., Impact of policy incentives on the promotion of integrated PV and battery storage systems: A techno-economic assessment. *IET Renew. Power Gener.*, 14, 1174, 2020.

12

State-of-the-Art in Electroceramics for Energy Storage

M. Rizwan[1]*, F. Seerat[2], A. Ayub[2] and I. Ilyas[2]

[1]School of Physical Sciences, University of the Punjab, Lahore, Pakistan
[2]Department of Physics, University of the Punjab, Lahore, Pakistan

Abstract
High-performance storage materials are an absolute necessity of the current ceramic industry due to the growing demand for efficient energy storage devices. Electroceramics are an astonishing class of energy storage materials. For a long period, lead-dependent ceramics, such as $PbZrTiO_3$-based ceramics, have ruled the ceramic industry as a consequence of their amazing energy storage properties. But the modern world requires lead-free, tremendous-performance ceramics for storage applications. The high requirements and urgent need for storage materials require new and enhanced ceramics. Some state-of-the-art ceramics, including lead-based, lead-free, multilayer ceramics, glass ceramics, and ceramic films, are discussed in detail along with ways to improve their storage properties.

Keywords: Electroceramics, breakdown strength, storage properties, storage density, glass ceramics, lead-free, bulk-ceramics

12.1 Introduction

Carbon dioxide (CO_2) discharges are to drop 45% by 2030 and reach zero by 2050 to accomplish the Paris arrangement's goal of restraining global warming to 1.50°C [1, 2]. To achieve these goals, technologies that depend on renewable properties like tides, sun, and wind will be essential. Although the expansion of renewable energy production is encouraging, there remain numerous difficulties in the replacement of conventionally

**Corresponding author*: rizwan.spr@pu.edu.pk

Inamuddin, Tariq Altalhi and Sayed Mohammed Adnan (eds.) Electroceramics for High Performance Supercapacitors, (269–296) © 2024 Scrivener Publishing LLC

high carbon dioxide-emitting areas dependent on gas and coal for power production. Because of the unpredictable nature of renewable energy sources, that is still a significant percentage of the energy supply. Hence, this is vital to combine energy-reaping technology with energy storage to instantaneously move gone from fossil fuels and avoid the unpredictable nature of fresh energy properties. As an outcome, energy storage is becoming a crucial enabler for supportable renewable technologies [3].

Batteries, electrostatic capacitors, and electrochemical supercapacitors are a few examples of technologies that are now available to store energy [4, 5]. The latter are electrical energy-storage units that fall within the inactive component group and are widely used in electronics [6–8]. Due to their more rapid charging/discharging characteristics (μs), dielectric capacitors or non-polarized electrostatic have a higher power density (104–105 W/kg) than Lithium-ion fuel cells or batteries. That is beneficial for pulse power applications and power electronics in electrical vehicles (EVs). For practical uses of dielectric capacitors, other qualities such as frequency/temperature stability, lifetime reliability, fatigue resistance, manufacturing cost, and equivalent series resistance are equally crucial. These qualities go beyond greater energy density and firm discharging/charging rates [9–12].

To permit engine power electronics, demonstrate superfast charging, and have additional lasting EV performance at high voltage and temperature, new electroceramics are consequently necessary. Future electroceramics must, therefore:

(i) Provide high conversion efficiencies and energy density,
(ii) Withstand a wider frequency range (1–1000 Hz) and temperature range (50–250°C)
(iii) Demonstrate greater fatigue resistance and reliability (>105 cycles)
(iv) Be companionable with internal electrodes that are affordable and simple to integrate with other components

Electrostatic capacitors have historically been made from a wide variety of dielectric materials, including plastic, paper, and ceramics.

Nowadays, capacitors are made of ceramics or polymers for the reason that they provide the optimum functionality in terms of breakdown strength (BDS), thermal stability, dielectric loss, and capacitance. The potential for using ceramic capacitors as energy storage devices dates back to research conducted by Jaffe from the USA, in the 1960s [13, 14]. Smyth and Burn assessed the energy-storing presentation in $BaTiO_3$ (BT) and

$SrTiO_3$ (ST) within the useful electric fields up to 400kVcm^{-1}. This was done ten years after the initial study [15]. Because of the comparatively smaller dielectric, BDS of the manufactured ceramics, quantifiable information on energy storage on these materials had up been restricted to fields typically smaller than 150kVcm^{-1} until that moment. They underlined that because of the lesser possibility of flaws, which are familiar causes of dielectric breakdown, thinner dielectric layers should be used to achieve the ceramic's maximal energy density.

Love suggested that while intermediate materials display higher BDS than high relative permeability (ε_r) materials, the greatest energy storage density may be reached in the latter. Higher energy-storing densities could be attained in ferroelectric (FE) materials, according to Fletcher and colleagues, who convincingly hypothesized this after adjusting the material's Curie temperature (Tc) to operate it in the Para-electric system [16, 17]. Energy storage device fabrication using referred to as weakly coupled relaxors, for example, 0.7 $BaTiO_3$ - 0.3 $BiScO_3$ (0.7 BT - 0.3BS), was suggested by Ogihara and colleagues in 2009 [18]. This innovative conceptual strategy is intended to take advantage of the exceptional thermal constancy of ε_r that this class of materials displays.

Once more, the huge dielectric BDS was crucial to this performance. The manufacture of chemically heterogeneous but electrically homogenous ceramics is a revolutionary strategy that Wang, Reaney, and colleagues [19] announced in 2019 to improve energy storage properties. Here, we give an overview of electroceramic for high energy performance as well as the concepts governing energy storing presentation in electroceramic. The state of the art for lead-free and lead electroceramics for energy-storing capacitors will then be reviewed, with separate assessments of ceramic multilayers (MLs), bulk ceramics, glass ceramics, and ceramic films. We will talk about ceramic multi-layers, ceramic films, and an overview of the state of the art in ceramics before we conclude.

12.2 Electroceramics for Energy-Storing Devices

12.2.1 Bulk-Based Ceramics

A. Lead-Based Ceramics

Due to their good energy conversion efficiency (η) and recoverable energy (W_{rec}), Pb-dependent ceramics are utilized commercially as energy-storing components for greater-power pulsed capacitors [20].

B. Pb-Dependent Relaxor-FE

There have been several reports of lead-based relaxor ferroelectrics (RFEs) as prospective candidates for energy storage capacitors, as well as $Pb(Mg_{1/3}Nb_{2/3})O_3$-$PbTiO_3$ (PMNPT), (and $Pb(Zn_{1/3}Nb_{2/3})O_3$-$PbTiO_3$ (PZN-PT), Sr, Pb, Bi) TiO_3 (SPBT)-dependent materials [21–23]. At room temperature, Zhang and colleagues looked into the energy-storing capabilities and easing behavior of (1-x) $PMN_{-x}PT$ ceramic [24]. Li and colleagues investigated how the domain structure of 0.2PMN-0.8Pb $(Sn_xTi_{1-x})O_3$ ($PMN\text{-}PS_xT_{1-x}$) ceramics affected W_{rec} and thermal stability.

C. Lead-Based Anti-Ferroelectrics

The first known anti-ferroelectric (AFE), $PbZrO_3$ (PZ), displays a double polarization electric polarization hysteresis loop under critical temperature, T_C. However, applications for energy storage are constrained by the high critical switching field needed for an antiferroelectric-ferroelectric phase transition at ambient temperature. A good solution to the issue is chemical replacement, which lowers the switching field [25, 26].

D. (Pb,La) $(Zr,Ti)O_3$ (PLZT)

Conferring to the previous knowledge, PLZT is present as homogenous composition [27, 28]. According to a Pb vacancy ionic recompense model, having an orthorhombic antiferroelectric period that resembles lead zirconate develops when lead ions are substituted on A-site through 30 mol% La. For energy storage applications, though, only PLZT within 10 mol % La is commonly used because larger applications have smaller polarization and, hence, lesser W_{rec} [28, 29].

Li and colleagues used a solid-state process to create $(Pb_{0.97}La_{0.02})(Zr_{0.95}Ti_{0.05})O_3$ porcelains, producing η~70% and W_{rec} of 0.83 J cm^{-3} in an electric field of 55kV cm^{-1}. Jo and colleagues discovered that the replacement of extra PbO and La in PLZT may both produce AFE and RFE behavior, which improves W_{rec} by encouraging a slanted and thin hysteresis loop. After 105 cycles, high η~92% and W_{rec} of 3.04 J cm^{-3} were reached through no performance decline. It is also proposed that Mn doping will increase the W_{rec} of PLZT by "increasing anti-ferro-electricity" [30–32].

E. (Pb, La)(Zr, Sn, Ti)O_3 (PLZST)

Tin can be replaced on the B-site of material to increase the compositional variety of AFE and further improve the energy-storing capabilities of PLZT porcelains [16, 33]. For concentrations of 15 mol% Ti, PLZST is AFE. W_{rec} in PLZST ceramics may be optimized by modifying the Sn/Zr/Ti ratio; however, when Sn concentration rises, the switching field and Ferroelectricity decrease [34, 38].

In contrast to Wang and coworkers, who observed better η of 82% with storage density (W_{rec}) of 4.2 J cm^{-3} for PLZST porcelains within strong temperature constancy in their research of the PLZST solid solution [20]. A ferroelectric (FIE) arrangement that comprises FE arrangement sectors with either angular modulation or magnitude of dipoles was recently disclosed in PLZST. By varying the Sn/Ti ratio, the total polarization of field-induced ferroelectric demand may be modified. The Pb/La ratio has an impact on PLZST ceramics' performance as well [36, 37].

As La concentration rises, the AFE stage becomes more steady, and the AFE-FE switching field also rises proportionally. Because of a high BDS and strong switching electric field, $(Pb_{1-1.5x}La_x)(Zr_{0.5}Sn_{0.43}Ti_{0.07})O_3$ ceramics' energy storage capabilities were improved (W_{rec} of 4.2 J cm^{-3}) for compositions with x = 0.03 by Dan and coworkers [3]. Additionally, doping with Sr and Ba (A-site) promotes energy storage, reduces stress sensitivity, and improves temperature stability and fatigue behavior [37–39]

F. (Pb, La), (Zr), and (Sn) O_3 (PLZS)

In PLZS, Wang and colleagues described a novel electric field-induced multiphase conversion for which an increase in polarization results from a normal antiferroelectric-ferroelectric phase conversion at small E, charted through a second ferroelectric to ferroelectric phase conversion at a greater E [40]. For $(Pb_{0.98}La_{0.02})$ $(Zr_{0.55}Sn_{0.45})_{0.995}O_3$ porcelains, η of 87% and W_{rec} of 10.4 J cm^{-3} were obtained at 400 kV cm^{-1}, coupled with bigger discharge current density of 1640Acm^{-2} and ultra-fast discharge speed. Then, in $(Pb_{0.98-x}La_{0.02}Sr_x)(Zr_{0.9}Sn_{0.1})_{0.995}O_3$ porcelains, a greatest high storage density, W_{rec} of 11.2 J cm3 and a high 82% were achieved. The performance of energy storing was significantly enhanced through the replacement of Sr for Pb due to the growth in FE/AFE BDS and switching fields [41–43].

12.2.2 Lead-Free Ceramics

In recent years, due to massive energy consumption, the need for clean, eco-friendly, and renewable energy storage sources has increased massively. The vastly used clean storage devices nowadays are batteries, dielectric capacitors, fuel cells, and electrochemical capacitors. The great interest in storage density has led to the development of new and innovative storage materials such as ceramics, glass, and polymers. Lead-based ceramics have dominated the industry for quite some time now such as PZT ceramics. But there is a dire need for clean and lead-free storage materials that do not pose harm to humans and environmental health. Although lead-based ceramics possess superior storage properties, such as high storage density and efficiency, the lead-based ceramics have ampt energy density, but the energy density of lead-free ceramics has been amplified up to 12.2 J cm^{-3}.

Despite the high-performance characteristics, the lead-toxic nature of these materials led to a shift towards lead-free ceramics. There has been increasing attention toward lead-free ceramics [1]. The extensive research on lead-free ceramics has led to continuous enrichment in the storage properties of lead-free electroceramics and has also led to the development of new lead-free ceramics. Some new lead-free ceramics have astounding properties and the ability to replace well-established lead-based ceramics. A few of the prominent lead-free ceramics that are considered quintessential for storage applications are discussed ahead [2]. Some lead free ceramics are (K, Na) NbO_3 (KNN), $Bi_{1/2}Na_{1/2}TiO_3$ and (Ba,Ca)(Zr,Ti)O3(BCZT).

A. Barium Titanate Based Ceramics

Electroceramics are very important for energy storage and conversion as a result of their special electrical and Opto-magnetic properties. These ceramics have subcategories such as ferroelectrics, dielectrics, pyroelectrics, and magnetic ceramics. Presently the market of electroceramics is conquered by $BaTiO_3$ (BT) ceramics. BT ceramics have great applications in storage applications such as in the production of multilayer capacitors. $BaTiO_3$ is primitive lead-free ferroelectric and piezoelectric material that had a high piezoelectric constant and dielectric constant. It was reported that introducing substitutions such as Ca^{+2}, and Zr^{+2} can improve energy storage density and efficiency. $(Ba_{0.7}Ca_{0.3})TiO_3$ (BCT) and $Ba(Zr_{0.20.3})TiO_3$ (BZT) have an energy density of 1.41 and 0.71 Jcm^{-3} [3].

The storage properties of barium titanate-based ceramics can be heightened via various methods such as via oxides (Al_2O_3, MgO, SiO_2) substitution to enhance breakdown strength. It has also been suggested that opting for diverse sintering techniques such as cold sintering, citrate precursor and spark plasma sintering will help in controlling grain growth and ceramic density. The ceramic density can also be increased by adding sintering aids. The introduction of further end members in solid solutions will also lead to relaxor ferroelectric behavior. Some end members for solid solutions are $Bi(Mg_{1/2}Ti_{1/2})O_3$, BMN, and NBT. Table 12.1 summarizes the storage properties of some prominent BT-ceramics.

The most operative way to enrich the storage properties of BT-based ceramics is via the inclusion of a bismuth-based perovskite which has multiple cations at the B-site. The polarization can also be improved with the substitution of a bismuth ion that has a lone pair at the Ba site. When

Table 12.1 Energy storage properties of BT-based ceramics

BT-ceramics	E ($kVcm^{-1}$)	ΔP (μCcm^{-2}0	W_{rec} (Jcm^{-3})	η (%)	Reference
0.9BT-0.1BMN	143.5	16	1.13	95	[4]
0.88 $(Ba_{0.8}Sr_{0.2})TiO_3$-0.12$Bi(Zn_{2/3}Nb_{1/3})O_3$	225	17	1.62	99.8	[6]
0.9BT-0.1BMN-0.3wt%$MnCO_3$	205	16.28	1.7	88.5	[7]
0.88BT-0.12$Bi(Li_{0.5}Nb_{0.5})O_3$	270	19	2.03	88	[8]
$Ba_{0.85}Ca_{0.15}Zr_{0.1}Ti_{0.9}O_3$	20015	15	1.153		[5]
0.9BT-0.1$Bi(Li_{0.5}\ Ta_{0.5})O_3$	280	23	2.41	91.6	[9]
BT-0.06$Bi_{2/3}\ (Mg_{1/3}Nb_{2/3})\ O_3$	520	2li5	4.55	91	[10]

multiple ions are substituted at Ti-site, it disturbs the log range polar coupling, which in turn minimizes the remnant polarization owing to the formation of a weakly coupled relaxor state. Employing this technique Hu and Co. reported a storage density of 4.49 J cm$-^{3}$ with an efficiency of 93% for 0.6BT−0.4 Bi $(Mg_{0.5}Ti_{0.5})\ O_3$ (BT−BMT). Similarly, yang and Co. reported a much better BT-ceramic with commercial potential and similar properties, BT-0.06$Bi_{2/3}$ $(Mg_{1/3}Nb_{2/3})\ O_3$ (BT—0.06$B_{2/3}$MN). This composition was suitable with silver/Palladium electrodes due to the presence of 4mol% bismuth on the A-site and has similar properties but the highest breakdown strength.

$BaTiO_3$- $BaMeO_3$ (Me=trivalent cation) is one of the elementary BT-based ceramics which undergo a conversion from ferroelectric to relaxor ferroelectric as the concentration of Me is increased. It was reported that Me^{+3} radius increases the substitutions shifts from B site to A site. The maximum energy storage density is observed when the ionic radius of Me^{+3} is between 80 and 100 pm. Figure 12.1 explains the effect of Me ion on storage properties, such as breakdown strength and energy density [11].

B. Strontium titanate-based ceramics

$SrTiO_3$ (ST)is one of the aspiring lead-free ferroelectrics and is an important promising candidate for energy storage applications owing to its high permittivity of 300 and very low dielectric loss of less than 1 %. Many efforts have been contributed to improve the storage properties of $SrTiO_3$, such as via substitution on A-site or B-site with (Ba, Dy, Mg, Ce, Bi) [12]. The storage properties can also be enhanced via employing sintering aids such as oxides (ZnO, MgO, SiO_2, Al_2O_3) or mixed oxides (SrO-B_2O_3- SiO_2, ZnO-Li_2O) [13]. other methods include opting for different sintering techniques such as stark plasma sintering or microwave sintering and employing complex end members. Table 12.2 summarizes some ST-based ceramics and their energy storage properties.

C. $K_{0.5}Na_{0.5}\ NbO_3$ (KNN) based ceramics

KNN-based ceramics are another class of lead-free ceramics that were first investigated in 2016 in the context of storage properties. The storage density of 0.54 Jcm^{-3} was reported at 129kVcm^{-1} [20]. Like other lead-free ceramics, oxide sintering aids such as zinc oxide and copper oxide were also implemented here to enhance storage density by reducing porosity and decreasing grain growth in KNN-based ceramics. 0.8KNN-0.2Sr$(Sc_{0.5}Nb_{0.5})O_3$ with 0.5mol% of zinc oxide was reported to have breakdown strength of 400kVcm^{-1} [21]. Similarly, 0.9KNN-0.1BMN ceramics was reported to

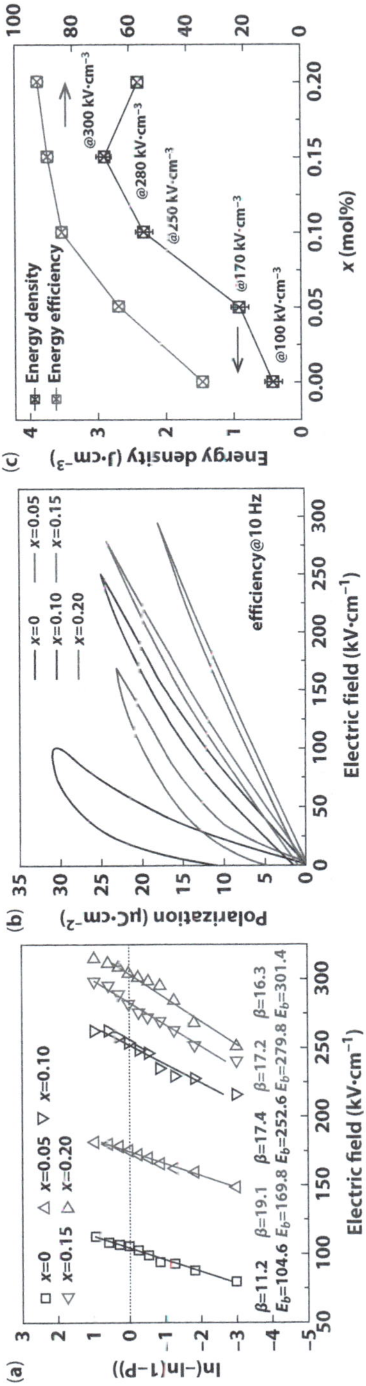

Figure 12.1 (a) dielectric breakdown strengths, (b) hysteresis loops, and (c) energy density and efficiency of (1-x)BT-xBMZ [11].

Table 12.2 Energy storage properties of ST-based ceramics.

ST-ceramics	**E ($kVcm^{-1}$)**	**ΔP (μCcm^{-2}0**	**W_{rec} (Jcm^{-3})**	**η (%)**	**Reference**
95wt%$Ba_{0.4}Sr_{0.6}TiO_3$-5wt%MgO	300	11.88	1.5	88.5	[14]
$(Sr_{0.99}Mg_{0.01})$ TiO_3	362	12	1.86	89.3	[18]
$Ba_{0.4}Sr_{0.6}TiO_3$-8MOL% SiO_2	400	9.11	1.6	90.9	[15]
0.6ST-0.4NBT	210	20	1.7	69.93	[16]
0.45 ST-0.2NBT-0.35 BT	170	25	1.78	77.06	[17]
0.9$(Sr_{0.7}Bi_{0.2})$ TiO_3 -$Bi(Mg_{0.5}Hf_{0.5})O_3$	360	22	3.1	93	[19]

Table 12.3 Energy storage properties of KNN-based ceramics.

KNN-Ceramics	E (kVcm^{-1})	ΔP (μCcm^{-2}0	W_{rec} (Jcm^{-3})	η (%)	Reference
0.93KNN-0.07BMN	150	22.5	1.3	58.8	[22]
0.9KNN-0.1BF	206	23.7	2	61	[23]
0.85KNN-0.15ST	400	26	4.03	52	[24]
0.9KNN-0.1BMN	300	34	4.08	62.7	[25]
0.9KNN-0.1BMN-1mol% CuO	400	21	4.02	57.3	[26]

have enhanced storage density due to CuO. Storage properties of some KNN-based ceramics are summarized in Table 12.3.

D. $BiFeO_3$ (BF) based ceramics

BF have major application as multiferroics but due to its large polarization, it is also being explored in piezoelectric applications. Its high leakage current rendered it suitable for storage applications. The volatilization of bismuth and the variation of Fe valencies limits the breakdown strength and storage density, but this can be solved by introducing dopants. BF-BT-based ceramics are alleged to be very suitable energy storage materials owing to their high polarization and breakdown strength. The storage properties of BF-BT-based ceramics can be improved by doping at A or B site, alloying with end member [27].

E. Glass Ceramics

These ceramics are made by dispersing one or more phases of ceramics in an amorphous phase. They display the hybrid properties of ceramics and glass. The assembly of glass ceramics is shown in Figure 12.2 [28].

The microstructure of glass ceramics is mostly construed as two- or three-dimensional defects in the free glass phase and ceramic phase. The absence of defects in glass ceramics gives high storage density and efficiency as well. The microstructure and properties of glass ceramics are

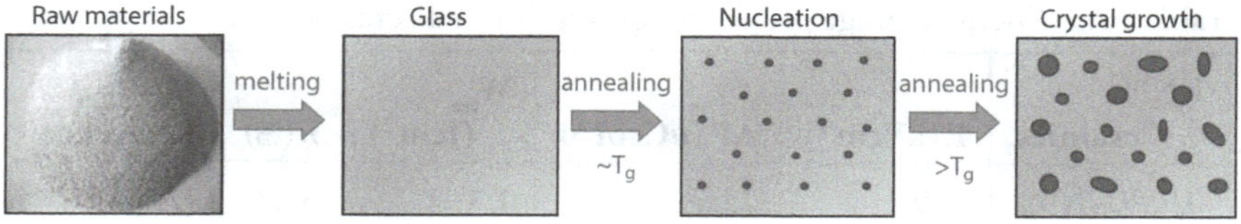

Figure 12.2 Diagram of the processing step of glass-ceramics [28].

measured by annealing techniques. Microwave treatment is described to increase the storage properties of glass ceramics [29].

There is a still conflict on whether lead-free ceramics can swap lead-based ceramics. Lead-based ceramics have superior properties to their counter-lead-free alternatives. Even though many an effort has been made to improve the properties of lead-free perovskites. But a large number of lead-free ceramics and their different formulations have been discussed and investigated to replace PZT ceramics. Lead-free ceramics have a large number of applications, but their promising application is the high energy density capacitors. Because the lead-free compositions have comparable properties to lead-based, moreover increasing breakdown strength leads to compensate for the reduction of electrical properties. The capacitors industry is ruled by BT-based ceramics and it is expected that more products will not contain lead. The comparison of storage properties of lead-based dead free ceramic is made in Figure 12.3.

12.3 Ceramic Multilayers and Films

In recent decades, growing population, social, and technical developments have demanded more energy and natural resources. Technologies associated with the utilization of non-renewable fossil fuels have been limited because of several challenges regarding serious environmental and ecological issues. There are also renewable energy resources like solar and wind energy that are encouraging but become periodic with the changings in the environment. For practical applications, energy storage appliances have got great research interest in having high-energy, high-power density, low cost, eco-friendly, and high conversion efficiency. Increasing demand for high energy density for electronic appliances has boosted the consumption of environmentally friendliness energy storage capacitors in applications. As compared to other energy storage electrochemical capacitors; dielectric capacitors have got a lot of attention because of having capability of generating ultra-high-power densities >10kWkg^{-1} with high charging and

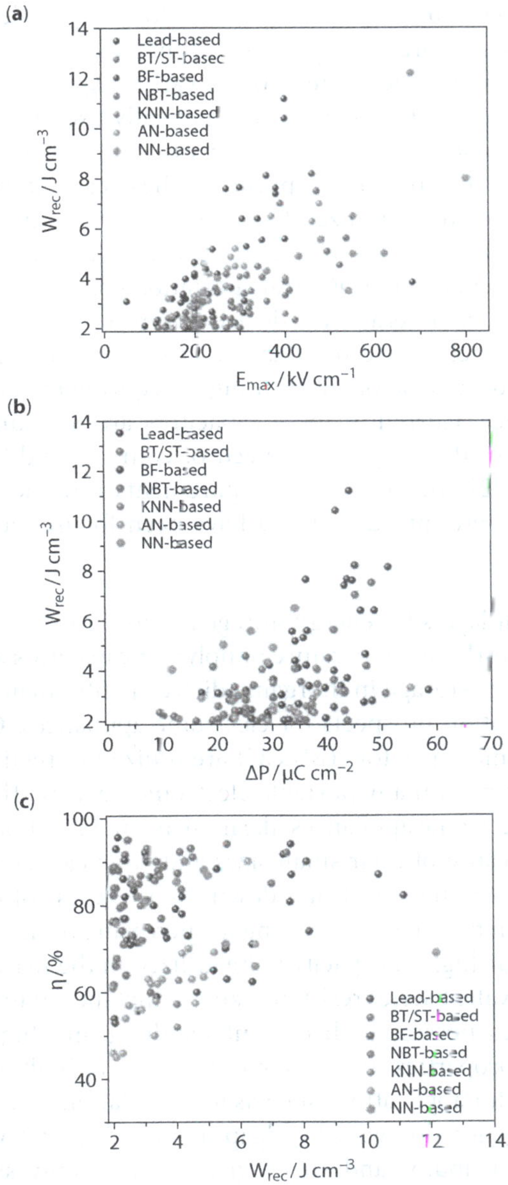

Figure 12.3 Contrast of (a) Emax vs Wrec; (b) ΔP vs Wrec; and (c) Wrec vs η for lead-based/lead-free bulk ceramics [28].

discharging speed [30], high pulse power, ultra-long cycle life, reliability, and ability to omit stored energy in small intervals of time like in micro or nanosecond time scale. Instead of its various applications in recently developed semiconductor devices; commercially used polymer dielectric capacitors still possess a low energy density of < 0.1 Whkg^{-1} in comparison with other fuel cells and supercapacitors. These capacitors call for more advanced methods to be utilized to increase their energy storage performance further. The weight of dielectric capacitors increases up to 50kg in high voltage direct current (DC) transportation converters for each transfer of high-speed train. As a result, device volume up to ~50.0% is occupied by a capacitor which may cause damage to semiconductor devices when quickly switched because of substituting an equivalent series inductance (ESL) in a device. Currently, these capacitors are not suitable for those electronic devices that require the need of compact and light-integrated capacitors [31, 32]. To meet these requirements ceramic multilayer and film capacitors were introduced and have been focused a lot on further investigations.

A. Ceramic multilayers for energy storage in capacitors

The low stable working temperature of polymer capacitors and low potential of total energy storage in inorganic dielectric film materials have limited their application prospects for electronic appliances. Comparatively, multilayer ceramic capacitors (MLCC) are utilized to retain electricity or to stabilize current in many portable electronic devices. These are widely used in many electronic appliances like in many mobile phones, PMPs, and MP3 players because of their small sizes and large capacitance. In recent years, there is more need to bring down the thickness of ceramic sheets and laminate it in multilayers by seeing its increasing trends toward miniaturization and the highest capacity to be utilized in the market. Because of having low equivalent series resistance and inductance; multilayer ceramic capacitor devices possess high current handling and high-temperature stability. These properties fulfill the requirements of high integration and miniaturization for applications such as in base stations, clean energy generations, third-generation wide bandgap semiconductor devices including fast switching capability, and smart grids [33]. Energy storage characteristics of commercially utilized multilayer capacitors are introduced in table-01 after performing several efforts by many researchers to get highly reliable MLCC devices via simulations and experiments. The realization of high capacitance and dielectric breakdown strength for MLCC is attributed to thinner ceramic dielectric layers between them. After optimizing and accomplishing the manufacturing process for the composition and structure of dielectric materials and appliances; the application area of MLCC will be broad in the field of energy storage.

From Table 12.4, it is evident that C0G type capacitors having high breakdown strength (BDS) can achieve energy storage of 1 Cm^{-3} and are manufactured with a dielectric material that has low relative permittivity (ε_r). BDS becomes significant for K7R-type capacitors that are fabricated from high ε_r (BT) materials to achieve high energy storage. While comparing the energy storage capacities of Z5U and K7R-type capacitors; it was notified that ε_r is not the only parameter that affects energy storage but also BDS of ceramics significantly alters the energy storage characteristics in ceramic capacitors. Fabrication of MLCCs takes place after following some steps of processing that contain slurry mixing of ceramic powder, tape casting, sheet cutting, fabrication, dicing, termination and shipping as possessed in Figure 12.1. This manufacturing is a powdered dependent that is scaled up from laboratory to market applications. Commercially, the scaling of ceramic capacitors MLs in the market has reached ~\$5.3 billion till 2017 which will reach up to ~\$7.8 billion by 2024 not only limited to mobile phones, electronic vehicles, and laptops but for many electronic applications [36]. About three trillion MLCCs are manufactured utilizing perovskite ($BaTiO_3$ (BT)) that possess properties of ferroelectric (FE) material. Classical ferroelectric materials such as BT possessed a high remanence whose charging capacity is soaked up by domain shifting and continued as (P_r). This high remanence can be reduced with chemical doping such as for doped (BT) is minimized to make it characteristic for relaxor ferroelectrics (RFEs).

Remanence-free materials are recommended to achieve high recoverable energy density (W_{rec}) that corresponds to the area covered above a polarization-electric (P-E) loop. Anti-ferroelectrics (AFEs) afford the advantages of high energy storage by displaying low remanence for low values of E but high BDS at large E to obtain AFE-FE transition. Conventionally, energy dissipation happens in all nonlinear dielectric-based materials like ferroelectrics (Fes), relaxor ferroelectrics (RFEs), and anti-ferroelectrics (AFEs). On the other hand, recently developed high energy density ceramic AFEs and RFEs multilayer materials are used in those high-power hybrid electric vehicles that require high operating temperatures and recoverable energy density. The highest performance MLCCs can be achieved after several types of research on low-cost internal electrodes [28].

Lead-based ceramic MLs with different internal electrodes possess prominent energy storage properties because of exhibiting small size and field-induced multiphase transitions. Different lead-based ceramic materials have been studied in the literature that possessed ultra-high W_{rec} and

Table 12.4 Energy storage characteristics of commercially utilized MLCCs.

MLCCS	Energy	Dielectric breakdown field E_b (MVm^{-1})	Energy efficiency η (%)	References
PLZT-based (B5803115105 M002)	93mJ, 500V (0.690 J cm^{-3})	–	89.5	[34]
BT-based (C1812C334KCRACTU)	10.7mJ, 500V (0.38 J cm^{-3})	–	63.0	[34]
C16 (C0G)	0.88J, 1kV	65	–	[35]
C11 (Z5U)	0.02J, 1kV	13.2	–	[35]
PMN-a (Z5U)	0.02J, 1kV	10	–	[35]
PMN-b (Z5U)	0.02J, 1kV	11	–	[35]
PLZT (X7T)	0.71J, 1kV	16	–	[35]
C08 (X7R)	1.40J, 1kV	30	–	[35]
C20 (X7R)	1.34J, 1kV	40	–	[35]
Exp (X7R)	4.82J, 1kV	90	–	[35]

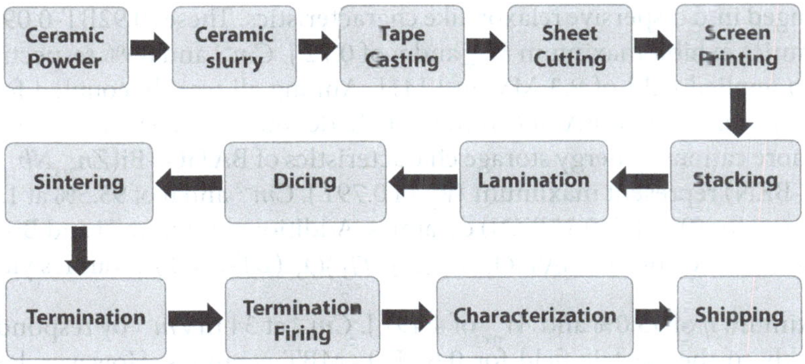

Figure 12.4 A series of ceramic multilayers (MLs) fabrication processing steps [37].

efficiency up to ~11.18J. Cm^{-3} and 87% [38] under different conditions, respectively. Even some lead-based antiferroelectric ceramic materials possess W_{rec} and efficiency values to such an extent that are not achieved by lead-free energy storage ceramic materials. However toxic nature of lead elements in these dielectric materials causes serious environmental issues that limit their applications. There is need a to develop lead-free ceramic materials that exhibit the highest energy storage capacities in capacitors covering all FEs, PFEs, and AFEs ceramics. Some compositionally optimized lead-free nonlinear dielectric ceramics have been discussed here.

B. $BATiO_3$-based

Barium titanate $BATiO_3$ (BT) is greatly studied lead-free dielectric ceramic material that exhibits two phase transitions; one at 125°C and the other at room temperature and transforms into a paraelectric cubic phase and ferroelectric tetragonal phase respectively. Many studies have attempted to decrease remanent polarization in BT to improve the E_b by reducing grain size, or by doing appropriate doping at its cationic site ions. By substituting (La, Ca, Zr, and Sr) at A/B site ions of $BATiO_3$ compositions changes to Ba(Zr, Ti) O_3, (Ba, La)TiO_3, and (Ba, Ca, Sr)(Ti, Zr) O_3 that cannot yield a storage density, storage density, W_{rec} of > 1.0 J. Cm^{-3} [30, 39]. Relaxor ferroelectric like $BATiO_3$- $BAScO_3$ (BT-BS) ceramics have high activation energy and are also termed "weakly coupled relaxors". The polar nano regions in these ferroelectrics minimize remanence polarization by possessing a fast response to an applied electric field, narrow hysteresis loop, and higher η. The storage density of 2.29 J. Cm^{-3} and E_b of 23.0 MV. m^{-1} are noticed for 0.7BT-0.3BS ferroelectric ceramics [40]. With increasing $BiYbO_3$ content in $BATiO_3$- $BiYbO_3$ (BT-BY) ceramics their normal ferroelectric behavior changed into dispersive relaxor-like characteristics. These (0.92BT-0.09BY) ceramics exhibit maximum W_{rec} and η of 0.72 J. Cm^{-3} and 83% respectively at an applied field of 9.3 MV. m^{-1} [41]. Among all weakly coupled ferroelectric ceramics of BATiO_3-BiMeO_3 (Me denotes tri-valent B-site of two or more cations); energy storage characteristics of BATiO_3-Bi$(Zn_{2/3}Nb_{1/3})O_3$ (BT-BZN) represent maximum W_{rec} of 0.791 J. Cm^{-3} and η of 93.5% at 13.11 MV. m^{-1} for (0.85BT-0.15BZN) ceramics. Additionally, many Ti and Bi-rich polar nano regions in $BATiO_3$- Bi$(Mg_{\frac{1}{2}}Ti_{\frac{1}{2}})O_3$ (BT-BMT) ceramics yield a maximum η of 93.0% and W_{rec} of 4.491 J. Cm^{-3} at 34 mVm^{-1} by responding quickly to the electric field for 0.6BT-0.4MBT ceramics. However, larger grain size > 8μm in these ceramic materials was detrimental to the miniaturization of MLCCs [30]. A decrease in grain size and an increase in both bulk density and E_b were liable for the enhancement of W_{rec} up to 2.90 J. Cm^{-3} at 30.14 MV. m^{-1} for $BATiO_3$- Bi$(Mg_{\frac{1}{2}}Zr_{\frac{1}{2}})O_3$ (0.85BT-0.15BMZ) ceramic. To decrease MLCCs cost in BaTiO_3-based dielectric ceramics; Ni internal electrodes must be co-fired for anti-reduction properties in them in a decreasing atmosphere. The powder form of BaTiO_3 is doped with rare earth oxides for sintering in a decreasing atmosphere; coating of Al_2O_3 on BaTiO_3 provides not only smaller size up to grain but also more η, W_{rec}, and E_b values at ambient temperature. BaTiO_3 based electrodes would possess practical importance for various device applications in energy storage Ni-electrode MLCCs via these anti-reduction properties [42]. In summary, BaTiO_3-based dielectric ceramics have achieved higher W_{rec} and η values that are responsible for high energy storage capacitors. Specifically, BaTiO_3 ceramics co-fired with base metal internal electrodes (Ni, Cu) have raised anti-reduction properties that are promising for the reduction in cost of MLCCs and are suitable for pulsed power technology and power electronic applications.

C. $K_{0.5}Na_{0.5}NbO_3$-based

Potassium-sodium niobate $K_{0.5}Na_{0.5}NbO_3$ (KNN) is found between ferroelectric (KNbO_3) and antiferroelectric (NaNbO_3) that with increasing temperature possess several phase transitions. The large ferroelectricity and good piezoelectric properties of KNN-based ceramics are not acceptable for various energy storage device applications. A KNN-based solid solution is formed by adding SrMO_3 (M denotes tetravalent metallic ions) or BiMeO_3 (Me symbolizes trivalent ions). By increasing the content of the second element; relaxor properties of KNN-based solutions are enhanced because of the enriching of dielectric permittance peak and shifting of T_c toward low temperature. Energy storage characteristics in KNN-based ferroelectric materials were improved after several modifications in composition, E_b, grain size engineering, and the correlation between polarization (P) and applied field (E) [23]. By adding $Sr(Zn_{1/3}Nb_{2/3})O_3$ in KNN with an amount of 0.94KNN-0.06SZN not only leads to uniform grain size < 200nm and high optical transparency but also storage density, W_{rec} of 1.51 J. Cm^{-3} with an η of 50.0% under 18.0 MV. m^{-1}. Similarly, for $0.80KNN\text{-}0.20Sr(Sc_{\frac{1}{2}}Nb_{\frac{1}{2}})O_3$(0.80KNN-0.20SSN) ceramic W_{rec} of 2.03 J. Cm^{-3} with an η of 81.40% under 29.51 MV. m^{-1} with a uniform grain size of ~ 500nm [43]. The introduction of 0.5 mol% ZnO into the 0.80KNN-0.20SSN enhance the E_b up to 40 MV. m^{-1} with lower porosity and higher storage density, W_{rec} of 2.60 J. Cm^{-3} with an η of 73.3%. With increasing ST content in (1-x)KNN-xSr-TiO_3 (KNN-ST); average grain size was reduced up to 0.35μm and 0.28μm for 0.85KNN-0.15ST and 0.85KNN-0.2ST respectively having properties of ferroelectric and large E_b, W_{rec} and η values. The addition of $BiFeO_3$ (BF) in KNN with 0.9KNN-0.1BF reduced the grain size up to 150nm with W_{rec} and η values of 2.0 J. Cm^{-3}, 61% respectively under 20.60 MV. m^{-1}. Furthermore by adding BF; properties like compression strength, binding strength, and elastic modulus increase in KNN-based ceramics making them beneficial for the lifetime and reliability of capacitors [30]. In summary, studies of KNN relaxor ferroelectrics have achieved E_b > 40.0 MV. m^{-1} and W_{rec} within 2.0-4.0 J. Cm^{-3}. However, ferroelectric and remanent polarized (P_r) behavior in these ceramic materials limits η < 75.0% which is not appropriate for energy storage capacitors applications. Reduction in P_r achieve more energy efficiency and energy density in KNN ceramics, is the main challenge for MLCCs applications.

D. $BiFeO_3$-based

$BiFeO_3$-based (BF) ceramics are considered desirable candidates for various storage applications due to possessing giant saturation polarization P_S ~ 100μC. cm^{-2}, low sintering temperature, and high curie temperature. There are still some difficulties that should be overcome to increase their energy storage applications such as high P_r, undesirable large dielectric losses, high breakdown strength, and conductivity that arises during the process of sintering. To minimize these major issues main focuses were paid on multivalent elements to reduce defects and to enhance polar nano regions for improving breakdown strength. Developed BF relaxor ferroelectric ceramics have enhanced energy storage properties because of presenting excellent comprehensive properties such as wide bandgap, heterogeneous nanodomain structure, and high spontaneous polarization gene. W_{rec} of 8.13 J. Cm^{-3} with an η of 90.0% under 36.0 MV. m^{-1} with extraordinary thermal stability has been achieved for 0.571 $BiFeO_3$-0.33 $BiTiO_3$-0.1$NaNbO_3$(0.571BF-0.33BT-0.1NN) ceramic material [44]. Some BF-made ceramics are ideal components for some storage device applications under low electric fields because of demonstrating giant polarization in these regions. The introduction of $BiMeO_3$ in BF-based ceramics has improved poor electrical insulation by frustrating long-range ferroelectric orders. Resultantly, with 0.35$BiFeO_3$-0.65(0.85 $BaTiO_3$-0.15$Bi(Sn_{0.5}Zn_{0.5})O_3$) ceramic, optical energy storage properties like excellent η of 92%, W_{rec} of 3.06 J. Cm^{-3} at a low field of 18.50 MV. m^{-1} have been obtained [30]. So, BF-relaxor ferroelectric ceramics are a potential element for future energy storage applications both at high field and low fields.

E. $AgNbO_3$-based

$AgNbO_3$ (AN) based ceramics being lead-free antiferroelectric materials have attained great attention for storage MLCCs applications. Energy storage characteristics of AN ceramics were improved after doping of Ta at the A-site, and W at the B cationic site of AN ceramic or by adding MnO_2 as a sintering aid. The addition of Ta in $Ag(Nb_{1-x}Ta_x)O_3$ (ANT) solid solutions effectively reduce the size and improve the antiferroelectric behavior in these ANT studied materials. Consequently, due to this antiferroelectricity, W_{rec} of 4.20 J. Cm^{-3} and η of 69.0% under an applied field of 24 MV. m^{-1} was obtained in ANT-15 based ceramics that was about 260% more than pristine AN ceramic [45]. La-doping in AN-ceramics also enhanced antiferroelectric phase stability and E_b by minimizing the grain size from 5.30 to 3.3μm with an increase in La^{3+} content. AgO should place in a dark environment because of its sensitivity to light and heat. The AN should be sintered in oxygen (O_2) atmosphere to form AgO compound that will further decompose into silver and O_2 at high temperatures. These properties of AN ceramics prefer the AN-MLCCs to be used expensive metals to make inner electrodes those will upsurge the cost of MLCCs. Moreover, the energy efficiency of AN-multilayer ceramic capacitors is <75% [30]which decreases their application area as energy storage capacitors. Despite these, many other ceramic materials have been studied, observed, and modified for energy storage capacitors and still are understudies.

12.4 Ceramic Films for Energy Storage in Capacitors

Ceramic film ferroelectric capacitors having large storage density, good high-temperature resistance, and electric field endurance have attracted intensive research interest for highly integrated designed capacitive energy storage applications. Reduction of occupied space and electromagnetic (EM) interference are some demands for highly integrated and miniaturization of electronics that is accomplished by implanting dielectric film-based capacitors within interior layers of PCB (printed circuit boards). It is encouraging to use a multilayer ceramic film for finding an appropriate design for high energy density pulse power capacitors. The energy storage characteristics of these materials have been improved after utilizing the design concept of different layers of dielectric-based materials. Dielectric ceramic films have owned not only W_{rec} of 50-150 J. Cm^{-3} with an efficiency of 60-90% under a breakdown field strength of 10.0 MV. Cm^{-1} but also, attractive temperature stability within the range of -50 to 200°C and energy storage properties [46, 47]. Various modifications have been adopted to control the parameters that alter the energy storage performance of ceramic films. Ferroelectric materials are greatly dependent upon nonlinear hysteresis curves with higher dielectric losses and lower BDS values. Significant research efforts on some ferroelectric (FE) ceramic films to improve energy storage characteristics have been discussed here.

A. Pb-Based FE films

Doped-$PbTiO_3$ have been discussed greatly in the past decade for energy storage applications using different preparation methods. Processing of (100)-oriented La and co-doped Ca with PT films at the temperature of 450°C with the composition of $Pb_{0.8}La_{0.1}Ca_{0.1}Ti_{0.975}O_3$ (PLCT) leads to low loss of Pb, dielectric, and leakage current because of the formation of oxygen vacancies. Films with these minimum losses displayed a small hysteresis loop with large saturation polarization and small P_r making them favorable for energy storage applications having W_{rec} of 14.90 J. Cm^{-3} and η of 77.57%. Thin film capacitors like $Pb(Zr_{0.53}Ti_{0.47})O_3$ have improved capacitance density by utilizing a large area electrode of 9mm^2 with W_{rec} of 12.5 J. Cm^{-3} at the field of 1.3 MV. Cm^{-1} [48]. When $Pb(Zr_{0.52}Ti_{0.48})O_3$ (PZT) thin films along distinct orientations ((001), (111), (011)) are deposited on the substrate of $SrRuO_3$ (SRO)/$SRTiO_3$(STO) utilizing pulsed layer deposition then all films possessed the same saturation polarization but fluctuating P_r along (001) and (111) oriented films. Different orientations were representing different hysteresis loops yet energy densities and efficiencies along all orientations were similar with W_{rec} of 9.20 J. Cm^{-3} and η of 56.4% under the field of 1 MV. m^{-1}. Using a sol-gel technique to deposit (111) PZT films on Pt/Si [49] has enhanced W_{rec} up to 15.60 J. Cm^{-3} and η of 58.8%. (001)- oriented PZT films have also enhanced energy storage characteristics of capacitors with faster discharge speed (4.1μs) by the chemical deposition method.

B. Bismuth-Based layer-structured FE films

Bismuth layer-based ferroelectric materials like $Bi_4Ti_3O_{12}$ (BIT), and Ca$Bi_2Nb_2)O_9$ (CBNO) because of possessing excellent endurance to an electric field and high curie temperature are suitable candidates for non-volatile random access memory applications. La-doped BIT films such as $Bi_{3.25}La_{0.75}Ti_3O_{12}$ (BLTO) were modified to get high capacitive storage density after suppressing large P_r, controlling grain size, and optimizing annealing temperature. Very slim hysteresis loop having high W_{rec} of 44.67 J. Cm^{-3} and η of 78.4% under an applied field of 2.05 MV. m^{-1} was achieved after utilizing these BLTO films. Moreover, improvements were made by preparing bi-layered and tri-layered films that were showing W_{rec} values of 54.86 and 65.46 J. Cm^{-3} [50] respectively with the same efficiency of 74.0% with an applied field of 2.75 MV. m^{-1}. High polarization of BFO, low leakage current, and increase in BDS factors was responsible for these energy storage characteristics. A natural superlattice ferroelectric thin film structure CBNO-BIT (like Ca$Bi_6Nb_2Ti_3O_{21}$) was modified to have high values of W_{rec}, and η with 76.0 J. Cm^{-3} and 66.4% respectively [49]. This superlattice structure was revealed on a nanoscale because of having lattice parameters the same as the lattice parameters of CBNO and BIT. A trim P-E hysteresis loop, low P_r with the low coercive field, enhanced dielectric constant, and high saturation polarization were attributed to this increase in energy storage properties of MLCCs.

C. Bi($Ni_{0.5}Ti_{0.5})O_3$ (BNT)-Based FE films

Compositions of solid solutions of Bi-based perovskite ferroelectric films (0.5Bi($Ni_{0.5}Ti_{0.5})O_3$)-0.5PbTiO$_3$) are adjacent to MPB (morphotropic phase boundary) compositions. These Bi-based films were reflecting a great impact of PbO- substitutions (0%, 10%, 20%) and of annealing temperature (600-850°C) on composition, piezoelectric and dielectric properties, and capacitive storage characteristics. With the increasingly strong influence of PbO, films were representing preferred orientation along (100) and good stability of storage properties within a temperature range of -190 to 250°C [51]. Moreover. Phase transitions were observed at different temperatures such as the pure perovskite phase being detected under 750°C and the addition of the pyrochlore phase above 800°C. In addition, high W_{rec} of 45.10 J. Cm^{-3} and η of 43.5% under an applied field of 2.25 MV. m^{-1} was achieved for these dense (0.5Bi($Ni_{0.5}Ti_{0.5})O_3$)-0.5PbTiO_3) films. Such as Pt which is so much expensive for mass production. From a practical perspective, major attention has been paid to modified BT compositions that are more effective with low-cost electrodes like Ag, Ni, and Ag/Pb. MLCCs should be further investigated to move forward in the market industry for the synthesis of low-cost electrodes, to maintain high BDS, and to get fatigued and reliable characteristics for the fabrication of more industrial applications energy dissipation, and associated defect dipoles and varies significantly with changes in composition for all bulk, MLs, and ceramic films. Commercially, in the past few years, lead-free MLCCs like BF and NBT, have prevailed over lead-based MLCCs by delivering high-energy storage performance W_{rec} > 15.0 J. Cm^{-3} under a field of ~ 1000 kV. m^{-1} [28]. However, for these materials, inner electrodes must be made with precious metals 21 J. Cm^{-3} and field of ~ 1000.0 kV. m^{-1} and bulk ceramic of W_{rec}~12.0 J. Cm^{-3} and field ~ 649.6 kV. m^{-1} . W_{rec} values in ceramic films can also be enhanced by utilizing ceramic-based MLs up to ~70μCcm^{-2} and bulk ceramic of ~60μCcm^{-2}. η of MLCCs depend upon factors such as domain switching, leakage current, polarization rotation, and ceramic films were reviewed by explaining benefits and design ideas within various layers of dielectric-based materials.

12.5 Conclusion

In this chapter, we have discussed many state-of-the-art ceramics candidates for capacitive storage applications. Among these is lead-based ceramics, which has the utmost potential in modern microelectronics due to its energy storage properties. Lead-based antiferroelectric is one of the candidates which has superior energy density and efficiency. Lead-free ceramics are more in demand nowadays and the amount of research in lead-free ceramics outweighs the research in lead-based ceramics. Many successful methods have been introduced to enhance the storage characteristics of lead-free-based ceramics, which have been briefly discussed here.

Although significant progress has been made for MLCCs still there is a large promotion space to enhance and improve their energy storage characteristics. Lead-free storage density MLCCs like BT, BF, NNT, and NBT are extensively studied to obtain the desired practical demands of current device applications showing storage density of 50 to 150 J. Cm^{-3} and r_{i} of 60.0-90.0%. Despite many breakthroughs, ceramic MLs and ceramic films still face many difficulties that contain high capability, high reliability, compatibility of low-cost metal-based electrodes, and industrial application-oriented measurement. Besides these challenges, lead free multilayer film capacitors are expected to become part of great future industrial research and development to empower a more energy-efficient and eco-friendly world.

References

1. Zhang, H., Wei, T., Zhang, Q., Ma, W., Fan, P., Salamon, D., Zhang, S.-T., Nan, B., Tan, H., Ye, Z.-G., A review on the development of lead-free ferroelectric energy-storage ceramics and multilayer capacitors. *J. Mater. Chem. C*, 8, 16648–16667, 2020.
2. Wang, D., Wang, G., Murakami, S., Fan, Z., Feteira, A., Zhou, D., Sun, S., Zhao, Q., Reaney, I.M., $BiFeO_3$-$BaTiO_3$: A new generation of lead-free electroceramics. *J. Adv. Dielectr.*, 8, 1830004, 2018.
3. Puli, V.S., Pradhan, D.K., Riggs, B.C., Chrisey, D.B., Katiyar, R.S., Investigations on structure, ferroelectric, piezoelectric and energy storage properties of barium calcium titanate (BCT) ceramics. *JALCOM*, 584, 369–373, 2014.
4. Wang, T., Jin, L., Li, C., Hu, Q., Wei, X., Relaxor ferroelectric $BaTiO_3$–Bi $(Mg_{2/3}Nb_{1/3})$ O_3 ceramics for energy storage application. *ACS*, 98, 559–566, 2015.
5. Yang, H., Yan, F., Zhang, G., Lin, Y., Wang, F., Dielectric behavior and impedance spectroscopy of lead-free $Ba_{0.85}Ca_{0.15}Zr_{0.1}Ti_{0.9}O_3$ ceramics with B_2O_3-Al_2O_3-SiO_2 glass-ceramics addition for enhanced energy storage. *JALCOM*, 720, 116–125, 2017.
6. Zhang, L., Pang, L.-X., Li, W.-B., Zhou, D., Extreme high energy storage efficiency in perovskite structured $(1\text{-}x)(Ba_{0.8}Sr_{0.2})TiO_3\text{-}xBi(Zn_{2/3}Nb_{1/3})O_3 (0.04 \leq x \leq 0.16)$ ceramics. *J. Eur. Ceram. Soc.*, 40, 3343–3347, 2020.
7. Li, W.-B., Zhou, D., Pang, L.-X., Enhanced energy storage density by inducing defect dipoles in lead free relaxor ferroelectric $BaTiO_3$-based ceramics. *Appl. Phys. Lett.*, 110, 132902, 2017.
8. Li, W.-B., Zhou, D., Pang, L.-X., Xu, R., Guo, H.-H., Novel barium titanate based capacitors with high energy density and fast discharge performance. *J. Mater. Chem. C*, 5, 19607–19612, 2017.
9. Zhou, M., Liang, R., Zhou, Z., Dong, X., Novel $BaTiO_3$-based lead-free ceramic capacitors featuring high energy storage density, high power density, and excellent stability. *J. Mater. Chem. C*, 6, 8528–8537, 2018.
10. Yang, H., Lu, Z., Li, L., Bao, W., Ji, H., Li, J., Feteira, A., Xu, F., Zhang, Y., Sun, H., Novel $BaTiO_3$-based, Ag/Pd-compatible lead-free relaxors with superior energy storage performance. *ACS*, 12, 43942–43949, 2020.
11. Yuan, Q., Li, G., Yao, F.-Z., Cheng, S.-D., Wang, Y., Ma, R., Mi, S.-B., Gu, M., Wang, K., Li, J.-F., Simultaneously achieved temperature-insensitive high energy density and efficiency in domain engineered $BaTiO_3$-$Bi(Mg_{0.5}Zr_{0.5})O_3$ lead-free relaxor ferroelectrics. *Nano Energy*, 52, 203–210, 2018.
12. Wu, T., Pu, Y., Gao, P., Liu, D., Influence of Sr/Ba ratio on the energy storage properties and dielectric relaxation behaviors of strontium barium titanate ceramics. *J. Mater. Sci.*, 24, 4105–4112, 2013.
13. Song, Z., Liu, H., Hao, H., Zhang, S., Cao, M., Yao, Z., Wang, Z., Hu, W., Shi, Y., Hu, B., The effect of grain boundary on the energy storage properties

of $(Ba_{0.4}Sr_{0.6}M)TiO_3$ paraelectric ceramics by varying grain sizes. *IEEE*, 62, 609–616, 2015.

14. Huang, Y.H., Wu, Y.J., Qiu, W.J., Li, J., Chen, X.M., Enhanced energy storage density of $Ba_{0.4}Sr_{0.6}TiO_3$–MgO composite prepared by spark plasma sintering. *J. Eur. Ceram. Soc.*, 35, 1469–1476, 2015.
15. Huang, Y.H., Wu, Y.J., Liu, B., Yang, T.N., Wang, J.J., Li, J., Chen, L.-Q., Chen, X.M., From core–shell $Ba_{0.4}Sr_{0.6}TiO_3$@SiO_2 particles to dense ceramics with high energy storage performance by spark plasma sintering. *J. Mater. Chem. A*, 6, 4477–4484, 2018.
16. Cui, C., Pu, Y., Gao, Z., Wan, J., Guo, Y., Hui, C., Wang, Y., Cui, Y., Structure, dielectric and relaxor properties in lead-free ST-NBT ceramics for high energy storage applications. *JALCOM*, 711, 319–326, 2017.
17. Cui, C., Pu, Y., Shi, R., High-energy storage performance in lead-free (0.8-x) $SrTiO_3$-0.2 $Na_{0.5}Bi_{0.5}TiO_3$-x$BaTiO_3$ relaxor ferroelectric ceramics. *JALCOM*, 740, 1180–1187, 2018.
18. Yao, Z., Luo, Q., Zhang, G., Hao, H., Cao, M., Liu, H., Improved energy-storage performance and breakdown enhancement mechanism of Mg-doped SrTiO3 bulk ceramics for high energy density capacitor applications. *J. Mater. Sci.*, 28, 11491–11499, 2017.
19. Kong, X., Yang, L., Cheng, Z., Zhang, S., Bi-modified $SrTiO_3$-based ceramics for high-temperature energy storage applications. *ACS*, 103, 1722–1731, 2020.
20. Tao, H., Wu, W., Wu, J., Electrical properties of holmium doped (K,Na) $(Nb,Sb)O_3$-(Bi, Na)HfO_3 ceramics with wide sintering and poling temperature range. *JALCOM*, 689, 759–766, 2016.
21. Qu, B., Du, H., Yang, Z., Liu, Q., Liu, T., Enhanced dielectric breakdown strength and energy storage density in lead-free relaxor ferroelectric ceramics prepared using transition liquid phase sintering. *RSC Adv.*, 6, 34381–34389, 2016.
22. Qiao, X., Zhang, X., Wu, D., Chao, X., Yang, Z., Influence of Bi nonstoichiometry on the energy storage properties of 0.93KNN–0.07Bi_xMN relaxor ferroelectrics. *J. Adv. Dielectr.*, 8, 1830006, 2018.
23. Yang, Z., Gao, F., Du, H., Jin, L., Yan, L., Hu, Q., Yu, Y., Qu, S., Wei, X., Xu, Z., Grain size engineered lead-free ceramics with both large energy storage density and ultrahigh mechanical properties. *Nano Energy*, 58, 768–777, 2019.
24. Yang, Z., Du, H., Qu, S., Hou, Y., Ma, H., Wang, J., Wang, J., Wei, X., Xu, Z., Significantly enhanced recoverable energy storage density in potassium–sodium niobate-based lead free ceramics. *J. Mater. Chem. C*, 4, 13778–13785, 2016.
25. Shao, T., Du, H., Ma, H., Qu, S., Wang, J., Wang, J., Wei, X., Xu, Z., Potassium–sodium niobate based lead-free ceramics: Novel electrical energy storage materials. *J. Mater. Chem.* 5, 554–563, 2017.
26. Wang, J., Chen, X., Wang, J., Wang, G., Nie, H., Cao, F., Dong, X., Improved dielectric breakdown strength of $Pb_{0.99}(Zr_{0.95}Ti_{0.05})_{0.98}Nb_{0.02}O_3$ ferroelectric ceramics with the addition of CuO. *J. Mater. Chem. A*, 26, 8207–8211, 2015.

27. Li, Y., Cao, M.-S., Wang, D.-W., Yuan, J., High-efficiency and dynamic stable electromagnetic wave attenuation for La doped bismuth ferrite at elevated temperature and gigahertz frequency. *RSC Adv.*, 5, 77184–77191, 2015.
28. Wang, G., Lu, Z., Li, Y., Li, L., Ji, H., Feteira, A., Zhou, D., Wang, D., Zhang, S., Reaney, I.M., Electroceramics for high-energy density capacitors: Current status and future perspectives. *ACS*, 121, 6124–6172, 2021.
29. Liu, S., Shen, B., Hao, H., Zhai, J., Glass–ceramic dielectric materials with high energy density and ultra-fast discharge speed for high power energy storage applications. *J. Mater. Chem. C*, 7, 15118–15135, 2019.
30. Zhao, P., Cai, Z., Wu, L., Zhu, C., Li, L., Wang, X., Perspectives and challenges for lead-free energy-storage multilayer ceramic capacitors. *J. Adv. Ceram.*, 10, 1153–1193, 2021.
31. Hao, X.J., A review on the dielectric materials for high energy-storage application. *J. Adv. Dielectr.*, 3, 1330001, 2013.
32. Zou, K., Dan, Y., Xu, H., Zhang, Q., Lu, Y., Huang, H., He, Y., Recent advances in lead-free dielectric materials for energy storage. *Mater. Res. Bull.*, 113, 190–201, 2019.
33. Liang, Z., Liu, M., Shen, L., Lu, L., Ma, C., Lu, X., Lou, X., Jia, C.-L., All-inorganic flexible embedded thin-film capacitors for dielectric energy storage with high performance. *ACS Appl. Mater. Interfaces*, 11, 5247–5255, 2019.
34. Xu, R., Feng, Y., Wei, X., Xu, Z., Analysis on nonlinearity of antiferroelectric multilayer ceramic capacitor (MLCC) for energy storage. *IEEE*, 26, 2005–2011, 2019.
35. Love, G.R., Energy storage in ceramic dielectrics. *J. Am. Ceram. Soc.*, 73, 323–328, 1990.
36. Wang, X., Fan, Y., Zhang, B., Mostaed, A., Li, L., Feteira, A., Wang, D., Sinclair, D.C., Wang, G., Reaney, I.M., High discharge energy density in novel $K_{1/2}Bi_{1/2}TiO_3$-$BiFeO_3$ based relaxor ferroelectrics. *J. Eur. Ceram. Soc.*, 42, 7381–7387, 2022.
37. Pan, M.-J. and Randall, C.A., A brief introduction to ceramic capacitors. *IEEE*, 26, 44–50, 2010.
38. Liu, X., Li, Y., Hao, X., Ultra-high energy-storage density and fast discharge speed of $(Pb_{0.98-x}La_{0.02}Sr_x)(Zr_{0.9}Sn_{0.1})_{0.995}O_3$ antiferroelectric ceramics prepared via the tape-casting method. *J. Mater. Chem. A*, 7, 11858–11866, 2019.
39. Chao, S. and Dogan, F., $BaTiO_3$–$SrTiO_3$ layered dielectrics for energy storage. *Mater. Lett.*, 65, 978–981, 2011.
40. Ogihara, H., Randall, C.A., McKinstry, S., High-energy density capacitors utilizing 0.7 $BaTiO_{3-}$ 0.3 $BiScO_3$ ceramics. *J. Am. Chem. Soc.*, 92, 1719–1724, 2009.
41. Shen, Z., Wang, X., Luo, B., Li, L., $BaTiO_3$–$BiYbO_3$ perovskite materials for energy storage applications. *Mater. Chem. A*, 3, 18146–18153, 2015.

42. Zhao, Q., Wang, X., Gong, H., Liu, B., Luo, B., Li, L., The properties of Al_2O_3 coated fine-grain temperature stable $BaTiO_3$-based ceramics sintered in reducing atmosphere. *J. Am. Chem. Soc.*, 101, 1245–1254, 2018.
43. Qu, B., Du, H., Yang, Z., Lead-free relaxor ferroelectric ceramics with high optical transparency and energy storage ability. *J. Mater. Chem. C*, 4, 1795–1803, 2016.
44. Qi, H., Xie, A., Tian, A., Zuo, R., Superior energy-storage capacitors with simultaneously giant energy density and efficiency using nanodomain engineered $BiFeO_3$-$BaTiO_3$-$NaNbO_3$ lead-free bulk ferroelectrics. *Adv. Energy Mater.*, 10, 1903338, 2020.
45. Zhao, L., Liu, Q., Gao, J., Zhang, S., Li, J.F., Lead-free antiferroelectric silver niobate tantalate with high energy storage performance. *Adv. Mater.*, 29, 1701824, 2017.
46. Zhang, T., Li, W., Zhao, Y., Yu, Y., Fei, W., Structure-property relationships: High energy storage performance of opposite double-heterojunction ferroelectricity–insulators. *Adv. Funct. Mater.*, 28, 1870066, 2018.
47. Fan, Z., Li, L., Mei, X., Zhao, F., Li, H., Zhuo, X., Zhang, X., Lu, Y., Zhang, L., Liu, M.J., Multilayer ceramic film capacitors for high-performance energy storage: Progress and outlook. *J. Mater. Chem. C*, 9, 9462–9480, 2021.
48. Sigman, J., Brennecka, G.L., Clem, P.G., Tuttle, B.A., Fabrication of perovskite-based high-value integrated capacitors by chemical solution deposition. *J. Am. Chem. Soc.*, 91, 1851–1857, 2008.
49. Palneedi, H., Peddigari, M., Hwang, G.T., Jeong, D.Y., Ryu, J., High-performance dielectric ceramic films for energy storage capacitors: Progress and outlook. *Adv. Funct. Mater.*, 28, 1803665, 2018.
50. Xiao, S., Sun, H., Liu, X., Sui, H., High-performance $(Na_{0.5}Bi_{0.5})(Ti_{0.97}Fe_{0.03})O_3$-based heterostructure thin films for energy storage capacitors. *Ceram. Int.*, 15, pp. 214448–21456, 2022.
51. Xie, Z., Peng, B., Meng, S., Zhou, Y., Yue, Z.J., High-energy-storage density capacitors of $Bi(Ni_{1/2}Ti_{1/2})O_3$–$PbTiO_3$ thin films with good temperature stability. *J. Am. Chem. Soc*, 96, 2061–2064, 2013.

13

Lead-Free Ceramics for High Performance Supercapacitors

Asma Farrukh[1], Sara Yaseen[1], Abdul Ghafar Wattoo[1*], Adnan Khalil[1], Muhammad Sohaib Ali[1], Kamran Ikram[2] and Muhammad Bilal Tahir[1]

[1]*Institute of Physics, Khwaja Fareed University of Engineering and Information Technology, Rahim Yar Khan, Pakistan*
[2]*Department of Agricultural Engineering, Khwaja Fareed University of Engineering and Information Technology, Rahim Yar Khan, Pakistan*

Abstract
Supercapacitors are one of the most intriguing devices for storing electrical energy because of their fast storage capabilities, higher power density, long cycle stability, and environmental friendliness. Nanomaterials have been the subject of extensive research to develop high-efficiency, low-cost and stable electrodes. For SCs electrodes, ceramic materials are attractive candidates. On the other hand, low surface activity and low specific surface area of ceramic materials; significantly limit the performance of supercapacitors. To make it possible efficient electron transportation and high electrical conductivity, as well as achieve economically viable ceramic electrodes in industry, the fundamental insight of ceramic materials, development in search of ceramic electrodes, and method of optimization are critical phases.

Keywords: Supercapacitors, ceramic capacitors, Pb-based ceramics, piezoelectric activity

13.1 Introduction

The most hazardous heavy metal in the environment is lead. Because of its important physicochemical qualities, it has been used since ancient times.

**Corresponding author*: abdul.ghafar@kfueit.edu.pk

Inamuddin, Tariq Altalhi and Sayed Mohammed Adnan (eds.) Electroceramics for High Performance Supercapacitors, (297–314) © 2024 Scrivener Publishing LLC

On a global scale, it is a widely distributed, essential, but dangerous environmental chemical [1]. Its significant qualities include ductility, resistance to corrosion, softness, weak conductivity, and malleability, making it not easy to abandon. Because of its long-term use and non-biodegradable nature, its concentration accumulates in the environment posing increasing risks. Lead and its compounds are largely exposed to humans in lead-related activities as a result of several resources such as leaded gasoline, industrial methods for example Pb-based painting, lead combustion and smelting, pottery, Pb comprising pipes, grids, the arms industry, battery recycling, pigments, book printing, and so on. Even though it is no longer commonly used in numerous countries, and yet utilized in a range of manufacturing industries for example battery recycling and production, automobile maintenance, refining, and smelting, etc. The nervous system is the most generally affected organ in both adults and children who have been exposed to lead.

Following the industrial revolution, technology advanced quickly in several countries resulting in an economic boom [2]. Medical electronic equipment and mobile communications stand out as important modernizing areas among technological advancement innovations. Nevertheless, we paid a significant price for these benefits which included harmful effects on the environment, impacting health and employment problems caused by huge utilization of fossil fuels (gas, oil, coal) [3]. The overall global need for fossil fuels was around 13.7 BTOE in 2012, and it is expected to rise to 18.3 BTOE by 2035 [4]. The increase in CO_2 emissions per year from 1.09 billion tonnes in 2011 to 36.58 billion tonnes in 2018 is one of the detrimental consequences. The demand for sustainable and renewable energy sources (for example, solar, wind, tidal, geothermal, and biofuels) [5] is driving the development of relevant energy storage, generation, and conservation technologies. Thermochemical energy storage (for example, solar hydrogen, heat storage) and thermal energy, chemical energy storage and conversion (for example, fuel cells, water splitting), electrical energy storage (i.e., electric double layer capacitors, physical capacitors), mechanical energy storage (such as flywheels), and electrochemical energy storage have all been developed so far (like batteries, pseudocapacitors) [6]. Between them, SCs also referred to as electrochemical capacitors or ultracapacitors have a high capacity of storage (small discharge time of 1 to 10 s), easy operation mode, better reversibility, environmental friendliness, long-term stability (>30,000 h and > 10^5cycles), enhanced energy density and higher power density (around 10 kW/kg) [7]. Because of these properties, supercapacitors can cover the energy/power gap between higher energy density fuel cells or batteries and larger power density capacitors [8]. Moreover, because the charge storage mechanism is simple, it produces less thermochemical heat [9], allowing SCs to be used in a wider range of applications including memory backup systems, consumer electronics, and industrial power [10]. For supercapacitor electrodes, a variety of materials have been developed including materials based on carbon (CNTs, conducting polymers, GO, activated carbon) [11], carbides [12], oxides [13], sulfides [14], hydroxides [15], nitrides [1], MOF [16, 17] and MXene [18]. In general, operating voltage, capacitance, and equivalent series resistance are used to evaluate the performance of supercapacitor electrodes, from which power density and energy density may be computed [19]. Also, cycling stability is an important parameter for electrodes [20]. Electrolytes, electrode materials, and potential windows all play a role in the electrochemical properties of SCs [21]. Nevertheless, much of the present research has concentrated on the component design and structure of electrode-based materials, which leads to good conductivity, specifically higher surface area, and ample pores, allowing for ion diffusion capabilities and electron transport [22]. For SC electrode materials, a range of materials (for example, MOF, ceramics, metals, COF, polymers) have been developed [23]. Despite their low surface activity and low specific surface area, ceramic materials are nevertheless appealing for supercapacitor electrode development due to their thermal shock resistance, corrosion resistance, high temperature resistance and radiation resistance [24]. Jiang and coworkers, for example, made all ceramic V_2O_3/MnO_2hybrid electrode for highly efficient pseudocapacitors [25], where interpenetrating nanopores provide abundant V_2O_3/MnO_2 interfaces as well as quick ion transportation channels, through V–O–Mn chemical bond this considerably improves interfacial electron transport. Liu and his colleagues homogeneously loaded CuO NPs (10 mg/cm^2) over a highly conducting $La_{1-x}Sr_xCoO_{3-\delta}$ ceramic substrate [26], this results in effective ion diffusion and quick electron transmission, and therefore a supercapacitor without standing performance in quasi solid state. Chang and coworkers reported flexible all solid-state supercapacitors utilize hard B_4C@C core shell ceramics as electrodes [27]. Carbon shell enhanced B_4C ceramic's electric conductivity; while ceramics itself stabilized particles during discharging and charging. Generally, implementing techniques to improve microstructure and components of ceramic materials can help them have faster electron transportation and better ion diffusion. As a result, the electrode performance of supercapacitors is improved.

13.2 Ceramics

Ceramics is a non-metallic inorganic substance made primarily of crystalline oxide, nitride, or carbide. The word Ceramic derives from the Greek word keramos which means "potter's clay." Many modern ceramic compounds, on the other hand, do not contain clay. Metal and non-metal compounds are the building blocks of modern ceramics. The atomic bonds between them are usually ionic. Insulating materials, abrasives, glass, refractories, and enamels are all examples of traditional ceramics. Metal oxides, nitrides, carbides, borides, and silicates are among them. Tungsten carbide, alumina, silicon carbide, and magnesia are some of their examples.

13.2.1 General Classification of Ceramics

13.2.1.1 Ceramic-Based Capacitors

The dielectric in a ceramic capacitor is made of ceramic. In modern electronics, there are two categories of ceramic capacitors: ceramic disc and multilayer ceramic (MLCC). Ceramic capacitors are nonpolarized and have modest capacitances ranging from 1 nF to 1 μF. In comparison to electrolytic capacitors, they have a low maximum rated voltage. Surface mount devices use MLCCs because they are significantly smaller than disc capacitors. The most common form of the capacitor is ceramic capacitors used throughout many electrical devices. Figure 13.1 shows the general classification of ceramics. They are more durable and less expensive to fabricate. The ceramic material is regarded as an excellent dielectric and a good supporter of electrostatic fields due to its poor conductivity. These

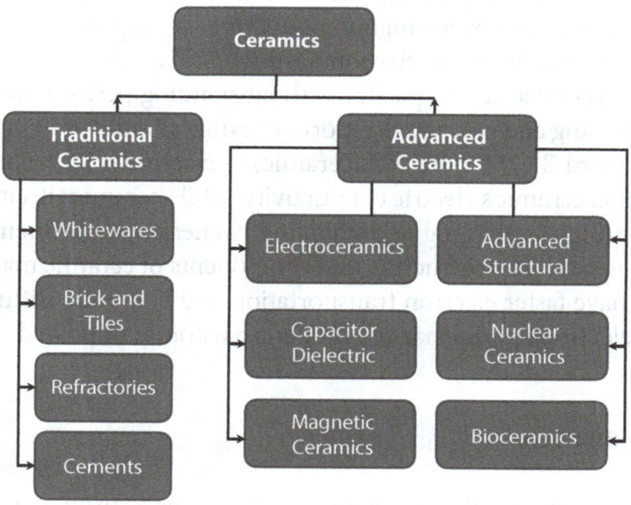

Figure 13.1 General classification of ceramics.

capacitors are utilized in a variety of applications. Ceramic or porcelain discs are used to make them.

13.3 Types of Ceramic Capacitors

Ceramic capacitors are divided into two types:

1. Multi-layered Ceramic Capacitors (MLCC): These are commonly used and produced capacitors utilized in electronic devices. They are utilized in RFI/EMI suppression systems, and larger-scale systems as control capacitors in transmitters and feed-through capacitors and come in a range of shapes and styles.
2. Ceramic Disc Capacitors: These are sometimes used as protective capacitors in electromagnetic interference reduction applications. They are manufactured in small sizes. They can be safely connected to an AC source. MLCC and ceramic discs capacitors as shown in Figures 13.2 (a) and (b).

13.4 Overview of Ceramics for Supercapacitors

Ceramic is a versatile material with good chemical and thermal stability, hardness and high mechanical strength, and significant electrical, magnetic, and optical properties making it widely used in a variety of fields such as construction [28], energy (e.g. fuel cells, supercapacitors, solar cells, and batteries) [29], catalysis (for example, electrocatalysis,

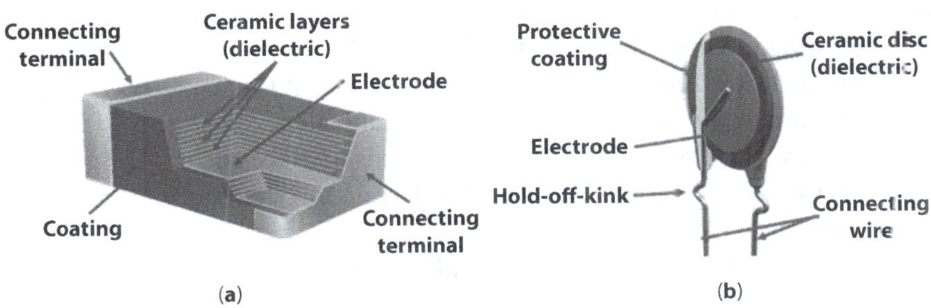

Figure 13.2 (a) Diagram representing construction of multilayer ceramic capacitor. (b) Ceramic disc capacitor. Reproduce with permission from Reference [67].

heterogeneous catalysis, and photocatalysis) [30], machinery, chemical industry [31], aerospace, electronics [32], laser [33], biomedical engineering [34] and dental implant [35]. Ceramic materials have a variety of uses, but they are becoming more and more essential in applications related to energy. The fundamental cause is that the energy problem has gotten more severe as nonrenewable energy resources like natural gas, oil, and coal are decreasing and fossil energy is being excessively exploited and consumed. As a result, researchers are continuing to develop new materials to reduce emissions and save energy while adhering to the principle of sustainable development. Ceramic material advancement is one of them. Evidently, corrosion resistance, higher temperature resistance, thermal shock resistance, and high temperature resistance of ceramic material still make it a viable candidate for use as an electrode material in SCs. Numerous papers describe interesting strategies to optimize size (nanoclusters, quantum dots, single atoms, nano-particles), internal structure (arrays, hollow, yolk-shell, porous, frames, core-shell),shape (rods, wires, plates, spheres, sheets, cubes), and composition (multi-component, bi, or mono) of ceramic materials to attain abundant pores and higher specific surface area along with fast electron transfer and better dispersion of ions. As a result, a wide range of ceramic electrode materials has been developed for SCs including carbide and nitride ceramics, metal oxide ceramics, ceramics based on carbon, ceramics based on metal hydroxide, multi-elemental oxide ceramics, and other special ceramics.

13.4.1 Metal Oxide Ceramics for Supercapacitors

Metal oxides (MO) such as supercapacitors [36], fuel cells, lithium batteries, and electrocatalysis are extensively employed in the energy transformation and storage field due to their low cost, eco-friendliness, natural abundance, easy fabrication, and multiple valences [37]. Between them, Transition metal oxides have gotten a lot of interest owing to their low cost and a high potential for being environmentally friendly [38]. Charge storage procedures of MO-based electrodes (for example, Co_3O_4, NiO, MnO_2,) in aqueous electrolytes are commonly considered to be based on valence changes of metallic species via surface redox reactions with anions, surface adsorption/desorption or Faradaic proton/alkali metal intercalation/deintercalation. Metal oxide ceramics, like transition metal oxide ceramics (Co_3O_4, Mn_3O_4, NiO, ZrO_2, MnO_2, V_2O_5), Al_2O_3ceramics, and SnO_2 ceramics have become more popular as SC electrode materials in recent years. Ceramics based on transition MO are utilized to hold larger density energy in quick surface redox reactions. Table 13.1 shows the metal oxide based ceramics for supercapacitors.

Table 13.1 Metal oxide based ceramics for supercapacitors.

Materials	Method	Morphology	Capacitance
CuO-Co_3O	Electrospinning	Nanowires	1277 F/g at 2 A/g
MnO_2	Electrophoretic deposition	Film	0.34 F/cm² at 2 mV/s
MnO_2-MWCNT	Liquid-liquid extraction method	Nanocomposites	5.7 F/cm² at 2 mV/s
V_2O_5	Sol-gel method and freezing	Scaffold's lamellar structure	
Al_2O_3	Selective laser etching	Micropillars	5.5 mF/cm² at 5 mV/s
V_2O_3/MnO_2	Pulsed electrodeposition	Corundum-type crystalline	1172 F/cm³ at 10 mV/s

13.4.2 Multi-Elemental Oxide Ceramics for Supercapacitors

13.4.2.1 Spinel Oxide Ceramics

Two metals are present in spinel oxide ceramics, resulting in more complex redox chemistry than single constituent oxides [39]. Single-component oxides frequently have high electrochemical activity and stronger electrical conductivity than binary oxides. MFe_2O_4, (Spinel ferrites) for example, have been employed as supercapacitor electrodes. The properties of $NiFe_2O_4$ ceramic powders made by several methods (sol-gel synthesis, polyol-mediated synthesis, and combustion synthesis) were studied [40]. Morphology that could be modified by the synthesis method influenced double-layer capacitors and their behavior observed in $NiFe_2O_4$ ceramic powder. Finally, because of the better micro and high porosity of the electrode, $NiFe_2O_4$ ceramic synthesized using the sol-gel technique had the highest specific capacitance of 97.5 F/g. Kovalenko and colleagues reported the synthesis of $NiCo_2O_4$ as potential electrode material for SCs [41]. Nanocrystalline-based material with 25-30% exposed porosity was fabricated by combining crystallization of nitrate solution with resultant ultrasonic and thermal treatment. The variable valence of Co and Ni, like other spinel oxides, enhanced the electrode's pseudo-capacity and electrical conductivity, making it promising electrode material [41]. Example of Multi-elemental oxide ceramics for SCs is $BaTiO_3$ ceramics.

13.5 Lead-Based Ceramics

Environmental issues have been a major source of concern throughout the world in recent years [42]. Glass, batteries, and gasoline are just a few examples that contain lead [43]. The most extensively employed piezoelectric material PZT has about 60% PbO [44].To reduce the use of dangerous compounds in final products, the Restriction of Hazardous Substances Directive was enacted [45]. As a result, research into lead-free piezoelectric materials is critical right now [46]. Among numerous Pb-free piezoelectric materials, like $BiFeO_3$-based piezoelectric materials, $BaTiO_3$, and (Bi, Na)TiO_3-based piezoelectric materials with higher piezoelectric properties and larger Curie temperatures are regarded as a possible candidate for lead zirconate titanate-based materials in the industrial sector [47].

To get appreciable piezoelectric capabilities, $PbTiO_3$ is infrequently utilized in its pure state, preferring to be mixed or converted into solid solutions [48]. $PbTiO_3$ belongs to the ABO_3 perovskite family. At ambient temperature, it is tetragonal and ferroelectric but at 490°C, it experiences a phase transition and transforms into the cubic paraelectric form [49]. The short-range repulsions are decreased by the hybridization of the Ti-O bond. In $PbTiO_3$, this is required for ferroelectricity. It possesses a low dielectric anisotropy and a large permittivity perpendicular to the polar axis. With a high temperature for phase transition, lead titanate has a low dielectric constant. These characteristics make them a good fit for high-end applications. Curie temperature and spontaneous strain are reduced when $PbTiO_3$ is doped. This is advantageous because it helps to protect the structure from cracking when the temperature is reduced from sintering levels. Electrical resistance is also increased [50]. ABO_3 perovskite structure of (a) cubic and (b) tetragonal phases has been illustrated in Figure 13.3.

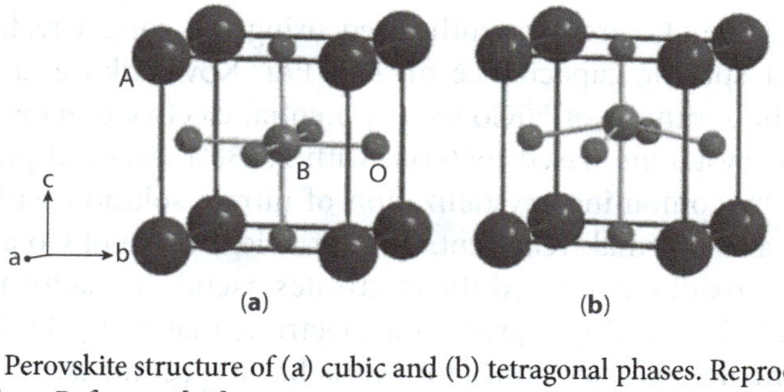

Figure 13.3 Perovskite structure of (a) cubic and (b) tetragonal phases. Reproduced with permission from Reference [50].

Lead zirconate is antiferroelectric and it lacks piezoelectric characteristics. On the other hand, pure lead titanate has restricted piezoelectric response. Unexpectedly, PZT, a solid solution of lead titanate and lead zirconate, has a high piezoelectric response and is widely used in industry, transportation, communication, medicine, and science and information technology. Because of the toxicity of lead, questions about its use as a piezoelectric material have been raised. Consequently, there is a push to produce Pb-free piezoelectric materials with qualities comparable to or better than those of existing Pb-based piezoceramics. Potassium sodium niobate is also known as KNN is an intriguing Pb-free candidate. As it offers similar piezoelectric properties to the PZT while posing no environmental risks. However, the claim that KNN is more environmentally friendly than PZT is still debatable. Ibn Mohammed *et al.* evaluated the environmental issues of KNN and PZT in a study [51].

13.6 Lead-Free Ceramics

PZT which is recognized for its outstanding electroactive characteristics has paved the way for Pb-based piezoelectric materials. However, because of growing issues about the environment and ecosystem, Pb-based piezoelectrics are being phased out in favor of lead-free alternatives, owing to the negative effects of lead on humans and the environment. The piezoelectric potential of Pb-free materials, both inorganic and organic, has been investigated. The piezoelectric properties discovered were comparable to, and in some cases even better than, those of existing PZTs. Furthermore, because of their environmental friendliness and biocompatibility, they are capable of replacing Pb-based piezoelectric materials shortly. Many Pb-free piezoelectric devices have been developed as a result of technological advancements, with applications in energy, military, bioengineering, and optoelectronic information [52]. The KNN-based ceramic system has been recognized as one of the most interesting Pb-free piezoelectric materials due to its high Tc (420°C), large k_p, and high Pr (33 μC/cm^2) [53]. KNN ceramics can be made in a variety of ways including the wet chemical method, solid-state method, and so on. The latter methods are designed to compensate for the inadequacies of the former methods. To address issues like volatilization of alkali metal, deliquescence, etc. modified sintering procedures have been devised [54] KNN-based materials have a large piezoelectric constant (d_{33}). New phase boundary construction (for example, R–O–T, R–T, etc.) and chemical modification (e.g., Sb^{5+}, Ta^{5+}, Li+, $SrTiO_3$, $CaZrO_3$, Ba^{2+}, $Bi_{0.5}Na_{0.5}ZrO_3$)

have been used in general. One such Pb-free piezoelectric system is based on barium titanate (BT) [54]. The structure of this system is perovskite, having A-site atoms containing barium, strontium, calcium, though B-site atoms are titanium, niobium, and tantalum, etc. Despite benefits like good electromechanical coupling, stable electrical properties, and low dielectric loss, low d_{33} and TC of BT-based ceramic systems limit its application. Modification via doping leads to the formation of new MPB and therefore better piezoelectric performance. Bismuth layer-structured piezoelectric ceramics are another lead-free alternative. The ceramic's structure is made up of two layers: $(Bi_2O_2)^{2+}$ and $(A_{m-1}B_mO_{3m+1})^{2-}$ [54]. These have a low tan δ, low ε_T aging resistance, and high Tc. This class also has several drawbacks, such as polarization difficulties owing to the higher coercive electric field and lower piezoelectric action because of spontaneous polarization limitations. Pb-free ceramics based on$SrTiO_3$ (ST), $(K_{0.5}Na_{0.5})NbO_3$, $BaTiO_3$, and $(Bi_{0.5}Na_{0.5})TiO_3$, have received a lot of attention recently for storage applications relevant to high energy [55]. Because of their large P_{max}, BNT and BT-based Pb-free ceramics have been extensively explored for storing energy. However, most Pb-free ceramics do not exhibit higher η (> 80 percent) and high W_{rec} (> 2 J/cm^3) at the same time due to large P_r and low BDS [56]. Potassium sodium niobate-based ceramics raw materials are too costly to be marketed, and they are complicated to attain due to their extremely narrow sintering temperature range [57]. $SrTiO_3$ requires relatively low-cost raw ingredients, has a wide sintering temperature range, and can be mass-produced for high-voltage capacitors in large quantities [58]. Also, ceramics based on ST are predicted to be utilized in higher energy-storage capacitors.

13.6.1 Analysis of Pb-Free Hybrid Materials for Energy Conversion

Ceramics (both Pb-based and Pb-free), composites, and polymers are three types of piezoelectric materials. Because of the possible environmental risk caused by lead in Pb-based piezoelectric materials, the focus has steadily switched to Pb-free piezoelectric materials. Piezoelectric characteristics can be found in a variety of ceramics, polymers, and composites. Ceramics may again be Pb-free or Pb based. When compared to Pb-free materials, Pb-based piezoelectric compounds exhibit superior piezoelectric characteristics. However, due to the environmental risks caused by Pb in ceramics with Pb content, the focus is now increasingly turning to Pb-free ceramics [54]. KNN (Pb-free piezoelectric) has emerged as a possible substitute for Pb-based ceramics. Other Pb-free piezoelectric materials contain bismuth multi-layer-based systems, barium titanate-based systems, etc. Despite their excellent piezoelectric performance, ceramics are not the best choice for applications that demand flexibility. Ceramics are typically brittle and inflexible. For flexible applications, polymers with piezoelectric properties like PVDF are utilized. Composites take advantage of the benefits of both polymers and ceramics. Polymers constitute the matrix, which gives composites flexibility, while ceramic fillers improve the overall piezoelectric capabilities of the composite. Lead-free fillers are preferred in composites because lead-based fillers have environmental consequences. Bismuth layer-based fillers, Sodium potassium niobate-based fillers, molybdenum sulfide-based fillers, and barium titanate-based fillers, are the most frequently utilized lead-free ceramic fillers. Ceramics have high values of d_{33}. They are, as a result, the most frequently utilized piezoelectric energy harvesting materials. Conversely, PVDF is a polymer that has a higher voltage constant g_{33}. Thus, these are more suited for acoustic sensors and pressure purposes. Restrictions of ceramics regarding brittleness, processing ease, and flexibility have limited their use in situations when their constraints are critical. In the meanwhile, ceramic-based filler materials are categorized into two groups: Pb-based and Pb-free. Pb-based ceramics have been shown to offer excellent piezoelectric characteristics and have thus been used in a variety of applications. The leading lead-based piezoceramic lead zirconium titanate (PZT), has a large number of applications. Due to the hazardous nature of lead, questions have been raised about the recyclability and disposal of lead-containing devices, particularly those for consumer goods such as sound generators and other smart systems. Electromechanical properties are excellent in compositions close to MPB. Furthermore, the long-term presence of Pb in the environment, as well as its accumulation in important internal organ systems of organisms, that results in nervous system difficulties and brain damage, has led to the formation of rigorous restrictions prohibiting the utilization of Pb and Pb-based materials. Concerns are being lifted regarding the biocompatibility of Pb-based materials. As a result, Pb-free ceramics have been developed as an alternative to Pb-containing materials. To adapt to the environmentally responsible approach, Pb-free ceramics are increasingly being employed as fillers in composites. The lower density of Pb-free materials is advantageous in applications such as medical imaging and underwater transducers, etc. Materials suited for higher temperature purposes that are primarily Pb-free are being researched. Some Pb-free systems appropriate for piezoelectric uses are alkali niobates and barium titanate-based systems. Potassium-sodium niobate has appeared as interesting Pb-free piezoelectric material among alkali niobates. Other advantages include higher piezoelectric constant, higher coupling coefficient, biocompatibility, and higher Curie temperature. Alternatively, the thermal, mechanical, physical, and piezoelectric properties of lead-free ceramic filler are limited. As a result, there is a growing research trend toward adding fillers to these lead-free materials to develop composites with improved piezoelectric performance.

13.7 Comparison of Pb-Based Ceramics and Pb-Free Ceramics

Owing to their toxicity, Pb-based piezoelectric materials are currently subject to international limitations. As a result, it is critical to producing Pb-free replacement with higher temperature and piezoelectric stability, the most promising of which is potassium-sodium niobate. In KNN-based systems, achieving high piezoelectric performance while maintaining stable stability is extremely difficult. Higher-performing piezoceramics have found widespread use in electronic types of equipment like sensors, actuators, and transducers [59]. Because of its higher TC and excellent piezoelectricity, lead zirconate titanate-based ceramics have gotten a lot of attention. Alternatively, Pb-based piezoceramics will be forbidden in the future as environmental issues and human health become more prominent. As a result, one of the most significant goals is to produce Pb-free piezoceramics to replace PZT. Numerous studies of Pb-free materials, like BT, $Bi_{0.5}Na_{0.5}TiO_3$, $BiFeO_3$, and potassium sodium niobate-based ceramics have been carried out in recent years. However, various limitations such as weak piezoelectricity for BNT-based ceramics, low TC for BT-based ceramics, and higher leakage current for BFO-based ceramics have limited their continued development. Because of their high Curie temperature and enormous piezoelectricity, KNN-based ceramics have emerged as the most probable materials to substitute Pb-based ceramics [60]. Much emphasis has been paid to constructing phase boundaries driven by composition modifications to increase the piezoelectric action of Potassium Sodium Niobate-based ceramics [61]. The construction of orthorhombic–tetragonal phase boundaries to increase d33 of potassium sodium niobate-based ceramics is common, although d33 is often restricted to 200–300 pC N^{-1} [60], which is insufficient to replace PZT. A novel phase boundary (R–T) was constructed to increase their piezoelectric activity (d33 = 425–570 pC N^{-1}) [62]. Though, the physical or structural cause of high piezoelectricity is still unknown, which has hampered development of new Pb-free materials with improved characteristics for a long time. For practical applications, outstanding piezoelectric activity and temperature/field-cycling stability are compulsory. Owing to intrinsic properties of MPB, PZT-based ceramics have been shown to have good temperature stability of d33. Conversely, Potassium Sodium Niobate-based ceramics contain PPB rather than MPB, resulting in a high-temperature sensitivity of piezoelectric response [63]. The inverse piezoelectric coefficient (d_{33}*) in 0.948KNN-0.052$LiSbO_3$ ceramics, for example, can fall from 355 pm V^{-1} at ambient temperature to 250 pm V^{-1}at 50 °C (30 percent variation) [64]. Calcium titanate was added to increase temperature consistency by lowering the matching T_{O-T} below room temperature; however, their d_{33} was severely affected as a result [65]. Therefore, achieving both good temperature stability and high piezoelectric response in KNN-based ceramics is difficult. For industrial applications, consistency of electrical properties in Pb-free piezoelectric materials is critical. Because of their PPBs that are reliant on not only temperatures but also compositions, it was previously thought that potassium sodium niobate-based ceramics have insufficient temperature consistency of d_{33}.

13.8 Conclusion

Developing effective ways to optimize the shape, size, composition and internal structure of ceramic materials is critical to achieving abundant pores and specifically high surface area along with fast electron transfer and efficient ion dispersion abilities. Despite the wide variety of Supercapacitors applications for ceramic nanocomposites, there is however a long way to go before they can fully penetrate the commercial sector. Advancement of Pb-free materials as well as the necessity to improve their qualities for practical use, has resulted in the progress of new processing methods that aim to be cheaper substitutes to costly crystal growth methods in the pursuit of higher polarization alignment with electric field in ceramics. Nonetheless, it becomes evident that there are no Pb-free solutions that can immediately substitute commercial PZT that can be suitably doped to enhance the qualities necessary in each application. Instead, the current strategy is to create the most suitable Pb-free composition for each application. Finally, antiferroelectric and ferroelectric Pb-free polar perovskites play a significant role in the search for suitable piezoelectric materials for applications related to energy. Energy harvesting and storage are examples of applications where there is currently a lot of study going on.

References

1. Mahaffey, K.R., Environmental lead toxicity: Nutrition as a component of intervention. *Environ. Health Perspect.*, 89, 75, 1990.
2. Raza, W., Ali, F., Raza, N., Recent advancements in supercapacitor technology. *Nano Energy*, 52, 441, 2018.
3. Chu, S., Cui, Y., Liu, N., The path towards sustainable energy. *Nat. Mater.*, 16, 16, 2017.
4. Singh, S., Jain, S., Venkateswaran, P., Hydrogen: A sustainable fuel for the future of the transport sector. *Renewable Sustain. Energy Rev.*, 51, 623, 2015.
5. Azcarate, C., Mallor, F., Mateo, P., Tactical and operational management of wind energy systems with storage using a probabilistic forecast of the energy resource. *Renew. Energy*, 102, 445, 2017.
6. Noori, A., El-Kady, M.F., Rahmanifar, M.S., Kaner, R.B., Mousavi, M.F., Towards establishing standard performance metrics for batteries, supercapacitors and beyond. *Chem. Soc. Rev.*, 48, 1272, 2019.
7. Zeng, X., Yang, B., Li, X., Three-dimensional hollow CoS_2 nanoframes fabricated by anion replacement and their enhanced pseudocapacitive performances. *Electrochim. Acta*, 240, 341, 2017.
8. Zhai, S., Karahan, H.E., Wang, C., 1D supercapacitors for emerging electronics: Current status and future directions. *Adv. Mater.*, 32, 1902387, 2020.
9. Kurzweil, P. and Chwistek, M., Electrochemical stability of organic electrolytes in supercapacitors: Spectroscopy and gas analysis of decomposition products. *J. Power Sources*, 176, 555, 2008.
10. Xue, Q., Sun, J., Huang, Y., Recent progress on flexible and wearable supercapacitors. *Small*, 13, 1701827, 2017.
11. Miller, E.E., Hua, Y., Tezel, F.H., Materials for energy storage: Review of electrode materials and methods of increasing capacitance for supercapacitors. *J. Energy Storage*, 20, 30, 2018.
12. Chen, T., Li, M., Song, S., Biotemplate preparation of multilayered TiC nanoflakes for high performance symmetric supercapacitors. *Nano Energy*, 71, 104549, 2020.
13. Abdah, M.A.A.M., Azman, N.H.N., Kulandaivalu, S., Review of the use of transition-metal-oxide and conducting polymer-based fibres for high-performance supercapacitors. *Mater. Des.*, 186, 108199, 2020.
14. Zhao, Y., Shi, Z., Li, H., Designing pinecone-like and hierarchical manganese cobalt sulfides for advanced supercapacitor electrodes. *J. Mater. Chem.*, 6, 12782, 2018.
15. Gonçalves, J.M., da Silva, M.I., Toma, H.E., Trimetallic oxides/hydroxides as hybrid supercapacitor electrode materials: A review. *J. Mater. Chem.*, 8, 10534, 2020.
16. Wang, H., Li, J., Li, K., Transition metal nitrides for electrochemical energy applications. *Chem. Soc. Rev.*, 50, 1354, 2021.

17. Li, Q., Dai, Z., Wu, J., Fabrication of ordered macro-microporous single-crystalline MOF and its derivative carbon material for supercapacitor. *Adv. Energy Mater.*, 10, 1903750, 2020.
18. Hu, M., Zhang, H., Hu, T., Emerging 2D MXenes for supercapacitors: Status, challenges and prospects. *Chem. Soc. Rev.*, 49, 6666, 2020.
19. Allagui, A., Freeborn, T.J., Elwakil, A.S., Review of fractional-order electrical characterization of supercapacitors. *J. Power Sources*, 400, 457, 2018.
20. Mohanty, A., Jaihindh, D., Fu, Y.-P., An extensive review on three dimension architectural Metal-Organic Frameworks towards supercapacitor application. *J. Power Sources*, 488, 229444, 2021.
21. Zhao, H., Liu, L., Vellacheri, R., Recent advances in designing and fabricating self-supported nanoelectrodes for supercapacitors. *Adv. Sci.*, 4, 1700188, 2017.
22. Wang, F., Wu, X., Yuan, X., Latest advances in supercapacitors: From new electrode materials to novel device designs. *Chem. Soc. Rev.*, 46, 6816, 2017.
23. Zhang, Y.-Z., Wang, Y., Cheng, T., Printed supercapacitors: Materials, printing and applications. *Chem. Soc. Rev.*, 48, 3229, 2019.
24. Shen, Z.-Y., Wang, Y., Tang, Y., Glass modified barium strontium titanate ceramics for energy storage capacitor at elevated temperatures. *J. Materiomics*, 5, 641, 2019.
25. Lang, X.Y., Liu, B.T., Shi, X.M., Ultrahigh-power pseudocapacitors based on ordered porous heterostructures of electron-correlated oxides. *Adv. Sci.*, 3, 1500319, 2016.
26. Liu, P., Weng, X., Liu, Z., High-performance quasi-solid-state supercapacitor based on CuO nanoparticles with commercial-level mass loading on ceramic material $La_{1-x}Sr_xCoO_3$-δ as cathode. *ACS Appl. Energy Mater.*, 2, 1480, 2019.
27. Chang, Y., Sun, X., Ma, M., Application of hard ceramic materials B_4C in energy storage: Design B_4C@C core-shell nanoparticles as electrodes for flexible all-solid-state micro-supercapacitors with ultrahigh cyclability. *Nano Energy*, 75, 104947, 2020.
28. Faseeva, G., Nafikov, R., Lapuk, S., Ultrasound-assisted extrusion of construction ceramic samples. *Ceram. Int.*, 43, 7202, 2017.
29. Li, D., Shen, Z.-Y., Li, Z., PE hysteresis loop going slim in $Ba_{0.3}Sr_{0.7}TiO_3$-modified $Bi_{0.5}Na_{0.5}TiO_3$ ceramics for energy storage applications. *J. Adv. Ceram.*, 9, 183, 2020.
30. Liu, X., Xiao, L., Zhang, Y., Significantly enhanced piezo-photocatalytic capability in $BaTiO_3$ nanowires for degrading organic dye. *J. Materiomics*, 6, 256, 2020.
31. Cheng, Z., Ye, F., Liu, Y., Mechanical and dielectric properties of porous and wave-transparent Si_3N_4-Si_3N_4 composite ceramics fabricated by 3D printing combined with chemical vapor infiltration. *J. Adv. Ceram.*, 8, 399, 2019.
32. Jiang, C.S., Dunlap, N., Li, Y., Nonuniform ionic and electronic transport of ceramic and polymer/ceramic hybrid electrolyte by nanometer-scale

operando imaging for solid-state battery. *Adv. Energy Mater.*, 10, 2000219, 2020.

33. Li, W., Huang, H., Mei, B., Fabrication and characterization of polycrystalline Ho: CaF_2 transparent ceramics for 2.0 μm laser application. *Mater. Lett.*, 207, 37, 2017.
34. Shu, L., Liang, R., Rao, Z., Flexoelectric materials and their related applications: A focused review. *J. Adv. Ceram.*, 8, 153, 2019.
35. Reveron, H., Fornabaio, M., Palmero, P., Towards long lasting zirconia-based composites for dental implants: Transformation induced plasticity and its consequence on ceramic reliability. *Acta Biomater.*, 48, 423, 2017.
36. Xiong, C., Li, M., Zhao, W., Flexible N-Doped reduced graphene oxide/carbon nanotube-MnO_2 film as a multifunctional material for high-performance supercapacitors, catalysts and sensors. *J. Materiomics*, 6, 523, 2020.
37. Hu, M., Yang, W., Tan, H., Template-free synthesis of mesoporous and crystalline transition metal oxide nanoplates with abundant surface defects. *Matter*, 2, 1244, 2020.
38. Liu, Y., Tian, D., Biswas, A.N., Transition metal nitrides as promising catalyst supports for tuning CO/H_2 syngas production from electrochemical CO_2 reduction. *Angew. Chem. Int. Ed.*, 59, 11345, 2020.
39. Hirakawa, T., Shimokawa, Y., Tokuzumi, W., Multicomponent spinel oxide solid solutions: A possible alternative to platinum group metal three-way catalysts. *ACS Catal.*, 9, 11763, 2019.
40. Anwar, S., Muthu, K.S., Ganesh, V., A comparative study of electrochemical capacitive behavior of $NiFe_2O_4$ synthesized by different routes. *J. Electrochem. Soc.*, 158, A976, 2011.
41. Kovalenko, A., Shilova, O., Morozova, L., Features of the synthesis and the study of nanocrystalline cobalt-nickel spinel. *Glass Phys. Chem.*, 40, 106, 2014.
42. Zheng, K., Quan, Y., Zhuang, J., Achieving high piezoelectric performances with enhanced domain-wall contributions in < 001>-textured Sm-modified PMN-29PT ceramics. *J. Eur. Ceram. Soc.*, 41, 2458, 2021.
43. Wu, J., Xiao, D., Zhu, J., Potassium–sodium niobate lead-free piezoelectric ceramics: Recent advances and perspectives. *J. Mater. Sci. Mater. Electron.*, 26, 9297, 2015.
44. Jiang, L., Xing, J., Tan, Z., High piezoelectricity in (K, Na)(Nb, Sb) O_3–(Bi, La, Na, Li) ZrO_3 lead-free ceramics. *J. Mater. Sci.*, 51, 4963, 2016.
45. Saito, Y., Takao, H., Tani, T., Lead-free piezoceramics. *Nature*, 432, 84, 2004.
46. Zhao, J., Zhang, N., Ren, W., Polar domain structural evolution under electric field and temperature in the $(Bi_{0.5}Na_{0.5})$ TiO_3-0.06 $BaTiO_3$ piezoceramics. *Am. Ceram. Soc.*, 102, 437, 2019.
47. Zhang, S., Xia, R., Shrout, T.R., Lead-free piezoelectric ceramics vs. PZT. *J. Electroceramics*, 19, 251, 2007.
48. Zhu, L., Wang, L., Pan, C., Enhancing the efficiency of silicon-based solar cells by the piezo-phototronic effect. *ACS Nano*, 11, 1894, 2017.

49. Damjanovic, D., *Lead-based piezoelectric materials*, 59, 79, Springer, US, 2008.
50. Cheng, L.-Q. and Li, J.-F., A review on one dimensional perovskite nanocrystals for piezoelectric applications. *J. Materiomics*, 2, 25, 2016.
51. Mohammed, T., Koh, S., Reaney, I., Integrated hybrid life cycle assessment and supply chain environmental profile evaluations of lead-based (lead zirconate titanate) versus lead-free (potassium sodium niobate) piezoelectric ceramics. *Energy Environ. Sci.*, 9, 3495, 2016.
52. Maeder, M.D., Damjanovic, D., Setter, N., Lead free piezoelectric materials. *J. Electroceramics*, 13, 385, 2004.
53. Lin, D., Xiao, D., Zhu, J., Piezoelectric and ferroelectric properties of $[Bi_{0.5}(Na_{1-x-y}K_xLi_y)_{0.5}]TiO_3$ lead-free piezoelectric ceramics. *Appl. Phys. Lett.*, 88, 062901, 2006.
54. Wei, H., Wang, H., Xia, Y., An overview of lead-free piezoelectric materials and devices. *J. Mater. Chem. C*, 6, 12446, 2018.
55. Yao, M., Pu, Y., Zhang, L., Enhanced energy storage properties of (1− x) $Bi_{0.5}Na_{0.5}TiO_{3-x}Ba_{0.85}Ca_{0.15}Ti_{0.9}Zr_{0.1}O_3$ ceramics. *Mater. Lett.*, 174, 110, 2016.
56. Xu, Q., Xie, J., He, Z., Energy-storage properties of $Bi_{0.5}Na_{0.5}TiO_3$-$BaTiO_3$-$KNbO_3$ ceramics fabricated by wet-chemical method. *J. Eur. Ceram. Soc.*, 37, 99, 2017.
57. Mohammed, T., Koh, S., Reaney, I., Are lead-free piezoelectrics more environmentally friendly. *MRS Commun.*, 7, 1, 2017.
58. Xiong, Z., Zhou, X., Kishi, K., Development of ferroelectric ceramics with high dielectric constant and low dissipation factor for high-voltage capacitors. *J. Electroceramics*, 3, 239, 1999.
59. Park, K.-I., Xu, S., Liu, Y., Piezoelectric $BaTiO_3$ thin film nanogenerator on plastic substrates. *Nano Lett.*, 10, 4939, 2010.
60. Wu, J., Xiao, D., Zhu, J., Potassium–sodium niobate lead-free piezoelectric materials: Past, present, and future of phase boundaries. *Chem. Rev.*, 115, 2559, 2015.
61. Wang, X., Wu, J., Xiao, D., Giant piezoelectricity in potassium–sodium niobate lead-free ceramics. *J. Am. Chem. Soc.*, 136, 2905, 2014.
62. Zheng, T., Wu, J., Xiao, D., Strong piezoelectricity in $(1-x)(K_{0.4}Na_{0.6})(Nb_{0.96}Sb_{0.04})O_3$-x $Bi_{0.5}K_{0.5}Zr_{1-y}Sn_yO_3$ lead-free binary system: Identification and role of multiphase coexistence. *ACS Appl. Mater. Interfaces*, 7, 5927, 2015.
63. Shrout, T.R. and Zhang, S.J., Lead-free piezoelectric ceramics: Alternatives for PZT. *J. Electroceramics*, 19, 113, 2007.
64. Zhang, S., Xia, R., Shrout, T.R., Piezoelectric properties in perovskite 0.948 $(K_{0.5}Na_{0.5})NbO_3$–0.052 $LiSbO_3$ lead-free ceramics. *J. Appl. Phys.*, 100, 104108, 2006.
65. Zhang, S., Xia, R., Shrout, T.R., Modified $(K_{0.5}Na_{0.5})NbO_3$ based lead-free piezoelectrics with broad temperature usage range. *Appl. Phys. Lett.*, 91, 132913, 2007.

Index

Printed in the USA/Agawam, MA
September 16, 2026

910661.090